NIGHT VISION

basic, clinical and applied aspects

NIGHT VISION

basic, clinical and applied aspects

EDITED BY

R F Hess

L T Sharpe

K Nordby

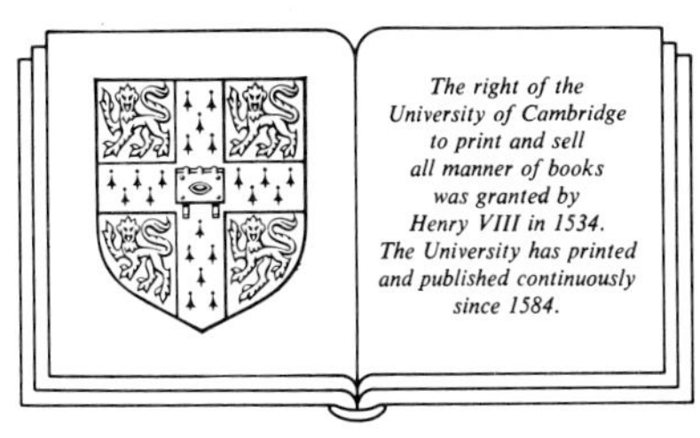

CAMBRIDGE UNIVERSITY PRESS

Cambridge

New York   Port Chester   Melbourne   Sydney

Published by the Press Syndicate of the University of Cambridge
The Pitt Building, Trumpington Street, Cambridge CB2 1RP
40 West 20th Street, New York NY 10011, USA
10 Stamford Road, Oakleigh, Melbourne 3166, Australia

First published 1990

Printed in Great Britain at the University Press, Cambridge

British Library cataloguing in publication data

Night vision.
1. Man. Night vision.
I. Hess, R. F. II. Sharpe, L. T. III. Nordby, K.
612′.84

Library of Congress cataloguing in publication data

Night vision: basic, clinical, and applied aspects /
edited by R. F. Hess, L. T. Sharpe, K. Nordby.
p. cm.
Includes bibliographical references.
ISBN 0 521 32736 9
1. Night vision. I. Hess, Robert Francis
II. Sharpe, Lindsay Theodore, 1951–
III. Nordby, Knut, 1942–
QP482.N54 1990
612.8′4–dc20 89–25439 CIP

ISBN 0 521 32736 9

CE

Contents

Contributors ix
Preface xi

PART I NORMAL VISUAL SENSITIVITY 1

1 Rod-mediated vision: role of post-receptoral filters 3
Robert F. Hess

1.1 Introduction 3
1.2 Detection sensitivity 4
1.3 Discrimination sensitivity 37
1.4 Concluding remarks 47

2 The light-adaptation of the human rod visual system 49
Lindsay T. Sharpe

2.1 Introduction 49
2.2 The absolute sensitivity of the rods 57
2.3 The desensitization of the rods 68
2.4 The influence of the cones upon rod desensitization 98
2.5 The saturation of the rods 117
2.6 Conclusions 122

3 Physiological mechanisms of visual adaptation at low light levels 125
Maureen K. Powers and Daniel G. Green

3.1 Introduction 125
3.2 Effects of background light on luminance detection 127
3.3 Effects of background light on spatial vision 138
3.4 Summary 144

4 Absolute sensitivity 146
Walter Makous

4.1 Basic concepts 146
4.2 Light as a noisy carrier 147
4.3 Quantum detector with light loss 147
4.4 Poisson noise 148
4.5 Non-Poisson noise 160
4.6 The nature of the centrally acting noise 167
4.7 Neural noise 173
4.8 Summary 175

5 Dark adaptation: a re-examination 177
T. D. Lamb

5.1 Introduction 177
5.2 Psychophysics 180
5.3 Receptor physiology 193
5.4 A model of dark adaptation 210
5.5 Summary 219

6 Invertebrate vision at low luminances 223
Simon B. Laughlin

6.1 Introduction 223
6.2 Responses of invertebrate photoreceptors at low luminances 224
6.3 Photoreceptor intrinsic noise 226
6.4 The efficiency of transmission of single photon signals 235
6.5 Sampling and processing 239
6.6 Optical trade-offs 239
6.7 Neural sampling and processing 245

PART II ACHROMATOPSIA 251

7 Total colour-blindness: an introduction 253
Lindsay T. Sharpe and Knut Nordby

7.1 Early observations about colour-blindness 256
7.2 Theories of total colour-blindness 268
7.3 A short taxonomy of achromatopsias 278
7.4 Conclusions 288

8 Vision in a complete achromat: a personal account 290
Knut Nordby

8.1 Introduction 290
8.2 A short biography 290
8.3 Rod vision 304
8.4 Closing remarks 315

9 Clinical aspects of achromatopsia 316
Egill Hansen

9.1 Classification 316
9.2 Heredity 318
9.3 Associated somatic defects 319
9.4 Natural history 319
9.5 Clinical findings 321
9.6 Electrophysiological examinations 324
9.7 Colour vision tests 325
9.8 Tests for incomplete achromatopsia 329
9.9 Diagnosis 331
9.10 Visual habilitation 333
9.11 Prognosis 334

10 The photoreceptors in the achromat 335
Lindsay T. Sharpe and Knut Nordby

10.1 Introduction 335
10.2 The histology 337
10.3 The scotoma 338
10.4 The photopigment: fundal reflectometry and spectral sensitivity 339
10.5 Saturation 346
10.6 Directional sensitivity 348
10.7 The psychophysics 353
10.8 The electroretinogram 376
10.9 Concluding remarks 380
10.10 Appendix 382

11 Post-receptoral sensitivity of the achromat 390
R. F. Hess

11.1 Introduction 390

11.2 Are there high intensity receptors in the achromat's retina? 391
11.3 Do the rods in the achromat's retina make normal post-receptoral connections? 393
11.4 Mesopic vision 397
11.5 Concluding remarks 412

PART III CLINICAL AND APPLIED 415

12 The loss of night vision: clinical manifestations in man and animals 417
Harris Ripps and Gerald A. Fishman

12.1 Introduction 417
12.2 Non-invasive tests of visual function 418
12.3 Vitamin A in night vision 427
12.4 Inherited night blindness in man and animals 429
12.5 Summary 450

13 Aided vision at low luminances 451
A. van Meeteren

13.1 Introduction 451
13.2 Night-glasses 459
13.3 Image intensifying devices 464

References 473
Index 538

Contributors

Dr Gerald A. Fishman (Chapter 12)

Lions of Illinois Eye Research Institute, Department of Ophthalmology, University of Illinois College of Medicine, 1855 West Taylor Street, Chicago, Illinois 60612, USA

Dr Daniel G. Green (Chapter 3)

Neuroscience Laboratory, University of Michigan, Ann Arbor, Michigan 48109, USA

Dr Egill Hansen (Chapter 9)

University Eye Clinic, Rikshopsitalet, 0027, Oslo 1, Norway

Dr Robert F. Hess (Chapters 1, 11)

Physiological Laboratory, Downing Street, Cambridge CB2 3EG

Dr Trevor D. Lamb (Chapter 5)

Department of Physiology, University of Cambridge, Downing Street, Cambridge CB2 3EG

Dr Simon B. Laughlin (Chapter 6)

Department of Zoology, University of Cambridge, Downing Street, Cambridge CB2 3EJ

Dr Walter Makous (Chapter 4)

Center for Visual Science & Department of Psychology, University of Rochester, River Campus Station, Rochester 146727, USA

Dr Arrt van Meeteren (Chapter 13)

TNO Institute for Perception, PO Box 23, 3769 Soesterberg, Kampweg, The Netherlands

Dr Knut Nordby (Chapters 7, 8, 10)

Norwegian Telecom Research Department, Postboks 83, N-2007 Kjeller, Norway

Dr Maureen K. Powers (Chapter 3)
Department of Psychology, Vanderbilt University, Nashville, Tennessee, USA

Dr Harris Ripps (Chapter 12)
Lions of Illinois Eye Research Institute, Department of Opthalmology, University of Illinois College of Medicine, 1855 West Taylor Street, Chicago, Illinois 60612, USA

Dr Lindsay T. Sharpe (Chapter 2, 7, 10)
Neurological University Clinic, 7800 Freiburg.i.Br, FRG.

Preface

The last major resumé of work about night vision was published by Jayle & Ourgaud in 1950, entitled *La Vision Nocturne et ses Troubles*, later translated by Baisinger & Holmes into English (1959) as *Night Vision*. It contained in its chapters the beginnings of what we now know to be fundamental advances in the field. Appropriately, Sir Stewart Duke-Elder, in his introduction, praised the authors for bringing order to a subject, which previously was 'difficult, vague and chaotic, weighed down with theories and complicated by experimental work'.

The content of Jayle, Ourgaud, Baisinger & Holmes's book is informed, to a great extent, by research strategies and developments originating from specific concerns during the Second World War about night aerial activities and dark sensitivity. However, its importance, then and now, resides more in fundamental theoretical and clinical issues than in practical ones. Firstly, the link between biochemistry and behaviour emanating from the work of Wald and co-workers on vitamin A is outlined as are some initial objections to the biochemical theory of Hecht. Secondly, the link between physics and behaviour is examined by a discussion of the work of Hecht, Shlaer & Pirenne on quantal detection. Thirdly, the various manifestations of congenital night-blindness and its converse (roughly speaking), congenital total colour-blindness, are enumerated. Finally, the initial attempts are reported of Granit and co-workers to establish a link between physiology and behaviour by recording mass evoked potentials from the retina and optic nerve under condition for which the psychophysics was known.

The content of our book represents the thinking forty years on in all of these fundamental areas. In particular, there has been rapid advance in the techniques of electrophysiology such that the response properties of single neurones in most parts of the visual pathways can now be examined. This has forged a solid link between physiology and function which was so tentative even four decades ago. We now have a much clearer idea of the role that the visual photoreceptors play in adaptation and as a consequence the importance of post-receptoral mechanisms in this process. This has also lead to the development of more refined psychophysical tools with which to examine the sensitivity of night vision in normal and pathological eyes.

In this book along with the more usual approaches there is emphasis placed on the usefulness of studying the visual function of the typical, complete achromat in helping to disentangle the rod from cone contributions to our vision at night. Unlike the original book *Night Vision*, in the present book the topics of biochemistry, electrophysiology and psychophysics are much more interrelated, which is in itself an index of progress in the field.

R. F. Hess
L. T. Sharpe
K. Nordby

PART I

Normal visual sensitivity

1

Rod-mediated vision: role of post-receptoral filters

Robert F. Hess

1.1 Introduction

The histological studies of Max Shultze (1866) laid the foundations for what we now call the Duplex theory of visual function. It is one of the cornerstones of visual physiology founded as it was on correlating anatomy and behaviour. It is one of the first pieces of information a teacher in visual physiology must impart yet even today many questions remain unanswered about this basic aspect of physiology. As a first step towards answering some of these we need to develop a clearer idea of the properties of rod-mediated vision. It is only then that we can move towards an understanding of the rules that govern the combination or interaction of rod and cone signals.

In this chapter I will discuss what is known about rod-mediated vision as if such interactions do not exist, in an attempt to understand the capabilities of the rod mechanism in isolation. This involves drawing together pieces of the rod puzzle obtained not only from different psychophysical techniques but also from very different methods of isolation. This turns out to be more a strength than a weakness, for in some cases the information gathered from different methods is complementary and in other cases where there are conflicts, their resolution makes its own contribution to completing the picture.

Historically, rod and cone function have been teased apart in the Duplex retina by comparing scotopic with photopic function. This relies on the fact that rods saturate at lower photopic retinal illuminances and do not contribute to vision at mid to high photopic levels whereas cones do not operate under scotopic conditions due to their restricted adaptation range. This type of comparison is not wholly satisfactory because we are comparing cone vision at its optimal retinal illuminance with rod vision well below its optimal retinal illuminance. Another approach that has been adopted is to produce stimulus conditions that, owing to the different spectral sensitivity and directional sensitivity of cones, puts these receptors at a disadvantage so that the rod mechanism determines threshold (Aguilar & Stiles, 1954; Conner, 1982; D'Zmura & Lennie, 1986). This isolation by psychophysical means has allowed rod function to be investigated at more mesopic levels where its contrast sensitivity is better, but where, under normal circumstances, cones would determine threshold. The shortcomings of this approach are two-fold. First, such isolation is never perfect, and so absolute sensitivity of the rod mechanism is difficult to determine and second, it applies only to threshold. One way to supplement these inadequacies is to use the genetic isolation produced in humans who have no functional cone mechanism (i.e. the total and complete achromat). The validity of this step relies on achromats being functionally equivalent to rod monochromats. Since this approach helps to complete the picture of rod function the evidence that this step can be made is presented in Chapters 10 and 11.

There are pitfalls in each of these approaches, but their information is, to a large extent, complementary, and when taken together go some way towards giving us a clearer outline of the capabilities of rod vision.

One important notion which has emerged over the last two decades is that the initial stages of vision involve spatial, temporal and contrast filtering. This aspect of organization itself plays an important role in extending our range of stable vision to low light levels because the adaptation mechanism which is a filter-based operation can vary independently along each of these filtering dimensions. The acceptance of the concept of a stage of early filtering in vision leads to a reinterpretation of some of the more classical findings using spot stimuli. This chapter will concentrate on examining the role of visual filters in extending our dynamic range.

1.2 Detection sensitivity

1.2.1 Difference approaches

There have been two different experimental approaches used in the investigation of rod sensitivity. Originally, the information on scotopic sensitivity and on the isolation of rod vision in the Duplex retina at higher light levels has come from increment threshold experiments. In such experiments, the stimulus is a sharply focused spot of light of luminance ΔI which is abruptly presented on a much larger steady background field

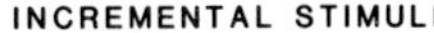

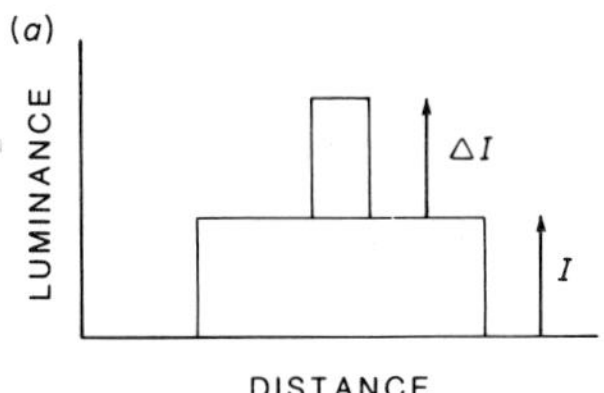

GRATING STIMULI

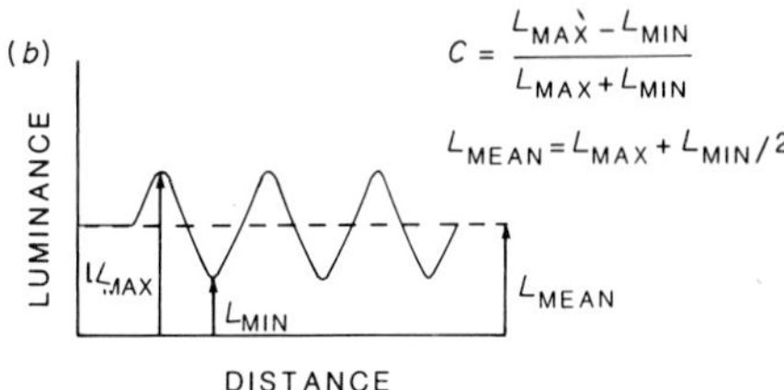

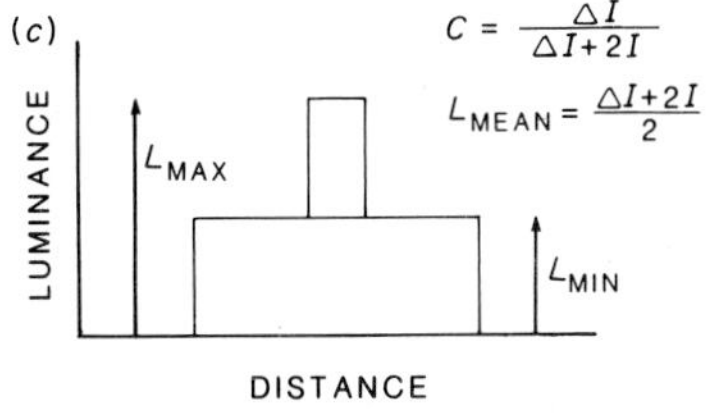

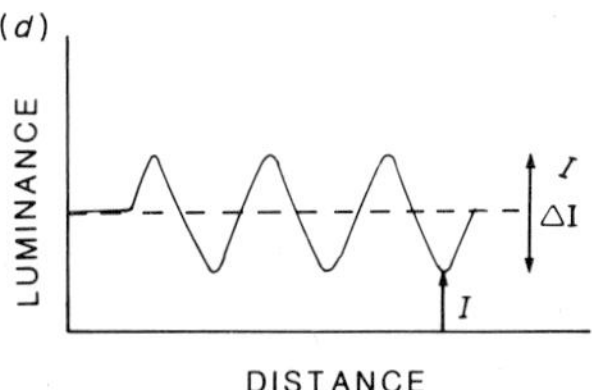

Fig. 1.1. Luminance profiles for incremental threshold stimuli (*a*) and grating stimuli (*b*) are depicted. In (*c*) an equivalent contrast is derived for the increment threshold stimulus and in (*d*) equivalent increment threshold measures are derived for the grating stimuli.

of luminance I (Fig. 1.1*a*). What is measured is the smallest value of ΔI that can be detected and this is plotted as a function of I (increment threshold or t.v.i. curve).

More recently, scotopic function has been investigated using a different approach. The stimuli are periodic in space and time so that they contain restricted spatial and temporal frequency components. These stimuli are useful because there is both psychophysical (Blakemore & Campbell, 1969; Stromeyer & Julesz, 1972) and neurophysiological evidence (Hubel & Wiesel, 1977; Enroth-Cugell & Robson, 1966) for the role of different spatial and temporal filters in early visual processing. For such a stimulus the modulation depth or contrast (defined as $(L_{max} - L_{min}/(L_{max} + L_{min}))$ is varied (Fig. 1.1b) until the spatial or temporal structure is detected. The reciprocal of the contrast needed for threshold detection is then plotted as contrast sensitivity (contrast sensitivity function). This can be repeated over a range of mean luminances $((L_{max} + L_{min}/2))$. One advantage of this stimulus is that the light adaptation state of the eye can be kept constant, independent of contrast. This will hold as long as the spatio-temporal properties of the adaptation mechanism are poor relative to the spatio-temporal properties of the stimulus. Each of these different approaches has made important contributions to our knowledge of rod sensitivity but, as we will see, there are also some important conflicts that need to be resolved.

1.2.2 Range and form of the rod-mediated response of unitary cortical mechanisms

The range of rod vision can be best seen in the increment threshold results of normal observers as found by Aguilar & Stiles in 1954. They used a 9 deg diameter spot on a 20 deg background field and took advantage of the difference in spectral and directional sensitivity of rods compared with cones (Stiles & Crawford, 1933; Stiles, 1939; van Loo & Enoch, 1975) to isolate the rod response in the normal Duplex retina. In Fig. 1.2*a* their averaged result is plotted in the usual way, that is ΔI as a function of I (solid curve) on log coordinates. Under these conditions the visual system is in adaptational equilibrium for all thresholds. The incremental sensitivity of rod vision exhibits a linear relationship with background intensity from 10^2 scotopic trolands to 10^{-2} scotopic trolands, a range of 4 log units. This has traditionally been considered in terms of the adaptation properties (Weber behaviour, $\Delta I/I$ = constant) of unitary visual mechanisms. However, as we will see later more recent psychophysics and cortical neurophysiology suggest a different interpretation. The rapid rise in threshold at higher illuminances is due to saturation of the rod photoreceptors whereas the asymptote at lower illuminance is thought to be due to the intrinsic noise in the photoreceptors themselves (Barlow, 1957, 1977). Using these types of stimuli, cone-mediated vision can usually be followed down to around 1–10 Ts after which rods determine sensitivity, thus extending the visual range by 4–5 log units. A similar picture, although plotted in a slightly different way is seen when contrast sensitivity is plotted against mean retinal illuminance (solid curve in Fig. 1.2*b*), for a periodic stimulus of low spatial and temporal frequency (0.4 c/deg, 1Hz). These results are for a total and complete achromat whose sensitivity was solely determined by rods (for evidence see Chapters 10 and 11). The total sensitivity range obtained by extrapolation is 6–7 log units with saturation beginning at 200 Ts and complete by 2000 Ts.

There are, however, important differences when one compares the shape of the rod response across illuminance using these two approaches (compare solid curve in Fig. 1.2*a* with solid curve in Fig. 1.2*b*). The incremental threshold curve (Fig. 1.2*a*) is defined by three regions; a saturating response at high retinal illuminance, a large region where $\Delta I/I$

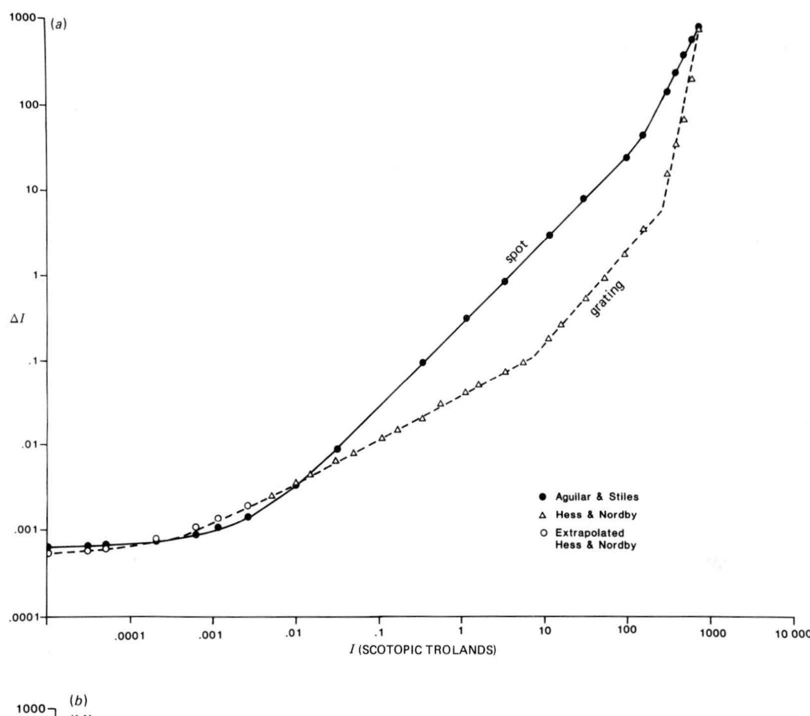

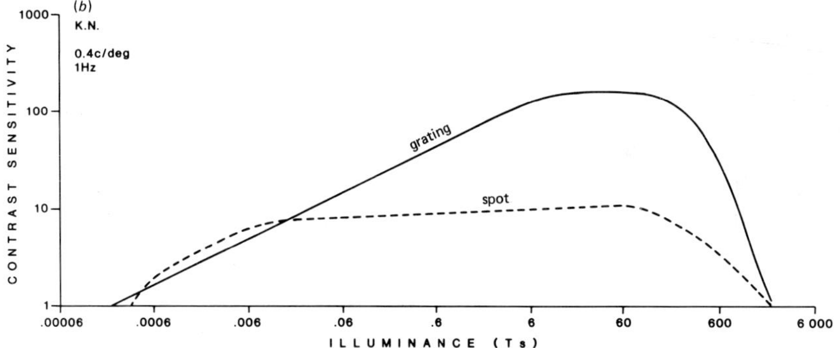

Fig. 1.2. In (*a*) the just detectable increment ΔI is plotted against the background retinal illuminance I for the rod mechanism of normal vision (solid curve) from the averaged results of Aguilar & Stiles (1954). The dashed curve is the result obtained with grating stimuli for a rod monochromat according to the transformation in Fig. 1.1*d*.

In (*b*) the contrast sensitivity of the rod monochromat is plotted against the mean retinal illuminance (solid curve). The dashed curve is the incremental result from normal vision (solid curve in (*a*)) transformed into the contrast metric according to the transformation in Fig. 1.1*c*.

is constant (so-called Weber region) and a lower illuminance asymptote. The contrast sensitivity response (solid curve in Fig. 1.2*b*) can also be defined by three regions; a saturating response, a Weber response and a large region where sensitivity varies as the square root of the retinal illuminance (so-called Rose–de Vries region). The increment threshold curve does not display a slope of both 1 *and* 0.5 on these coordinates (as the contrast sensitivity measurements do) and the contrast sensitivity curve does not exhibit an obvious low illuminance asymptote so characteristic of incremental threshold result. Let us first ask to what extent is this discrepancy in the shape of these curves dependent on the fact that in one case an incremental measure is used whereas in the other a contrast measure is used? To assess this, one can replot the grating data (solid curve in Fig. 1.2*b*) in incremental terms (dashed curve in Fig. 1.2*a*) and compare it with the incremental result (solid curve in Fig. 1.2*a*). Likewise, the original increment threshold results can be replotted in contrast terms (dashed curve in Fig. 1.2*b*) and compared with the contrast sensitivity result (solid curve in Fig. 1.2*b*). These equivalent transforms are described in Fig. 1.1*c*, *d*. When this is done the increment threshold and contrast data are similar in form in the saturating region but still different at intermediate illuminances. In this region grating stimuli produce a Weber *and* Rose–de Vries region whereas sharply focused spots above 0.5 deg in diameter only exhibit a Weber relation. Thus one cannot explain this discrepancy in terms of the different metrics used. This issue is worth resolving because the form of the function relating rod sensitivity to illuminance may have important implications for what limits rod sensitivity. For example, the square-root response has been interpreted by some as evidence that sensitivity is limited by the quantal nature of the stimulus (Rose, 1942; De Vries, 1943).

An explanation based on filters

Since it is now accepted that the initial stage of vision involves an array of space-time separable filters it would seem reasonable to suggest that stimuli which are sinusoidal in space and time will activate only a limited subset of this array at threshold. This being the case, a spatio-temporally broad band stimulus such as a sharply focused spot, abruptly presented will activate many filters. Thus the relationship between contrast sensitivity and retinal illuminance seen for sine gratings (slope of zero and 0.5) is then likely to reflect the response of *unitary* visual filters whereas the response found for spots is likely to represent the involvement of different visual filters (the most sensitive ones) at different retinal illuminances. The latter response will be an *envelope* not a unitary response.

This case rests on two different pieces of evidence. The first concerns the fact that the form of the incremental response depends on the spatio-temporal properties of the stimuli. This is not the case for sinewave stimulation. The second involves more direct evidence that broad band spatial stimuli are detected by different visual filters at different illuminances.

One type of evidence

If the form of the relationship for spots is determined by different visual filters at different illuminance one would expect it to critically depend on the spatio-temporal properties of the stimuli. On the other hand if the form of the response for sinewave gratings represents the unitary response of visual filters this would not be expected to vary for different spatio-temporal frequencies of stimulation (which would isolate different filters having the same unitary response, i.e. slope of zero and 0.5). This prediction is borne out.

The slopes of unity *and* square-root are universally found for gratings. The results of van Nes & Bouman (1967) and van Nes *et al.* (1967) show that this is a feature of both receptor systems. Their results which are depicted in Fig. 1.3*a* also show that the retinal illuminance at which Weber-like behaviour changes to square-root behaviour varies with spatial frequency. Since their results span the spatial frequency range 48 c/deg to 0.5 c/deg (Fig. 1.3*a*) and since the rod mechanism cannot resolve above 7 c/deg (see Fig. 1.9), we can safely conclude that this form of response is characteristic of rods as well as cones. Hess & Howell (1988) have extended these findings to spatial frequencies below 0.5 c/deg (Fig. 1.3*b*) and found evidence for similar behaviour. Indeed the shape of the response when normalized for both contrast sensitivity and retina illuminance is similar for all spatial frequencies and always shows *both* a Weber and Rose–de Vries region (Fig. 1.3*c*). Similar results have also been found for the rod monochromat where the rod response can be tested in isolation (Hess & Nordby, 1986*a*, *b*). These results for a wide range of spatial and temporal frequencies are seen in Fig. 11.1 (Chapter 11).

On the other hand the form of the relationship between incremental sensitivity and retinal illuminance for spot stimuli is critically dependent

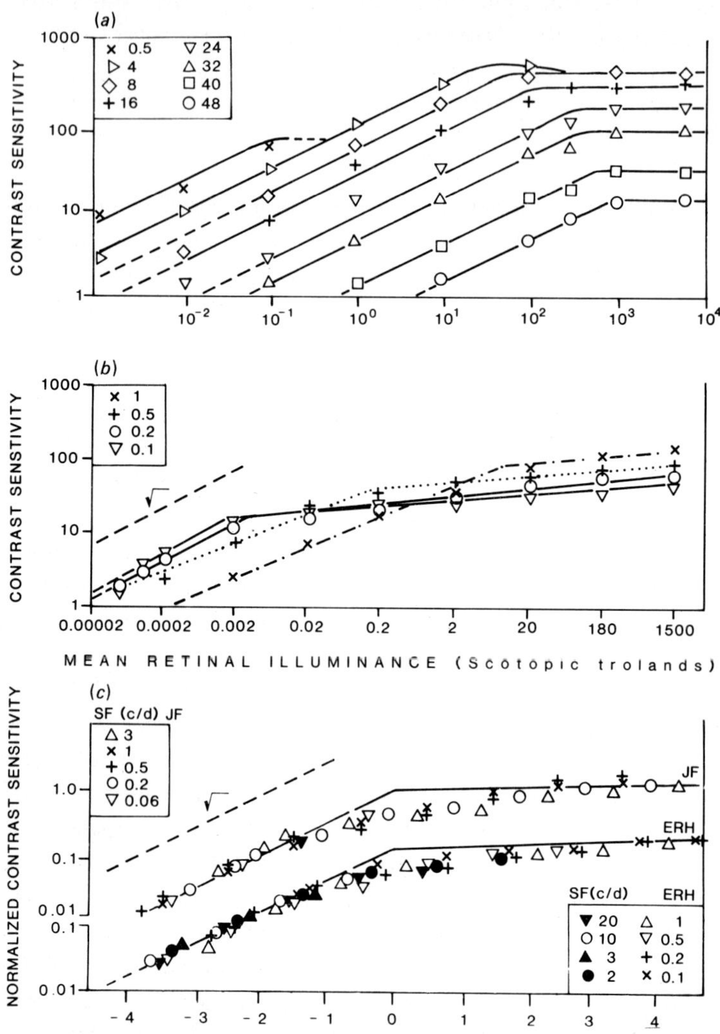

Fig. 1.3. In (*a*) contrast sensitivity is plotted against the mean retinal illuminance for grating stimuli for a normal observer. The data are from van Nes & Bouman (1967) and cover the range 48–0.5 c/deg. In (*b*) a similar pattern is seen for spatial frequencies down to 0.1 c/deg from the data of Hess & Howell (1988). In (*c*) the contrast sensitivity dependence on retinal illuminance has been normalized to show that the function is of similar form from 20 to 0.1 c/deg.

on the spatio-temporal properties of stimulation. The slope of this relationship changes between the limits of unity and 0.5 when large, long duration stimuli are changed for small, short duration stimuli (Ten

Doesschate, 1944; Bouman, 1952; Barlow, 1958*b*, 1972). This suggests that the result for spot stimuli is the composite response of different visual filters at different illuminances.

Another type of evidence

One important difference between sharp edged spots presented abruptly and sinusoidal gratings presented gradually in time is that in the latter case the spatio-temporal spectrum of the stimulus is more confined. Since there is evidence from both human psychophysics (Blakemore & Campbell, 1969; Campbell & Robson, 1968; Stromeyer & Julesz, 1972; Stromeyer *et al.*, 1982; Watson & Robson, 1981; Wilson & Bergen, 1979) and from neurophysiology (Hubel & Wiesel, 1977; Enroth-Cugell & Robson, 1966) that the visual system has a number of spatial and temporal filters which can participate in vision, this difference may be important. A spot stimulus may in principle be detected at high retinal illuminances by high frequency filters via the components contributing to its edge, while at lower illuminances by low frequency components which contribute to its overall width. If one assumes that the most sensitive filter determines threshold at any illuminance, then the overall response would ride on the Weber regions of lower and lower filters and slopes of close to unity would be seen over most of the illuminance range (see dashed curve in Fig. 1.2*b*). Evidence in favour of this suggestion is seen in Fig. 1.4. Here, contrast sensitivity is compared for a 0.1 and 1 c/deg sinewave grating with that of a 0.1 c/deg squarewave grating as a function of retinal illuminance. The sinewave responses are similar to those of van Nes & Bouman (1967) where the illuminance (termed the transition illuminance by van Nes & Bouman) at which the Weber response changes to a square-root response is shifted to lower values for this low spatial frequency stimulus. Notice however, that for the squarewave stimulus, sensitivity at high illuminances, initially follows that of its higher frequency components (being similar to the 1 c/deg sensitivity) whereas at lower illuminances it follows that of its low frequency component (being similar to the 0.1 c/deg sinewave sensitivity). The resultant overall response exhibits a slope which is fairly flat (and hence just slightly shallower than unity when plotted as an increment threshold) over most of the retinal illuminance range. Furthermore only for illuminances above the arrow in Fig. 1.4 can the low frequency squarewave be reliably discriminated from the low frequency sinewave at threshold. Thus it seems more than a distinct possibility that this discrepancy in the

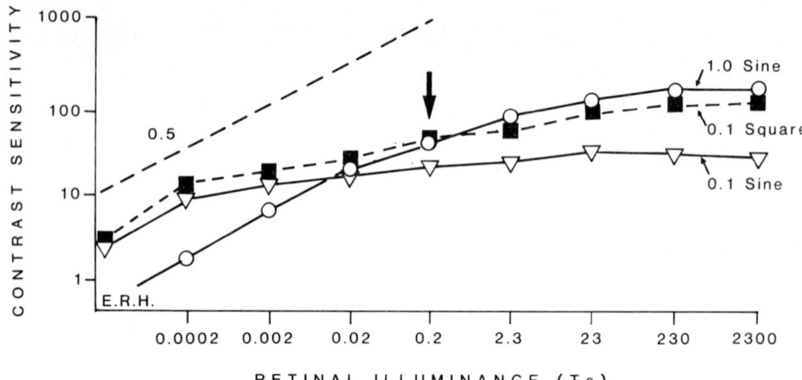

Fig. 1.4. Contrast sensitivity is plotted against retinal illuminance for a low spatial frequency squarewave grating (■) compared to sinewave gratings of 0.1 c/deg (▽) and 1 c/deg (○). Note that sensitivity initially follows the 1 c/deg sinewave at photopic illuminances and later the 0.1 c/deg sinewave at scotopic illuminances.

shapes of the functions relating rod sensitivity to retinal illuminance occurs because in the increment threshold approach we may be measuring the envelope of the sensitivities of many *different* visual filters as illuminance is reduced. Hence in terms of visual mechanisms it is not a unitary response. Further confirmation comes from increment threshold measurements for very small spots presented very briefly. This stimulus manipulation effectively spatially and temporally filters the stimulus and favours detection by mid–high spatially and temporally tuned mechanisms whose sensitivity is highest. Barlow (1965) shows some schematic results for such a stimulus indicating the presence of both square-root and Weber regions for normal vision.

However, the exact picture in normals as presented by Aguilar & Stiles might be further complicated by rod–cone interactions. There is now evidence to suggest that (1) the slope of the second limb of the increment threshold curve can occupy any one of a number of values between 0.5 and 0.8 (Stabell, Nordby & Stabell, 1987) and that (2) this could result from a cone–rod interaction due to the long wavelength nature of the background field (Makous & Peeples, 1979; Buck & Makous, 1981; Stabell *et al.*, 1987). Such an interaction must have also contributed to the original results of Aguilar & Stiles (1954) and this emphasizes the importance of the rod monochromat's contribution to this question (Stabell *et al.*, 1987).

If this is the case, the more informative result concerning *individual* visual mechanisms comes from the grating experiments and especially those from the monochromat because here we can see (1) the depend-

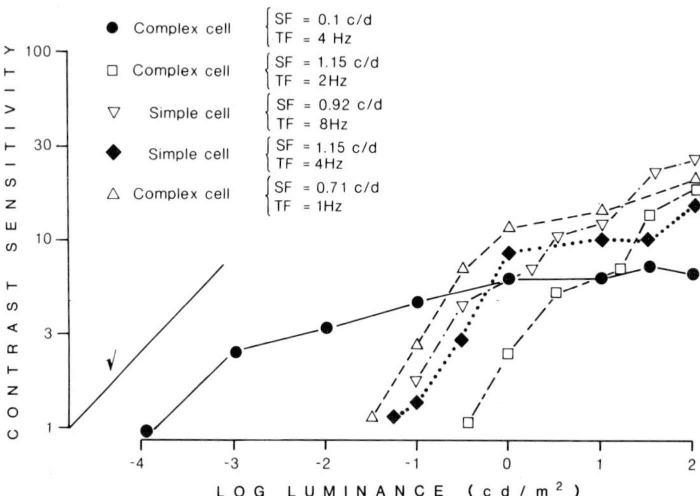

Fig. 1.5. Steady-state contrast sensitivity is plotted against mean luminance for five cat striate neurones. The stimulus used at all luminances was optimal for the neurone and thresholds were set using an auditory criterion. Compare this with the psychophysics of Fig. 1.3 for gratings. (Data from Lillywhite & Hess, unpublished).

ence of sensitivity of individual filters on illuminance rather than for the population of filters as a whole and (2) possible rod–cone interactions need not concern us.

Three interesting conclusions emerge from these results. Firstly, the fact that the transition illuminance changes progressively to lower values as the spatial frequency is lowered suggests that larger summation areas are being used and that adaptation is a filter-based operation (Enroth-Cugell & Shapley, 1973*b*). The results below 0.5 c/deg suggest that summation areas as large as 5 deg with separate adaptation properties are available to rod vision. This is not due to a changeover from cone to rod function as a similar effect can be seen for rod vision in isolation (see Fig. 11.1, Chapter 11). The second point involves the square-root response. This is a characteristic feature of the psychophysical results and is also seen in the responses of single neurones in striate cortex of the cat. In Fig. 1.5 results are given for five striate neurones in cat cortex (Hess & Lillywhite, unpublished data). The peak spatial and temporal response functions for each cell are given in the figure inset (top left). For each neurone a contrast threshold was set using an auditory criterion for a stimulus of optimal spatio-temporal frequency (this did not change as a function of luminance) at each of a number of mean luminances once adaptation equilibrium had been reached. The pupil was dilated and a 4 mm artificial pupil used. Notice that individual neurones exhibit a similar response form to the psychophysical results for gratings depicted in Fig. 1.3. Each neurone has both a characteristic Weber region and a Rose–de Vries region. The neurones tuned to lower space frequencies exhibit responses which extend to lower luminances. Low frequency neurones have reduced photopic sensitivity but extend to lower scotopic levels. It was Rose (1942, 1948) and De Vries (1943) who first pointed out that because of the inevitable fluctuations about a mean value in the number of absorbed quanta per unit area and per unit time, that in order for a signal ΔI to be detected above the noise due to these statistical fluctuations in I (determined by Poisson Statistics) it must exceed a value proportional to $(I)^{0.5}$. Thus if sensitivity is limited solely by the quantal fluctuations of the light itself, one would expect a square-root relationship between sensitivity and mean retinal illuminance (in other words a slope of 0.5 on log/log coordinates). If we assume that each of these grating stimuli which are at least a factor of two apart in spatial frequency is detected by different neural filters at threshold, and that the same mechanism is responsible as retinal illuminance is lowered (see Fig. 1.19 of this chapter and Fig. 3.6 of Chapter 3) then the results in Fig.1 3 suggest that each of these filters exhibits a square-root response with illuminance. This is substantiated for individual neurones in cat cortex (Fig. 1.5) and this finding in itself adds further weight to the previous argument that the slopes of zero and 0.5 from the grating psychophysics represent the response of *unitary* visual filters at the *cortical level*. It is tempting to conclude that the sensitivity of each is limited by the quantal nature of light rather than just depending on it, but there is another possibility. If there were internal neural noise that was multiplicatively related to the input signal then this would also have Poisson statistics and result in a square-root behaviour (see Teich *et al.*, 1982). This has been found to be the case in the locust by Lillywhite & Laughlin (1979, and see Chapters 4 and 6). The fact that the quantum efficiency of the eye (for definition see Chapter 13 by van Meeteren) is so low, i.e. between 1% (Cohn, 1976; van Meeteren, 1973) and 5–10% (Barlow, 1962; Hallett, 1969) argues against sensitivity being *solely* limited by the inherent statistics of the photon catch (see Chapter 13, Section 13.1 for opposite view).

Finally let us consider the retinal illuminance region of the rod response (see solid curve in Fig. 1.2*b*) where contrast sensitivity is relatively independent of illuminance. This is usually assumed to be the result of an active process whereby the visual system adjusts its gain to maintain a constant contrast sensitivity in the face of reducing retinal illuminance. There is neurophysiological support that the gain of ganglion cells and other retinal neurones changes as a function of the background illuminance so as to maintain the contrast sensitivity of individual neurons constant as background retinal illumination is varied (Enroth-Cugell & Shapley, 1973*b*; Shapley & Enroth-Cugell, 1984; and results of Fig. 1.5). Furthermore, the shift that occurs in the extent of this so-called Weber region (i.e. transition illuminance) as spatial frequency is changed may have its neurophysiological counterpart in the fact that larger summation areas are relatively more light adapted than small ones since it is the background light flux (luminance × area) that determines the gain control (Enroth-Cugell & Shapley, 1973*b*). According to this view, thresholds being representative points on the sensitivity curve merely reflect this gain control (see section on discrimination sensitivities in this chapter). However, there are other possibilities (see Bouman, Vos & Wolrareen, 1963, and Teich *et al.*, 1978) one of which is that the Weber region in the psychophysics (Fig. 1.2*a*, *b*) is a purely threshold phenomenon and nothing to do with the maintenance of a constant contrast perception. Psychophysical threshold sensitivity, unlike suprathreshold performance in this region, could be limited by additive noise, the absolute value of which varies with the spatial frequency of the target used (or size of summation area). This would suggest that the noise source occurs at or before the point of summation of photoreceptor signals. The transition illuminance as defined by van Nes and Bouman (1967) would then represent the illuminance at which the external noise (see Teich *et al.*, 1982, for counter argument) equals the internal noise. This highlights the importance of measuring the full performance of visual neurones. A recent report by Troy, Enroth-Cugell & Robson (1987) suggest that the Weber response of ganglion cells in cat is reflected equally in *threshold and suprathreshold* measures of performance. However, this is not the case for cortical cells (see Fig. 1.6). In this figure we see the contrast response functions of four cat striate neurones. For each the response is plotted against the stimulus contrast with mean luminance as the parameter. The stimulus used was independently verified to be optimal in its spatio-temporal frequency at each adaptation level for each neurone. In the inset, threshold and gain measures are derived for each neurone's response. Two points are noteworthy. First, threshold and gain measures differ in their relationship with mean

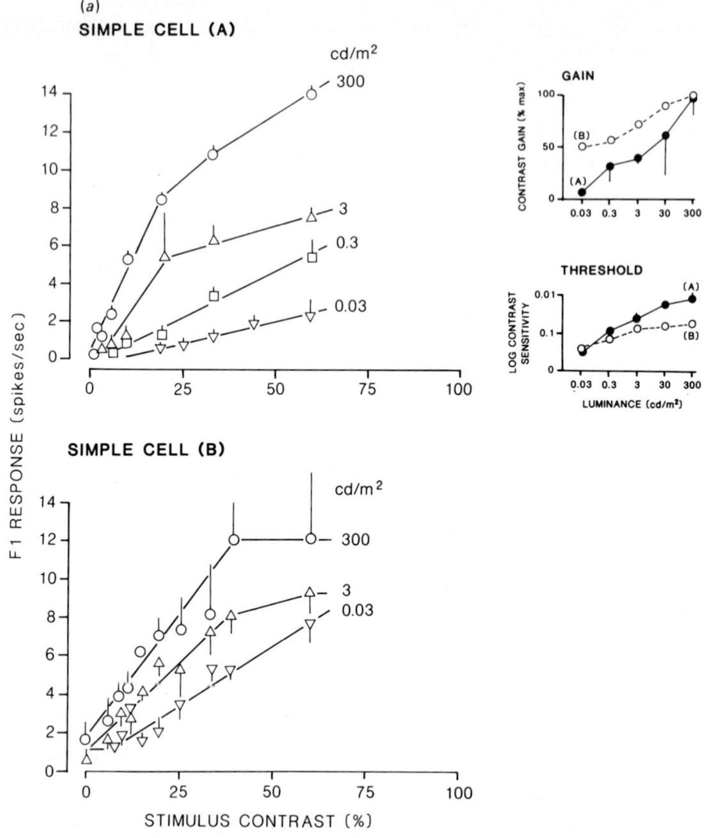

Fig. 1.6. Cat cortical neuronal response in spikes per second is plotted against stimulus contrast for a range of different adaptation levels ranging from photopic to scotopic. The stimulus is a drifting sinewave grating of optimal spatio-temporal frequency. Gain and threshold measures are derived and compared.

luminance for individual neurones and secondly, saturation occurs at neither a constant response nor a constant contrast level at different adaptation levels. Thus for neurones thresholds and suprathreshold performance may be quite different at the level of the striate cortex.

The low illuminance asymptote

The second point of initial discrepancy between grating and increment threshold studies involves the slope of the increment threshold curve at low scotopic levels (see dashed curve in Fig. 1.2*a*). This is a constant feature of increment threshold experiments occurring at about the same

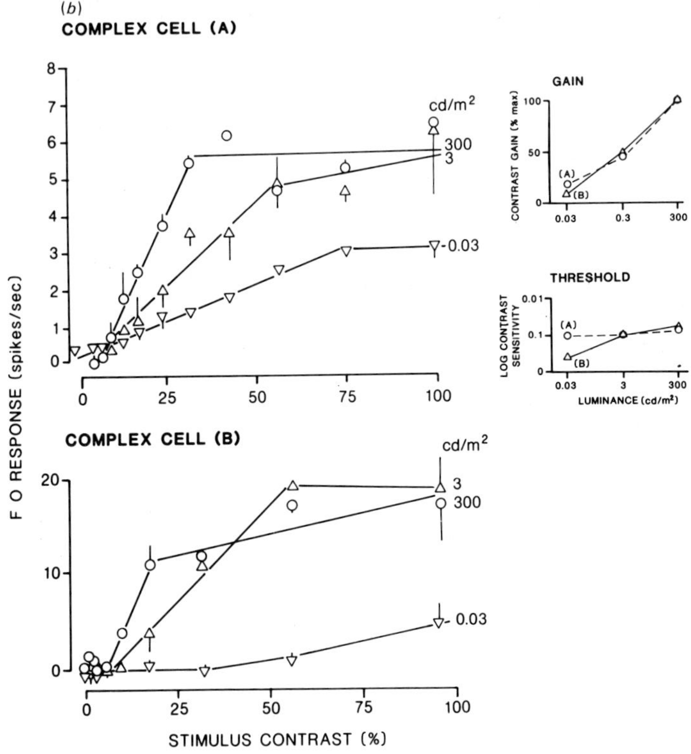

(Data from Hess & Lillywhite, unpublished.) Gain is plotted as a percentage of the slope found at the highest luminance and threshold is plotted as the lowest contrast at which the response reaches an asymptotic level.

illuminance irrespective of the stimulus size (Barlow, 1958*b*). This asymptotic behaviour has been interpreted as evidence for an added source of photoreceptor noise, termed 'dark light', which is indistinguishable from real light (summates over space and time like real lights) and adds to it to produce a physiological background pedestal (Barlow, 1977). Since this internal 'light' is larger than the external background light at these levels it dominates and produces an asymptote in performance.

Various estimates can be derived from the literature for the magnitude of this dark light (see also Section 2.2.5 in Chapter 2). Psychophysical estimates are of the order of 0.016 quanta/s/rod at the retina (Barlow, 1977) whereas individual primate rod photoreceptors have been measured to contain noise equivalent to 0.0063 isomerizations (Baylor,

Nunn & Schnapf, 1984). Although Barlow (1957) has put forward a compelling case (see also Aho *et al.*, 1988) it is not yet clear whether the noise that is now known to be present in individual photoreceptors actually sets the limit of psychophysical absolute sensitivity (see Teich *et al.*, 1982, and also Chapter 4 for greater detail, and also Chapters 2 and 5). The reason why a similar discontinuity is not seen in the relationship of contrast sensitivity to mean retinal illuminance is because of the way it is plotted as can be seen by the equivalence transformation in Fig. 1.2*a*. Incremental measures do not take into account any contribution from the increment to the physiological background. If an incremental measure is derived from contrast sensitivity measurements such that the increment and background are no longer independent (as is the case for increments on backgrounds) then a similar lower illuminance asymptote is seen. This is done by taking L_{min} as the equivalent background illuminance.

In conclusion, the main difference between the form of rod sensitivity as measured via the increment threshold method for spots and the contrast sensitivity method for sinewave gratings can be ascribed to the fact that when the stimulus in the former case is spatially and temporally broadband, the rod post-receptoral mechanism has a range of spatial and temporal filters at its disposal and by using different filters at different luminances, see also Ross & Campbell (1978), it maintains its sensitivity across a wider illuminance range. This highlights the importance of the post-receptoral contribution to extending our operating range. The fact that we have visual neurons with independent spatio-temporal filtering properties and gain control allows the visual system as a whole to detect different aspects of a broad-band stimulus and hence register its presence over a range of light levels exceeding a million to one. Let's begin with the spatial aspects of this organization.

1.2.3 Spatial sensitivity

Spatial summation

Historically, spatial influences on threshold have been assessed by varying the size of a test stimulus and adjusting its intensity to threshold. The stimulus has been invariably a sharply focused spot. This was first investigated by Ricco (1877) who made such measurements for the absolute threshold of the dark adapted eye. He found that for circular targets of up to approximately 42 min in diameter threshold luminance was inversely proportional to area. This relationship, which is now known as Ricco's law, means that the threshold luminous flux is independent of its spatial distribution. The stimulus areas over which Ricco's law holds increases as the stimulus is moved to more eccentric positions in the visual field (Hallett, Marriott & Rodgers, 1962), and as the background luminance is reduced (Barlow, 1958*a*). Piper (1903) was the first to investigate the nature of this relationship for areas outside the range where Ricco's law holds. He found that for circular stimuli of diameter between 2 and 26 deg threshold varied inversely with the square-root of the area. This has become known as Piper's law. It is rather limiting to think of the spatial influences on threshold as determined solely by these two laws. They are better thought of as two hypotheses which usually offer only approximate fits to data. When plotted in terms of log threshold intensity versus stimulus area, Ricco's hypothesis is given by a slope of -1 and Piper's by a slope of $-1/2$. Piper's hypothesis in particular often does not well describe the data obtained for large stimulus areas. In some cases such data cannot be described by a straight line of any slope (Graham, Brown & Mote, 1939; Barlow, 1958*a*). Since Ricco's hypothesis is more successful it has been generally interpreted that the largest area over which it holds indicates the *greatest* degree of spatial summation and hence the *largest* summation pool available to the visual system under those particular conditions. The dependence of spatial summation on background intensity and presentation duration are clearly seen in Barlow's results (1958*a*) which are reproduced in Fig. 1.7. Log threshold intensity for circular spots is plotted against log area of the stimulus for a range of background intensities (expressed quanta/s. deg^2) from photopic to absolute threshold (no background). Results are displayed for two durations of presentation so that the degree of temporal interaction can be gauged. The straight lines have a slope of -1 and represent Ricco's hypothesis. Piper's hypothesis can be rejected since the data not described by Ricco's hypothesis are best fit by a curve rather than a straight line. If one takes the area at which the data just depart from Ricco's hypothesis as an estimation of the greatest degree of physiological spatial summation and hence the largest neural summation area, one might be prompted to conclude that the degree of spatial summation increases at low light levels especially for long durations of presentation. At intensities at and above $10^{5.94}$ quanta/s.deg^2, complete spatial summation extends only to 0.025 deg whereas at intensities at and below $10^{5.94}$ quanta/s.deg^2 summation extends to 0.3 deg. A similar though less dramatic effect is seen for the short presentation duration. However, since the background

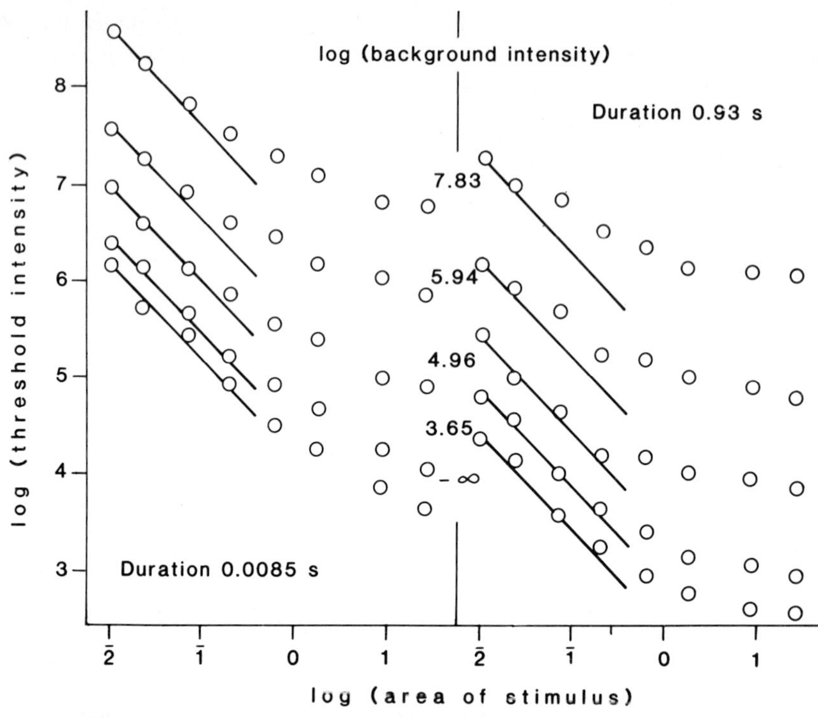

Fig. 1.7. Spatial summation for spot stimuli from the results of Barlow (1958*a*). Log (increment threshold intensity) plotted against log (area) for a short (8.5 ms) and long (930 ms) stimulus duration at five different background intensities. The straight lines have a slope of -1 and are continued to 0.4 deg. Intensities are in quanta (507 nm)/s. deg^2; areas in deg^2.

intensity at which this change occurs roughly corresponds to where cone vision is giving way to rod vision, the increase in spatial summation may be solely due to the intrusion of the rod mechanism. Hence there is no evidence from these results that spatial summation increases within the rod mechanism itself as a function of decreasing background intensity.

Furthermore there is even a problem in interpreting these results to mean that the rod mechanism has available to it larger neural summation areas (or lower spatial frequency filters) than the cone mechanism. As discussed earlier, spots have broad spatial frequency spectra and there is evidence that the visual system can analyse the retinal image over different spatial scales, that is, different sized filters or summation areas can be used at any one illuminance. The combination of these two factors makes the interpretation a little more involved than Ricco first thought. This is also suggested by the findings that the summation function for rectangular stimuli (Lamar *et al.*, 1947) and double stimuli (Sakitt, 1971) do not

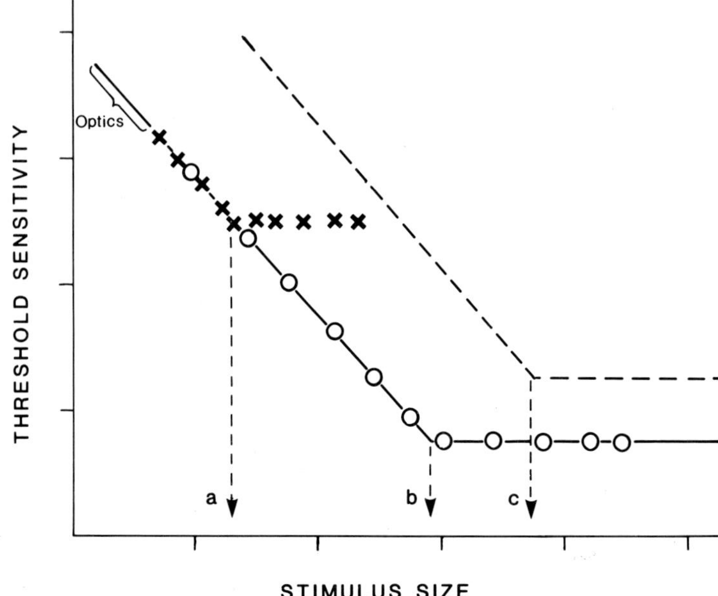

Fig. 1.8. Schematic representation of the contribution of different sized receptive fields to a spot summation experiment of the type depicted in Fig. 1.7. The threshold performance is dominated by the properties of the neurones with the most sensitive receptive fields regardless of whether they are the largest ones or not.

follow Ricco's prediction. In Fig. 1.8, Ricco's response is broken down into hypothesized components. For extremely small spots of light Ricco's hypothesis must be true as a trivial consequence of optical factors. As the size of the test spot increases beyond the optical spread function one would expect, on a signal-to-noise consideration that larger and larger neural summation areas would contribute to its threshold detection. The most *sensitive* summation area would eventually determine where Ricco's hypothesis begins to fail psychophysically. Assuming that this mechanism has some intermediate value of around 2 c/deg, its threshold would progressively fall as the stimulus energy at that spatial frequency increased and this would follow the prediction (open circle in Fig. 1.8) approximating a slope of unity. For larger stimulus areas the edges of the stimulus could be used to enable its detection to be roughly independent (i.e., within the limits of probability summation) of its area. If there are larger summation areas, but with reduced threshold sensitivity (dashed curve in Fig. 1.8), their contribution would not be seen. Thus what is being measured in such experiments is not the *greatest degree* of spatial summation and hence the *largest* neural summation pool under some particular condition, but instead the degree of spatial summation associated with the *most sensitive mechanism*. Therefore one can reinterpret the results of Fig. 1.7 to suggest that the spatial properties of the most sensitive neural mechanism is a factor of 10 or so larger for the rod as compared with the cone mechanism.

Spatial modulation transfer function

Another way of assessing the spatial sensitivity of the rod mechanism is to measure threshold sensitivity for spatially periodic targets that have a sinusoidal intensity profile (see Fig. 1.1*b*). At any particular background luminance the spatial periodicity or spatial frequency can be set and the contrast determined for detecting it. This can be done for a range of different spatial frequencies to obtain the overall spatial sensitivity function. Such an approach offers two advantages. First, the stimuli favour detection by equivalent sized summation areas and second, the overall extent of the stimulus does not change. This allows a better estimate of the overall threshold sensitivity of the different size summation areas that subserve rod vision within a fixed region of the visual field. The results of the threshold sensitivity for detecting relatively small two-dimension Gaussian patches of gratings of different spatial frequency are seen in Fig. 1.9 for central (*b*) and peripheral (*a*) parts of the visual field. The results are plotted as contrast sensitivity (threshold^{-1}) versus spatial frequency on log/log coordinates. The filled symbols in (*a*) are for the isolated rod mechanism of the Duplex retina (D'Zmura & Lennie, 1986) whereas those in (*b*) are for the achromat (Hess, Nordby & Pointer, 1987). Rod sensitivity is shown for two mean retinal illuminances, one mesopic and the other scotopic. The unfilled symbols and dashed curve are for the mesopically adapted cone mechanism of a normal trichromat. Notice that for both rod and cone mechanism, as the spatial frequency is increased, contrast sensitivity rises until a peak is seen at intermediate levels. For the cone system the falloff in sensitivity at high spatial frequencies is mainly due to neural factors although there is also a significant optical contribution at high illuminances (Campbell & Green, 1965; Campbell & Gubisch, 1967). For rod vision, it is limited solely by neural factors, rod acuity being around 7 c/deg. As the spatial frequency is further lowered, sensitivity begins to decline and it is here that rod and cone mechanisms have equal contrast sensitivity. It has been shown that the photopic cone curve is made up of a number of more

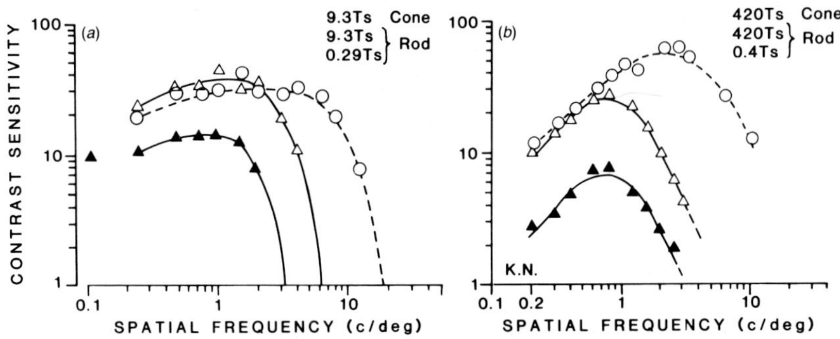

Fig. 1.9. Spatial contrast sensitivity functions for the rod mechanism of normal vision at an eccentricity of 10 deg (*a*) and from the central field of the rod monochromat (*b*) are compared at mesopic and scotopic levels of illumination. The results in (*a*) are from D'Zmura & Lennie (1986) and in (*b*) from Hess *et al.* (1987). The results depicted with open circles are for the cone mechanism under mesopic levels. Note that the rod spatial function is just displaced vertically as illumination is reduced.

spatially selective mechanisms or neural summation areas (Campbell & Robson, 1968; Blakemore & Campbell, 1969; Watson & Robson, 1981) and so the spatial sensitivity curve should be considered as the envelope of their individual sensitivities. Likewise the rod contrast sensitivity function is also the envelope of the sensitivities of a number of summation areas subserving rod vision (Kranda & Kulikowski, 1976; Hess & Nordby, 1986*b*). In comparing the rod and cone spatial sensitivity functions a number of points are noteworthy. The rod mechanism does not possess the high frequency filters that underlie the cone mechanism's superior sensitivity at high spatial frequencies. Optimum sensitivity is found for intermediate size stimuli under mesopic and scotopic conditions. This is crucial as far as the argument outlined in Fig. 1.8 is concerned. The size of the most sensitive summation area for rod vision is a factor of 5–10 larger than for cone vision. The largest summation areas accessible to rod vision may be no larger than those accessible to cone vision. The results for the rod monochromat (Fig. 1.9*b*) are in good agreement with the isolated rod response of the Duplex retina (Fig. 1.9*a*). There is also evidence that spatial bandwidths of individual low frequency mechanisms for rod and cone vision are similar (Kranda & Kulikowski, 1976; Hess & Nordby, 1986*b*). Thus there is no evidence to suggest that there is any substantial difference between the characteristics of individual low spatial frequency mechanisms for rod and cone systems. For the rod mechanism alone, the size of the most sensitive summation area does not change greatly with either eccentricity or luminance (compare Fig. 1.9*a*, *b*). Thus the main difference between the spatial properties of the rod and cone mechanism is not that the rods are connected to make larger summation areas but that the cones are connected to make small as well as large ones. The most sensitive summation area is a factor of 10 or so larger for rod vision as compared with photopically adapted cone vision (in general agreement with the results of Fig. 1.7). The reduced sensitivity of the larger summation areas for both rod and cone vision highlights the caution with which the spot summation results should be interpreted. Lastly, it is interesting to note that one extension of a rather strict interpretation of the Duplex theory of two independent visual systems, is that they may have no overlap in the size of the summation areas. This is not so, the large summation areas are shared and most probably involve common pathways (D'Zmura & Lennie, 1986), it is only the smaller ones that the rod mechanism lacks.

1.2.4 Temporal sensitivity

Temporal summation

As for spatial sensitivity, temporal sensitivity has also been traditionally viewed in terms of temporal summation which in turn has been measured by varying presentation duration (abrupt presentation) and adjusting the luminance of test stimuli (usually spots) to threshold. For sufficiently brief presentations the product of luminance and duration determine threshold. This implies that the visual system performs as a simple first order low pass filter. This is analogous to Ricco's law for spatial summation and is known as Block's law for temporal summation. For stimuli of very long duration, threshold is independent of exposure duration.

Among others, Bouman (1950, 1952) and Barlow (1958*a*) have examined temporal summation for stimuli of different size and at different adapting luminances. Barlow's results are reproduced in Fig. 1.10. Log threshold intensity is plotted against log duration for spot stimuli of diameter 7.1 min and 5.9 deg over a range of background intensities (quanta/s.deg^2). The straight lines have a slope of -1 and describe complete temporal summation (Block's law). It is only for large spatial stimuli that the results can be described by Block's law followed by a region of zero summation. For small stimuli, the data initially follow Block's law but then exhibit only partial summation. Under photopic conditions, the region of complete temporal summation extends from 30 to 50 ms depending on the spatial characteristics of the stimulus. Under

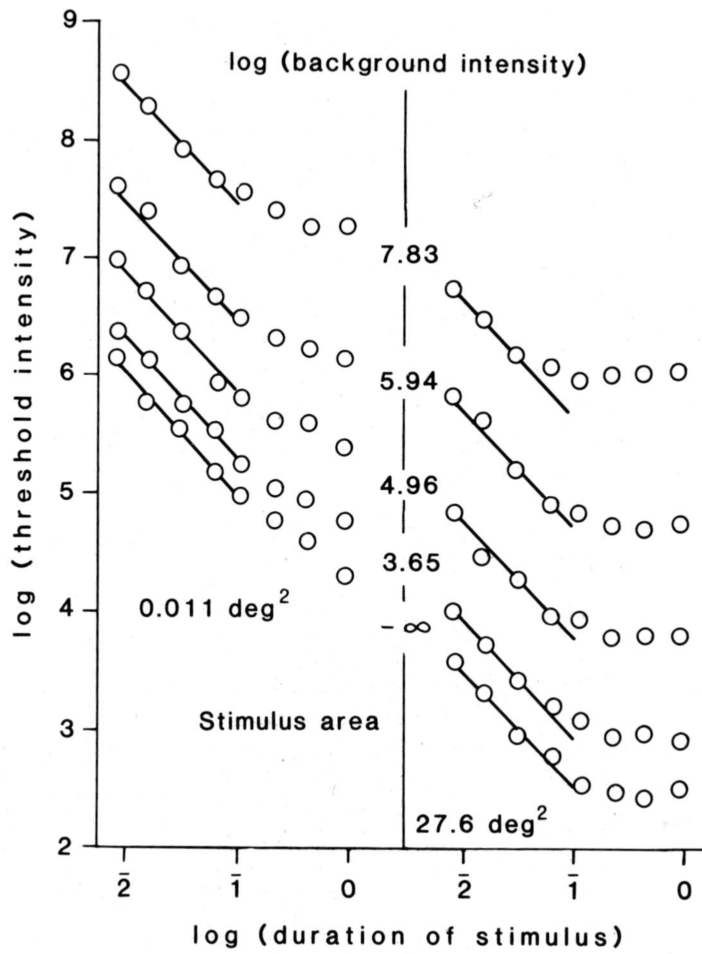

Fig. 1.10. Temporal summation for abruptly presented stimuli from the results of Barlow (1958*a*). Log (increment threshold intensity) plotted against log (stimulus duration) for a small (0.011 deg) and a large (27.6 deg) area of stimulus at five levels of background intensity. The straight lines have a slope of −1 and are continued down to 0.1 s. Intensities are in quanta (5;7 nm)/s.deg^2; areas in deg^2.

scotopic conditions this is increased to 100 ms. Two differences can be seen between these results and the corresponding ones for spatial summation (Fig. 1.7). The change in temporal summation is small (factor of 2–3) compared with the correspondingly larger change in spatial summation (factor of 10) as one goes from photopic to scotopic conditions. Second, this change does not take place abruptly across some luminance boundary unlike its spatial counterpart.

As for spatial summation one needs to exercise care in interpreting these results simply in terms of the largest temporal integration time available to the rod mechanism. Firstly there is evidence for bandpass temporal filtering in the visual system (Ikeda, 1965; Rashbass, 1970) and for probability summation over time (Watson, 1979). Furthermore there is also ample evidence for a covariation of the temporal filtering properties with the spatial structure of the stimulus (Robson, 1966; Watson & Nachmias, 1977, Tolhurst, 1975; Hess & Plant, 1985). Again the most likely interpretation is that this sort of measure reflects not the activity of the mechanism with the largest temporal summation, but the summation characteristics of the most sensitive mechanism. Therefore Barlow's results suggest that the temporal properties of the most sensitive filter gradually changes to lower values for both rod and cone mechanisms as the luminance decreases.

Temporal modulation transfer function

Another approach is to measure the contrast sensitivity for stimuli which vary sinusoidally in time (Robson, 1966). The results in Fig. 1.11*a* are from the work of Conner (1982) for the isolated rod response of a normal observer at 16 deg eccentricity. The stimulus is a spot of light sinusoidally modulated in time. The modulation amplitude is plotted against temporal frequency of the stimulus on log/log coordinates. Each curve represents a different background illuminance which span the rod range. Notice that the mesopic response displays a peak around 10 Hz on either side of which sensitivity falls off. Temporal acuity, obtained by extrapolation of the high frequency limb of this curve, is around 30 Hz under mesopic conditions. As illuminance is reduced, sensitivity is lost more rapidly at higher temporal frequencies resulting in a shift of the peak of the function to lower temporal frequencies. In other words, reducing the luminance not only reduces sensitivity but reduces the dynamics of rod vision. Compare this with the spatial sensitivity function in Fig. 1.9 where there is only a sensitivity change. In Fig. 1.11*b* similar results are seen for the central field of a rod monochromat for stimuli varying sinusoidally in space as well as time. Included in this figure as open symbols and a dashed curve is the temporal sensitivity function of the mesopically adapted cone mechanism of the trichromat. Its peak sensitivity and acuity are a factor of 2 higher than seen for the rod response under similar mesopic conditions. Notice also that the peak of the rod function has shifted by a factor of 2–3 from mesopic to scotopic conditions in agreement with the results in Fig.1 10.

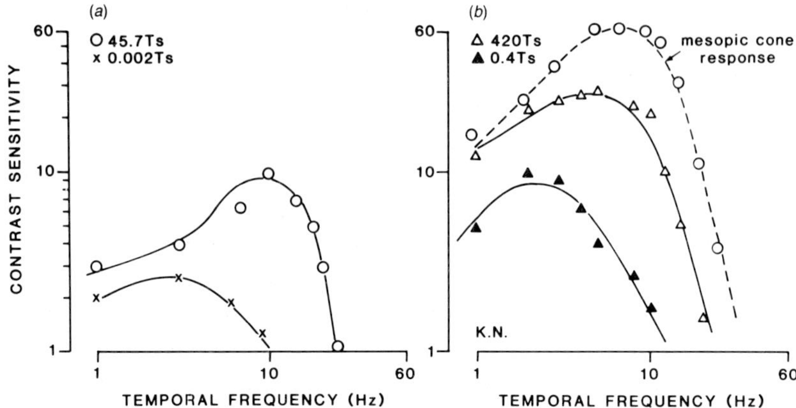

Fig. 1.11. Temporal contrast sensitivity functions for the rod mechanism of normal vision at 16 deg eccentricity (*a*) and for central field of the rod monochromat (*b*) are compared at a mesopic and a scotopic level of illumination. The results in (*a*) are from Conner (1982) and in (*b*) from Hess *et al.* (1987). The results depicted by open circles are for the cone mechanism of normal vision under mesopic conditions. Note that the rod curve is displaced down and to the left as illuminance is reduced.

There is now evidence of a duplicity of temporal function within the rod mechanism itself, comprising fast mesopic and slow scotopic sub-mechanisms (Conner & MacLeod, 1977; Conner, 1982). There are three pieces of evidence for this. First, rod temporal acuity exhibits a double-branched function with illuminance. This is shown in Fig. 1.12*a* from the results of Conner (1982). The function relating temporal acuity to illuminance exhibits a discontinuity around 3 Ts (corresponding to a temporal acuity of 15 Hz). Similar results are seen in Fig. 1.12*b* from the rod monochromat (Hess & Nordby, 1986*a*). The more extended scotopic limb seen in Connor's results is due to the peripheral location of his stimulus. The evidence suggests that both segments of this curve are determined by rods (Hecht *et al.*, 1948). The second piece of evidence relies on the change in shape of the temporal sensitivity function from bandpass (open symbols in Fig. 1.11*a*) to lowpass (crosses in Fig. 1.11*a*) on either side of 3 Ts discontinuity. This is not a large effect and is not present for the rod monochromat when more spatially confined stimuli are used (Fig. 1.11*b*). The third piece of evidence is more convincing as it involves interaction between these two hypothesized rod temporal mechanisms across the 3 Ts boundary when their signals are out of phase (Conner, 1982; Sharpe, Stockman & MacLeod, 1989).

We are left wondering what determines the shape and position of these

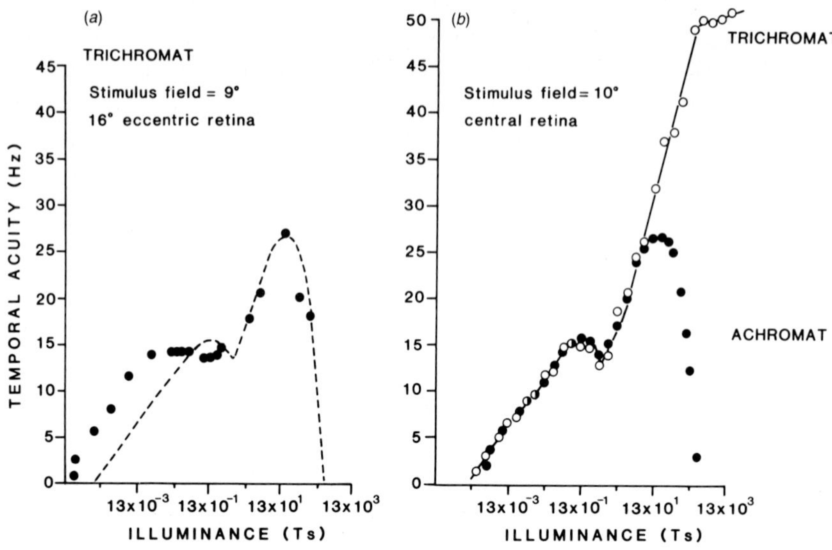

Fig. 1.12. Temporal acuity is plotted as a function of mean illuminance for the isolated rod mechanism (filled symbols) of normal vision (in (*a*) from the results of Conner, 1982) and for the rod monochromat (in (*b*) from the results of Hess & Nordby, 1986*a*). The results depicted with open circles are for the normal Duplex retina. Note that rod temporal acuity is around 28 Hz. The dashed curve in (*a*) represents the rod monochromats results from (*b*).

temporal responses for the rod and cone mechanism. Is it the receptors themselves or their post-receptoral pathways? Brindley (1962) tried to answer this for cone vision by seeing how high a flickering light needed to be to produce visible beats with alternating current passed directly through the eye. The flickering light could be raised to 120 c/s (the critical flicker frequency was 90 c/s when presented alone) and still produce visible beats. Brindley proposed that the highest frequency point on the cone temporal sensitivity function was not solely limited by the receptors (more correctly by the transduction process up to the point where light-induced neural signals and his electricity interacted). He suggested that there were two or more post-receptoral high frequency attenuators. Although a similar experiment has not yet been done for rod vision, Brindley (1970) has argued that the reduced temporal resolution of rod vision is likely to be due to the rod receptors themselves. His argument relies on the assumption that rods and cones share the same neural pathway which Brindley's results suggest can transmit cone signals to 90 c/s. Since it is now known, at least in cat, that the rod pathway involves an A II amacrine cell not shared by cone signals, a lot depends on its temporal properties. Furthermore, there is also evidence that rods can send signals via gap functions to cone terminals and into the cone pathway (Kolb, 1977; Nelson, 1977). The fact that there are two routes for rod signals offers a possible post-receptoral explanation for the duplicity of rod-mediated vision. A more direct comparison between the overall temporal response of rod vision and the temporal response of rod receptors is seen in Fig. 1.13. Here the recent electrophysiological step response data of Baylor *et al.*, from isolated rod photoreceptors (see Fig. 5.5) of the primate has been transformed into the frequency domain.

The amplitude ratio of the frequency response has the form

$$\frac{A(f)}{A(0)} = \frac{1}{[1+(2\pi f\tau)^2]^{n/2}}$$

where Baylor *et al.* (1984) found that $n = 6$ and $\tau = 40$ ms for isolated rods irrespective of background illuminance (Nunn, personal communication). Since the psychophysical temporal acuity does reduce with reducing luminance, the high frequency limb of the receptoral response (solid line in Fig. 1.13*a*, *b*) has been fitted to the highest frequency point of the mesopically adapted rod-mediated psychophysical response for the normal observer (from the data of Conner, 1982; Fig. 13*a*) and for the achromat (from the data of Hess *et al.*, 1987; Fig. 1.13*b*). It seems clear that most of the post-receptoral attenuation occurs at intermediate and low temporal frequencies as has also been deduced for the cones (Kelly, 1971, Lamb, 1984). Thus the post-receptoral shaping of the step response is mainly in terms of its duration rather than its initial rising portion. Also the reduced dynamics of the psychophysical response as luminance is reduced must be post-receptoral in nature since it is not found in isolated primate photoreceptors (Nunn, personal communication).

1.2.5 Regional sensitivity of rod vision

So far we have considered rod vision along the dimensions of illuminance, spatial sensitivity and temporal sensitivity. Another important dimension is retinal eccentricity. Little is known about how rod sensitivity is distributed across the retina except under extreme scotopic conditions. Under these conditions rod sensitivity is reduced in the central field and in far periphery. This has been known since the early astronomers who noticed that very faint stars could be best observed by looking to one side of them, and thus imaging them on the parafoveal

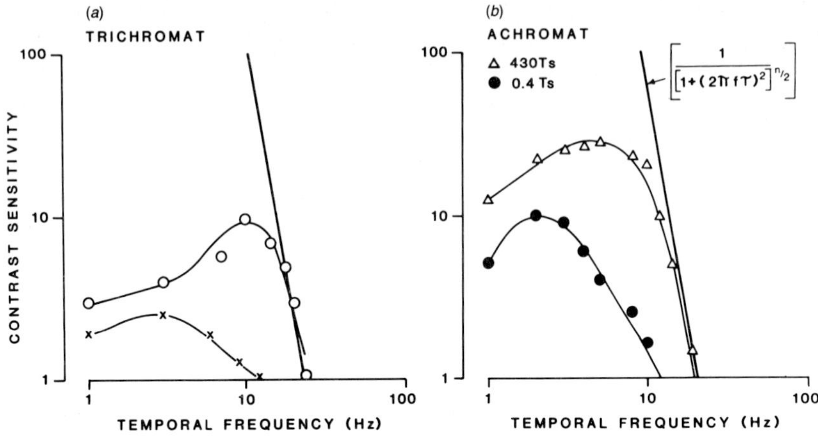

Fig. 1.13. Mesopic and scotopic temporal sensitivity functions for the rod mechanism of normal vision (in (*a*) from the results of Conner, 1982) and the rod monochromat (in (*b*) from the results of Hess *et al.*, 1987) are compared with the frequency response derived from the step response data of individual rod photoreceptors from the data of Baylor *et al.* (1984). The transformed step response and the psychophysical result have been equated in terms of temporal acuity.

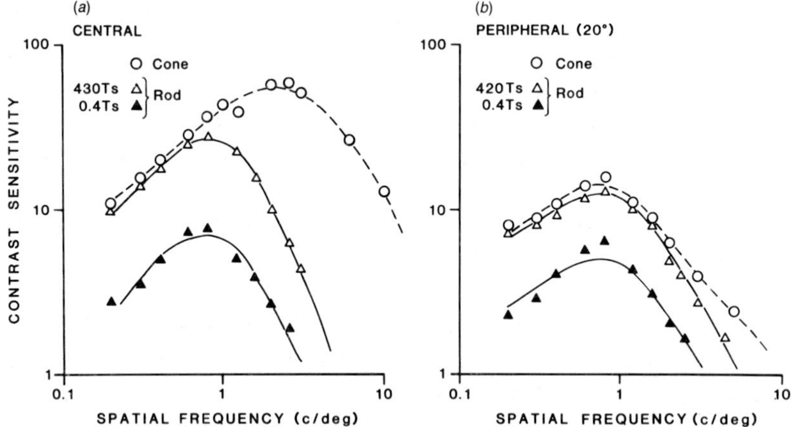

Fig. 1.14. Central (*a*) and peripheral (*b*) spatial sensitivity functions are compared for the rod monochromat at mesopic and scotopic levels of illumination. The results depicted by open circles are for the cone mechanism of normal vision under mesopic illumination. Note that for both central and peripheral regions, the rod spatial sensitivity curve is displaced vertically with reduced illuminance.

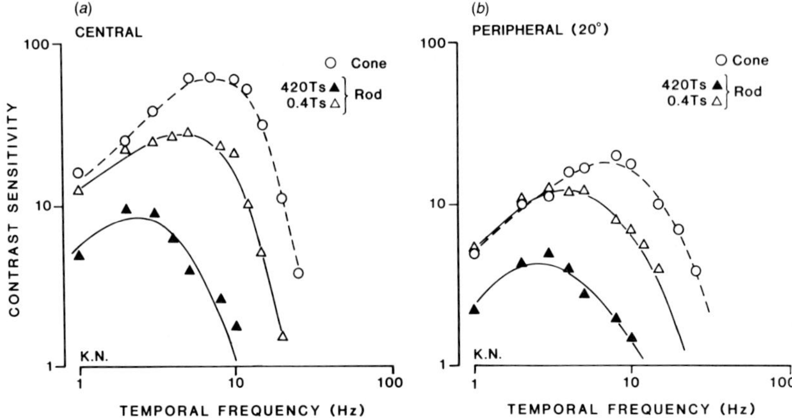

Fig. 1.15. Central (*a*) and peripheral (*b*) temporal sensitivity functions are compared for the rod monochromat at mesopic and scotopic levels of illumination. Open circles are for the cone mechanism of normal vision under mesopic conditions. Note that for central and peripheral vision rod temporal sensitivity is displaced down and to the left.

retina. It would be clearly useful to examine this in a little more detail. For example, if scotopic *sensitivity* is better in the mid-periphery of the retina, is this also true for *acuity*? Also, does the rod mechanism have a similar sensitivity distribution under all levels of illumination? An answer to the former bears upon the rules that govern receptor to ganglion cell convergence, whereas an answer to the latter would determine whether the rod mechanism behaves in a unitary manner as illuminance is reduced.

The only results that are available on how mesopic spatial and temporal sensitivity and acuity vary with retinal eccentricity come from a recent study of the rod monochromat (Hess *et al.*, 1987). These results are displayed in the following three figures (Figs 1.14–1.16). In Fig. 1.14 we see how spatial contrast sensitivity varies as a function of both retinal eccentricity and illuminance for small, Gaussian patches of gratings. The dashed curve indicates the mesopic sensitivity of the cone mechanism. These results for central viewing are identical to those already described in Fig. 1.9*b*. Peak rod sensitivity is around 0.8 c/deg and acuity is 5–6 c/deg. Reducing the illuminance from mesopic (420 Ts) to scotopic (0.4 Ts) reduces sensitivity evenly by about a factor of 3. In the mid periphery (Fig. 1.14*b*) the spatial sensitivity curve is of a similar shape but is lower in sensitivity for all spatial frequencies. For cone vision, a lateral as well as vertical shift occurs. Under scotopic conditions the rod peripheral

(a)

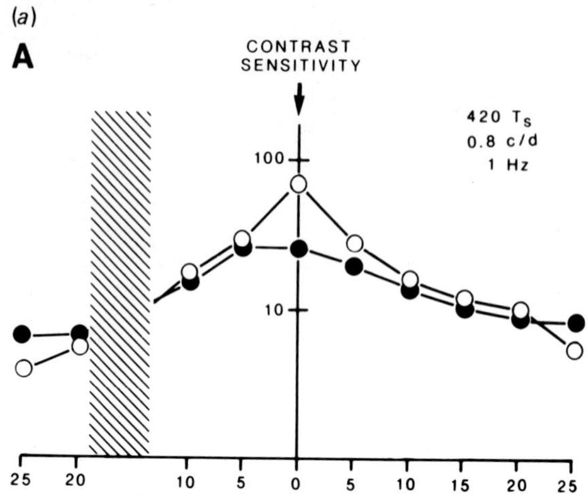
A
CONTRAST SENSITIVITY
420 T_s
0.8 c/d
1 Hz
100
10
25 20 10 5 0 5 10 15 20 25

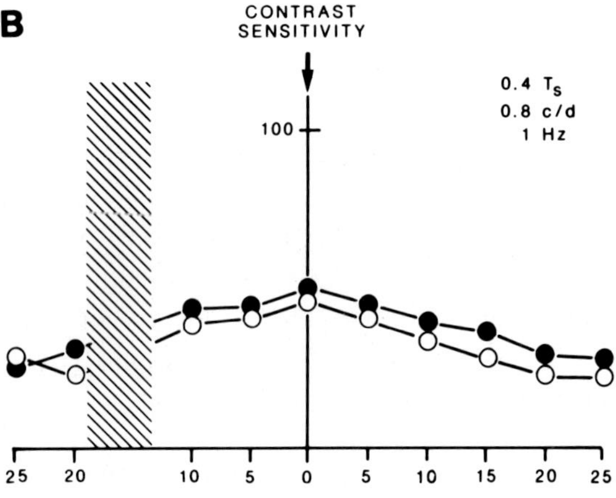
B
CONTRAST SENSITIVITY
0.4 T_s
0.8 c/d
1 Hz
100
25 20 10 5 0 5 10 15 20 25

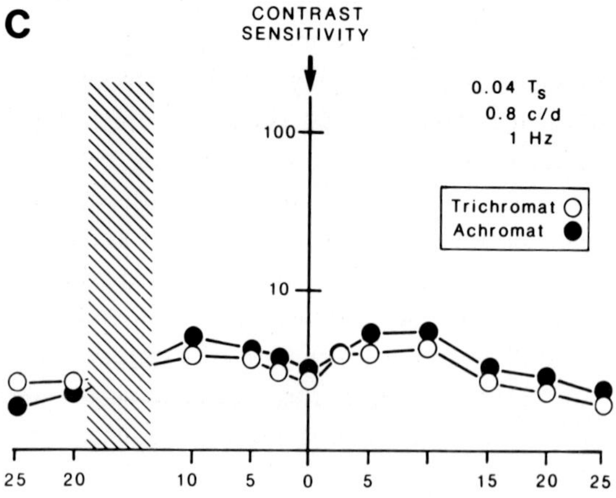
C
CONTRAST SENSITIVITY
0.04 T_s
0.8 c/d
1 Hz
Trichromat
Achromat
100
10
25 20 10 5 0 5 15 20 25

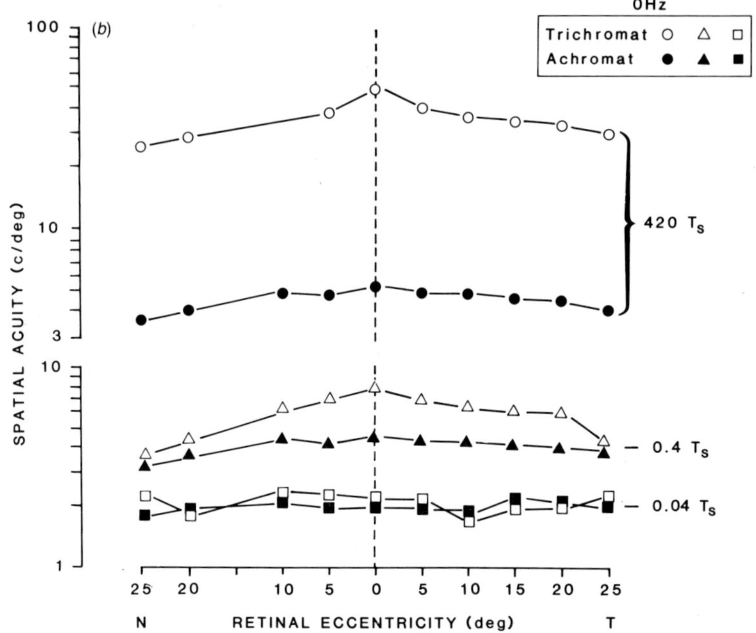

Fig. 1.16. In (*a*) contrast sensitivity is plotted against retinal eccentricity for a spatial frequency stimulus which optimally stimulates the rod mechanism of a rod monochromat (filled symbols). The open circles are for the normal Duplex retina. Note that for the rod mechanism the distribution of sensitivity varies with the mean level of illumination (Results from Hess *et al.*, 1987). In (*b*) the fall-off in spatial acuity for the rod monochromat and normal observer are measured under comparable conditions. A flat acuity profile is seen under scotopic conditions (results from Hess *et al.*, 1987).

sensitivity curve maintains its shape and shifts down vertically in sensitivity. Two factors emerge; under mesopic conditions spatial sensitivity for all sized targets is best in the central 10 deg of the visual field whereas under scotopic conditions the regional sensitivity profile is relativcly flat. The corresponding result for temporal sensitivity is displayed in Fig. 1.15. As described previously (Fig. 1.11), the peak of the temporal sensitivity function shifts to lower temporal frequencies (sensitivity curve shifts laterally as well as vertically) as illuminance is reduced. These slower dynamics may be another reflection of the temporal duplicity within the rod mechanism (Conner, 1982). In the mid periphery, the temporal sensitivity function for the rod system has the same shape but is progressively displaced in sensitivity as the temporal frequency is lowered (Fig. 1.15*b*). A similar effect is seen for cone vision (dashed curves of Fig. 1.15*a*, *b*). Under scotopic conditions the temporal sensitivity functions for central and peripheral regions are of similar shape, and overall sensitivity. Again temporal sensitivity is best in the central 10 deg for the optimal stimulus and falls off with eccentricity under mesopic conditions but is invariant with eccentricity under scotopic conditions.

Are these gains in spatial sensitivity across the retina seen in Fig. 1.14 at the expense of losses in spatial acuity or do both functions behave similarly? Fig. 1.16 compares the fall-off in rod sensitivity across the retina for the rod monochromat and trichromat (open circles) for 3 illuminances (*a*) with that of spatial acuity (*b*). The rod spatial sensitivity profile (Fig. 1.16*a*) is seen to undergo a continuous change as the illumination is reduced. Initially at mesopic levels it is peaked in the centre of the retina, under upper scotopic conditions it is relatively flat and then under lower scotopic conditions it exhibits a mid peripheral peak. Rod spatial acuity exhibits a shallow peak in the centre of the visual field under both mesopic and upper scotopic levels but is relatively flat under the lower scotopic conditions (Fig. 1.16*b*). These results do not suggest that the relative sensitivity gains in the centre of the retina under mesopic conditions and in the mid periphery under scotopic conditions are at the expense of acuity. It would seem that the rules that govern receptor convergence do not elect to endow different retinal regions with different functions. For example, it would seem that the small rod summation areas or the ganglion cells receiving least convergence are equally distributed at all eccentricities independent of illuminance. For some reason the sensitivity of the larger summation areas is greater in the central retina at mesopic conditions and in the mid periphery at scotopic conditions.

The mesopic–scotopic duplicity in the regional distribution of rod vision could also be explained by the two pathways through which rod signals can travel to a ganglion cell. The mesopic, cone-like distribution may reflect the organization of the post-receptoral layout of the cone pathway through which rod signals can travel (Kolb, 1977; Nelson, 1977; Sterling, Freed & Smith, 1986).

1.2.6 Rod–cone interactions

A great variety of stimulus situations have been reported where the rod–cone independence as put forward by the Duplex theory is violated. It is beyond the scope of this chapter to go into the details that would be necessary to do justice to these many and varied reports (see Chapter 2 for discussion on this topic). Although important, they represent excep-

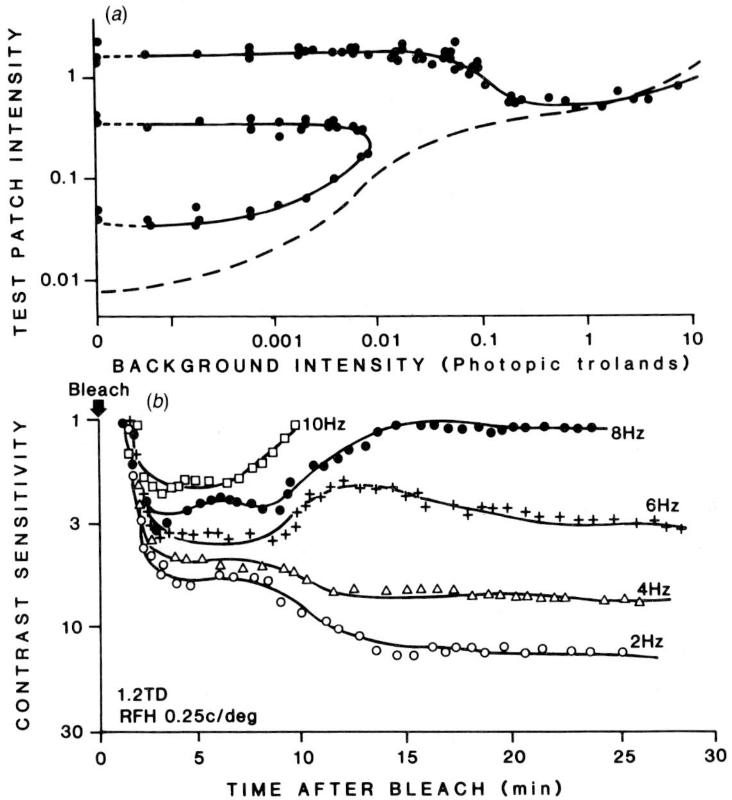

Fig. 1.17. In (*a*) flicker detectability contours from MacLeod (1972). The points show the test patch intensities at which 7.5 Hz flicker can be just detected against blue-green backgrounds of various intensities. At very low test patch intensities flicker is never seen whereas at high test patch intensities it is always visible. The upper and lower data set are separated by a region in which flicker is never seen. Intensities are in photopic trolands. In (*b*) the time course of recovery in contrast sensitivity after a 90% bleach is plotted for a low spatial frequency grating whose contrast was counterphasing at rates between 2–10 Hz. At 2 Hz sensitivity recovers in the expected way with the typical cone and rod branches whereas above 6 Hz the longer one waits in the dark after a bleach, the poorer vision becomes. (From Hess & Mullen – see Hess & Mullen, 1982).

tions to Duplex behaviour rather than serious challenges to it as a general rule. Their effects on visual sensitivity are small and the range of conditions over which they operate is rather limited. Thus their effect on night perception is slight.

They can be divided into linear and non-linear interactions. In the linear category, constructive (complete or physiological summation) and destructive (out of phase cancellation) interference of rod and cone signals have been reported by psychophysicists (MacLeod, 1972; Frumkes *et al.*, 1973; van den Berg & Spekreijse, 1977; Bauer, Frumkes & Nygaad, 1983) and neurophysiologists (Donner & Rushton, 1959; Rodieck & Rushton, 1976). MacLeod demonstrated that under the appropriate conditions rod and cone signals could exactly cancel producing a perceptual null for flicker at a mesopic level. This is illustrated in Fig. 1.17*a*. A temporal frequency of 7.5 Hz was such that the rod delay became equivalent to a 180 deg phase shift. A variety of non-linear interactions have also been reported. These can be subdivided into four groups. First, detection thresholds and colour discrimination thresholds can be elevated near the rod–cone transition of the typical dark adaptation curve (Wooten & Butler, 1976; Spillmann & Conlon, 1972; see also Chapter 5 for more basic details on 'bleaching adaptation'). Secondly, another possibly related type of rod to cone interaction involves the central/parafoveal cone-mediated flicker perception being suppressed as the rods dark adapt and enhanced as rods light adapt (Goldberg, Frumkes & Nygaad, 1983; Hess & Mullen, 1982; Alexander & Fishman, 1984; Goldberg & Frumkes, 1983; Coletta & Adams, 1984, 1985, 1986). This is thought to be due to rod modulation of horizontal cell feedback onto cones (Frumkes & Eysteinsson, 1988). Thirdly, there are conditions under which there is only partial summation of rod and cone signals (Benimoff, Schneider & Hood, 1982; Drum, 1982) for which inhibitory models have been invoked (Levine & Frishman, 1984). Lastly, there is also evidence for cones affecting rod sensitivity (Blick & MacLeod, 1978; Makous & Boothe, 1974; Makous & Peeples, 1979; Latch & Lennie, 1977; Buck, Peeples & Makous, 1979; Frumkes, Sekuler & Reiss, 1972; Buck & Makous, 1981; Alexander & Kelly, 1984). This is particularly interesting because it has been recently shown that such interactions may have been present in the rod isolation procedures of Aguilar & Stiles (1954). If this is true, then the shape of their increment threshold curve for rod vision may be contaminated in the mesopic background range (see Fig 1.2 in this chapter and Stabell *et al.*, 1987). In terms of its perceptual effect the suppression of cone-mediated flicker by dark adapting rods is noteworthy because it is the only case where the longer one dark adapts the worse vision becomes. An illustration of this effect is seen in Fig. 1.17*b*. Sensitivity has been measured as a function of time in the dark after a substantial bleach. Temporal sensitivity above 4 Hz recovers initially, but then declines. Perceptually the effect is quite dramatic for flicker above 10 Hz. Initially nothing is seen, then the visibility of flicker increases and then later declines. It occurs only in the parafoveal region and its origin is not understood (Hess & Mullen, 1982).

1.3 Discrimination sensitivity

1.3.1 Veridical perceptions

Thresholds are the least troublesome quantities to assess for any sensory system, being reasonably easy to define and the most straight forward to relate to single cell neurophysiology. However, they do not represent the whole story and may at times give a misleading picture of vision as a whole. A good example is the spatial sensitivity function seen in Fig. 1.9. This is the threshold picture of how contrast sensitivity varies and does not accurately reflect what happens above threshold. Above threshold, different spatial frequencies are seen to be perceptually equivalent in contrast when their physical contrast is equal (Georgeson & Sullivan, 1975). The same is true of loudness perception for the auditory system. In vision, apart from optical considerations at very high spatial frequencies (a matter not yet resolved; see Georgeson & Sullivan, 1975, and Lillywhite, Hess & Parker, 1982) this can be simply thought of as thresholds being limited by noise which, while of small amplitude is strongly dependent on some stimulus parameter, for example spatial or temporal frequency. At high signal strengths, since the relative magnitude of the noise is small, its effect is not seen. More elaborate explanations have also been proposed (Georgeson & Sullivan, 1975).

Whatever the explanation, suprathreshold measures of vision can often be more important for understanding perception than threshold ones, but unfortunately, they pose added difficulties in that they are more difficult to relate to the underlying physiology. Scotopic vision is a good example. Although *threshold sensitivity* for detecting spatial and temporal targets varies with luminance producing severe distortions to the sensitivity curve, suprathreshold perceptions of the spatial, temporal and contrast variables remain fairly stable. This is illustrated in Fig. 1.18 where results are displayed which show how well spatial (0.5 c/deg and 6 c/deg) and temporal targets (2 Hz and 10 Hz) can be psychophysically matched between photopic and scotopic luminances. The absolute thresholds for these targets are marked by arrows. Over most of the range, spatial and temporal *perceptions* are veridical to within 15% although their detection thresholds vary by up to 3 log units (see Fig. 1.3 for threshold results). The difference in the size of the effect between

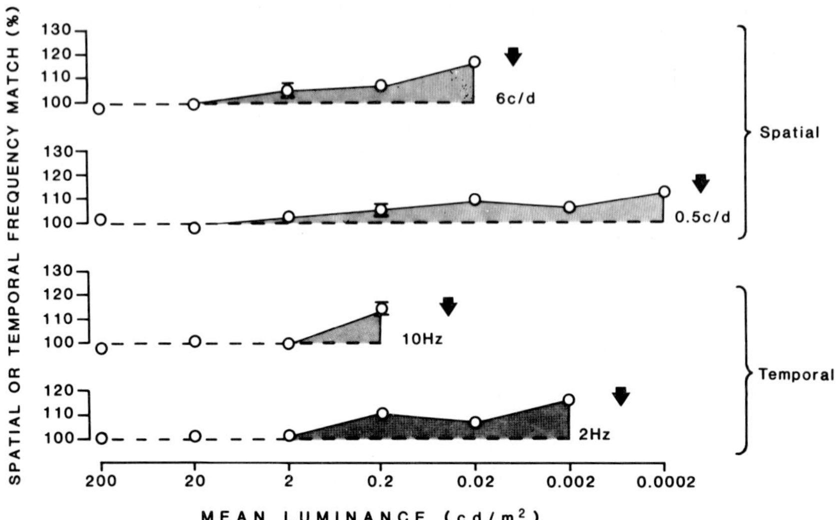

Fig. 1.18. Apparent spatial and temporal frequency is plotted as a function of mean retinal illumination. The dashed line represents veridical matches between one eye at photopic levels and the other at reduced lumination. Arrows indicate the illuminance at which this particular stimulus was no longer detectable. Perception is veridical to within 15% over 6 log units of reduced lumination (Hess, unpublished). The contrast was set to 90% – for reason, see results in Fig. 1.20. Veridical matches are represented by the horizontal dashed link.

these results and a previous report (Virsu, 1974) are due to a higher contrast level being used for the present results. This compensates for a contrast-dependent effect which is illustrated in Fig. 1.19. The fact that spatial and temporal perceptions are veridical or nearly so is probably due to the finding that the overall sensitivity functions are composed of more spatially and temporally selective mechanisms whose individual properties do not vary with luminance (Graham, 1972). These maybe the psychophysical counterpart of single cells in striate cortex as it has also been found that the spatial and temporal properties of these neurones unlike their retinal counterparts (Robson, unpublished) do not change with luminance (Bisti *et al.*, 1977). The results illustrated in Fig. 1.19 (Hess & Lillywhite, unpublished) show that the temporal properties of striate neurones do not change when luminance is reduced. For an illustration of the comparable results for spatial frequency see Fig. 3.6 of Chapter 3.

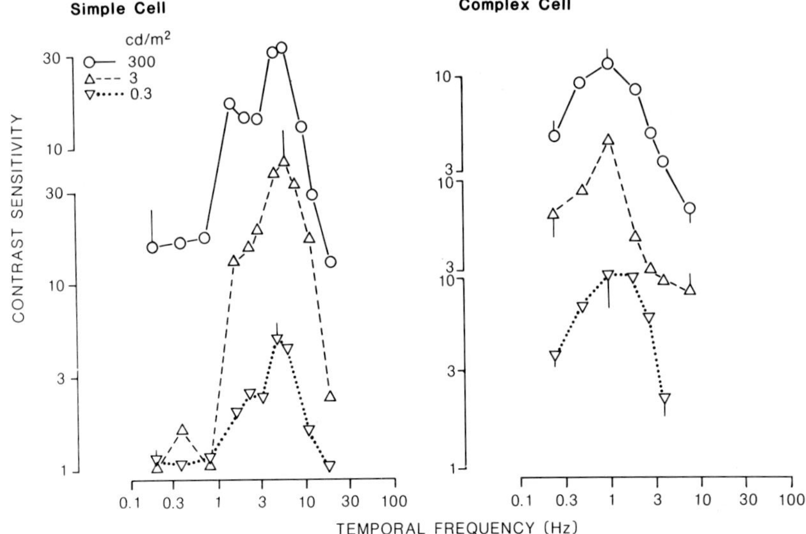

Fig. 1.19. Temporal tuning curves for two striate neurones in cat cortex for a range of different mean luminances. These were measured using an auditory criterion. Note that the ordinate is discontinuous. (Results from Hess & Lillywhite, unpublished.) Reducing the luminance does not change the neurone's filtering properties, only its sensitivity. See Fig. 3.6 for comparable spatial results.

Contrast perception

It could be argued that if elevated contrast thresholds are going to affect anything (except for contracting the range), they should affect the perception of contrast. But then the question becomes, is contrast perception affected in direct proportion to the threshold elevation produced by reducing the light level? The answer is, no. If one matches contrasts between the two eyes where each eye is adapted to different light levels, then the reduction in perceived contrast becomes less, the more suprathreshold it is. At contrasts above 30% very little perceptual effects are seen and yet threshold for these targets can be raised 2 log units or more. Results showing this effect are seen in Fig. 1.20 for three different spatial scales (0.25 c/deg; 2.5 c/deg and 10 c/deg). Although in each case the luminance range is different, the same rules apply. A power law best describes the relationship between physical contrast and perceived contrast. Its exponent increases as illuminance is reduced and detection thresholds become progressively more elevated. Thus there is a world of difference between '*threshold contrast sensitivity*' and '*contrast sensitivity*' *per se*.

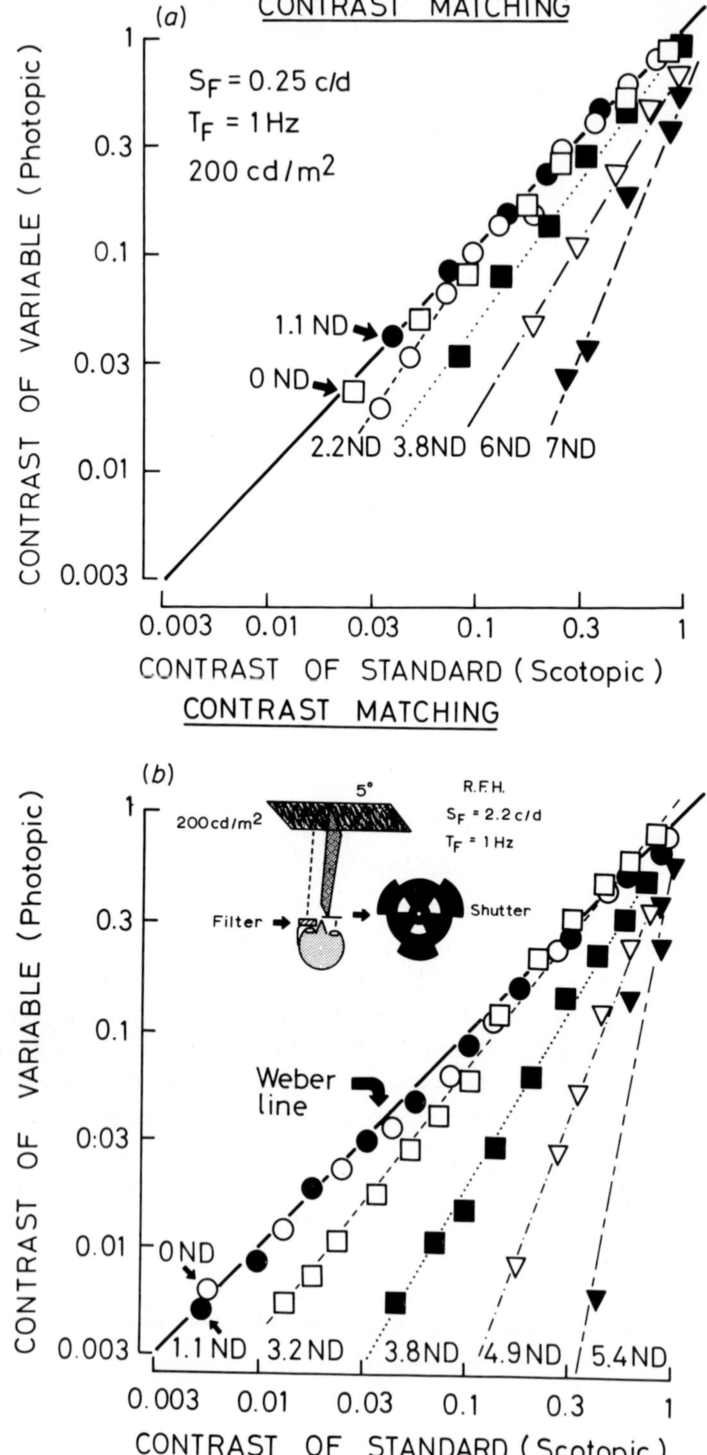
CONTRAST MATCHING
(a)
S_F = 0.25 c/d
T_F = 1 Hz
200 cd/m²
1.1 ND
0 ND
2.2ND 3.8ND 6ND 7ND
CONTRAST OF VARIABLE (Photopic)
1
0.3
0.1
0.03
0.01
0.003
0.003 0.01 0.03 0.1 0.3 1
CONTRAST OF STANDARD (Scotopic)
CONTRAST MATCHING
(b)
5°
200cd/m²
R.F.H.
S_F = 2.2 c/d
T_F = 1 Hz
Filter
Shutter
Weber line
0 ND
1.1 ND 3.2ND 3.8ND 4.9ND 5.4ND
CONTRAST OF VARIABLE (Photopic)
1
0.3
0.1
0:03
0.01
0.003
0.003 0.01 0.03 0.1 0.3 1
CONTRAST OF STANDARD (Scotopic)

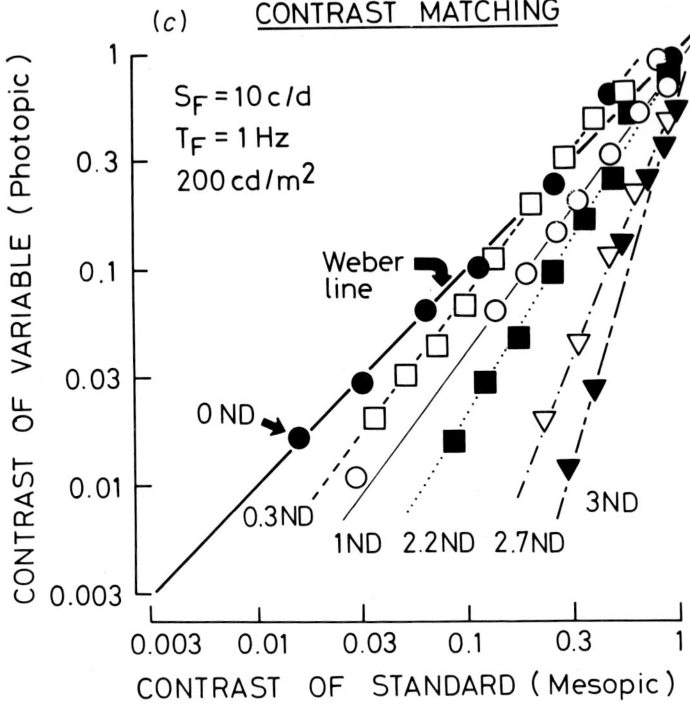

Fig. 1.20. Contrast matching data for three different spatial frequencies. The eye which viewed the standard was kept under scotopic levels whereas the eye which viewed the adjustable contrast test stimulus was kept under photopic conditions (see inset in (*b*) for experimental set up). The higher the contrast the less perceptual reduction due to reduced illumination. The results are described by a power law whose exponent varies with mean retinal illumination (Hess & Lillywhite, unpublished).

This is very similar to what has been termed auditory recruitment in audition (see Moore *et al.*, 1985). This threshold/ suprathreshold departure for contrast perception may be explained by the fact that individual cortical neurones respond over different contrast ranges. Thus there are, to a lesser extent, contrast filters operating in vision. This means that different neural populations are responsible for threshold and suprathreshold vision. Since adaptation is a filter-based operation it can also be arranged to vary across this filtering dimension. There is also evidence that for individual cortical neurones threshold and suprathreshold measures may differ (see Fig. 1.6) and that individual neurones display contrast adaptation (Ohzawa, Sclar & Freeman, 1985). These factors all make contributions to allowing our suprathreshold perceptions to be more stable than we might have thought by just considering threshold measures.

Motion sensitivity

Very little quantitative work has been done on how our sensitivity to image motion changes as a function of luminance. The two-flash apparent motion task for random dot stimuli (Braddick, 1974) has been used to isolate the short range motion process at photopic levels and it would be interesting to know how the scotopic and photopic short range processes differ. The reason why it hasn't been done yet is because with the present means of stimulus generation changes in luminance and contrast are confounded. The dots would need to be modulated about a mean level which could then be reduced with neutral density filters.

Even without doing the experiment one could hazard a guess at the result. Some recent findings suggest that there is an optimal spatial displacement (Dopt) for velocity discrimination and that this corresponds to a constant (about 1/6) fraction of the spatial wavelength of the stimulus (Boulton & Hess, forthcoming). This would mean that in the case of two-flash apparent motion for random dots (whose spatial spectrum is broad) high spatial frequency tuned neurones may subserve small displacements and lower spatial frequency tuned neurones may subserve larger displacements. If this is so then the effects of reducing luminance are more predictable. Since high spatial frequency neurones are selectively disadvantaged in catching quanta, then the two-flash apparent motion performance should be selectively affected for small displacements. There is also evidence that the dynamics of more peripheral neurones is reduced as a function of reducing luminance and this should reduce the highest velocities able to be detected. In other words at scotopic levels we should selectively lose our ability to detect slow as well as fast motion while maintaining our performance in the intermediate velocity range. There is some indication from the velocity discrimination results of Orban, Wolf & Maes (1984) that, while the influence of reduced luminance is not great, it does selectively affect our ability to encode the slowest and the fastest image motion thereby leaving the mid range intact. The fact that striate neurones do not change their spatial or temporal tuning as the retinal illuminance is reduced offers the advantage of veridical velocity judgements within this intact mid range at scotopic levels (see Fig. 1.19 of this chapter and Fig. 3.6 of Chapter 3).

1.3.2 Incremental sensitivities

Contrast discrimination

A similar threshold/suprathreshold dissociation can be seen for the discrimination of contrast differences. The form of the relationship for ΔC, the smallest contrast difference that can be discriminated as a function of the contrast level (usually termed pedestal contrast) is seen in Fig. 1.21*a* (from the results of Bradley and Ohzawa, 1986). The photopic results (unfilled symbols) show a straight line relationship where ΔC is roughly proportional to C (called Weber response; but also see Legge, 1981) and a minimum at background contrasts equivalent to the contrast threshold. At this minimum the contrast needed for discrimination is up to a factor of 3 lower than that needed to detect the increment when presented by itself (Nachmias & Sansbury, 1974).

Under mesopic conditions, the position of this minimum changes but there is little or no change in contrast discrimination in the upper contrast range. The solid curve which best fits the photopic data is also seen to fit the mesopic data (dashed line) if scaled along a diagonal by the contrast threshold difference (marked by arrows in Fig. 1.21*a*). It is as if the visual system changes its contrast calibration for both increment and pedestal by a value equal to the threshold elevation. Whatever the explanation, the result is that contrast discrimination at high contrasts is more resistant to changes in luminance. The results in Fig. 1.21*b* are from a similar experiment (Hess, unpublished) and extend the picture to scotopic levels for a lower spatial frequency stimulus. Note that now the increment that can be discriminated is plotted against the background light level for each of a number of representative contrast levels (5.6%, 31%, 63%). Notice that the threshold (marked by arrows) begins to change at 20 cd/m^2 and displays a square-root response with luminance. The luminance at which each pedestal contrast is first affected varies with the contrast level. The higher the pedestal contrast the more resistant is its discrimination as luminance is reduced. In the region where discrimination is falling with luminance its values always represent lower contrasts than are needed for detection.

One plausible explanation for the form of the photopic result in terms of what we know of single cell neurophysiology is given by considering the finding that single cells display thresholds and their response variance increases with contrast (Tolhurst, Movshon & Thompson, 1981). The mesopic and scotopic results of Fig. 1.21*a*, *b* respectively can also fit

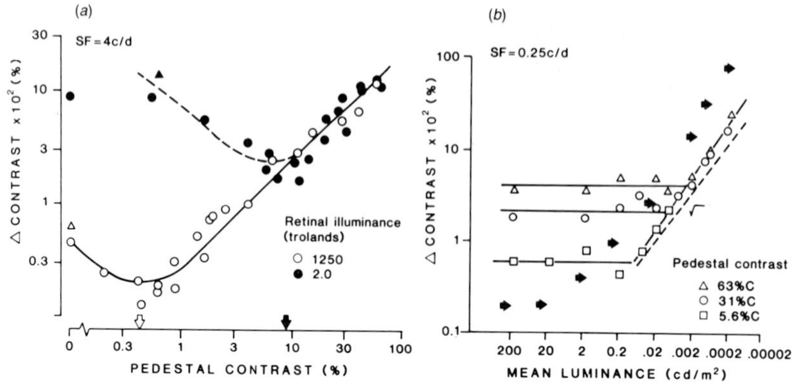

Fig. 1.21. In (*a*) contrast discrimination data are plotted at a photopic and mesopic level of illumination from the results of Bradley & Ohzawa (1986). The arrows indicate the contrast threshold for the stimuli. In (*b*) contrast discrimination at three representative pedestal contrasts is plotted as a function of mean luminance. The filled arrows indicate the contrast threshold for the stimulus. Note that for high pedestal contrasts, contrast discrimination is very resistant (as compared with contrast thresholds) to change of mean luminance over 4 or 5 log units. (Hess & Lillywhite, unpublished.) Thresholds begin to change at 20 cd/m^2 where as suprathreshold measures can remain stable down to 0.002 cd/m^2.

into this framework because the reduced scotopic responses of neurones at a given contrast level are associated with reduced variance (see Fig. 1.22). Therefore, at photopic and scotopic levels discriminating differences in the output distribution of a single cell would vary in proportion to the signal strength (Weber-like response) over most of the range, but would display a minimum due to the threshold non-linearity. It should also be realized that the fact that neurones operate over different contrast ranges means that different neurones determine performance at low and high contrasts. This alone may account for the above difference in contrast discrimination at low and high pedestal contrasts.

Spatial and temporal discrimination

Very little is known about spatial and temporal discrimination at scotopic levels. What is known involves the performance of the rod-monochromat at mesopic conditions and this gives an estimate of the upper limit of discriminable sensitivity for the rod mechanism. These results, which are referred to in detail in Chapter 11 (Figs 11.12–11.17), suggest that threshold and suprathreshold discrimination is similar for the rod and cone mechanism over their common spatio-temporal range. What differ-

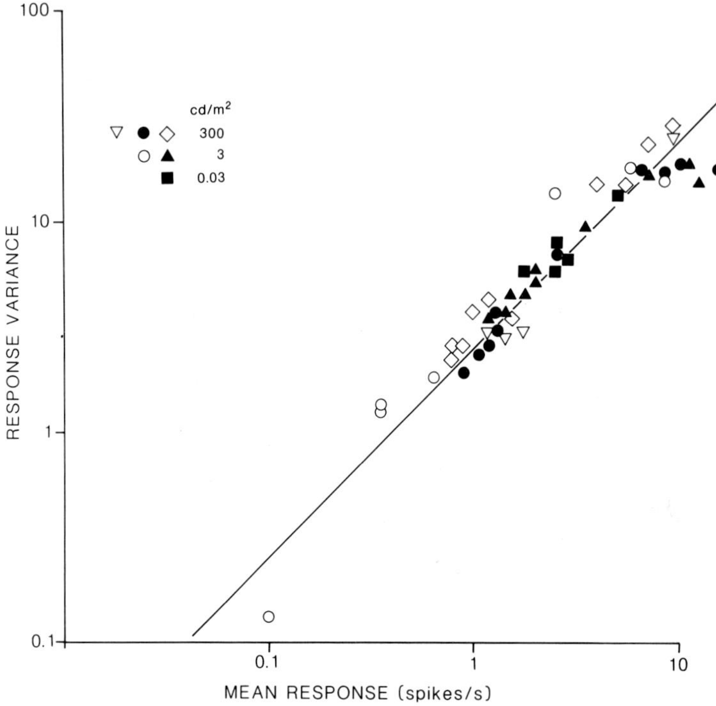

Fig. 1.22. Relationship between mean response and response variance over a range of luminances for a simple cell in cat striate cortex. (Lillywhite & Hess, unpublished.)

ence there is results from the fact that the cone mechanism works over a wider spatio-temporal range. Recently similar results have been reported for normal spatial discriminations under scotopic conditions (Pandey Vimal & Wilson, 1987).

Blur perception and discrimination

Is vision blurred at night? Unfortunately, blur has a rather specific optical connotation which is likely to mislead in this case because, as we have already seen, the suprathreshold contrast loss at low light levels is very different to that expected from optical degradation (see Fig. 1.20). It might be better to ask whether sharp edges appear less sharp at night. This can be assessed by psychophysically equating edge sharpness at different luminances in a similar dichoptic experiment to that already described for contrast matching. The results of such matches are seen in

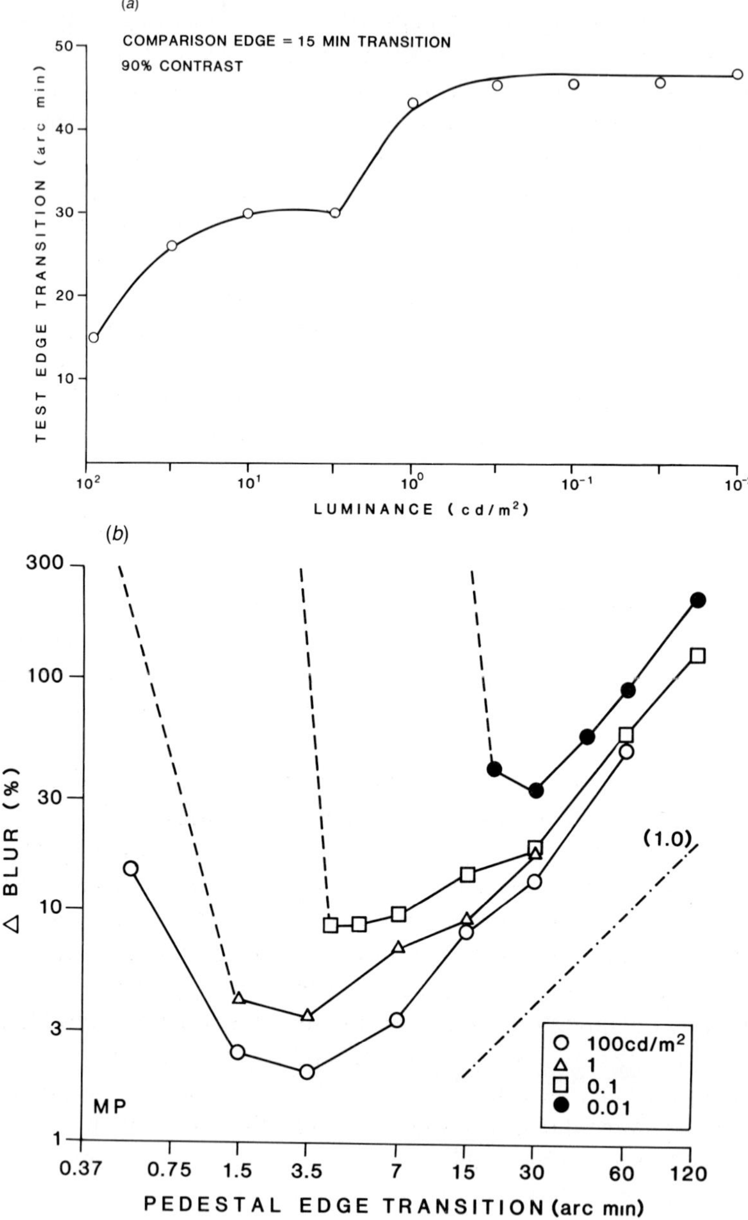

Fig. 1.23. In (*a*), edge matching data between eyes at different mean luminances. The stimulus is an edge with a sinusoidal transition (that is a half cycle of a sinewave). The comparison edge has a sinusoidal transition of 15 arc minutes. The transition of the test edge is varied to match the comparison edge. Initially as luminance is changed from photopic to mesopic, sharp edges look more blurred but this does not continue to be the case under scotopic conditions. In (*b*),

Fig. 1.23*a*. The perceptual sharpness of this particular edge transition falls rapidly until the upper mesopic illuminance is reached after which it stabilizes. Blur perception has a duplex-like character. In Fig. 1.23*b*, results are shown for blur discrimination as a function of pedestal blur at each of a number of fixed mean luminances. The dashed lines represent discrimination that could not be performed at the 300% level. As luminance is reduced blur discrimination is degraded particularly for sharp edges (i.e. for low pedestal blurs). At any luminance, best edge blur discrimination is obtained for intermediate edge translations. As the luminance is lowered the position of optimal performance is shifted to edges having larger transitions. This suggests that one of the reasons why we do not see things as 'blurred' at night as we might expect is because our sensitivity for discriminating a difference in 'blur' is also reduced at low light levels.

1.4 Concluding remarks

The examination of vision under low light levels dates back to the early astronomers yet we still know so little. Over the past thirty years we have learnt much about how receptors respond at different retinal illuminances and how the gain of individual visual neurones depends upon the ambient retinal flux. However, only preliminary attempts have been made at understanding how their outputs are combined into different spatial, temporal and contrast post-receptoral filtering channels which by their very existence allow the visual system to respond over a wide operating range with minimal loss in sensitivity. This follows from the fact that (1) most visual objects are spatially broad band and that their presence can be registered by neurones with different filtering properties over different parts of the operating range, and (2) adaptation is a filter-based operation. Similarly, because neurones operate over different contrast ranges and also exhibit contrast adaptation it is now becoming obvious that an understanding of scotopic vision involves more than just assessing thresholds, suprathreshold discrimination of one sort or another must also be considered.

Fig. 1.23 (*cont.*)

edge-blur discrimination functions at different mean luminances. Best blur discrimination occurs for edges that are already slightly blurred. As luminance is reduced the position of this maximum sensitivity is displaced to higher pedestal blurs (edges with wider transitions) but blur sensitivity at the higher pedestal blurs is little affected by reduced luminance.

Our present knowledge can be summarized as follows. At night we are restricted to a lower range of spatial, temporal and contrast filters. The filters which subserve rod vision are a subset of those that subserve cone vision. Within this range the quality of visual discrimination is little affected by reduced light level. The fact that we have neurones with different spatial, temporal and contrast filtering properties combined with an adaptation mechanism that is filter-based must be one of the main reasons why we can perform so well over such a large operating range. The stability of our spatial, temporal and contrast perceptions above threshold result from the fact that reducing the light level changes only the sensitivity of individual filters not their individual filtering properties.

Acknowledgements

I am grateful to all of my colleagues for helpful discussions especially Fergus Campbell, Horace Barlow, John Robson and Ted Sharpe. I am especially indebted to Ed Howell and Peter Lillywhite for allowing me to discuss some of the experiments that we have done together over the past decade and never published. I would also like to thank Mary Hayhoe for taking the time to discuss the appropriate contrast metric with which to compare increment threshold results. It is always a pleasure to acknowledge the financial support of the Wellcome Trust and Medical Research Council of the United Kingdom and the National Health and Medical Research Council of Australia. A Wellcome–Remiciotti travel grant helped to get this chapter written up.

2

The light-adaptation of the human rod visual system

Lindsay T. Sharpe

'Eh bien, oui: il a pu faire tout ça, mais ce n'est pas prouvé: je commence à croire qu'on ne peut jamais rien prouver. Ce sont des hypothèses honnêtes et qui rendent compte des faits: mais je sens si bien qu'elles viennent de moi, qu'elles sont tout simplement une manière d'unifier mes connaissances.'

(Jean-Paul Sartre, *La Nausée*, Editions Gallimard, 1938, p. 30)

2.1 Introduction

From the 'dark, dark, dark' of night to the 'blaze of noon', the prevailing light can vary over 10 decades of intensity. It is the wondrous ability of the eye to regulate its sensitivity within this enormous range that allows us to see not only the dull glimmer of starlight, but also the full sheen of sunlight. How the eye administers its control in the seven or so lowest decades of that range – the range in which the rods control visual sensitivity, either alone, in isolation, or jointly, in consort with the cones – is what will concern us here.

The term 'rod light-adaptation' is conventionally used to refer to the desensitization of the rod visual system that occurs during exposure to steady, adapting fields. The phenomenon is also known as 'rod field adaptation' (after Rushton, 1965*b*). The usage, which implies that the light-adaptation of the 'rods' is independent from that of the 'cones', is honoured by tradition and follows directly from the duplicity theory (Duplizitätstheorie) of vision (Schultze, 1866; Parinaud, 1881; von Kries, 1894, 1895). However, it obscures an important truth: in the normal eye, at light levels where rods and cones are simultaneously active, the sensitivity regulation of the rod visual system cannot be strictly independent of that of the cone systems. In fact, evidence to the contrary is manifest in the morphology, physiology and psychophysics; and was apparent even to those who conceived the Duplizitätstheorie

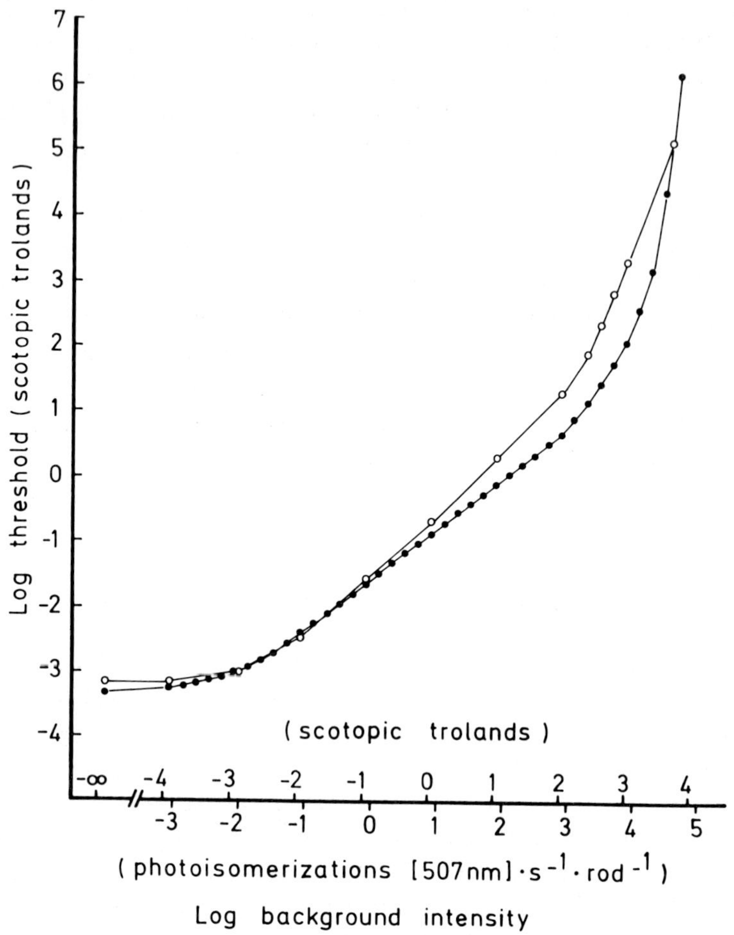

Fig. 2.1. Increment threshold as a function of background intensity for the achromat observer K.N. (filled circles). The test flash and adapting field parameters were chosen to favour the rods relative to the cones – an unnecessary precaution in the achromat. The target was large (6 deg), long (200 ms), and short in wavelength (520 nm). It was presented 12 deg extrafoveally in the centre of a long-wavelength (640 nm), 18 deg diameter, adapting field; and it entered the edge of the dilated pupil (3 mm off-centre) to take advantage of the Stiles–Crawford effect. The open circles indicate increment thresholds averaged from four normal observers by Aguilar & Stiles (1954). They were measured under essentially the same conditions as used for K.N.; only the target was slightly larger, 9 deg instead of 6 deg in diameter. The two curves are in their correct positions on the $\log_{10}$ threshold and $\log_{10}$ background intensity axes. The $\log_{10}$ background intensity is given in both scotopic trolands and photoisomerizations (507 nm) per second per rod (see text and Table 2.1 for details of how the effective quantum absorptions at the retina were estimated).

(Ramon y Cajal, 1893; von Kries, 1929; cf. Polyak, 1941). Complete autonomy of rod function is only intrinsic to the typical, complete achromat or functional rod-monochromat, for whom the cones neither mediate vision nor affect rod-mediated vision. (For the proof that the achromat K.N., whose curves are shown below, essentially lacks cone vision, see Chapter 10.)

Therefore, when describing the process of light-adaptation in the rod visual system, it makes sense to use a typical, complete achromat as guide (cf. Blakemore & Rushton, 1965; Rushton, 1965*a*, *b*). By comparing the achromat's results with those of the normal observer, it is possible to separate out the intricate contribution of the cones to the 'rod' light-adaptation process. The need for doing so will become clear from an inspection of the threshold versus intensity or increment threshold curve; the earliest (Bouger, 1760; Fechner, 1860) and the most frequently used means of psychophysically studying the adaptation process.

2.1.1 The increment threshold curve of the rods

Figs 2.1 and 2.2 show how log increment threshold increases as a function of log background (or adapting) intensity for the achromat K.N. (filled circles) and a normal observer (triangles), respectively. Both curves were obtained under the 'classic' rod-isolation conditions of Aguilar & Stiles (1954). These conditions refer to target and background parameters chosen to favour the response of the rods relative to the responses of the three cone systems. (For the achromat who lacks cone vision such conditions are obviously unnecessary.) Basically the idea is to light-adapt the cones and thus desensitize them as much as possible relative to the rods so that the rod thresholds can be followed up to higher levels where they are normally obscured by the cone thresholds. Specifically, this involves: (i) selecting a target wavelength, for which the ratio of rod to cone sensitivity is as large as possible (in Fig. 2.1, 520 nm was chosen; for why see Fig. 2.3); (ii) selecting an adapting field wavelength, for which the ratio of rod to cone sensitivity is as small as possible (640 nm; see Fig. 2.3); (iii) making the target large (6 deg in diameter) and long (200 ms in duration) to take advantage of the greater spatial and temporal summation of the rod system (Sharpe, Fach & Nordby, 1988); (iv) imaging the target onto the peripheral retina (12 deg temporal to fixation, in the nasal field of view), where the rods are optimally sensitive (Cabello & Stiles, 1950); (v) directing the target rays so that they enter at

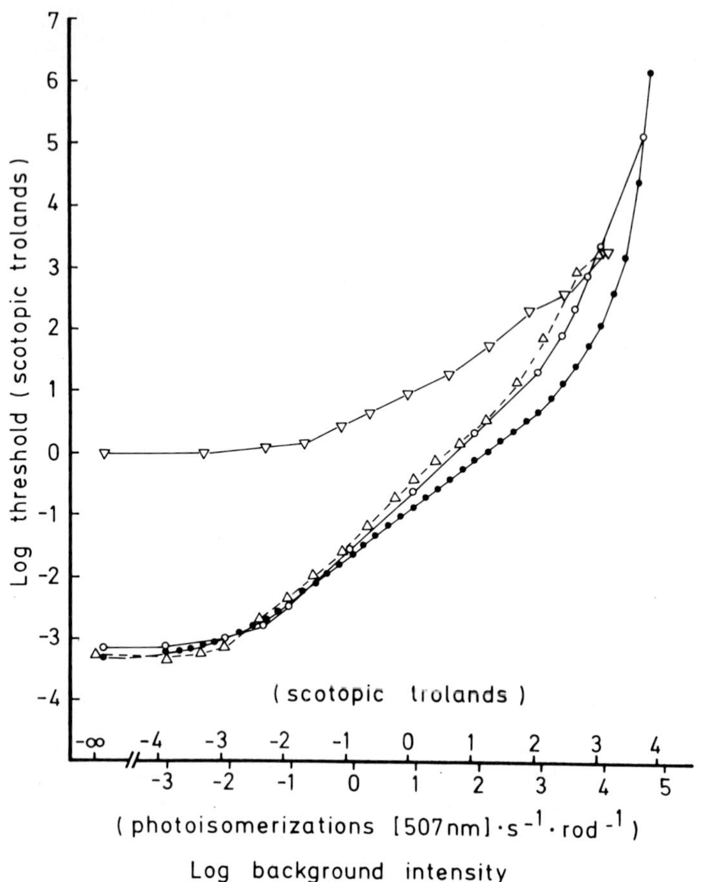

Fig. 2.2. Increment threshold (triangles) as a function of background intensity for a normal observer, measured for the same test flash and background conditions as in Fig. 2.1. The inverted triangles indicate the normal observer's cone thresholds measured during the plateau terminating the cone phase of recovery from a white (3100 K) bleaching light of 7.7 $\log_{10}$ photopic td-s. The filled and open circles are the increment thresholds, respectively, for the achromat K.N. and the average observer of Aguilar & Stiles, as in Fig. 2.1.

the edge of the pupil (3 mm from the centre of the fully dilated pupil) in order to exploit the reduced sensitivity of the cones to obliquely entering light (Stiles & Crawford, 1933; Stiles, 1939; Flamant & Stiles, 1948; Westheimer, 1967; Alpern, Ching & Kitahara, 1983; Nordby & Sharpe, 1988); and (vi) using a large adapting field (18 deg in diameter) to desensitize the rods over a substantial retinal area and thus reduce the influence of stray light on target detection.

The effectiveness of these 'rod isolation' conditions in securing the

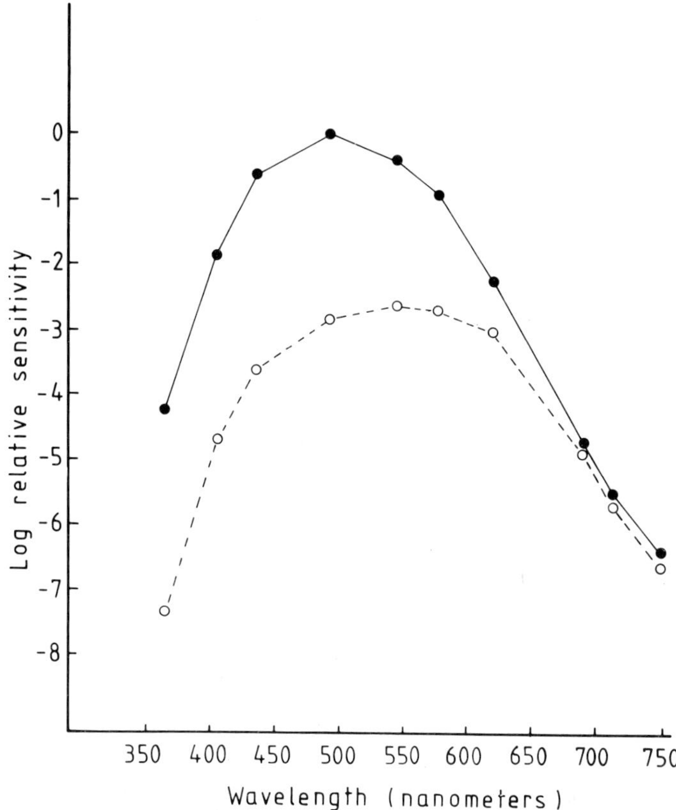

Fig. 2.3. $\log_{10}$ relative sensitivity as a function of wavelength for the peripheral rods and cones of the normal dark-adapted eye. The target was a 1 deg diameter field exposed for 40 ms and imaged 8 deg above the fovea. Data are expressed relative to the maximum sensitivity of the rods. Both the rod (mean of 22 observers) and cone (mean of 10 observers) values are from Wald (1945, Table 2.1).

detection of the target by the rods is undeniable. It can be assessed by comparing, in the normal observer, the thresholds measured during field adaptation (Fig. 2.2, triangles) with those measured during the plateau terminating the cone phase of recovery from a 7.7 $\log_{10}$ photopic troland-s bleaching light (inverted triangles). Over almost the entire range of adapting intensity, the rod thresholds are much lower than the cone thresholds. Only at the very highest backgrounds, where the two curves intersect, are the cones more sensitive to the target than the rods (i.e. the highest triangle is a cone threshold). The transition takes place at a background intensity near 3.0 $\log_{10}$ scotopic trolands (td), which is about 3.0 $\log_{10}$ units higher than the background at which the rods normally yield the increment threshold to the cones.

The effectiveness of the 'rod isolation' conditions in securing an independent measure of rod field adaptation is another matter, however. It can be assessed by comparing the field adaptation curve of the normal with that of the achromat. In the region below where the cones are detecting the target in the normal, the shape of the curve should be the same in the normal and the achromat, if rod light-adaptation proceeds independently of the cones. But the two curves clearly differ in slope; and this is not due to individual differences, as proven by comparing the achromat and normal thresholds with the mean thresholds obtained by Aguilar & Stiles (1954) under essentially the same conditions (Figs 2.1 and 2.2, open circles; the average data are taken from Wyszecki & Stiles, 1982, p. 547). The Aguilar & Stiles curve, which has not been shifted along either axis, provides an excellent fit to the normal trichromat's data, but not to the achromat's. This is an important discrepancy and will be discussed in detail below (Sharpe *et al.*, 1989*a*). For the moment, we will set it aside and look at what the normal and achromat curves have in common.

Both the normal and achromat curves have three aspects, each reflecting different problems faced by the visual system in sensitivity regulation. First, there is the absolute sensitivity asymptote (the foot of the curve). Here, where the rods function in true isolation, the system faces the problem of extracting information amid the 'black mist low creeping' (Milton). The task is to detect the obscure object; to make the most of each quantum caught. As we will see, the result is an exquisite sensitivity closely following the limits imposed by intrinsic noise in the physical stimulus and in the phototransduction process (see also Chapter 4).

Second, there is a section of constant ascending slope. In this region, where the rods function partly alone and partly together with the cones, the quanta, 'through utter and through middle darkness borne' (Milton), are more plentiful. The emphasis of the visual system changes; discrimination becomes more important than detection; and sensitivity is sacrificed for enhanced resolution and improved reliability (Craik, 1938; Barlow, 1962). More quanta are required to detect dim lights than are compelled by physical and physiological noise limitations. This higher adjustment of sensitivity is enforced by system dynamics: the visual system must scale down the enormous range of input levels to the much smaller range that its neurones can handle. So the problem of extracting a signal from the noise – the major problem at low intensities – is eclipsed by the problem of being able to respond at all at higher intensities.

Third, there is the upper, 'rod saturation' asymptote, evinced by a sudden upsurge in threshold. In this region, the quanta are abundant; and the visual system's goal is fine discrimination; a job which the cones, with their higher spatial and temporal resolution, are much better at than the rods. In fact, here, the rule of the rods 'blasted with excess of light' (Thomas Gray) collapses under the heavy rain of photons. But, the mandate of vision is preserved and sublimed by full transfer of function to the cones. For the achromat, this is a catastrophe; in effect, his vision extinguishes.

2.1.2 The decrement threshold curve of the rods

The curves shown in Figs 2.1 and 2.2 were measured for increments of light. Threshold curves may also be measured for decrements (Gildemeister, 1914). One might well expect, for the same target conditions, the two types of curve to be identical; i.e., the amount of light needed to see a small deviation above the prevailing luminance level to be symmetrically equal to the amount needed to see a small deviation below it. But experiments show that this is not the case (Stiles & Lambert, see Short, 1966; Blackwell, 1946; Herrick, 1956; Aulhorn, 1964; Short, 1966; Patel & Jones, 1968; Cohn, Weissman & Wasilewsky, 1972; Ehrenstein & Spillmann, 1983; Whittle, 1986; Sharpe, Whittle & Nordby, 1990).

In Fig. 2.4, the increment and decrement thresholds of achromat K.N. are given for a 520 nm, 1.85 deg in diameter, 200 ms test flash superimposed on a 520 nm, 11 deg in diameter background (except for the background wavelength, these are essentially the same conditions as those used in Figs 2.1 and 2.2). Clearly, at the lowest background (−2.2 $\log_{10}$, scotopic td) from which a 100% decrement can be subtracted, it is easier to see a decrement (filled circles) than an increment (open circles) of equal magnitude. In fact, up to backgrounds of about 2.0 $\log_{10}$ scotopic td, the decremental threshold is on average 0.2 $\log_{10}$ unit lower than the incremental threshold (other investigators have reported a difference of as much as 0.4 $\log_{10}$ unit). At higher backgrounds, the two curves converge and the onset of saturation (see Section 2.5) occurs in both near the same background intensity, 2.6 $\log_{10}$ scotopic td.

The measured discrepancy cannot be attributed to a change of criterion for detecting increments and decrements, nor to using linear steps to compare logarithmic threshold differences (Short, 1966); for these

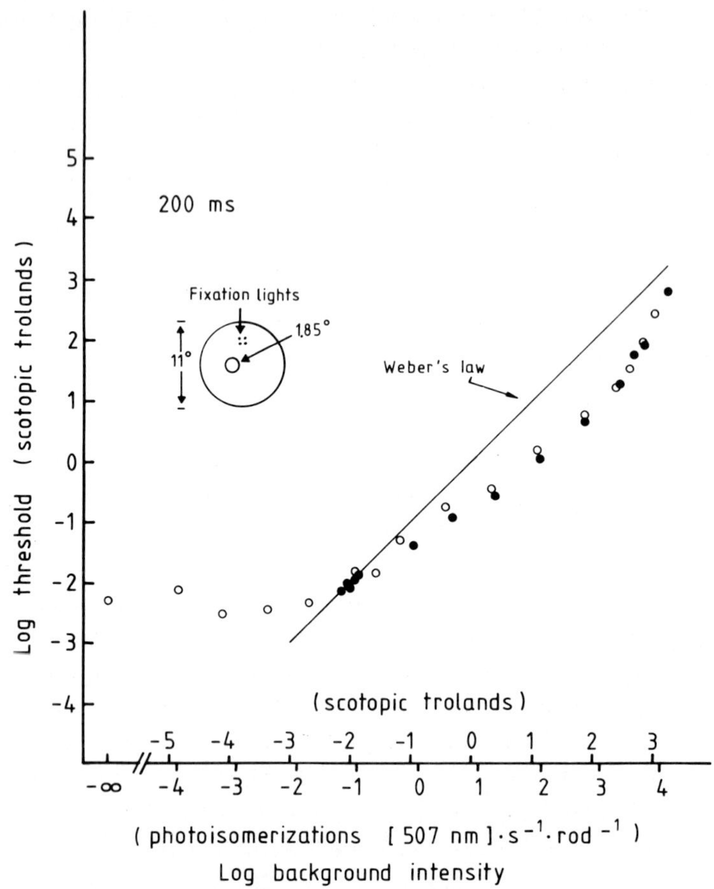

Fig. 2.4. Increment (open circles) and decrement (filled circles) thresholds for achromat K.N., measured as a function of background intensity. The target was a 520 nm, 1.85 deg diameter flash exposed for 200 ms on a 520 nm, 11 deg diameter background. Fixation was 6 deg eccentric in the peripheral retina. The increment threshold curve has a slope of 0.73; the decrement threshold curve, 0.75. For comparison, Weber's law (slope = 1.0) is shown. (From Sharpe *et al.*, 1990.)

factors are small compared with the standard errors of the thresholds. Nor can it be simply explained by an asymmetry of sensitivity due to physiological factors; such as 'off-centre' retinal ganglion cells being more sensitive than their 'on-centre' counterparts (cf. Cohn, 1974).

Rather, it has been hypothesized that a decrement is easier to see than an equal-sized increment, particularly at low background intensities, because of the Poisson nature of the fluctuations in photon capture (Cohn *et al.*, 1972; Cohn, 1974, 1976). In short, the number of quanta in the adapting field is not constant, but follows a Poisson distribution, with a mean of n and a standard deviation of $n^{0.5}$. As a consequence, the quanta in the background are liable to be confused with the quanta in the target for the spatio-temporal interval corresponding to the target or to the summation limits of the rod visual system, whichever is smaller. This means the target can only be distinguished from the background when the number of quanta in the target (the signal) exceeds the square root of the mean number in the background (the noise). Since the variance of the stimulus distribution during the luminance change is greater for an increment than for a decrement (i.e. quanta are added rather than subtracted) the distribution for the former is broader and will overlap more with the background distribution. The greater overlap causes the observer to make more errors, thus decreasing detectability.

This argument predicts that the magnitude of the difference between the increment and decrement thresholds should decline with background intensity – as seems to be the case in Fig. 2.4 – because at higher levels (those causing more than a 100 photon isomerizations in the effective space-time interval of the target) the difference in the Poisson statistic becomes negligible. But the incremental and decremental thresholds coincide at background intensities between 1.0–2.0 log scotopic td, corresponding to a rate of isomerization between 2.0–3.0 log quanta (507 nm) s^{-1} rod^{-1}. This is 3.0–4.0 log units higher than the quantum fluctuation hypothesis predicts (Cohn, 1974). (An alternative hypothesis is that the measured discrepancy is due to the presence of multiplicative intrinsic noise in the visual system; Lillywhite, 1981; see below.)

2.2 The absolute sensitivity of the rods

2.2.1 The minimum threshold

The absolute threshold of the rod visual system is defined by the minimum energy required to detect the test flash. Far from being constant, it depends strongly on the size and duration of the target. Fig. 2.5 shows the increment threshold curves measured for the achromat K.N. for three different target sizes and durations: 200 ms, 6 deg (from Fig. 2.1); 100 ms, 1 deg; and 10 ms, 10 min. K.N.'s absolute thresholds for these three targets are −3.30, −2.48 and −0.30 $\log_{10}$ scotopic td, respectively. The three values fall within the range established for normal observers under similar conditions. For example, the value measured with the 6 deg, 200 ms target is very close to the mean value measured by

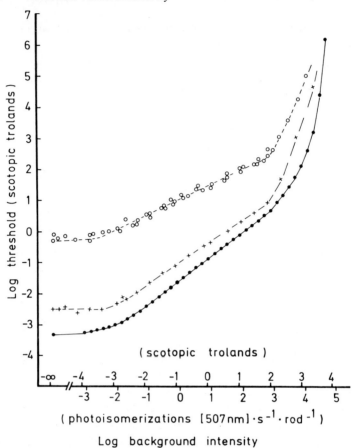

Fig. 2.5. The effect of target size and duration on the increment threshold of the achromat K.N. The filled circles represent the thresholds measured with a 200 ms, 6 deg diameter test flash (same conditions as in Fig. 2.1); the crosses, the thresholds measured with a 100 ms, 1 deg diameter test flash; the open circles, the thresholds measured with a 10 ms, 10 min diameter test flash. Otherwise the test flash and background conditions are the same as those used in Fig. 2.1.

Aguilar & Stiles for their four observers (−3.23), and is encompassed by the values measured for five normal observers (−3.22 to −3.97) in the same apparatus under the same conditions (see Table 2.6).

The absolute threshold in scotopic trolands can be expressed in terms of the number of quanta caught by the rods; i.e. the number of molecules of rhodopsin photoisomerized per second per rod. This requires making assumptions about the number of quanta incident at the cornea that: (i) are reflected, absorbed or scattered by the ocular media; (ii) are absorbed by the cones or fall into the interspaces between receptors;

Table 2.1. *The proportion of quanta at the cornea that excites the human rods*

	Source of loss	Best estimate	Range (Barlow, 1977)	Range (Hallett, 1987)	References
Fraction transmitted by ocular media	Reflection absorption and scattering	0.67	0.50–0.75	0.69–0.75	Said & Weale (1959) Tan (1971) Van Norren & Vos (1974) Wyszecki & Stiles (1982)
Fraction entering rods	Spaces between rod receptors	0.80	0.70–0.80	0.70–0.80	Hecht *et al.* (1942) Denton & Pirenne (1954)
Fraction absorbed by rhodopsin	Self-screening	0.55	0.50–0.55	0.55–0.80	Alpern & Pugh (1974) Zwas & Alpern (1976) Bowmaker & Dartnall (1980) Wyszecki & Stiles (1982)
Fraction exciting	Heat degradation	0.67	0.60–1.00	0.63–1.00	Dartnall (1972) Barlow (1977)
	Product:	0.20	0.11–0.33	0.17–0.48	

(iii) pass the visual pigment uncaught; and (iv) are degraded into heat. The conversion is simplified by expressing the quanta at a wavelength of 507 nm, the maximum of the scotopic luminosity function (see Wyszecki & Stiles, 1982, pp. 789–90). This does not alter the result because whatever the actual spectral composition of the target, it will produce the same number of absorbed quanta in the rods as a 507 nm target of the same scotopic luminance.

For a wavelength of 507 nm, one scotopic td is equal to 5.66 $\log_{10}$ quanta s^{-1} deg^{-2} (see Wyszecki & Stiles, 1982, p. 103); so at achromat K.N.'s dark-adapted threshold about 1200 quanta are incident on his cornea from the 0.2 s, 6 deg (28.27 deg^2) target, about 120 from the 0.1 s, 1 deg (0.79 deg^2) target and about 45 from the 0.01 s, 10 min (0.022 deg^2) target. According to the best available correction factors for the loss of photons (see Table 2.1), only 20% of the incident quanta probably produce photoisomerizations. Since there are roughly 12 500–15 000 rods per square degree of external field in the retinal region where the targets were imaged (Osterberg, 1935; Aguilar & Stiles, 1954; Denton & Pirenne, 1954; Curcio, Hendrickson & Kalina, 1985; Curcio *et al.*, 1987), it follows that the 260 or so quanta isomerized from the 6 deg

Table 2.2. *Absolute thresholds for the achromat observer K.N. for three target conditions*

Target	Threshold (scotopic trolands)	Threshold[a] (quanta (507 nm) s^{-1} deg^{-2})	Total quanta[b] (incident on cornea)	Total quanta[c] (absorbed at retina)	Total rods[d] (in imaged area)
200 ms 6 deg dia. (28.27 deg^2 area)	0.000 50 (−3.30 $\log_{10}$)	229	1295	259	353 375–424 050
100 ms 1 deg dia. (0.79 deg^2 area)	0.003 31 (−2.48 $\log_{10}$)	1,513	120	24	9875–11 850;
10 ms 10 min dia. (0.022 deg^2 area)	0.501 19 (−0.30 $\log_{10}$)	229,088	50	10	387–465[e]

[a] For a wavelength of 507 nm, one scotopic troland is equal to 457 800 quanta s^{-1} deg^{-2}.
[b] Multiplied by the area and duration of the target.
[c] The fraction of quanta at the cornea assumed to excite the rods is 0.2 (see best estimate, Table 2.1).
[d] The lower estimate is from Osterberg (1935); the upper from Curcio *et al.* (1987).
[e] These estimates have been corrected for optical spreading due to diffraction effects. Owing to the wave properties of light, the optical image of the 10 min diameter target on the retina will be a diffraction pattern, the main, central part of which will have a diameter of 12 min of arc (an area of 0.031 deg^2). Hence the target is spread over 387–465 rods rather than 275–330 rods. The spread of light beyond the geometrical image is of little importance in the case of the larger targets (cf. Pirenne & Marriot, 1959).

diameter target are spread over some 354 000–424 000 rods; the 24 from the 1 deg diameter target over some 9900–11 900 rods; and the 10 from the 10 min diameter target over some 400–500 rods (these are rounded values, see Table 2.2 for the exact calculations).

Thus the smallest energy threshold required to see the test flash is obtained with the small (10 min), brief target. In fact, the value found for K.N. falls within the 'classic' values reported over forty years ago in normal observers by Hecht, Shlaer & Pirenne (1942). Their target was also 10 min diameter in target, but it was 1 ms in duration. They estimated that between 5 and 14 quantal absorptions were required for threshold. Actually, the number required is probably double that, closer to between 10 and 30 absorptions; because they assumed that only 9.6% of the quanta incident at the cornea were actually absorbed by the rods. Twenty per cent is more reasonable and may even be an underestimate (see Table 2.1).

Since the 10 or more quanta exciting the rods from the 10 min target are distributed over some 400–500 rods (Hecht *et al.*, 1942, assumed a round value of 500), the chance of any rod receiving two or more quanta is very small. In point of fact, the probability that two of the ten quanta will be absorbed by a single rod is at most 12% (see Brindley, 1970, p. 187):

$$1 - [e^{-10} (1 + 10/387)^{387}]$$

a value substantially less than the 73% threshold-for-seeing criterion chosen for the experiments with achromat K.N. and the 60% threshold chosen by Hecht *et al.* (1942). Thus one can reasonably conclude, as Hecht *et al.* (1942) did, that at absolute threshold each quantum is absorbed by a separate rod and further that a single isomerization suffices to initiate a rod signal (for a detailed treatment of this theme, see Denton & Pirenne, 1954; Barlow, 1956; see also Chapter 4). This, in fact, has now been reliably demonstrated by suction-electrode recordings from individual rod photoreceptors in the macaque, whose rod outer segments are very similar to the human's. The absorption of a single quantum, regardless of its wavelength – which only affects the probability of absorption – triggers a 0.7 picoampere (peak amplitude) response. The quantal signal corresponds to a 3% reduction in the rod's circulating dark current and it exceeds the continuous noise level (0.0288 ± 0.0089 pA^2) by a factor of about five (Baylor, Nunn & Schnapf, 1984).

2.2.2 *Detective quantum efficiency*

If each quantum absorbed from the target generates a rod signal, why is it that more than 10 absorptions are required to detect a dim light? The reason is that noise within the visual system limits the dark-adapted rod sensitivity (cf. Barlow, 1956, 1957; see also Chapter 4). The signals associated with the target must be large enough so that the visual system can 'disambiguate' them from the intrinsic signals arising from spontaneous physiological events, which cannot be subsequently averaged or filtered out. The detectability of the target, then, depends on whether the visual signal exceeds the associated noise level or is drowned by it.

Sakitt (1972), on the basis of rating judgments, has argued that some subjects may be able to do better than chance at seeing a single rod signal. However, her argument requires that only 3% of the quanta incident at the cornea (at 7 deg eccentricity) give rise to a rod signal; a value at odds with the value given above. Moreover, the fact that the threshold quantity of light depends on the area and duration of the test flash, as illustrated in Fig. 2.5, tends to undermine her argument; for these factors do not affect the number of quanta that are on average absorbed per rod (for a re-analysis and discussion of Sakitt's data, see Chapter 4).

As a means of estimating the degradation of the apparent photon catch as the visual signal travels along the visual pathway, the detective quantum efficiency – or the minimum proportion of quanta actually used by the observer to detect the target – can be calculated. This involves comparing the performance of the rod visual system with that of a theoretically perfect system (Rose, 1948, 1973). Detective quantum efficiency has sometimes been called quantum efficiency, but the simpler term has also been used in at least two other contexts; both of which are concerned only with the energy of photons and not with their uncertainty properties (see Barlow, 1977). In particular, 'quantum efficiency' has been used to mean the average proportion of quanta absorbed in rhodopsin that cause isomerization or bleaching (this corresponds to the value given in the fourth row of Table 2.1; which is better referred to as 'isomerization efficiency'). It has also been used to mean the average proportion of quanta entering the eye that is absorbed in the rods (this corresponds to the overall value given in the bottom row of Table 2.1; which is better referred to as 'transduction efficiency').

Estimates of the detective quantum efficiency of the dark-adapted human retina vary because they depend strongly on target conditions and task requirements and involve several unknowns such as integration time and area and threshold criterion (for a discussion, see Hallett, 1987). Nevertheless, they always yield figures less than the 20% of the photons incident at the cornea believed to be absorbed by the rod pigment and to cause the crucial chromophore change of the rhodopsin molecule. Table 2.3 (after Hallett, 1987) summarizes estimates of the detective quantum efficiency made under experimental conditions similar to those used in Fig. 2.5 (i.e. with a small, brief target). The estimates range between 5% (Barlow, 1962) and 11% (Hallett, 1969). That is, the observer seems to act as if only 5–11 photons were available, despite having 100 incidents at the cornea and at least 20 causing a photoisomerization. In other words, after ocular media and photopigment losses have been taken into account, it appears that only one in two quanta

Table 2.3. *Absolute threshold and detective quantum efficiency of dark-adapted human vision*[a] *(after Hallett, 1987)*

Source of data	Absolute threshold (quanta (507 nm) s^{-1} deg $^{-2}$)	Detective quantum efficiency	Number of subjects
Long experiments[b]			
Hecht *et al.* (1942)	112	0.054	3
Barlow (1962*a*, *b*)	78	0.069	1
Baumgardt (1960)	102	0.073	4
Hallett (1969)	97	0.042	3
Hallett (1987)	107	0.064	3
Average	99	0.060	
Short experiments[c]			
Hallett (1969)	97	0.103	3
Hallett (1987)	86	0.090	3
Average	92	0.097	

[a] Target conditions: 495–530 nm, 0.13–0.67 deg subtense, 1–25 ms duration, 18–20 deg retinal eccentricity, monocular viewing, and central or peripheral pupilary entry. No background.

[b] Conventional long experiments in which thresholds were collected in blocks of 50 or more flashes.

[c] Short experiments in which thresholds were collected in blocks of 5 flashes.

signaled is used by the observer to detect the target. (The value can be raised to between 12 and 30 photons if the contribution of dark light to the overall efficiency is treated as system noise and discounted in the calculation; see Hallett, 1987.)

What is causing the degradation? Besides the noise attributable to the quantum fluctuations of light in the stimulus (referred to above), the system is susceptible to photon noise – due to random phototransduction events in the receptors – and to neural noise – due to random activity within the visual pathways. Moreover the inefficiency may also be due to the decision process of target detection (Burgess *et al.*, 1981; Cohn, 1981; van Meeteren & Barlow, 1981).

2.2.3 *Phototransducer dark noise*

The sources of noise intimately associated with the phototransduction process (Lamb, 1987) include the noise arising: (i) from the rapid, spontaneous opening and closing of single cyclic GMP-sensitive channels in the plasma membrane of the photo-receptor outer segment (the portion of the receptor that contains the photopigment); (ii) from fluctuations in biochemical intermediates in the chain of amplification (Baylor *et al.*, 1984); (iii) from photon-induced events in the presence of steady lights and flashes; (iv) from reversibility in the reactions that inactivate isomerized rhodopsin, following intense bleaching exposures (Lamb, 1987); and (v) from the spontaneous thermal activation of rhodopsin molecules. The last of these has been quantified. A primate rod gives spontaneous signals that are indistinguishable from a photon-elicited event at an average rate of once every 160 s (Baylor *et al.*, 1984; Baylor, 1987). (Although these spontaneous events are thought to be caused by thermal isomerization of rhodopsin in the primate, in the *Limulus* they can also be modulated by a circadian clock located in the brain; see Barlow & Silbaugh, 1989.)

The sources of phototransducer noise intrinsic to the primate eye are usually assumed to be additive in nature; that is, to be constantly present and/or to be independent of the strength of the light signal. However, multiplicative sources – proportional to the magnitude of the light signal – may also be present. Such sources have been demonstrated in the photoreceptors of the dark-adapted compound eye of the locust (Lillywhite & Laughlin, 1978; see also Chapter 6).

2.2.4 Neural noise

Noise limiting absolute threshold also originates from more central sources (see Chapter 4). These include the spontaneous release of neurotransmitter (synaptic noise), fluctuations in the thresholds for spike initiation (impulse quantization error) and threshold variation (instability of the criterion) (cf. Barlow, 1957, 1977). Such noise may be additive or multiplicative in nature (Lillywhite, 1981) and may be on the same order of magnitude as that arising in the photoreceptors (Barlow, 1977).

In the cat, noise has been identified in the irregularity of discharge of retinal ganglion cells. It is qualitatively different from that originating in random rod isomerizations and does not seem to follow a Poisson statistic (Frishman & Levine, 1983). Moreover, it is probably additive rather than multiplicative in nature; because the noise power (spectral density) at low frequencies – which is assumed to be the factor limiting the detectability of visual stimuli – remains roughly constant when the rate of the discharge of cat retinal ganglion cells is altered by visual stimulation (Robson & Troy, 1987). In the frog, neural noise in retinal ganglion cells adds to and is more prominent than the dark events in the rods. This extra noise grows when larger parts of the inhibitory zone surrounding the excitatory receptive field are included; implying that dark events are summed over extensive regions of the retina (Reuter, Donner & Copenhagen, 1986). In the monkey, neurons in the primary visual cortex (see also Figs 1.6 and 1.22 for cortical neuronal responses in cat) seem to have a response nonlinearity (i.e., a threshold), which occurs at about the level of the psychophysical threshold in man (Barlow *et al.*, 1987). The cortical threshold may be the visual system's way of avoiding false positive responses when there is much stimulus uncertainty; and it may help explain why quantum efficiencies calculated from detection thresholds are so poor compared with those estimated from the visual system's susceptibility to added noise (see Chapter 4).

2.2.5 Dark light

Psychophysically, it is possible to derive an overall value for the intrinsic limit to the absolute threshold by estimating what is variously known as the 'Augenschwarz' (Fechner, 1860), 'Eigengrau', 'dark light' (Barlow, 1956), 'self-light' or 'intrinsic light' of the visual system. This can be conceived as the stimulation from an imaginary light which is always illuminating the retina in addition to any light actually entering the eye (Barlow, 1957), or to employ Milton's stunning phrase about the illumination of Hell, as 'no light, but rather darkness visible'. The value of the dark light is determined graphically from the increment threshold curve. It is the background intensity corresponding to the intersection of the line of constant slope with the absolute threshold ordinate (Barlow, 1957).

When the extrapolation is made for the 200 ms, 6 deg target data, the dark light is estimated to be equal to a light sending into the eye of achromat K.N. 288 quanta (507 nm) s^{-1} deg^{-2} (-3.20 $\log_{10}$ scotopic td) or causing about one photoisomerization per rod every 217 s (assuming 12 500 rods per square degree). The value changes somewhat with target size and location. For the 1 deg, 100 ms target data, it is estimated to be 366 quanta (507 nm) s^{-1} deg^{-2} (-3.10 $\log_{10}$ scotopic td) or causing about one photoisomerization per rod every 171 s; and for the 10 min, 10 ms target data, it is estimated to be 115 quanta (507 nm) s^{-1} deg^{-2} (-3.52 $\log_{10}$ scotopic td) or causing about one photoisomerization per rod every 544 s.

The disparity between achromat K.N.'s dark light values for different target sizes and durations is not small (more than a factor of 4). The variability between observers for the same target conditions, however, is much larger and may be at least a factor of 16 (see Barlow, 1957, Table 1; Barlow gives values ranging from 200 to 16 000 quanta (507 nm) s^{-1} deg^{-2}, some of which are too imprecise to be reliable). For example, for the normal observer in Fig. 2.2, the dark light is estimated to be equal to a light sending into the eye 457 quanta (507 nm) s^{-1} deg^{-2} (-3.0 $\log_{10}$ scotopic td) or causing about one photoisomerization per rod every 137 s. And, the dark light estimates for the four observers whose thresholds make up the Aguilar & Stiles mean curve range from one photoisomerization every 48 s (1300 quanta (507 nm) s^{-1} deg^{-2}) to one every 313 s (200 quanta (507 nm) s^{-1} deg^{-2}). Barlow (1957) has suggested an average value equal to about 1000 quanta (507 nm) s^{-1} deg^{-2} at the cornea (-2.66 $\log_{10}$ scotopic td) or one photoisomerization every 62 s. More recent studies give values of 400 quanta (507 nm) s^{-1} deg^{-2} or about one photoisomerization every 156 s (Hallett, 1969) and 50–200 quanta (507 nm) s^{-1} deg^{-2} or one photoisomerization every 312 to 1250 s (Sakitt, 1972). Such additive dark noise can have a measurable influence on sensitivity, but only at or near absolute threshold. (Unlike multiplicative neural noise, at higher levels, it is swamped by the background.)

2.2.6 *The thermal limit to seeing*

The dark light values estimated psychophysically for achromat K.N. (and for other observers as well), it should be noted, are even smaller than the equivalent thermal isomerization rate (once every 160 s or about 390 quanta (507 nm) s^{-1} deg^{-2} at the cornea) measured in individual monkey rods (Baylor *et al.*, 1984). This is puzzling. One would expect his dark light to be larger if the dark noise in the photoreceptors is being compounded by photon fluctuations in the stimulus and dark noise in the retina and cortex.

That these additional factors do not seem to elevate threshold above the limit set by thermal isomerizations may be accidental, due in part to our uncertainty (and error) in estimating, psychophysically, dark light (noise estimates are highly dispersed) and in relating photons incident on the cornea to isomerizations per rod (see the range of estimates in Table 2.1). However, three intriguing lines of evidence go a long way to suggesting that the absolute threshold is set by thermal isomerizations (Barlow, 1956, 1988; Baylor *et al.*, 1984; Baylor, 1987).

First of all, recent measurements of ganglion cell thresholds in the amphibian retina (Reuter *et al.*, 1986; Copenhagen, Donner & Reuter, 1987; Aho *et al.*, 1987, 1988; Donner, 1989) indicate that the major factors limiting detection of dim lights by the most sensitive ganglion cells

– which are the neurones most likely to mediate vision at absolute threshold – are spontaneous dark events in rods. Not only do the most sensitive ganglion cells start to respond reliably at about the same level as the measured rates of rod dark events; but also their proportion suffices to ensure that behavioural performance in principle could reach the same level (Donner, 1989). This may also be the case for the cat. Barlow, Levick & Yoon (1971) found that the centre of the receptive field of dark-adapted retinal ganglion cells is so extremely sensitive that it can register and linearly sum the quantal signals arising in individual rods.

Second, the absolute threshold of the toad *Bufo bufo* for visually guided behaviour (i.e. for phototactic jumping) is as low as that allowed by the known spontaneous thermal isomerization rate in the toad's receptors (Aho *et al.*, 1987, 1988). And, in the frog *Rana temporaria*, the threshold for phototactic jumping increases fourfold with an ambient temperature increase from 10 to 20°C; with the molecular rate of photoisomerizations at threshold being roughly equal to the calculated molecular rate of thermal isomerizations (Aho *et al.*, 1987, 1988).

Third, a comparison of different species (man, frog and toad) at different temperatures shows a linear correlation between absolute threshold intensities and the estimated thermal isomerization rates in their retinae (Aho *et al.*, 1988).

If, indeed, the dark events in rods set the limit to visual sensitivity, it implies that evolution has successfully optimized the other retinal and cortical factors, but cannot further improve the thermal stability of rhodopsin (Barlow, 1988). This would seem to confirm the prediction made solely on the basis of psychophysical measurements by Barlow (1956, 1957) more than 30 years ago, and prefigured by Autrum (1943) even earlier: 'Durch thermischen Zerfall des Sehpurpurs enstehen endogene Störungen, die der Leistungsfähigkeit des Auges eine Grenze setzen' (p. 234; 'From thermal decomposition of rhodopsin arises endogeneous disturbances, which determine a limit to the performance of the eye').

But how has the system devised the means for maintaining its sensitivity near the intrinsic thermal noise limit? And, how does it counteract the effects of synaptic and other noise in the visual system? Autrum (1943) suggested that inter-retinal summation compensates for the endogeneous noise level. But how? It may be that the information about threshold does not reside in a strong response by a single 'most sensitive' neuron, but in the temporally correlated weak firing of several cells receiving signals from the same group of rod photoreceptors (cf. Meister, Pine & Baylor, 1989). Or, it may be that the progressive divergence and partial reconvergence of the retinal pathways act to multiply the effects of a single quantal absorption, by initiating several extra impulses at the ganglion cell (Barlow *et al.*, 1971). In the cat retina, for instance, along the major rod bipolar pathway believed to handle the threshold signals, one rod projects to two rod bipolar cells, which project to five AII amacrine cells (Famiglietti & Kolb, 1975), which in turn project to eight cone bipolar cells (with axons ending in sublamina b of the inner plexiform layer), which terminate on two ON-beta ganglion cells (Sterling, 1983; Smith, Freed & Sterling, 1986; Sterling, Freed & Smith, 1986). Thus, for each original quantal signal from the rod photoreceptor, as many as eight independent copies may be generated and summed together at the ganglion cell. This arrangement would probably best serve to remove the effect of synaptic noise on the quantal signals arising from receptors in the centre of the ganglion cell receptive field; because the multiple pathways carrying the independent copies would converge within the same ganglion cell and/or its neighbour. For receptors near the margin of the receptive field centre, on the other hand, the multiple pathways might terminate on separate and/or non-adjacent ganglion cells, diminishing the efficacy of the quantal multiplication process (cf. Barlow *et al.*, 1971).

2.3 The desensitization of the rods

2.3.1 The Weber–Fechner fraction

The increment threshold curve of the rods (Fig. 2.1) begins to rise at adapting intensities above $-3.0 \log_{10}$ scotopic td. The change in sensitivity can be specified by what is known as the Weber–Fechner fraction, c. In its simplest form (after Weber, 1834), $c = \Delta I/I$, where ΔI is the increment intensity and I is the background intensity. In its more general form (after Fechner, 1860), $c = \Delta I/(I + I_0)$, where I_o is a dark noise constant added to account for the levelling off of the curve at low background intensities (i.e. below $-2.0 \log_{10}$ scotopic td).

The change in achromat K.N.'s Weber–Fechner fraction, as a function of background intensity, for the 6 deg, 200 ms target, is shown in Fig. 2.6. His values (filled circles) are plotted along with those of Aguilar & Stiles's mean observer (open circles) and those of two normal observers (crosses and triangles), to give an idea of how much variability there is among normal observers. At very low intensities (below $-3.0 \log_{10}$ scotopic td), in both the achromat and normal observers, I_0 dominates and the incremental threshold ΔI is constant, so c decreases

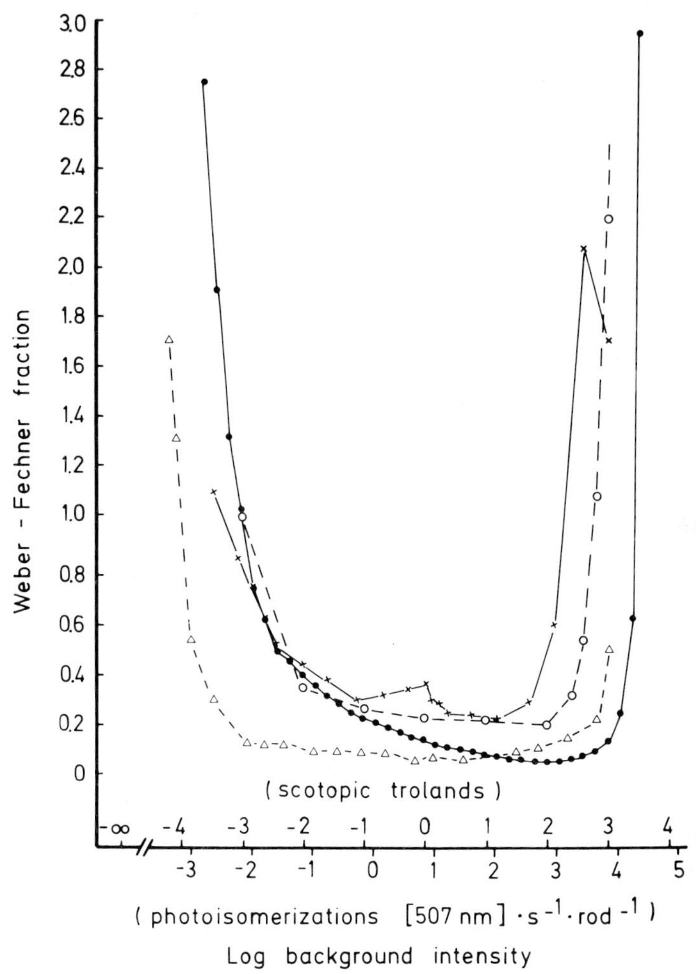

Fig. 2.6. The increment thresholds of the achromat K.N. from Fig. 2.1 (filled circles) are replotted to show the change in the Weber–Fechner fraction (the ratio of increment threshold to background intensity) as a function of background intensity. The open circles represent the Weber–Fechner fractions of the average observer of Aguilar & Stiles (1954). The crosses are the Weber–Fechner fractions of the normal observer in Fig. 2.2; the triangles are those of a second normal observer (his increment threshold curve is shown in Fig. 2.13).

according to I. At higher intensities (-3.0 to -2.0 $\log_{10}$ scotopic td), I is large enough to add significantly to I_0 and the threshold begins to rise; c decreases more slowly. At still higher intensities (-2.0 to 2.0 $\log_{10}$ scotopic td), I_0 becomes negligible compared to I. In the normal observers, but not the achromat, the threshold rises almost in direct

Table 2.4. *The slopes of increment threshold versus intensity curves*[a] *measured for achromat K.N.*

Target			Slope
diameter (deg)	area (deg^2)	duration (ms)	(log–log coordinates)
6.00[b]	28.30	200	0.77
1.85[d]	2.69	200	0.73
1 × 2[a]	2.00	1000	0.70
1 × 2[a]	2.00	125	0.67
1.85[d]	2.69	50	0.68
1.00[c]	0.79	100	0.67
1 × 2[a]	2.00	8	0.65
0.17[d]	0.02	200	0.63
0.20[a]	0.03	125	0.62
0.17[d]	0.02	50	0.59
0.17[c]	0.02	10	0.50

[a] From Stabell, Nordby & Stabell (1987).
[b] From Sharpe, Fach, Nordby & Stockman (1989).
[c] From Fach, Sharpe & Stockman (1990).
[d] From Sharpe, Whittle & Nordby (1990).

proportion to the intensity of the adapting field; *c* is approximately constant and the curve is said to obey Weber's (1834) law. In the achromat, however, *c* continues to decrease steadily with background intensity; indicating that there is an exponential relation between his threshold and intensity. Hence the value of his slope in logarithmic coordinates is not unity, as for the normal observers, but is significantly less, 0.77. (The difference is due to cone intrusion and will be explained below.) At the highest intensities (above 2.0 $\log_{10}$ scotopic td), Weber's law breaks down for the normal observers due to rod saturation. For them, as well as for the achromat, the threshold rises sharply and *c* explodes upwards.

As made explicit in Fig. 2.5, the value of the slope (and hence the rate of change in the Weber–Fechner fraction) depends upon target size and duration (Barlow, 1957, 1958): for achromat K.N., it is 0.67 for the 100 ms, 1 deg target; and 0.50 for the 10 ms, 10 min target. Table 2.4 gives the slopes of achromat K.N.'s increment threshold curve for various other target durations and sizes.

The change in achromat K.N.'s slope with target parameters implies that, unlike the absolute threshold, the Weber–Fechner relation has little or nothing to do with events inside the photoreceptor itself (see also

Chapter 1 for post-receptoral argument); if merely because the target size, at least within the range over which it is varied in Table 2.4, is many orders of magnitude larger than the rod outer segment. Still, there are processes within the photoreceptor which could contribute to the light-adaptation of the rod visual system, and which, in fact, do contribute to the light-adaptation of the cone visual system. These are photopigment bleaching and automatic gain control.

2.3.2 *Pigment depletion*

Does depletion of the photopigment within the outer segment provide sensitivity regulation in the rods? In principle, this is possible since its effect would be to decrease the quantal absorptions from the target, which is equivalent to decreasing the rod system's sensitivity. An analysis of the effects of bleaching on the sensitivity of the rod system is given in Fig. 2.7. The curve panel (*a*) indicates the proportion of rod pigment present (p) as a function of the intensity of a steady adapting field (I). It was calculated on the assumption that the rod photopigment obeys the laws of a first order photochemical reaction (Rushton, 1972*a*, *b*). That is, according to the equation: $p = I_0/(I_0 + I)$, where I_0 (4.4 $\log_{10}$ scotopic td) is the half-bleaching constant or the value of I that at equilibrium bleaches half of the rhodopsin (cf. Rushton, 1956; Ripps & Weale, 1969, Alpern, 1971). Although the proportion of molecules available to absorb light clearly decreases monotonically with intensity, it only does so at levels above 3.0 $\log_{10}$ scotopic td, where saturation is already extinguishing rod vision.

To picture how the rod threshold would rise if desensitization were due solely to the depletion of pigment molecules look at the curve at the far right in Fig. 2.6 (panel (*b*); open circles). The curve was calculated according to the equation, increment threshold (ΔI) = I_∞/p, where I_∞ is the absolute threshold (-3.30 $\log_{10}$ scotopic td). At the adapting intensity where saturation causes the threshold to rise above the Weber–Fechner line of constant slope in the experimental curve (filled circles), the predicted curve is in error by more than 5 $\log_{10}$ units of sensitivity. Pigment depletion, then, contributes in no important way to rod desensitization.

2.3.3 *Photoreceptor light-adaptation*

A process, variously termed photoreceptor light-adaptation, receptor gain control, cellular adaptation (Norman & Perlman, 1979), or σ-adaptation (Valeton & Van Norren, 1983), operates within invertebrate

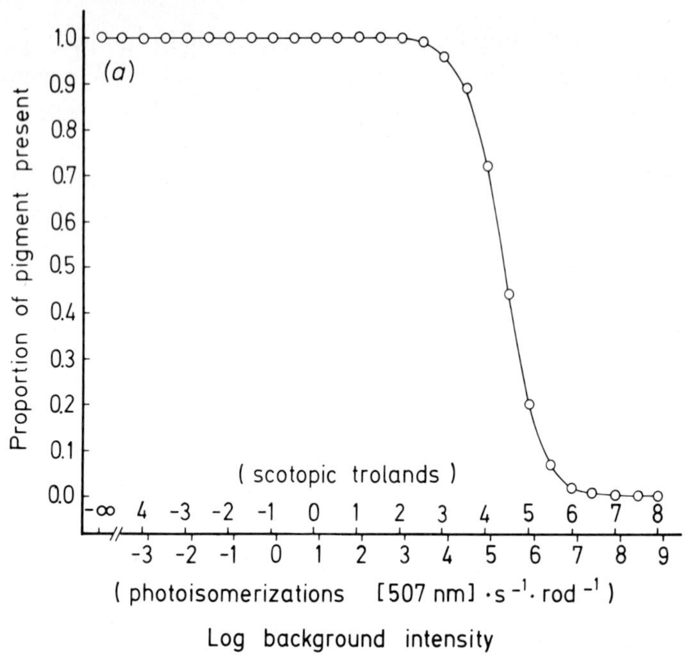

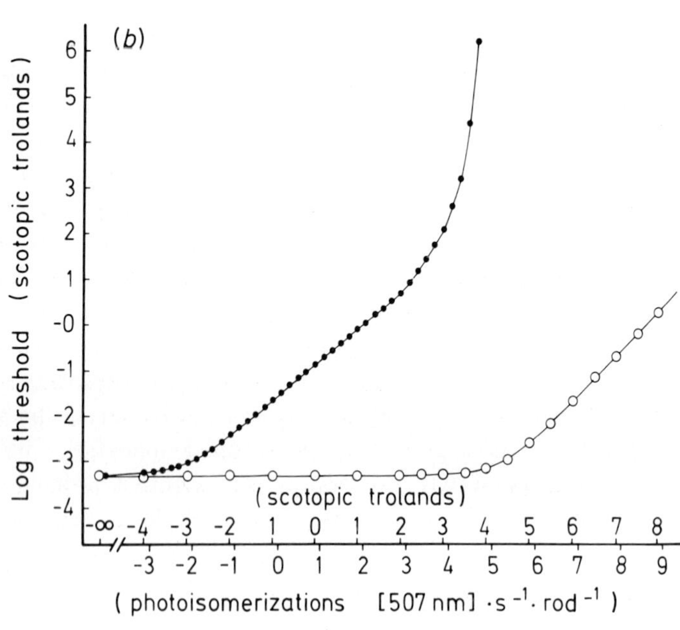

Fig. 2.7. The contribution of pigment depletion to sensitivity loss within the rod system. Panel (*a*) shows the proportion of pigment molecules available (open circles) as a function of background intensity (see text for details). Panel (*b*) shows achromat K.N.'s increment threshold function from Fig. 2.1 (filled circles) compared with the function that would be obtained if the only source of sensitivity loss was pigment depletion (open circles).

rods to counteract the loss in sensitivity resulting from the closing of sodium ion (or light-sensitive) channels in the outer segment. The closures occur whenever a photon is absorbed; and the number of closures determines the photoreceptor response. With increasing background intensity, more and more channels are closed by photons absorbed from the background, so fewer channels are available to be closed by photons absorbed from the test flash. Thus, if the relation between photon absorption, channel closure and the integration time of the light response is invariant, the maximum response amplitude of the photoreceptor will get smaller and smaller with increasing background intensity (once a critical number of channels have been closed). If, however, the relation changes with background intensity – as happens when the light response speeds up – the compression of the photoreceptor response may be completely or partially avoided, and there may be little or no loss in the photoreceptor dynamic coding range. Such a mechanism has been reported in the rods of the skate (Dowling & Ripps, 1972), the rat (Penn & Hagins, 1972), the turtle (Baylor & Hodgkin, 1974), the gecko (Kleinschmidt & Dowling, 1975), the toad (Fain, 1976; Baylor, Lamb & Yau, 1979; Baylor, Matthews & Yau, 1980), the salamander (Matthews *et al.*, 1988; Nakatani & Yau, 1988) and the cat (Tamura, Nakatani & Yau, 1989). Does it operate within primate rods?

We can determine the answer by plotting achromat K.N.'s increment threshold function from Fig. 2.1 (filled circles) along with a function constructed from the flash sensitivity data of primate (*Macaca fascicularis*) rod photoreceptors (various symbols). This is done in Fig. 2.8. The monkey data are redrawn from Baylor *et al.* (1984), and the theoretical curve fitted through them is derived from their equation 8 using the response property values listed in their Table 4. What is shown is the flash sensitivity of an individual rod outer segment S_F on a given steady background, relative to its flash sensitivity S_F^D in darkness (right ordinate). A comparison with the psychophysical data is possible because S_F is equal to $\Delta R/\Delta I$, or the peak amplitude of the criterion response (ΔR) divided by the flash strength (ΔI); and S_F^D is equal to $\Delta R/\Delta I_\infty$, or the peak amplitude of the criterion response (ΔR) divided by the flash strength in darkness (ΔI_∞). Thus $S_F/S_{F\max}^D$ equals $\Delta I_\infty/\Delta I$, and this corresponds to the quantity plotted in increment threshold functions (left ordinate).

Clearly, the two functions differ vastly in shape. Unlike the psychophysical function which increases monotonically over a wide range of $\log_{10}$ background intensity, the physiological function remains almost constant up to backgrounds causing about 42 (1.62 $\log_{10}$) photoisomerizations s^{-1} rod^{-1}, roughly the equivalent of 6 (0.78 $\log_{10}$) scotopic td

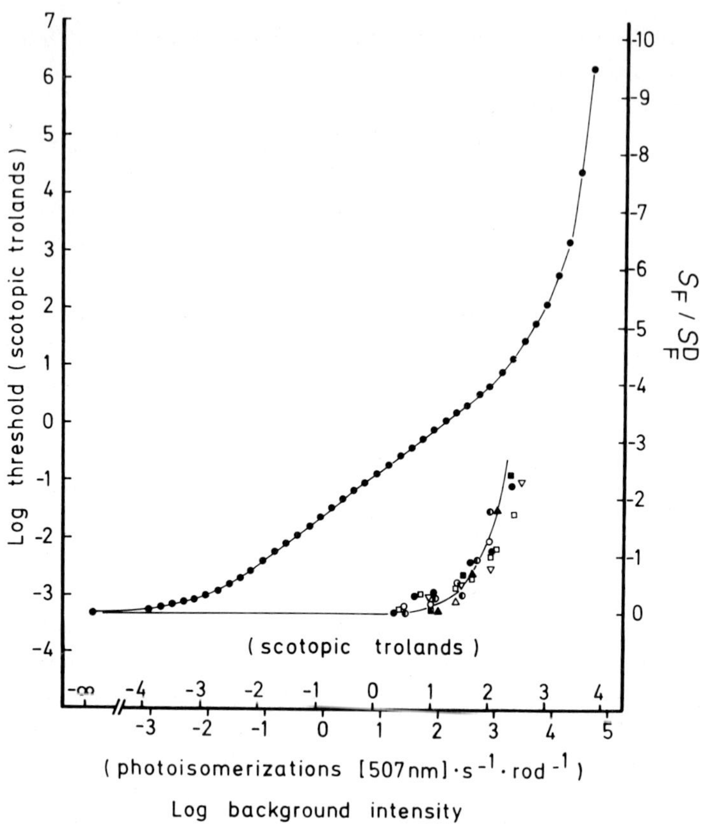

Fig. 2.8. Comparison of K.N.'s psychophysically measured increment threshold function (the 200 ms, 6 deg target data from Fig. 2.1; filled circles) with the physiologically derived increment threshold function for individual macaque rod outer segments from Baylor *et al.* (1984; various symbols). The left ordinate indicates the increment threshold sensitivity, while the right ordinate indicates the sensitivity to a flash relative to its value in darkness. The abscissa gives the background intensity in $\log_{10}$ scotopic td and $\log_{10}$ isomerizations (507 nm) per second per rod. The conversion was made according to the values given in the text and in Table 2.1. These differ slightly from the values given by Baylor *et al.*, 1984. (One can convert to their scale by subtracting 0.24 $\log_{10}$ unit from the photoisomerization s^{-1} rod^{-1} scale shown.) The solid line fitted through the outer segment data was calculated according to Baylor *et al.* (1984, eqn. 8): $S_F/S_F^D = e^{-k_s I_s}$; where S_F is the flash sensitivity in background light, S_F^D is the flash sensitivity in darkness, k_s (0.0123) is a scaling constant assuming that the outer segment has an effective collecting area of 0.0575 μm^2 and an effective collecting time of 217 ms, and I_s is the background intensity.

(Baylor *et al.*, 1984). Thereafter it surges upwards; indicative of severe response compression.

Four things should be noted. First, the scale of background intensity in photoisomerizations (507 nm) s^{-1} rod^{-1} given in Fig. 2.8 differs slightly from the scale given by Baylor *et al.* (1984). This is mainly because Baylor *et al.*'s for converting between scotopic trolands and photoisomerizations relies upon the light-collecting area of the rods; whereas the one used here relies on the spread of quanta over the receptor mosaic. One can convert to their scale of photoisomerizations s^{-1} rod^{-1} by subtracting 0.24 $\log_{10}$ unit from the scale shown. Second, the experiments of Baylor *et al.* (1984) were done with rods exposed to an artificial medium; whereas the rods in an intact eye interact metabolically with the pigment epithelium. Third, the story may be different when rods are continuously exposed to very intense lights. Yonemura & Kawasaki (1979) have made recordings from asparate-perfused human retinae, which suggest that rods may have some ability to regulate their sensitivity. Fourth, Tamura *et al.* (1989) have found light adaptation in the rods of cats and other mammalian species, including some primates. Thus the exact quantitative adaptation of single rods in pipettes must be interpreted with caution.

Setting these problems aside, it nevertheless seems that macaque rods, and presumably human ones as well, saturate without adapting and cannot explain the regular loss in sensitivity found for the intact human rod visual system. If the rods themselves were light-adapting, one would expect to find a decline in response amplitude and/or a significant speeding up of the rod response with backgrounds. (Besides reducing photoreceptor response amplitudes, adaptation affects the kinetics of the response.) But in macaque rods, there is 'little decline in the response to a bright step and little if any shortening in the time scale of flash responses in background light' (Baylor *et al.*, 1984, p. 591). The maximum reduction in light-integration time is about 1.4 times (the photoreceptors showing this speeding up are the ones lying to the right of the theoretical curve in Fig. 2.8; open squares and triangles).

Why macaque rods do not light-adapt may be due to an absence of calcium ion feedback in their outer segment (cf. Matthews *et al.*, 1988; Nakatani & Yau, 1988). Such ion feedback occurs in the rod photoreceptors of invertebrates, who depend upon rod vision at all levels of adaptation and who have very large rods, which may capture several quanta even at very dim intensities. Cats, too, may need such a mechanism because their cone system has a high light threshold and the rods must be prevented from saturating before the cones fully take over vision at higher light intensities. But it may not be imperative for the rod photoreceptors of the human and macaque, who do not depend on, or even need, rod vision at moderate and bright adaptation levels. At levels below cone absolute threshold, the shower of photons falling on the retina is so sparse that a rod only occasionally will absorb a photon. No internal regulatory mechanism is, therefore, required to counteract the effects of response compression. At higher levels, where the rain of photons is incessant and response compression comes into play, the cones are active. The rod signals – in all save the achromat, who has no alternative – only degrade the visual representation and are, arguably, better dispensed with (see below).

2.3.4 *Pupil constriction*

If sensitivity is not being regulated in the photoreceptor, then where? One factor that must be considered is the pupil aperture, whose diameter changes in proportion to the number of incident quanta. In the average adult eye, the diameter of the pupil ranges from 7.2 mm in the dark to 2.0 mm in bright sunlight. At the level where the rods are fully saturated in Fig. 2.1, it is about 2.4 mm (see De Groot & Gebhard, 1952; Alpern & Ohba, 1972), so the number of quanta reaching the rods is about 11% of the number that would reach the rods if the pupil area remained constant at its dark-adapted value. Normally it would be necessary to correct the desensitization curve of the rods for the change in pupil diameter as a function of background level. But this is unnecessary in Fig. 2.1 (and in all the other figures as well) because the curve was measured under conditions that controlled for pupillary variations. During the threshold measurements, the observer's pupil was fully dilated by a mydriatic and the cross-sections of the target and background beams entering the pupil were restricted to smaller than 2 mm. Thus, change in pupillary area, though it acts to control the number of quanta reaching the rods in other, everyday situations, cannot be used to explain the regular desensitization of the rods shown in Fig. 2.1.

Anyway, even if the pupil diameter were uncontrolled for, it would only reduce sensitivity by less than one $\log_{10}$ unit over the same background intensity range where target sensitivity, in fact, decreases by seven $\log_{10}$ units. And, more importantly, the one $\log_{10}$ unit influence of the pupillary reflex is ancillary to the light-adaptation process itself. It involves a feedback mechanism with a time constant that is considerably slower than those governing light adaptation. For moderately strong stimulation of the rod visual system (18 scotopic td), it has a latent period on the order of 320 ms and a peak time (i.e. time to maximum constriction) of more than 600 ms (see Sharpe & Nordby, The photoreceptors in the achromat, Chapter 10, Fig. A10.5; Sharpe *et al.*, 1988). For weaker stimulation, the latent period and peak times are even longer.

2.3.5 Physical noise (quantal fluctuations)

Another factor that must be considered in sensitivity regulation is noise. In addition to the noise limit upon performance imposed by electrical–chemical events within the visual system, there is a noise limit imposed by external physical events, which is a consequence of the Poisson nature of light. As described above, the number of quanta in the adapting field is not constant, but follows a Poisson distribution, with a mean of n and a standard deviation of $n^{0.5}$. So, as first recognized by Rose (1942, 1948) and de Vries (1943), the smallest possible threshold in a system that exhibits no intrinsic noise is set by the statistical fluctuations in the mean number of background photons entering the eye. (It is not clear whether the noise of photoreceptor transduction and synaptic transmission preserves or distorts the underlying Poisson statistics of photon capture; see Teich *et al.*, 1978, 1982; van Meeteren, 1978.) Thus the threshold intensity for detection of an increment light stimulus depends on the ability of the visual signals generated to reliably exceed the noise level associated with the background intensity. But do backgrounds raise the rod threshold only because of photon noise?

This can be answered by looking at Fig. 2.9, which shows achromat K.N.'s three increment threshold curves replotted from Fig. 2.5 along with predictions based on the quantal fluctuation theory of Barlow (1957). The theory assumes, first, that differential sensitivity is proportional to the square root of the number of quanta absorbed from the adapting field (i.e. that the increment threshold curve rises with a slope of 0.5 on log–log coordinates); and, second, that there is intrinsic (additive) noise in the visual pathway. If target detection were limited only by fluctuations in quantum noise, without a dark light component, then the increment threshold curve should start rising with even dim backgrounds; which it plainly does not. In fact, the thresholds on very dim backgrounds may even be slightly lower than those in the dark, due perhaps to summation of quanta contained in the background and quanta contained in the target (Baumgardt, 1959; Baumgardt & Smith, 1965) or to the visible background helping to lock-in fixation and attention.

The dashed curves in Fig. 2.9 are the predicted rise in threshold calculated according to Barlow's equation: $(\Delta I) = K\ (I + I_D)^{0.5}$

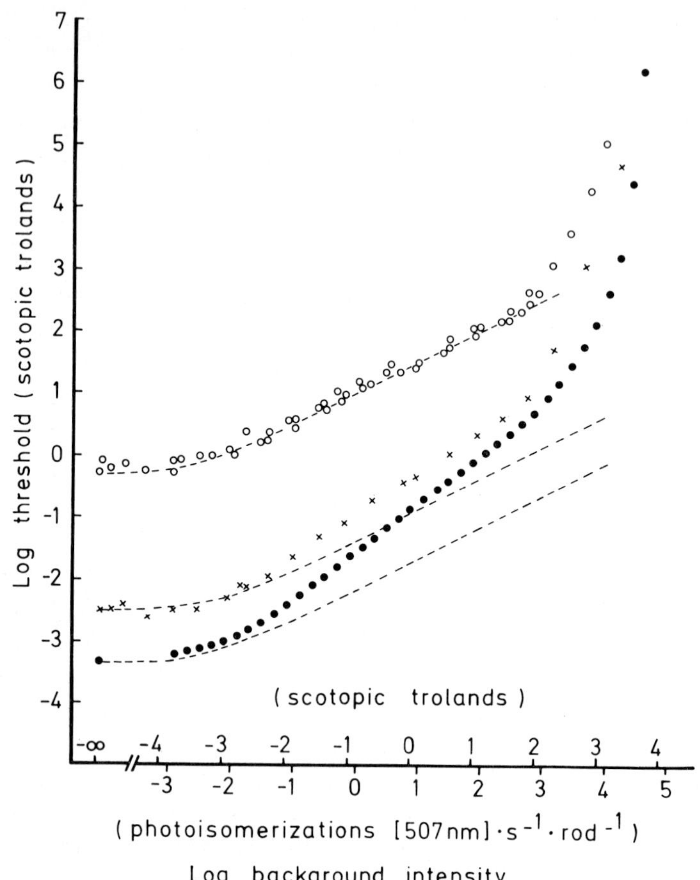

Fig. 2.9. The three rod increment threshold curves of achromat K.N. from Fig. 2.1 compared with theoretical curves derived from the Fluctuation Theory of Barlow (1957; dashed lines): 200 ms, 6 deg target (filled circles); 100 ms, 1 deg target (crosses); 10 ms, 10 min target (open circles). The theoretical curves are calculated according to the equation: increment threshold $(\Delta I) = K\,(I + I_D)^{0.5}\,(Q\,A\ \ t\,F)^{-0.5}$ (after Barlow, 1957); where K is the threshold signal-to-noise ratio; I is the adapting intensity in scotopic td; I_D is the 'dark light'; Q (4.5717×10^5) is the conversion factor for scotopic troland to quanta (507 nm) $s^{-1}\,deg^{-2}$; A is the rod summation area; t is the rod integration time; and F (0.2) is the fraction of quanta incident at the cornea that are effectively absorbed. The values of I_D were taken as −3.20, −3.10 and −3.52 $\log_{10}$ scotopic td, respectively, for the 200 ms, 6 deg; 100 ms, 1 deg and 10 ms, 10 min targets (see text for details). It was assumed that the other parameters, K, A and t, were constant for each target condition. Their values were determined as a lumped parameter by substitution in the formula, taking the absolute threshold values as −3.30, −2.48 and −0.30 $\log_{10}$ scotopic td for the 200 ms, 6 deg; 100 ms, 1 deg and 10 ms, 10 min targets, respectively.

$(Q\ A\ t\ F)^{-0.5}$; where ΔI is the increment threshold in scotopic td), K is the observer's internal criterion or reliability factor (see Baumgardt, 1972, p. 46; Rose, 1973), I is the adapting intensity in scotopic td, I_D is 'dark light', Q (4.5717×10^5) is the conversion factor for scotopic td to quanta (507 nm) s^{-1} deg^{-2}, A is the area of rod spatial summation or the area of the retina over which the background and the dark light are liable to be confused with the target, t is the integration time of the rods or the time during which the background and dark light is liable to be confused with the target, and F (0.2) is the fraction of quanta incident at the cornea that are effectively absorbed. For the theoretical curves shown, K, A and t were left as unknown constants and their combined value was determined as a lumped parameter by substitution in Barlow's equation (see the caption to Fig. 2.9).

Clearly, the predicted function provides a good fit only to the increment threshold curve measured with the small (10 min), brief (10 ms) test flash; which rises with a slope of 0.5 over almost the entire range of background intensity. The two other curves, obtained with larger, longer test flashes, rise with slopes of 0.69 and 0.77; indicating that sensitivity is decreasing more rapidly than can be accounted for simply in terms of an increase of noise due to quantum fluctuation. Thus quantum fluctuations cannot be solely responsible for the loss of rod sensitivity, though there is no denying that they define the rate of loss with small, brief targets and a lower limit to the loss with all other targets. Krauskopf & Reeves (1980), for instance, have shown that light detection threshold drops in proportion to the square root of the previous background intensity, when the background is turned off. This indicates that at least part of every dark adaptation curve is a component due to the removal of photon noise, and vice versa at least part of every light adaptation curve is a component due to the presence of photon noise.

Even for the small, brief target condition, it should be pointed out, rod sensitivity follows the photon-noise limit only at a certain distance. The need for the threshold criterion factor K in Barlow's equation implies that the visual system – even at its most efficient – is subject to intrinsic noise over and above that of photon fluctuations and photoreceptor transduction. One source compatible with the square-root law is multiplicative noise at the synapse, which would raise the incremental threshold and decrease detectability by the same proportion at all intensities (Lillywhite, 1981). However, there is as yet little evidence for this type of noise in the mammalian visual pathways.

2.3.6 Post-receptoral gain control: the adaptation pool

The absence of gain control and the belated onset of pigment depletion in primate (i.e. macaque) rods establishes that the first major site of rod sensitivity regulation is not the photoreceptors themselves. The same conclusion was reached by Rushton (1963, 1965*a*, *b*), 20 years earlier, on the basis of psychophysical experiments. Rod light-adaptation, he concluded, must be preceded by substantial interaction between signals from many rods. First, because the presence of a weak background field, which spares practically all the rods, elevates the threshold of rods which could not have absorbed a single quantum from it (Rushton, 1965*a*, *b*). And, second, because the loss of sensitivity brought about by a bleaching light is not confined to the area of the bleach, but also extends to adjacent non-bleached areas (Rushton & Westheimer, 1962; Rushton, 1965*a*, *b*).

To account for his findings, Rushton invoked a retinal network or areal process (this is developed further in Chapter 1), the automatic gain control (Rose, 1948; Fuortes & Hodgkin, 1964), which he called the adaptation pool (Rushton, 1963, 1965*a*, *b*). His idea was that rod signals sum linearly over a given retinal region before merging in a neural pool. Within the pool the incoming signals are attenuated by a factor according to their combined average; and the factor is used to reduce sensitivity in the area subserved by the pool.

The adaptation pool or gain control process offers two advantages. At low light levels, by integrating signals from many rods, it would counteract the effects of signal fluctuations caused by physical and photoreceptor noise; improving the rod system's sensitivity at the expense of its temporal and spatial resolution. In fact, at the lowest levels, it would provide the only means of representing light intensity at all because photoisomerizations in individual rods are too desultory to provide a reliable measure. At higher intensities where many photons are absorbed per rod, it would act as a floodgate, attenuating the signals to prevent them from overflowing the dynamic range of the visual neurones.

The site of the adaptation pool

To be effective, the adaptation pool ought to start its flood control in the retina as early as possible. The earliest possible site of action is at the receptors themselves, through chemical or electrical coupling. But, this seems to be a missed opportunity by the visual system. For one thing, adjacent receptors scarcely modify each other's sensitivity (Baylor, Fuortes & O'Bryan, 1971; Schwartz, 1975; Belgum & Copenhagen,

1988). Furthermore, although gap junctions between rods and cones are common in the primate, there is an apparent lack of gap junctions directly coupling rods with rods (Raviola & Gilula, 1973). And, the spatial spread of adaptation by electrical coupling between rod photoreceptors in the turtle, which has rod–rod gap junctions, is no greater than what can be accounted for by stray light (Copenhagen & Green, 1985). In short, the rod visual system seems to delay its major sensitivity control until a later stage. This may be for good cause. At moderate and high background levels, a large rod–cone electrical network would have obvious benefits for controlling visual sensitivity by dissipating large signals throughout the entire network. But in darkness and at low background levels, the tiny threshold signals arising in the rod outer segments would be drowned by the joint noise of all the receptors in the pool. Such an arrangement could only serve detection and sensitivity control if rod–cone gap junctions closed in the dark-adapted state, effectively disconnecting the rods from the combined electrical network. There is some evidence that this occurs in the tiger salamander retina, where background illumination enhances rod–cone coupling (Yang & Wu, 1989).

The next possible site for the adaptation pool is the horizontal cell in the outer plexiform layer. In the cat, these cells, when rod-driven, show a Weber–Fechner-like decline in incremental gain with background intensity (Steinberg, 1971). However, their sensitivity adjustments occur at relatively high background intensities, two to four $\log_{10}$ units higher than those at which comparable adjustments are found in rod-driven ganglion cells (Shapley & Enroth-Cugell, 1984). And the horizontal cell recordings are more nearly consistent with photoreceptor gain control – which may occur in cat rods (Tamura *et al.*, 1989) – than with adaptation pooling (Steinberg, 1971; Sakmann & Fileon, 1972).

In the primate, the best information places the adaptation pool at or before the bipolar-cell layer (Dowling, 1967, 1987; Shapley & Enroth-Cugell, 1984). This layer shows typical adaptation properties – as inferred from the b-wave of the electroretinogram (Fulton & Rushton, 1978) – and it has the requisite synaptic organization for supporting an inhibitory feedback mechanism (Boycott & Dowling, 1969). Moreover, on anatomical grounds, the rod bipolar cell is a natural candidate for the adaptation pool because of the convergence of many rods onto one bipolar. For instance, in the rhesus monkey retina, each rod bipolar cell connects to 30–50 rods and has a dendritic tree subtanding 3–6 min arc of visual angle in diameter (Kolb, 1970). This is the same order of magnitude as the best psychophysical estimates of the adaptation pool (see next section). The nonlinear feedback signal of the adaptation pool could arise in bipolar cells, with the reciprocal synapses between the terminals of the bipolar cells and the amacrine cell processes serving to laterally spread desensitization between bipolars (cf. Shapley & Enroth-Cugell, 1984). Regulatory feedback could also be provided by interplexiform cells, with their postsynaptic connexions in the inner plexiform layer and their presynaptic connexions in the outer plexiform layer.

The size of the adaptation pool

Rushton argued that the retinal region over which the rod adaptation pool summates signals is about 0.5 deg in diameter (Rushton & Westheimer, 1962; Rushton, 1963, 1965*a*, *b*). In support, he showed that rod desensitization effects were independent of whether the background light was homogeneously spread across the retina or concentrated in polka dots (separated by 24 min centre to centre) or the bright bars of gratings (30 min period). Rushton's findings, however, do not exactly square with other grating threshold experiments. Some yield much larger estimates of the rod adaptation pool (up to 3 deg in diameter; Spillmann & Coderre, 1973); while others indicate that it is small – 5–10 min of arc or less (Barlow & Andrews, 1967; Andrews & Butcher, 1971; Sternheim & Glass, 1975; MacLeod, Chen & Crognale, 1989) – and that its spread of desensitization is non-linearly weighted with distance (Barlow & Andrews, 1967; Andrews & Butcher, 1971). The strongest psychophysical evidence is that of MacLeod *et al.* (1989), who successively flashed bleaching and test gratings of slightly different spatial frequency. This caused the observer to view the test grating through a grid of sensitive (unbleached) and insensitive (bleached) stripes on his own retina. If the effect of desensitization were restricted to the bleached rods, the test and bleaching gratings should come in and out of register at the difference frequency and the observer should see a corresponding low-frequency grating even when the individual gratings themselves are not resolvable. MacLeod *et al.* (1989), however, failed to observe difference-frequency gratings above the resolution limit of rod vision; and estimated the adaptation pool size to be about 10 min of arc in diameter.

From the electrophysiology, it has been argued in the cat that, since there is areal summation of adaptive effects over the complete ganglion cell receptive field centre, rod adaptation pools could be coextensive with ganglion cell centres (Cleland & Enroth-Cugell, 1968; Enroth-Cugell & Shapley, 1973). (It is not being argued that the cat ganglion cell is the rod adaptation pool, only that its summing of

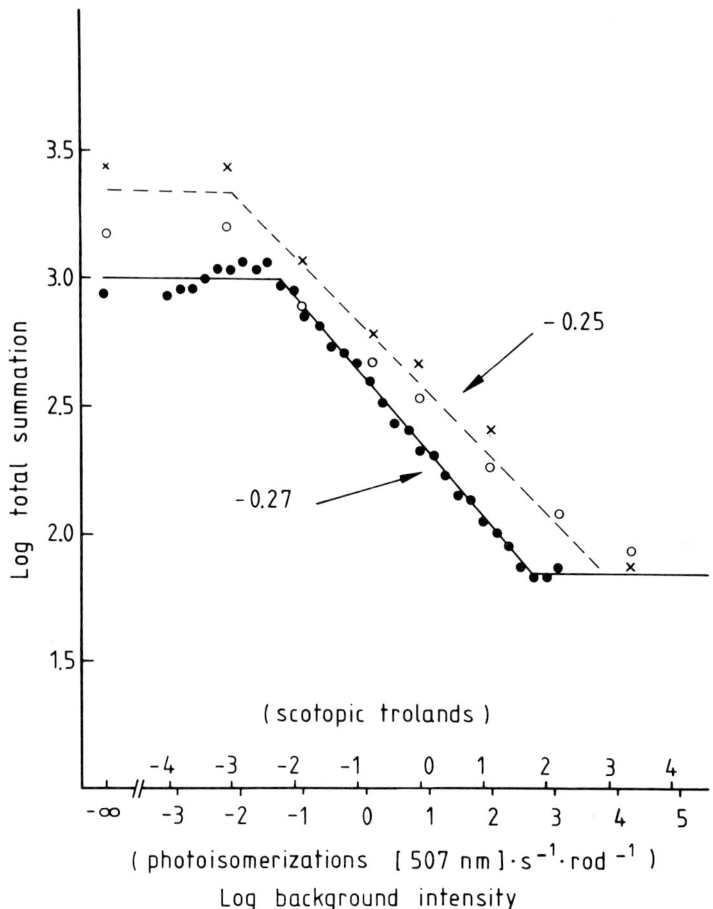

Fig. 2.10. Estimate of the change in the combined spatial and temporal summation of the rod visual system as a function of background intensity. Log_{10} total summation is the log ratio (filled circles) of achromat K.N.'s threshold quantity of light for the 10 ms, 10 min diameter target to his threshold intensity for the 200 ms, 6 deg target (from Fig. 2.5). The ratio decreases as the power 0.27. For comparison, the log ratios of two normal observers' (open circles and crosses) threshold quantity of light for a 7.5 ms, 6 min diameter target to their threshold intensity for a 935 ms, 4.92 deg target are shown (from Barlow, 1958). Their combined ratios decrease as the power 0.25.

signals must reflect the control of sensitivity in the cat preganglionic retina. Conceivably there are several pathways for the rod signals to take to the ganglion cells; and these may be optimized for increment detection at different levels of ambient illumination. Moreover, there is good evidence that the adaptation pool occurs before the site of spatial summation in the retina; see Hayhoe & Smith, 1989.) If this were also true of the primate – where comparable behavioural, but not electrophysiological measurements have been made (Ransom-Hogg & Spillmann, 1980; Oehler, 1985) – it would mean that the adaptation pools in the peripheral retina could be as much as 1.13–1.26 deg in diameter (Hubel & Wiesel, 1960; de Monasterio, 1978). Observations in the goldfish, frog and rat, however, speak against the adaptation pool coinciding with the central mechanism of the ganglion cell receptive field. In the goldfish, the pooling of adaptation is both larger or smaller than the ganglion cell centre size (Easter, 1968); and in the rat and frog, it is incomplete and confined to subareas of the receptive field (Burkhardt & Berntson, 1972; Green, Tong & Cicerone, 1977; Tong & Green, 1977; Cicerone & Green, 1980, 1981). So the major pooling of adaptive influences seems to occur prior to the combination of influences contributing to the centre response of ganglion cells (see Powers & Green Chapter 3).

2.3.7 *Spatio-temporal mechanisms of light-adaptation*

If adaptation pools are responsible for rod desensitization, are they invariant with background intensity? Or, does increasing the intensity reduce the area and time over which the pool integrates light? The steepening of the rod field adaptation curve with greater target size and duration can be taken as support for the latter conjecture; though it does not necessarily follow that the adaptation pool is the site where changes in integration area and time are taking place. After all, the neurons that set sensitivity may differ from the ones affecting visual resolution

Figure 2.10 provides an estimate of the change in the combined spatial and temporal summation of the rod visual system. It plots as a function of background intensity, the log ratio of achromat K.N.'s threshold quantity of light for the 10 ms, 10 min (0.022 deg^2) target to his threshold intensity for the 200 ms, 6 deg (28.27 deg^2) target (from Fig. 2.5). The comparison assumes that temporal and spatial summation does not affect the former – because it is measured with a target area and duration always within the ranges where complete temporal and spatial summation occur – while it affects the latter – because the target parameters are large enough for summation to overextend the ranges even on dim backgrounds. It can be seen that the amount of overall summation for the achromat K.N. is not constant but decreases as the power 0.27, as the background intensity is raised from about −3.0 to 2.0 $\log_{10}$ scotopic td. This value is nearly identical with the one (0.25) reported by Barlow

(1958) in his classic study, in which he compared thresholds for a 7.5 ms, 0.0077 deg^2 target and a 935 ms, 19 deg^2 target. And, it accords with much other evidence that the rod visual system's temporal and spatial limits vary with background intensity.

At absolute threshold in the peripheral retina, the spatial limit is typically assumed to be between 30 min and 2 deg in diameter (Graham, Brown & Mote, 1939; Bouman & Blokhuis, 1952; Barlow, 1958; Weale, 1958; Hallett, Marriott & Rodger, 1962; Hallett, 1963, 1969; Sakitt, 1971; Baumgardt, 1972; van Meeteren & Vos, 1972; Smith, 1973; Scholtes & Bouman, 1977; see also Chapter 1). And the temporal limit is assumed to be about 100 ms (Barlow, 1958; Baumgardt & Hillmann, 1961; Baumgardt, 1972; van Meeteren & Vos, 1972; Sharpe, Fach & Nordby, 1988; see also Chapter 1). But estimates of both spatial and temporal summation vary widely and depend upon stimulus configuration and retinal eccentricity (Bouman, 1953; Barlow, 1958; Hallett, 1963; Sakitt, 1971; Scholtes & Bouman, 1977). With light adaptation, the spatial limit of rod vision is thought to decrease by a factor of 4 (Barlow, 1958) and the temporal limit by a factor of 2–3 (Barlow, 1958; Conner & MacLeod, 1977; Conner, 1982; Hess & Nordby, 1986; Sharpe *et al.*, 1988). This yields an overall factor of 8 to 12; which accords very well with the 1.1 $\log_{10}$ unit change in rod increment detectability estimated from Fig. 2.10.

Changes associated with spatial organization are often assumed to have a larger effect on the rod threshold than those associated with temporal integration. But the evidence is somewhat equivocal. On the one hand, achromat K.N.'s rod-determined critical duration (a psychophysical measure of complete temporal summation; see also Chapter 1) decreases from 214 ms to 125 ms (a factor of 1.7) as he goes from scotopic to mesopic light levels (see Sharpe & Nordby, The photoreceptors in the achromat, Chapter 10, Fig. 10.15; Sharpe *et al.*, 1988). This suggests that spatial reorganization accounts for the greater part of the deviation from the de Vries–Rose law (see Chapter 1 for detailed discussion). On the other hand, comparisons between the slopes of his increment threshold curves (see Table 2.4) indicate that pure changes in target duration (when target area is always less than the spatial summation limit) and pure changes in target area (when target duration is always less than the temporal summation limit) have an equal influence upon the slope of the curve. Increases in both would seem to decrease detectability according to a power law of about −0.13. For a third alternative, there are yet other measurements suggesting that spatial changes may even be less important than temporal ones. For instance,

Table 2.5. *The slopes of increment threshold versus intensity curves*[a] *of normal observers as a function of stimulus diameter and temporal eccentricity. The values are given for* (i) *scotopic and mesopic and* (ii) *photopic adaptation levels*[b] *(after Scholtes & Bouman, 1977)*

(i)

Temporal eccentricity (deg)	Target diameter (deg)					
	0.12	0.27	0.47	1.13	2.28	4.67
7	0.52	0.55	0.57	0.58	0.59	0.60
10	—	—	—	—	0.62	0.62
15	—	—	0.60	0.63	0.65	0.66
18	—	—	—	0.66	0.68	—
20	—	—	—	0.64	0.66	0.64
25	0.39[c]	—	0.62	0.64	0.69	0.65
35	—	—	—	0.65	—	0.66
40	0.33[c]	—	0.64	—	0.64	0.66

(ii)

Temporal eccentricity (deg)	Target diameter (deg)					
	0.12	0.27	0.47	1.13	2.28	4.67
7	1.08	1.07	1.08	1.06	1.10	1.07
10	—	—	—	—	1.05	1.04
15	—	—	1.07	1.02	1.01	1.02
18	—	—	—	1.00	1.02	—
20	—	—	—	1.01	0.97	1.04
25	1.01	—	0.99	1.03	1.04	1.01
35	—	—	—	0.99	—	0.98
40	1.04	—	0.97	—	1.04	1.00

[a] Target conditions: 510 nm, 10 ms exposure. Background conditions: 510 nm, 10 deg diameter.

[b] Scholtes & Bouman estimated that the transition from scotopic/mesopic to photopic vision took place at all retina eccentricities within less than half a $\log_{10}$ unit of 10^{-10} W deg^{-2}. This corresponds to 2.7 $\log_{10}$ scotopic td (Wyszecki & Stiles, 1982).

[c] Slopes of less than 0.5 are presumably due to insufficient data.

Scholtes & Bouman (1977) found, at 7 deg in the temporal retina, that the effect of changing the target size from 0.12 to 4.67 deg in diameter, while holding target duration constant at 10 ms, is to increase the slope of the rod-detected increment threshold curve from 0.52 to 0.60; which suggests a decreasing power law of 0.08 (see Table 2.5(i)).

2.3.8 Local adaptation versus spatial reorganization

Although the threshold for a small target is of a higher intensity than the threshold for a large one, it does not follow that the change in the gradient of the increment threshold curve is necessarily due to changes in spatial integration. The change may be more parsimoniously explained by an adaptation-dependent non-linearity in the function relating local response to test flash intensity (Chen, MacLeod & Stockman, 1987). And, in fact, Chen *et al.* (1987) have convincingly demonstrated this to be the case for cone vision; finding that any reduction in sensitivity due to target size over and above that due to local adaptation was at most 28% in area or 15% in diameter (0.14 $\log_{10}$ unit). Does local adaptation also account for target size changes in rod vision?

To find out, Sharpe, Whittle & Nordby (1990) compared achromat K.N.'s small (0.10 deg) and large (1.85 deg) target increment threshold curves with large (1.85 deg) target suprathreshold (dichoptic) brightness matching curves. The intensity of the standard brightness matching field was chosen so that at low background intensities the intensity of the large target required to match it was the same as the threshold intensity of the small target. According to a pure spatial integration hypothesis, the brightness matching function should have the same slope as the large target increment threshold function; because the same sized target is used in the two types of measurements and the difference in brightness is held to be unimportant. According to the pure response–intensity non-linearity hypothesis, on the other hand, the brightness matching function should have the same slope as the small target increment threshold function; because the different sized targets are of the same brightness and will evoke the same local response.

Figures 2.11 and 2.12 show for measurements made with 200 ms and 50 ms target durations, respectively, that the brightness matching curve has a slightly steeper slope than the small test flash curve – for the 200 ms flash, the slopes are 0.67 versus 0.63 and for the 50 ms flash, 0.68 versus 0.59 – but that it has a slope equal to or less than that of the large test flash – for the 200 ms flash, the slopes are 0.67 versus 0.73 and for the 50 ms flash, 0.68 versus 0.68. Since the large target brightness matching intensities rise more steeply than the small target increment threshold intensity, there must be some loss of rod sensitivity with increasing background intensity due to spatial integration over and above that due to local adaptation.

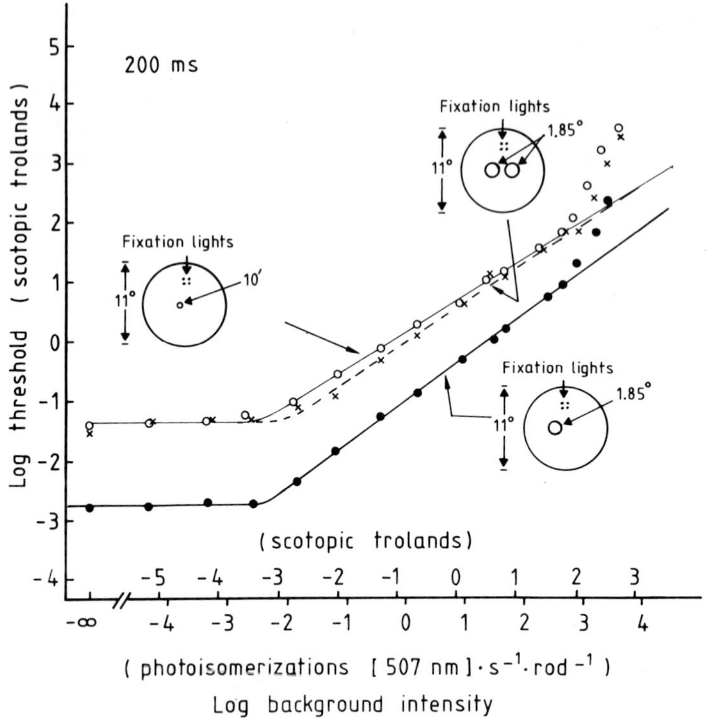

Fig. 2.11. The incremental thresholds and equal brightness matches of achromat K.N., for a green (Ilford 604; dominant wavelength approximately 518 nm), 200 ms target, plotted as a function of background intensity. All measurements were made on a red (Ilford 608; dominant wavelength approximately 600 nm), 11 deg diameter background. The filled circles are 1.85 deg test field incremental thresholds, the open circles are 10 min test field incremental thresholds and the crosses are 1.85 deg dichoptic brightness matches (see insets). For the brightness matches, the standard test field presented to the observer's right eye had an intensity approximately equal to that of the test field corresponding to the left-most data point of the 10 min test field. (From Sharpe, *et al.*, 1990.)

2.3.9 Electrophysiological correlates of spatio-temporal reorganization

The psychophysical evidence supports the hypothesis that in the rod visual system, sensitivity is regulated by changes in both spatial and temporal integration (see Chapter 1 for fitter-based description). What about the electrophysiological evidence? Are their retinal analogues of the psychophysically observed changes?

First consider changes in slope. There is good evidence in the cat that the slope of the increment threshold curve in rod-driven ganglion cells varies with target size. Barlow & Levick (1976) found, with a large area

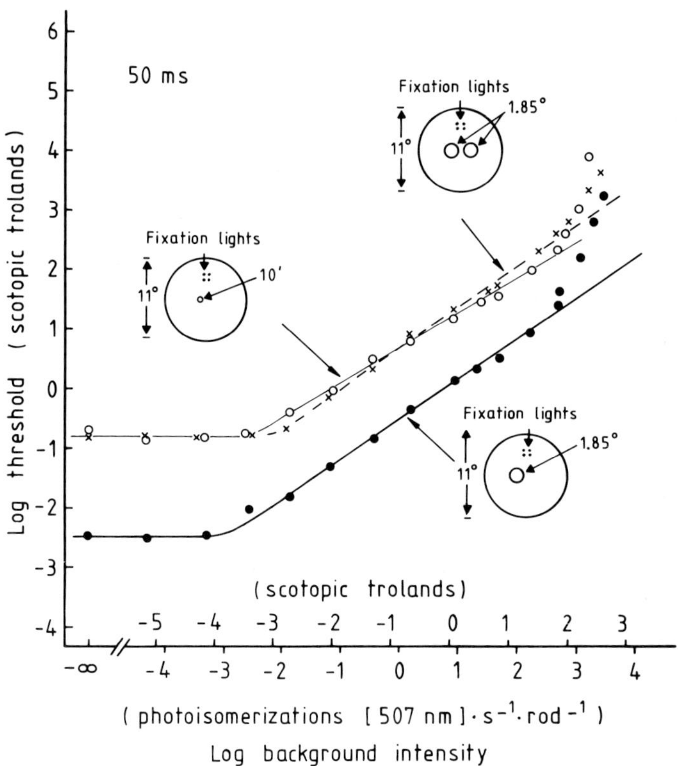

Fig. 2.12. The incremental thresholds and equal brightness matches of achromat K.N., for a 50 ms target, plotted as a function of background intensity. Otherwise same conditions as in Fig. 2.11. (From Sharpe *et al.*, 1990.)

(usually 4.6 deg), long duration (0.32–1.26 s) target, that slopes of single units averaged 0.82; whereas slopes, with a small (less than the receptive field centre size), brief (10 ms) or long (1 s) target, averaged about 0.53. These changes – though they confound temporal with spatial changes – conform almost exactly to what is shown in Fig. 2.4 for achromat K.N. (0.77 for a large, long test flash; 0.50 for a small, brief one). Lennie (1979), likewise, reported a consistent relation between target size and slope in cat retinal ganglion cells. But, he found that the curves for small stimuli (falling within the centre of the receptive field) were a little steeper (slope = 0.65) than those measured psychophysically in humans (slope = 0.5) under comparable conditions (0.2 deg target); while those for large stimuli (covering the whole receptive field) were much steeper (1.2–1.4) than the human curves (0.83, for a 7.5 deg target). The steeper slopes may reflect the activity of units that are stimulated sub-optimally; and they may point to the need to consider the responses of populations of retinal ganglion cells rather than the responses of individual units, when seeking physiological correlates of the psychophysical curves.

Allowing that there are changes in ganglion cell gain that are dependent upon background illumination, what is the physiological substrate of the change? In the frog, Donner (1987) has shown that the spatial summation of the excitatory receptive field centre of retinal ganglion cells decreases by 30–50% as the cells are light-adapted to a threshold some 4.0 $\log_{10}$ units above the dark-adapted one (a moderately strong background light). However, over the same range, temporal summation decreases by 90%. The rather modest reduction of the central summation area in the frog agrees well with values reported from rod-driven cat ganglion cells. Derrington & Lennie (1982) found a 32% reduction as background was raised by 5.0 $\log_{10}$ units; and Enroth-Cugell & Robson (1966) reported a 50% reduction over about 4.5 $\log_{10}$ units of background intensity. (Incidentally, this would seem to suggest that temporal changes are more influential than spatial ones.)

In the cat, lateral inhibitory influences, which may cancel the direct, excitatory effect of stimuli falling in the periphery of retinal receptive fields, become more prominent with background intensity (Barlow, Fitzhugh & Kuffler, 1957). True, the actual sizes of the centre and surround components of the receptive fields of rod-driven ganglion cells change very little, if at all, with adaptation (Cleland & Enroth-Cugell, 1968; Derrington & Lennie, 1982). But the antagonism from the surround of the receptive fields decreases appreciably in latency at higher adaptation levels; making the surround relatively more effective in exerting an inhibitory influence on the centre; and thereby reducing the effective size of the central summing area of each cell (Enroth-Cugell & Lennie, 1975; Barlow & Levick, 1976; Derrington & Lennie, 1982). The adjustment of sensitivity to a new level in rod-driven ganglion cells takes place within 100 ms after the onset of the adapting background (Enroth-Cugell & Shapley, 1973; Saito & Fukada, 1986). This value agrees well with human psychophysics; which suggests that gain changes take place within 100–200 ms (Crawford, 1947; Baker, 1963; Adelson, 1982; Shapley, 1986; Hayhoe, Benimoff & Hood, 1987) (Chapters 1 and 3 provide evidence that the spatial and temporal properties of cortical cells are independent of the adaptation level).

In the primate, very little is as yet known about how light-adaptation affects the temporal and spatial properties of the cells. Baylor *et al.*

(1984) have shown that the kinetic properties of individual rods speed up slightly, though only at relatively high luminances; and Purpura *et al.* (1988) have shown that the integration time of retinal ganglion cells shortens with increasing background level. Although light-dependent changes similar to those reported in the cat are assumed to occur, there seems to be a significant diversity in light-adaptation behaviour among ganglion cell types. In the macaque, ganglion cells projecting to the magnocellular layers of the dorsal lateral geniculate nucleus have a dark-adapted gain on average 100 times greater than that of cells projecting to the parvocellular layers; and their gain control mechanism requires one-tenth of the amount of light to be activated (Purpura *et al.*, 1988; Purpura, Kaplan & Shapley, 1989).

2.3.10 Multiple-sized adaptation pools

Although there is a good correspondence between area-dependent changes in human increment threshold curves and latency changes in ganglion cell receptive fields with light-adaptation, it may be unnecessary to rely on receptive field interactions, *per se*, to explain the psychophysical observations. As we have seen above, local adaptation may account for some of the gain change usually attributed to spatial integration. And, as we will see below, centre–surround antagonism may be better employed as an explanation for adaptation effects due to subtractive filtering than to multiplicative gain control.

Adaptation pools could be invariant, and there would be no need to invoke spatial summation changes, if there were more than one type of spatial organization of the rods at any given (nonfoveal) retinal eccentricity. In fact, there is some evidence for this contingency (Hallett, 1963; MacLeod, *et al.*, 1984; see also evidence provided in Chapters 1 and 11), which would explain the discrepancy between the psychophysical estimates of adaptation pool size, as well as the large inconsistencies between measurements of rod spatial summation (see Hallett, 1963, for a review).

The matter can be put in the context of selective adaptation of different sets of ganglion cells at any particular retinal locus. Observations in the cat indicate that rod-driven retinal ganglion cells with larger receptive field centres suffer more loss of sensitivity with increase in background than those with smaller receptive field centres (Enroth-Cugell & Shapley, 1973; Linsenmeier *et al.*, 1982; Shapley & Enroth-Cugell, 1984). The greater loss occurs because the cells with larger receptive field centres sum adaptive signals over a larger area and the loss in sensitivity in both types of cells depends upon the total flux (i.e. area times illumination). Thus, at higher adaptation levels, cells with smaller receptive field centres would be relatively less adapted and would be more sensitive than cells with larger receptive fields (Pirenne, 1967; Enroth-Cugell & Shapley, 1973).

2.3.11 Subtractive filtering

Steeper increment threshold functions cannot be the sole result of the continuous decrease in spatial and temporal summation and the increasing photon noise with intenser backgrounds. For if we use the total summation exponent from Fig. 2.10, we get a limiting slope of 0.64 $[(0.27 \times 0.5) + 0.5]$ for achromat K.N., which can be compared with his 0.77 slope measured with the 200 ms, 6 deg target. The shortfall indicates the difference in slope that cannot be explained by simple signal/noise considerations taking into account the decrease in spatio-temporal organization. Thus, some other factors must be affecting rod increment threshold.

In addition to multiplicative processes, there are subtractive processes controlling the sensitivity of the rod visual system to increments (Geisler, 1979, 1980; Adelson, 1982; Walraven & Valeton, 1984; Hayhoe *et al.*, 1987; Hayhoe & Smith, 1989). Such processes have been observed psychophysically in scotopic vision as high-pass filtering in both the spatial (Hayhoe & Levin, 1987; Hayhoe & Smith, 1989) and temporal (Adelson, 1982) domain. These processes have a much longer time constant than the multiplicative processes; requiring 30 s or more to be implemented (Geisler, 1979; Adelson, 1982; Hayhoe *et al.*, 1987). And, unlike gain control, they only attenuate signals from the mean background level, leaving transients, such as brief target flashes, unaffected.

Spatial filtering: centre–surround antagonism

Evidence for a role of spatial filtering in scotopic sensitivity control essentially derives from the observation that rod increment threshold is higher against small than against large backgrounds. This phenomenon has been quantified in the rod Crawford–Westheimer effect (Crawford, 1940; Westheimer, 1965, 1968, 1970). The effect shows that the rod threshold for a tiny, peripherally-viewed target at the centre of a moderately bright adapting field first rises (desensitization), as the diameter of the adapting field is increased from 10 min to 45 min, then gradually falls (sensitization) to a steady level with further enlargements (Westheimer, 1965; Westheimer & Wiley, 1970). (There is some evidence that the threshold may rise again when the field's diameter exceeds 2 deg.) Both the sensitization and desensitization effect are not large, usually on the order of 0.3–0.6 $\log_{10}$ unit, though they are sometimes reported as being larger. Their spatial dimensions change with eccentricity in accordance with the retino-cortical magnification factor (Ransom-Hogg & Spillmann, 1980). And, within the region of sensitization, the distribution of flux seems to be important: a constant quantal flux is less effective in lowering the threshold when concentrated in only part of the sensitization region than when distributed evenly over it (Teller, Matter & Phillips, 1970). Although the Crawford–Westheimer effect is typically demonstrated with small (5 min) targets, it can be obtained with targets at least as large as 2 deg in diameter (Alexander, 1974).

Three explanations have been offered for the rod Crawford–Westheimer effect: temporal transients generated by eye movements, effects of central origin, and centre–surround antagonism in the retina. The first of these gains plausibility because small eye movements occurring during normal fixation would tend to constantly sweep the edge of small backgrounds onto different sets of receptors, thereby artificially elevating threshold for the target. And, it accords with the fact that decreasing the size of bleaching fields – which by their nature are stationary on the retina and for which, consequently, there can be no possibility of transients from eye movements – does not affect threshold during rod dark-adaptation (Westheimer, 1968; Teller & Gestrin, 1969; Hayhoe, 1979). Nevertheless, when the retinal image of the background is stabilized during Crawford-Westheimer measurements themselves, a small, purely scotopic sensitization effect remains (Teller, Andrews & Barlow, 1966; Hayhoe & Smith, 1989). Thus it is incorrect to claim – as has been frequently done – that the added threshold elevation by the small field is reduced or abolished under stabilized viewing (Barlow & Sakitt, 1973; Tulunay-Keesey & Vassilev, 1974; Tulunay-Keesey & Jones, 1977). On the contrary, eye-movement transients seem to be a relatively minor artifact when measuring scotopic sensitivity on small backgrounds (Hayhoe & Smith, 1989).

The argument for a central origin of the rod-determined Crawford–Westheimer effect can similarly be dismissed. It has been advanced for several reasons. First because the extra loss in sensitivity caused by small backgrounds does not increase much with background intensity (Lennie

& MacLeod, 1973). Second because the loss is greatest when the background is nearly the same size as the target (Alexander, 1974). And, third because the loss is reduced, when the background is surrounded by an equiluminous annulus, but increases rapidly as the annulus is made brighter or dimmer than the background, increasing the distinctness of the border between them (Lennie & MacLeod, 1973). These effects are what one would expect if edge effects from small backgrounds, forming a border near the test flash, penetrate more effectively to central stages and modify sensitivity there (Lennie & MacLeod, 1973; Foster & Mason, 1977; Latch & Lennie, 1977; Blick & MacLeod, 1978; MacLeod, 1978; Hayhoe, 1979; Buss, Hayhoe & Stromeyer, 1982). And, indeed, there are physiological observations indicating that large, uniform backgrounds have little capacity to affect the maintained response of ganglion cells and more central neurons (Marrocco, 1972; Enroth-Cugell, Hertz & Lennie, 1977); whereas smaller or non-homogeneous backgrounds do.

Speaking against a central (non-retinal) site of the mechanism mediating the Crawford–Westheimer effect, however, are four findings. First, the processes involved in the desensitization of human rod vision by steady backgrounds must be largely retinal in origin because pressure-blinding the eye during light-adaptation, which temporarily blocks signal transmission along the optic nerve, does not affect the subsequent course of dark-adaptation (Craik & Vernon, 1941). Second, observers with inner retinal pathologies do not show the Crawford–Westheimer effect, while observers with more central pathologies do (Enoch & Sunga, 1969). Third, for steadily illuminated backgrounds, dichoptic presentation of the stimulus yields little, if any, effect (Westheimer, 1967; Fiorentini, Bayly & Maffei, 1972; Sturr & Teller, 1973); though for temporally modulated backgrounds, interocular transfer does occur (Markoff & Sturr, 1971; Fiorentini *et al.*, 1972; Sturr & Teller, 1973; Fuld, 1978). Fourth, since stabilization of the background does not eliminate the difference between small and large backgrounds, the sensitization effect must be occurring before a substantial reduction of the steady state signal has taken place (Hayhoe & Smith, 1989). This must be at or before the level of the retinal ganglion cells, whose maintained discharge at least in the cat is at best a poor index of sustained inputs (Barlow & Levick, 1969). Thus, more central cells in the lateral geniculate nucleus and the cortex can be effectively ruled out as a primary basis for the effect. The most likely physiological substrate of the filtering network is the outer plexiform layer (McKee & Westheimer, 1970; Teller *et al.*, 1971; Enoch, 1978; Hayhoe, 1979; Hayhoe & Smith, 1989).

This leaves the third (and original) explanation of the rod-determined Crawford–Westheimer effect holding the field: namely, that the effect parallels the centre–surround antagonism of single retinal neurons; with the initial desensitization reflecting summing within the receptive field centre mechanism and the subsequent sensitization reflecting antagonism on the centre mechanism by the surround mechanism (Westheimer, 1965; Westheimer & Wiley, 1970; Tulunay-Keesey & Vassilev, 1974; Tulunay-Keesey & Jones, 1977). According to this analogy, sensitivity should be greatest in regions remote from edges or in the centre of large backgrounds, since the signal from the adapting background in these regions is being removed by centre–surround antagonism.

However, whether this analogy stands or falls depends in part on how one defines sensitization. In the cat, which has served electrophysiologically as the primary model for mammalian adaptation and in which comparable electrophysiological measurements have been made, there is no exact analogue of the psychophysical observed effect of background size at the level of the retinal ganglion cell. True, the gain of the receptive field centre in rod-driven retinal ganglion cells does indeed decrease as the background encroaches upon more and more of the excitatory centre; indicating areal summation of the centre response. But it then levels off as the background diameter is enlarged beyond the excitatory centre (Barlow & Levick, 1969, 1976; Enroth-Cugell, Lennie & Shaply, 1975). So, if sensitization is taken to mean an increase in response of the cell's centre mechanism to the test flash, then neither desensitization, nor sensitization, of the centre mechanism occurs as the result of adapting light falling in the surround of the receptive field (Shapley & Enroth-Cugell, 1984; Saito & Fukada, 1986).

However, the psychophysics and physiology can be largely reconciled if the definition of sensitization is broadened to mean an increase in the ganglion cell's net response, rather than merely an increase in the cell's centre mechanism (Maffei, 1968; Essock *et al.*, 1985). This is because larger backgrounds, encroaching on the surround, serve to depress the responsiveness of the surround mechanism, such that the cell's net response to the test flash is larger due to a lessened antagonistic response from the surround. Thus it may be a change in surround responsiveness, rather than a change in centre sensitivity, *per se*, that is reflected in the Crawford–Westheimer effect (Enroth-Cugell *et al.*, 1975). This contention is supported by the psychophysical observation that beyond the central summation area, enlarging the adapting field does not alter the response to the incremental test flash, unless specific timing conditions are met between the onsets of the adapting field and the test flash (Tulunay-Keesey & Jones, 1977).

Temporal high-pass filtering

Evidence for temporal high-pass filtering in sensitivity control comes from increment threshold experiments in which the steady background is replaced with a flashed one. The flashed fields produce substantially greater threshold elevations than the steady fields (Crawford, 1947; Geisler, 1979, 1980; Adelson, 1982). Such effects are greater in magnitude than those produced by small backgrounds. For instance, with backgrounds bright enough to raise rod threshold by 2.0–2.5 $\log_{10}$ units the threshold difference between large and small backgrounds is only 0.3–0.6 $\log_{10}$ unit; whereas the difference between large steady and large flashed backgrounds (400 ms coincident with the onset of the target) is 1.0–2.0 $\log_{10}$ units.

The less effective sensitivity control for flashed as compared with steady backgrounds is shown in Fig. 2.13 for a normal observer (Fach, Sharpe & Stockman, 1990). Increment threshold curves are given for a 200 ms, 6 deg target presented either against a steady background (filled circles) or at the onset of a 400 ms flashed background (triangles). Whereas the thresholds measured on the steady background follow a slope of 0.96; those measured on the flashed background increase in accordance with an accelerating slope greater than one (1.10). Moreover, the onset of saturation in the flashed background curve (0.0 $\log_{10}$ scotopic td) occurs at many fewer quanta absorptions than those driving individual rod photoreceptors into response compression (lower curve; various symbols).

The difference between the increment threshold intensities measured against steady and flashed backgrounds can be explained by assuming that the signals from the flashed backgrounds are more effective in passing the temporal filtering control of the visual system unabated. Their sudden onset may deny the system the time it requires either to initiate feedback rescue measures at the receptor level or to forestall overloading at the neuronal sites downstream (cf. Geisler, 1979, 1980; Adelson, 1982; Walraven & Valeton, 1984; Alexander, Kelly & Morris, 1986). The horizontal cells have been suggested as the possible physiological substrate of such a temporal high-pass filtering network (cf. Werblin, 1974, 1977; Detwiler, Hodgkin & McNaughton, 1980).

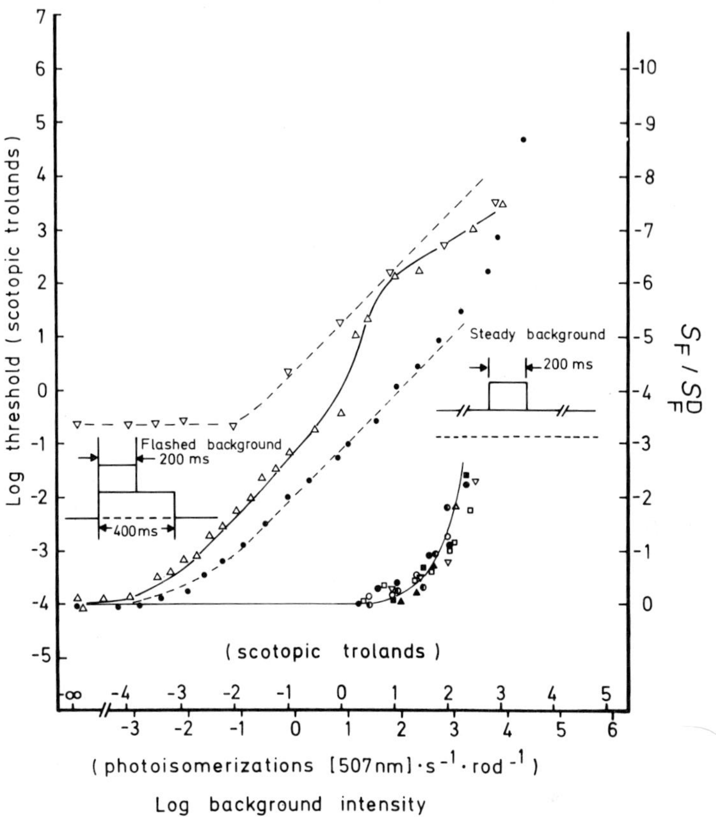

Fig. 2.13. Rod increment thresholds measured on a steady adapting field (filled circles) and flashed (400 ms) adapting fields (triangles) for a normal observer. The inverted triangles indicate the thresholds measured against the flashed backgrounds during the plateau terminating the cone phase of recovery from a white (3100 K) bleaching light of 7.7 $\log_{10}$ photopic td-s. The curve shown at the bottom (various symbols) is the physiologically derived increment threshold function for individual macaque rod outer segments from Baylor *et al.* (1984; as shown in Fig. 2.8). The thresholds measured on the steady background and the cone thresholds measured on the flashed background during dark-adaptation are fitted by functions (dashed lines) having a slope of 1.0 (Weber's law). The 'rod' thresholds measured on the flashed background are fitted by an accelerating function (solid line) that attains a slope of 1.10. Mean data from several sessions. The insets show the flash conditions. (From Fach *et al.*, 1990.)

However, other evidence would place it after the multiplicative gain control (see Hayhoe & Smith, 1989).

2.4 The influence of the cones upon rod desensitization

2.4.1 *The 'isolated' rod increment threshold function*

The Aguilar & Stiles conditions for isolating the rod response in the normal observer presuppose that rod desensitization is independent of the action of the test flash and background on the cone systems. The validity of this assumption was not supported by the comparison between the achromat and normal increment threshold curves in Fig. 2.2. Further disproof is given in Fig. 2.14 (Sharpe *et al.*, 1989*a*).

The figure shows the effect of background wavelength upon rod increment threshold for a 520 nm, 200 ms, 6 deg target. Curves measured against a background of 640 nm (the condition shown in Fig. 2.2) for five normal observers (A–E; filled circles), are juxtaposed with curves for the same observers measured against backgrounds of 450, 520 and 560 nm. If the assumption of receptor independence is valid, then the four curves should have the same shape below the region where the threshold is taken over by the cones; because backgrounds having the same intensity in scotopic td (i.e. equated for the rate of rod quantal absorptions) should have identical effects. But this clearly is not the case. For all four observers in Fig. 2.14, rod thresholds on the 640 nm field rise more steeply than those on the other fields. This is easy to see in Fig. 2.14. Each curve has been paired with the mean response function from Aguilar & Stiles (1954; see Figs 2.1 and 2.2), whose slope exactly matches that of the 640 nm data, but not those of the 450, 520 and 560 nm data.

The wavelength-dependency is quantified and confirmed by a one-way analysis of variance in Table 2.6. The table presents, for each background wavelength, for the five observers in Fig. 2.14, the slope of the curve between the background intensities −2.0 and 0.0 $\log_{10}$ scotopic td (Sharpe *et al.*, 1989*a*). The intensity limits were set to avoid a possible source of error: the slope of the rod increment threshold curve, rather than being constant, may slightly increase with background intensity. If so, the slope determined from the 640 nm background data would have a steeper value simply because more of the rod curve is revealed. The safest method, then, is to calculate the slope over the same region of background intensity for each wavelength. An upper limit of 0.0 $\log_{10}$

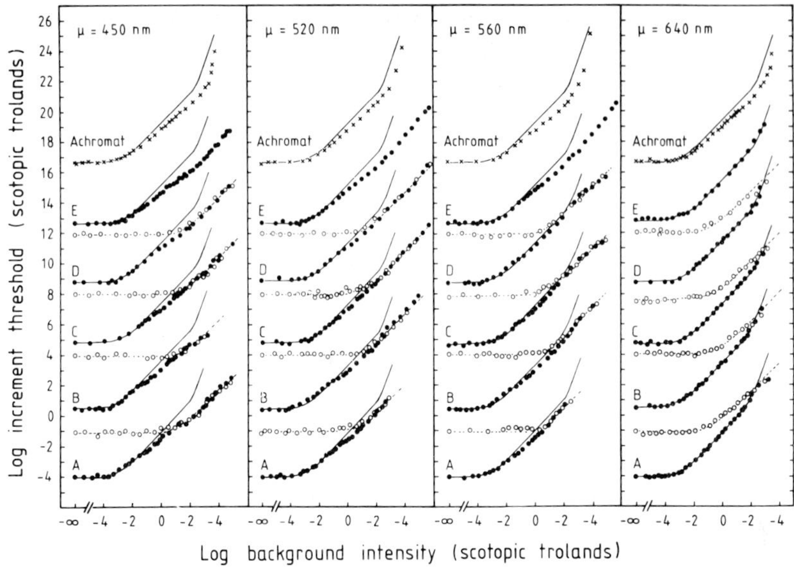

Fig. 2.14. The effect of background wavelength on the form of the rod increment threshold versus background intensity curve. The target and background conditions are the same as in Fig. 2.1, except the background wavelength (μ) was varied: (i) 450 nm, (ii) 520 nm, (iii) 560 nm and (iv) 640 nm. The filled circles (observers A–E) below where they intersect with the open circles are rod thresholds; above the intersection they are cone thresholds (or in some cases mixed rod and cone thresholds). The open circles are cone thresholds measured for the same stimulus conditions during the plateau terminating the cone phase of recovery from a white (3100 K) bleaching light of 7.7 $\log_{10}$ photopic td-s. (The cone plateau thresholds were not measured for observer E.) The crosses indicate the rod-only threshold responses of achromat K.N. All the curves are correctly placed with respect to the axis of the abscissae, but the axis of the ordinates is correct only for the lowest curve in each of the four panels; the other curves are displaced upwards in 4.0 $\log_{10}$ unit intervals. Each data point is a mean based on at least three sets of measurements made on different days. The solid line drawn through each increment threshold function is the mean function of Aguilar & Stiles (1954) shifted vertically to compensate for differences in absolute threshold. The function, which has a slope of 0.95, has also been fitted to the cone plateau thresholds (dashed line); demonstrating that for these target conditions, the cones, regardless of background wavelength, obey Weber's law. (From Sharpe *et al.*, 1989*a*.)

scotopic td (threshold intensity) was chosen because it was always at least 0.5 $\log_{10}$ unit below the intensity where the cones first detected the flash (open circles).

The dependency on wavelength is not restricted to the 200 ms, 6 deg target condition. It is also found for the briefer, smaller targets of Fig. 2.5; though, in general, the slopes are less steep than those measured with the 200 ms, 6 deg target (Markstahler & Sharpe, 1989).

Table 2.6. *Rod increment threshold responses for a 200 ms, 6 deg diameter target: absolute thresholds and slopes for five normal observers, achromat K.N. and the mean observer of Aguilar & Stiles (adapted from Sharpe et al., 1989)*

	Subject	Absolute threshold	Slope (wavelength) 450 nm	520 nm	560 nm	640 nm
	A	−3.97	0.69	0.69	0.71	0.95
	A (2AFC)[a]	−3.95	0.71	0.75	0.81	0.96
Normals	B	−3.60	0.76	0.80	0.72	0.97
	C	−3.23	0.78	0.81	0.86	0.99
	D	−3.22	0.73	0.71	0.76	0.92
	E	−3.27	0.78	0.77	0.79	0.95
	Mean	−3.46	0.75	0.76	0.77	0.96
	SD	0.33	0.04	0.05	0.06	0.03
	t-test	—	7.00[b]	6.73[b]	6.33[b]	—
	Achromat	−3.30	0.75	0.78	0.79	0.77
	Aguilar & Stiles	−3.23	—	—	—	0.95

[a] Temporal two-alternative forced-choice procedure. These values are not included in the mean and SD determinations.
[b] Scheffé *post hoc* comparisons $t(p = 0.01, df = 3, 16) = 3.98$.

In particular, curves measured for the normal observer with the 100 ms, 1.0 deg target have, on average, a slope of 0.75 on the 640 nm background as compared to a slope of 0.65 on the 450 nm background. And, curves measured with the 10 ms, 10 min target have a slope of 0.56 as compared to a slope of 0.50.

Such changes in slope by background wavelength, regardless of target size and duration, imply that the cones must have access to the postreceptoral sites where the rod system regulates its sensitivity (see also Makous & Boothe, 1974; Sternheim & Glass, 1975; Makous & Peeples, 1979; Stabell, Nordby & Stabell, 1987; Hayhoe & Smith, 1989). Just how is this interaction coming about?

2.4.2 *Rod–cone interaction in target detection*

Are cones influencing rod desensitization and distorting the 'rod' thresholds through the target? To answer this, we must consider the results of summation experiments based on bichromatic flashes, one component of which selectively stimulates the rods, while the other selectively stimulates the cones. The results of such experiments are generally interpreted as indicating that the signals from the rod and cone systems do not interact at all or only in a small excitatory manner at threshold (Bouman & van der Velden, 1948; Ikeda & Urakubo, 1969; Metz & Brown, 1970; Frumkes, Sekuler & Reiss, 1972; Frumkes *et al.*, 1973; Drum, 1982; Benimoff, Schneider & Hood, 1982; Levine & Frishman, 1984). Drum (1982), for instance, found that when rod and cone sensitivities were equal, the combined sensitivity was less than 0.2 $\log_{10}$ unit greater than it would have been for either rods or cones alone; and that when rod and cone sensitivities differed by 0.3 $\log_{10}$ unit, the less sensitive receptor type raised overall sensitivity by less than 0.1 $\log_{10}$ unit. This is less than linear addition of the signals; which would predict and 0.3 $\log_{10}$ unit increase for the equal sensitivity condition and a 0.18 $\log_{10}$ unit increase for the unequal sensitivity condition. (That is, where the sensitivities of the rods and cones are similar, one would expect sensitivity to the simultaneous stimulation of both systems to be equal to the sum of the sensitivities to stimulation of each alone or a 0.3 $\log_{10}$ unit increase in sensitivity.)

This apparent near-independence of threshold detection could be due to temporal phase differences between the rod and cone systems. In man, the rod signals may neurally lag the cone signals by 75–100 ms in complete darkness (Arden & Weale, 1954; Veringa & Roelofs, 1966; Frumkes *et al.*, 1972, 1973; MacLeod, 1972; Foster, 1976; van den Berg & Spekreijse, 1977); and by considerably more when the eye is light-adapted because cone signals speed up faster than rod signals with light-adaptation (Kelly, 1961; Baylor & Hodgkin, 1974; Sharpe, Stockman & MacLeod, 1989*b*). Such differences in the arrival time of rod and cone signals at say the retinal ganglion cells could largely preclude the two sorts of signals from interacting. First, because if one signal is delayed with respect to the other, the sum of the two signals will show an amplitude of oscillation of the neuron smaller than if the signals had arrived together. And, second, because the earliest signals to reach the ganglion cell may leave a transitory refractoriness in their wake (Gouras & Link, 1966). In accord with this delay hypothesis, Frumkes *et al.* (1972, 1973) have reported that, although rod and cone signals can summate to produce a threshold sensation, the degree of summation depends upon the temporal synchrony between the test flashes generating the two types of signals. Nearly complete summation occurs when the rod test flash (420 nm) precedes the cone test flash (680 nm) by 75 ms.

At other stimulus onset asynchronies, however, it falls off: for 0 ms delay or delays greater than 150 ms, virtually no summation is found.

However, what appears to be near-independence between the rod and cone signals at threshold detection may, in fact, be incomplete summation or inhibition; for the fact that less than linear addition is found could indicate small inhibitory interactions between the rod and cone systems prior to their summation into a final common pathway (Levine & Frishman, 1984). In accord with this interpretation, there is physiological evidence for antagonistic interaction between the rod and cone signals arriving at retinal ganglion cells in the goldfish (Shefner & Levine, 1977; Levine & Shefner, 1981) and cat (Rodieck & Rushton, 1976; Levine, Frishman & Enroth-Cugell, 1987). In the cat, for instance, when neighbouring rods and cones are stimulated, the signal in each is diminished by a quantity slightly greater than 30% of the signal in the other (Levine *et al.*, 1987). So the physiological sum of signals is smaller than a simple additive sum by about 0.15 $\log_{10}$ unit; which is similar to what Drum (1982) found in his bichromatic flash experiments.

Even allowing that rod and cone signals do interact at rod threshold by this small amount – whether in an excitatory or inhibitory manner – there is no evidence that they do so more than 0.5 $\log_{10}$ unit below the absolute sensitivity level of the cones. Yet changes in slope with background wavelength are first encountered in Fig. 2.14 far below this level (see the open circles, which are the cone absolute thresholds measured during the plateau terminating the cone phase of recovery from a full bleaching light). This is sufficient reason for discounting the target as an important source of rod–cone interactions. But there is another reason as well. If interactions were occurring through the target, it is dificult to explain why greater distortions in ‘rod’ increment threshold are reported when the threshold is measured against small backgrounds than against large ones (Lennie & MacLeod, 1973; Frumkes & Temme, 1977; Latch & Lennie, 1977; Buck, Peeples & Makous, 1979; Buck & Makous, 1981) and against flashed backgrounds than against steady ones (Frumkes *et al.*, 1972, 1973; Foster, 1976; Ingling *et al.*, 1977; Barris & Frumkes, 1978; Frumkes & Holstein, 1979; Alexander & Kelly, 1984). These sorts of effects are suggestive of high-pass temporal and spatial filtering, which act to attenuate signals from the mean background level, while leaving transients such as target flashes unaffected.

2.4.3 Rod–cone interaction in background adaptation

All in all, then, it seems the possibility that the cones are significantly influencing rod threshold through the target can be largely ruled out. If cones are having an effect, they must be mainly having it through the background. This could be in one of two ways. The cones excited by the background could be inhibiting the rods in raising the threshold; implying that the short-wavelength backgrounds in Fig. 2.14 are bending the rod desensitization curve downward. Or the cones could be facilitating the rods; implying that the 640 nm background is bending the rod desensitization curve upward.

Two lines of reasoning support the second alternative. First, one would expect the cone contribution to increase as the difference between the absolute spectral sensitivities of the rod and cone systems decreases. Since the absolute sensitivities of the rods and cones tend to converge at long-wavelengths (Fig. 2.3; Wald, 1945), long-wavelength fields will excite the cones much more strongly than scotopically-equated short- or middle-wavelength ones. Consequently such fields are more likely to influence rod threshold through their effects on cones. In fact, within the region used to calculate the rod threshold slopes (-2.0 to 0.0 $\log_{10}$ scotopic td), the short- and middle-wavelength fields have little effect on cone sensitivity. This can be seen in Fig. 2.14, where the cone thresholds (open circles) on the 450, 520 and 560 nm fields hardly differ from the absolute threshold value before the background exceeds 0.0 $\log_{10}$ scotopic td. In contrast, the cone thresholds on the 640 nm field have already begun to rise (which ironically is the reason why Aguilar & Stiles chose a long-wavelength adapting field for their 'rod-isolation' conditions). These thresholds, which are those of the middle-wavelength sensitive cones, hide those of the long-wavelength cones, which are even more strongly adapted by the 640 nm field.

The location of the long-wavelength sensitive cone thresholds is made explicit in Fig. 2.15. The figure shows a normal observer's increment thresholds for a 640 nm (instead of a 520 nm) test flash superimposed on the 640 nm background (otherwise the target and background conditions are the same as in Figs 2.1 and 2.2). The filled symbols are the thresholds measured when the eye was fully adapted to the background; the open symbols are the thresholds measured during the plateau terminating the cone phase of recovery from a white (3100 K) bleaching light of 7.7 $\log_{10}$ photopic td-s. Clearly, the dark-adapted sensitivity of the cones relative to that of the rods is considerably improved by changing the target

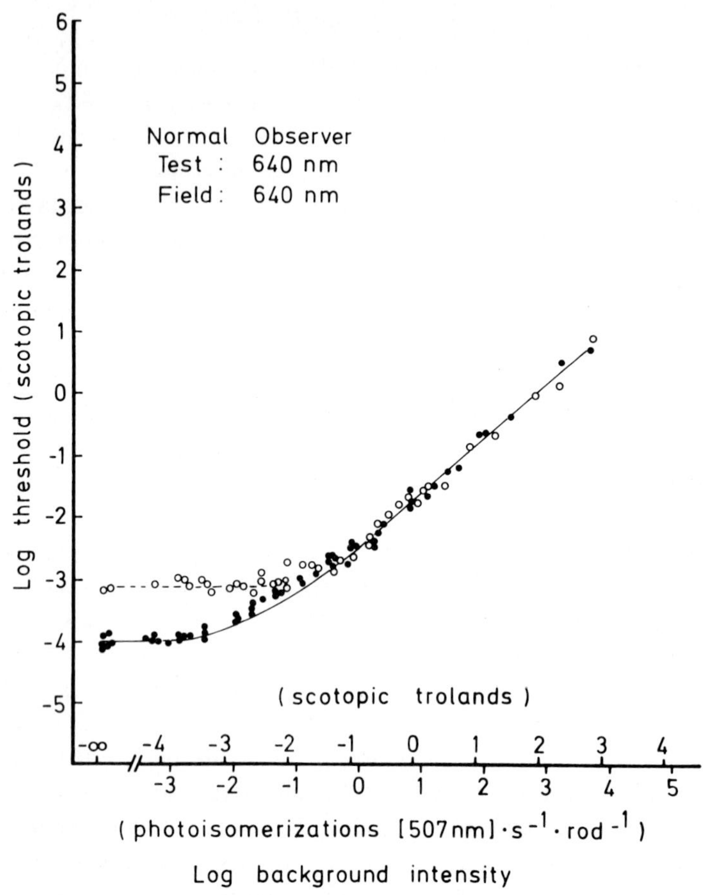

Fig. 2.15. The increment threshold as a function of background intensity for a normal observer. The thresholds were measured under the same conditions as those in Figs 2.1 and 2.2, except the test flash had a wavelength of 640 nm, instead of 520 nm (i.e. it was homochromatic with the background). The filled circles are thresholds measured when the eye was fully adapted to the background. The open circles are thresholds measured during the plateau terminating the cone phase of recovery from a white (3100 K) bleaching light of 7.7 $\log_{10}$ photopic td-s.

wavelength: the difference in threshold is less than 0.8 $\log_{10}$ unit, instead of more than 3.0 $\log_{10}$ units (compare Fig. 2.2). The difference would be even smaller (<0.3 $\log_{10}$ unit; see Fig. 2.3), if the target entered the pupil centrally instead of obliquely (the directional sensitivity of the cones disadvantages them relative to the rods).

But, what is more to the point, the adaptation of the cones can be seen to proceed in parallel with that of the rods. At background levels greater than -2.0 $\log_{10}$ scotopic td, the cone plateau thresholds (open circles) and the fully light-adapted thresholds (filled circles) run together (there is no rod–cone break in the curve). In fact, combined detection of the target by the rods and cones must be acting to lower threshold by summation; because the slope of the curve is 0.85. (A slope closer to 1.0 was expected, as in Fig. 2.2.)

The stronger activation of the cones by the 640 nm background as compared to that by shorter-wavelength backgrounds accords with two different sorts of observations. First it is paralleled by the phenomenological observation that there is virtually no photo-chromatic interval (i.e. the difference between the threshold for seeing and the threshold for seeing colour) for the 640 nm background (cf. Spillmann & Seneff, 1971). Almost as soon as the observer could see the 640 nm background, he could perceive its colour. This was not the case for the 450, 520 and 560 nm backgrounds.

Second, it is paralleled by the psychophysical observation that, for target wavelengths longer than 620 nm, the rod–cone break in the dark-adaptation recovery curve is absent (Kohlrausch, 1922) or reversed in direction; i.e. after an initial plateau, there follows at about 7 min an abrupt rise in threshold to a new plateau 0.15 $\log_{10}$ unit above the earlier one (Wooten, Fuld & Spillmann, 1975; Wooten & Butler, 1976). This suggests that for long-wavelength stimuli the fast-adapting cone and slower-adapting rod systems seek plateaux at nearly the same level of sensitivity and that their signals slightly interfere with each other to produce a net threshold increase. For shorter-wavelength stimuli, on the other hand, no interaction occurs because the rod–cone break comes at a time when the rod system is rapidly increasing in sensitivity (for an alternative explanation, see Latch & Baker, 1976).

A second – and more important – line of reasoning supporting greater rod–cone interactions with the 640 nm background hinges on the increment threshold functions of the achromat observer K.N. Because he lacks cone vision, K.N.'s thresholds for the same conditions (Fig. 2.14, crosses) can be used as a test to determine the nature of the cone influence. Regardless of background wavelength, this increment threshold curve has a slope of 0.77 ± 0.02 (see Table 2.4; Sharpe *et al.*, 1989*a*). This is much lower than the value found for the normal (average of five observers) with the 640 nm (0.96 ± 0.03) background and is almost identical to their values found with the 450 nm (0.73 ± 0.05), 520 nm (0.76 ± 0.05) and 560 nm (0.76 ± 0.07) backgrounds.

It follows, therefore, that cones excited by the 640 nm background are influencing the sensitivity of the rods to the test flash; a conclusion that is wholly consistent with other measurements of rod increment threshold made against backgrounds of differing wavelength (Makous & Boothe, 1974; Sternheim & Glass, 1975; Frumkes & Temme, 1977; Buck *et al.*, 1979; Makous & Peeples, 1979; Buck & Makous, 1981; Stabell *et al.*, 1987). Barlow (1957), unwittingly, may have foreshadowed this conclusion. Using homochromatic (blue–green) test and adapting wavelengths, he found that the 'rod' increment threshold curve for a long (935 or 945 ms), large (4.9 or 5.9 deg diameter), peripheral target had a slope of 0.75 (see his Table 1) and not 0.95!

2.4.4 *The nature of the cone influence*

Figure 2.16 shows the results from increment threshold experiments undertaken with various partially colour-blind observers in addition to the typical, complete achromat K.N. – blue-cone monochromats (who have, besides rods, only short-wave or S-cones), deuteranopes (who have only long-wave or L-cones, S-cones and rods) and protanopes (who have only middle-wave or M-cones, S-cones and rods) – to determine whether cone stimulation from all cone classes is equally effective in raising rod threshold (Fach, Sharpe & Stockman, 1990). The slopes are quantified in Table 2.7. The increment thresholds were measured with the same conditions as those used in Fig. 2.14.

It seems that quantum absorptions (from the adapting field) in both the M- and L-cones can raise rod increment threshold on the 640 nm background, in that the protanope and the two deuteranope thresholds are steeper than those of the achromat, though less steep than those of the normal observer. Although the protanope's slope is less steep than those of the deuteranopes, this cannot be taken to mean that M-cones are less effective than L-cones in raising the rod increment threshold because the difference is expected solely on the basis of quantum absorptions (i.e. from the relative M- and L-cone sensitivities). In short, it would require more intense 640 nm fields to cause enough quantal absorptions in the protanope's M-cones to equal the quantal absorptions in the L-cones of the deuteranope and in the M- and L-cones of the normal observers at a dimmer background.

The S-cones, on the other hand, seems to have little or no effect on threshold for these conditions, in that the blue-cone monochromat thresholds are similar to those of the typical, complete achromat and do

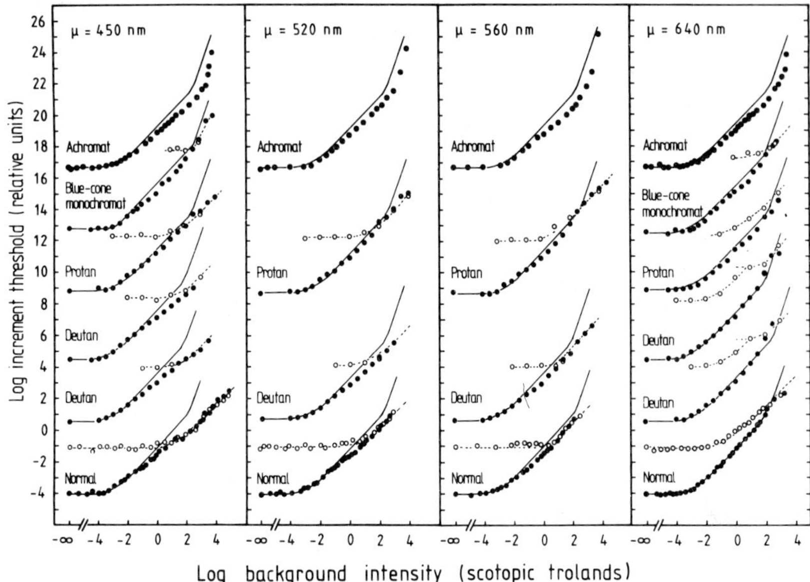

Fig. 2.16. The effect of background wavelength on the form of the rod increment threshold versus intensity curve for the achromat K.N., a blue-cone monochromat, a protanope, two deuteranopes, and a normal observer (observer D in Fig. 2.14). Same conditions as in Fig. 2.14. (From Fach *et al.*, 1990.)

Table 2.7. *Rod increment threshold responses for a 200 ms, 6 deg diameter target: absolute thresholds and slopes for a typical, complete achromat, a blue-cone monochromat, a protanope, two deuteranopes, and a normal observer*

Subject	Absolute Threshold	Slope (wavelength) 450 nm	520 nm	560 nm	640 nm
Achromat	−3.30	0.75	0.78	0.79	0.77
Blue-cone monochromat	−3.24	0.82	—	—	0.81
Protanope	−3.09	0.75	0.78	0.80	0.87
Deuteranope	−3.29	0.71	0.73	0.72	0.95
Deuteranope	−3.23	0.71	—	—	0.90
Normal (observer D from Table 2.6)	−3.22	0.73	0.71	0.76	0.92
Aguilar & Stiles	−3.23	—	—	—	0.95

not vary with wavelength. However, once again, it cannot be concluded that S-cones do not affect rod sensitivity because even on the 450 nm background – where one would expect the maximum stimulation – the S-cones are hardly light-adapted. This can be determined by looking at the S-cone cone-plateau measurements (open circles).

2.4.5 Other evidence for rod–cone interaction

The comparison between the achromat, deuteranope, protanope and normal increment threshold data forces the conclusion that the latter, despite being measured under 'rod-isolation' conditions, are influenced by cone absorptions from the background field. This confirms other psychophysical observations that cones interact with rods in light adaptation and threshold detection.

First, there is psychophysical evidence that cones make a contribution to the rod adaptation pools. In a procedure similar to Rushton's (1963, 1965*a*, *b*; Rushton & Westheimer, 1962), Sternheim & Glass (1975) measured luminance thresholds for test gratings presented in-phase and out-of-phase against background gratings of the same spatial frequency. The gratings had a 10.2 min period (Rushton's had a 30 min period) and their wavelengths and luminance levels were chosen to assure detection by the rods. In-phase and out-of-phase thresholds were essentially equal to each other, indicating that single adaptation pools were being sampled. But threshold elevation was significantly higher against long-wavelength (630 nm) background gratings than against shorter-wavelength ones (465, 540 and 570 nm), after adjustment for scotopic equivalence; implying that cones must be influencing threshold. The difference was particularly marked at higher levels of retinal illuminance.

Second, there is evidence that rod and cone signals are indistinguishable in contrast adaptation. Specifically, contrast adaptation to low-frequency gratings (2.77 c/deg^{-1}, moving at 4 Hz) that stimulate only rods subsequently raises thresholds for gratings of the same spatial-frequency that stimulate only cones, and vice versa (D'Zmura & Lennie, 1986). Moreover, the two kinds of gratings cannot be phenomenologically distinguished by the observer, when they are below the colour threshold.

Third, there is evidence that the photochromatic interval increases in the peripheral retina with dark adaptation and decreasing background luminance (Spillmann & Conlon, 1972). This can be attributed to chromatic desaturation of cone vision caused by rod intrusion. If, during the shift from photopic to scotopic vision, an increasing amount of white excitation from the rods were added to the perceived stimulus, its hue would be gradually diluted. Thus, there may be a swamping of the colour sense by the achromatic response.

Fourth, there is evidence that rod and cone signals summate to produce a perceptible flicker sensation. Rod and cone signals arising from a flickering, mesopic yellow target can combine to enhance the sensation of flicker, but at certain frequencies (7–8 Hz) they cancel it (MacLeod, 1972; van den Berg & Spekreijse, 1977). These results accord with those of Frumkes *et al.* (1972, 1973), suggesting that when rod and cone signals are corrected for phase delays between them, they can summate to produce a threshold sensation. The mesopic null can be attributed to a phase difference between the rod and cone signals, which destructively interfere with each other when the rod signal is equal in amplitude, but delayed by 180 deg relative to the cone signal (Veringa & Roelofs, 1966; MacLeod, 1972). Though MacLeod (1972) argued that he found no evidence for rod–cone inhibition, the summation between the rod and cone signals is probably not strictly linear. Small inhibitory interactions – similar in magnitude to the effects described by Levine & Frishman (1984) – may be taking place between the signals before they summate (cf. van den Berg & Spekreijse, 1977). Others, too, have found evidence for rod-cone interaction (and inhibition) in flicker sensitivity (Alexander & Fishman, 1984, 1985, 1986; Coletta & Adams, 1984; Nygaard & Frumkes, 1985; Frumkes, Naarendorp & Goldberg, 1986).

2.4.6 The site of rod–cone interaction

Such psychophysical evidence for the common pooling of rod and cone signals (see also Willmer, 1950; McCann & Benton, 1969; Trezona, 1970; McCann, 1972; Stabell & Stabell, 1975*a*, *b*; von Grünau, 1976) parallels abundant anatomical and physiological observations in the mammalian visual system indicating that signals from neighbouring rods and cones converge into the same common pathway before exiting the eye.

Not only has it been shown anatomically that vertebrate rods and cones are electrically coupled by gap junctions (Raviola & Gilula, 1973; Kolb, 1977) between the rod spherule and fine basal processes of the cone pedicle, it has also been shown, in the tiger salamander retina, that the coupling strengthens as a function of adaptation level (Yang & Wu, 1989). If this is also true of the cat – where about 50 rods converge on each cone via gap junctions (Smith, Freed & Sterling, 1986) – then rod signals could be conveyed to ganglion cells via rod-bipolar pathways at low light levels and via cone-bipolar pathways at higher light levels (Sterling, Freed & Smith, 1986).

Further, it has been demonstrated that primate and cat horizontal cells contact cones, through their dendritic trees, and rods, through their axon terminal system (Polyak, 1941; Dowling & Boycott, 1966; Boycott & Dowling, 1969; Steinberg, 1969*a*, *b*, *c*; Kolb, 1970; Niemeyer & Gouras, 1973). Physiologically in the cat a robust rod signal can be recorded in cones (Nelson, 1977), in all morphological varieties of horizontal cell receiving cone input (Steinberg, 1969*a*, *b*, *c*, 1971; Niemeyer & Gouras, 1973; Nelson, 1977) and in cone bipolars (Kolb & Nelson, 1983; Nelson & Kolb, 1984). The threshold for such rod signals lies about 3.0 log units higher than for rod signals recorded in the rod pathways. The rod and cone receptive fields are nearly coextensive and both are much larger than the dendritic fields of the horizontal cells (Nelson, 1977). So the rod and cone systems in the cat share a pathway to the ganglion cells and this may be one source of the common adaptation pool.

Two other means of rod–cone contact have been demonstrated in the inner plexiform layer of the cat. One is through the internuncial amacrine cells, which connect to the rod bipolar axons (Kolb & Nelson, 1981, 1983). Some of these – AII and A17 – receive major (95%) or exclusive rod bipolar input (Nelson, 1982), but others – A6, A13 and especially A8 – receive a mixed input from both rod bipolar and cone bipolar axon terminals. The other means is by way of the extensive gap junctions that join dendrites of the AII amacrine cell and the axon terminal processes of the cone bipolar (Kolb & Nelson, 1983).

In the primate, there is a lack of detailed information about retinal information processing. But it seems likely that the main locus of convergence of rod and cone signals – and possibly the source of the common adaptation pool – is in the inner plexiform layer, involving amacrine and bipolar cells. What is clear is that it must be before the ganglion cell level; because all ganglion cells receiving input from the rods also receive input from the cones in both cat (Enroth-Cugell *et al.*, 1977) and monkey (Gouras & Link, 1966; Wiesel & Hubel, 1966; Gouras, 1965, 1967; Kolb 1970). The convergence could occur earlier at the horizontal cell in the outer plexiform layer, but this seems unlikely for two reasons. First, there is no evidence for a horizontal cell feedback mechanism onto rods – though evidence is manifest in many species for a feedback of horizontal cells onto cones (Sterling, 1983). Second, there is a conspicuous lack of any antagonistic interaction between the rod and cone signals at this level. Since there is good evidence that rod and cone signals interact antagonistically before summing in a common pathway (Levine & Frishman, 1984), it would seem that the substrate for an influence of cones on rod sensitivity (or the substrate of the common adaptation pool) must be more central than the outer plexiform layer. In the inner plexiform layer, on the other hand, the opportunities for interaction are copious. For instance, in the rhesus monkey, there are at least 25 distinct types of amacrine cells; some of which resemble in their morphological features amacrine cell counterparts in the cat (Mariani, 1988).

2.4.7 The effect of subtractive filtering

Cones must be having an effect on rod threshold not only at the sites that multiplicatively transform the signal (i.e. the adaptation pool), but also at the sites that subtractively filter it. This is because the influence of the cones is more conspicuous against small backgrounds (or rod masking flashes) than against large ones of equal scotopic intensity (Lennie & MacLeod, 1973; Frumkes & Temme, 1977; Latch & Lennie, 1977; Blick & MacLeod, 1978; Buck & Makous, 1981; Bauer, Frumkes & Holstein, 1983*a*; Bauer, Frumkes & Nygaard, 1983*b*) and against flashed backgrounds than against steady ones (Alexander & Kelly, 1984; Fach, Sharpe & Stockman, 1989, 1990; Schenk, Volbrecht & Adams, 1989).

Consider first spatial filtering. Hayhoe & Smith (1989) found that thresholds on a small red background remain higher than those on a small green background, under both stabilized and unstabilized viewing. The difference is small (0.25–0.4 $\log_{10}$ unit) but reliable and is greater than the difference between thresholds measured on large red and green backgrounds. If cones only influenced rod sensitivity at the site of multiplicative gain control, then large backgrounds should be more than or at least as effective as small ones in stimulating cones. But since large backgrounds are less effective, the cones must be having an effect at the site of high-pass spatial filtering as well. The higher threshold elevations found with small backgrounds cannot simply be explained by differences in the size of the adaptation pool for rod and cone signals. For insofar as we can use cat ganglion cells as a guide, there is no marked change in the spatial organization of mammalian receptive fields during the transition from rod to cone vision (Gouras, 1967; Enroth-Cugell *et al.*, 1977).

Further evidence for cones influencing the site of subtractive interaction is given in Fig. 2.17 (Fach *et al.*, 1989, 1990). With flashed or

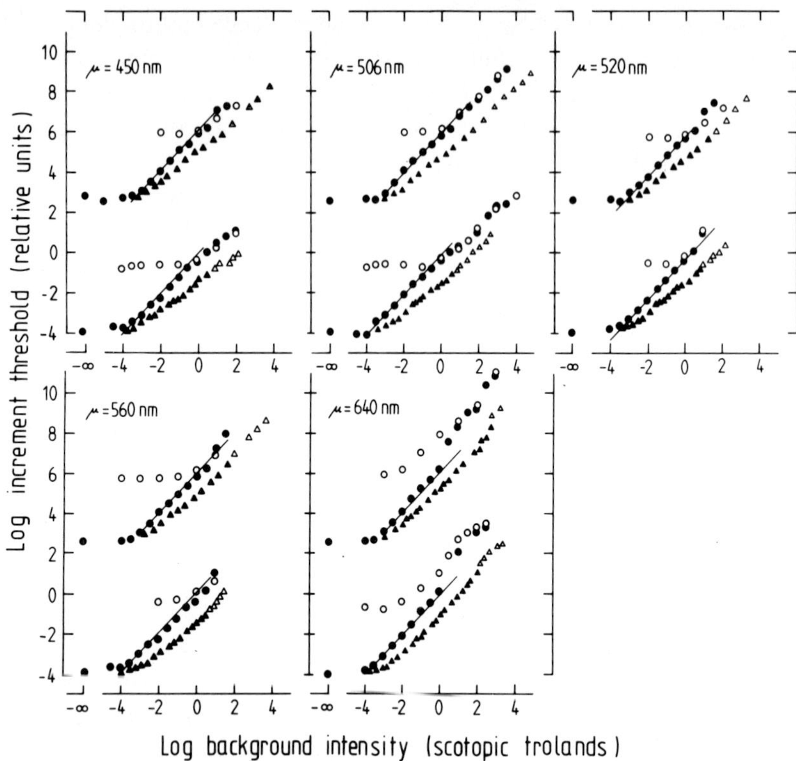

Fig. 2.17. Rod increment thresholds (two normal observers) measured on flashed adapting fields (filled circles) with a 520 nm, 200 ms, 6 deg diameter target. The adapting field wavelength (μ) was 450, 506, 520, 580 or 640 nm (400 ms exposure) backgrounds; its onset was simultaneous with that of the test flash (200 ms exposure). For comparison, the thresholds measured on the steady backgrounds triangles are shown (in their correct positions) to the right of each flashed background curve. The filled triangles are rod thresholds; the open triangles, cone thresholds. The open circles indicate the thresholds measured against the flashed backgrounds during the plateau terminating the cone phase of recovery from a white (3100 K) bleaching light of 7.7 $\log_{10}$ photopic td-s. The continuous line fit to the flashed background thresholds is Weber's law. (From Fach *et al.*, 1990.)

transient backgrounds, the rod increment threshold curve displays a steeper slope (as well as an earlier onset of saturation; see below) than with steady backgrounds. But the effect is greater on long-wavelength flashed backgrounds than on scotopically-matched short-wavelength ones. This is shown for thresholds measured with a 520 nm, 200 ms, 6 deg target (circles) superimposed upon 450, 506, 520, 580 and 640 nm flashed backgrounds (400 ms), whose onsets were simultaneous with that of the test flash (200 ms). For comparison, the thresholds measured on

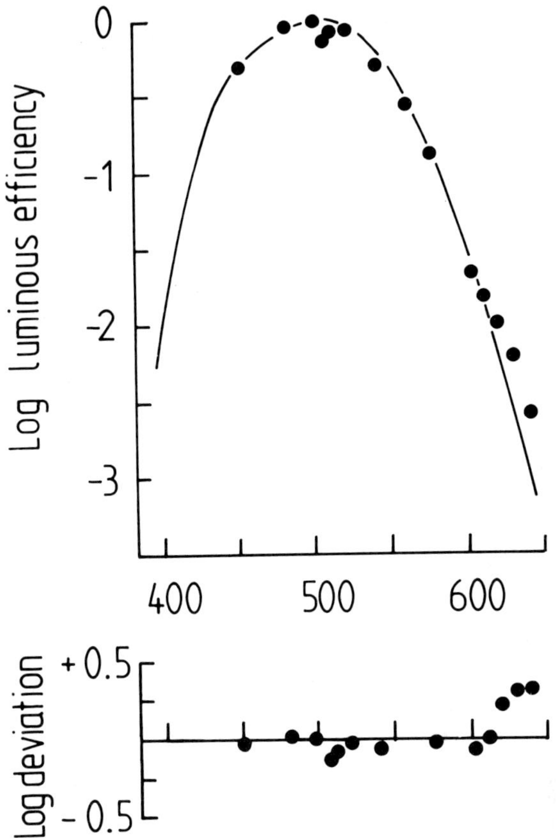

Fig. 2.18. The action spectrum (filled circles) of the receptors responsible for determining target sensitivity on the 400 ms flashed backgrounds. The upper panel displays the field sensitivity or the flashed background intensity, needed, as a function of background wavelength, to elevate target threshold by 1.0 $\log_{10}$ unit above the absolute threshold. The data have been plotted relative to the quantized CIE scotopic luminosity function (solid line). The lower panel displays the same data as $\log_{10}$ deviations from the scotopic luminosity function. (From Fach *et al.*, 1990.)

the steady backgrounds (crosses) are shown (in their correct positions) to the right of each flashed background curve.

Thus the transient effect cannot be rod-specific (Alexander & Kelly, 1984; Sharpe *et al.*, 1989; Schneck, Volbrecht & Adams, 1989), as has been argued by Adelson (1982). This is made explicit in Fig. 2.18, which displays, as a function of background wavelength, the action spectrum (filled circles) of the receptor responsible for determining flash sensitivity (i.e. the field sensitivity or the flashed background intensity needed to elevate test threshold to a criterion level). The solid curve is the quantized CIE scotopic luminosity function, which gives a good fit to the measured field sensitivity function except at long-wavelengths above 620 nm. This is made clearer in the lower panel, which indicates that the threshold is higher against long-wavelength backgrounds than would be predicted solely on the basis of quantal absorptions in the rods.

In short, the interaction effects between rod and cone systems observed with small backgrounds, which are preserved in stabilized vision and which also occur with flashed backgrounds, suggest that signals in the cone pathway are raising rod threshold by adding to the rod background signal where they converge at or before the level of the ganglion cell, before significant attenuation of the steady state response has occurred.

2.4.8 Why not Weber's law for the rods?

Figure 2.19 shows the achromat's increment threshold curve for the 200 ms, 6 deg target (slope 0.77) along with the predictions of the de Vries–Rose square-root law (slope 0.50) and Weber's law (slope 1.0). The former (lower dashed line) implies that only quantum fluctuations in the background and possibly multiplicative intrinsic noise in the visual system are limiting the detectability of the target; whereas the latter (upper dashed line) implies that additional neural mechanisms are raising the limit. We know from above that the achromat observer K.N., like the normal observer, achieves square-root law-like behaviour for a small (10 min), brief (10 ms) target; but that, unlike the normal observer, he never attains Weber law-like behaviour for a large (6 deg), long (200 ms) target. Why does his slope only reach a value of 0.77? Does the higher threshold in the normal observer depend specifically upon the cone contribution arising from long-wavelength backgrounds? Cone stimulation, for instance, could speed up the shrinking of temporal summation. Or, does it depend simply upon the level of the adaptation pool (i.e. the total number of incoming signals) and not upon how it is made up?

It is quite clear that the cones achieve Weber's law on their own under the same conditions where the rods fall short. This is not only true when the target is long and large (see Fig. 2.14, where all the cone bleach thresholds, regardless of background wavelength, are well fit by the

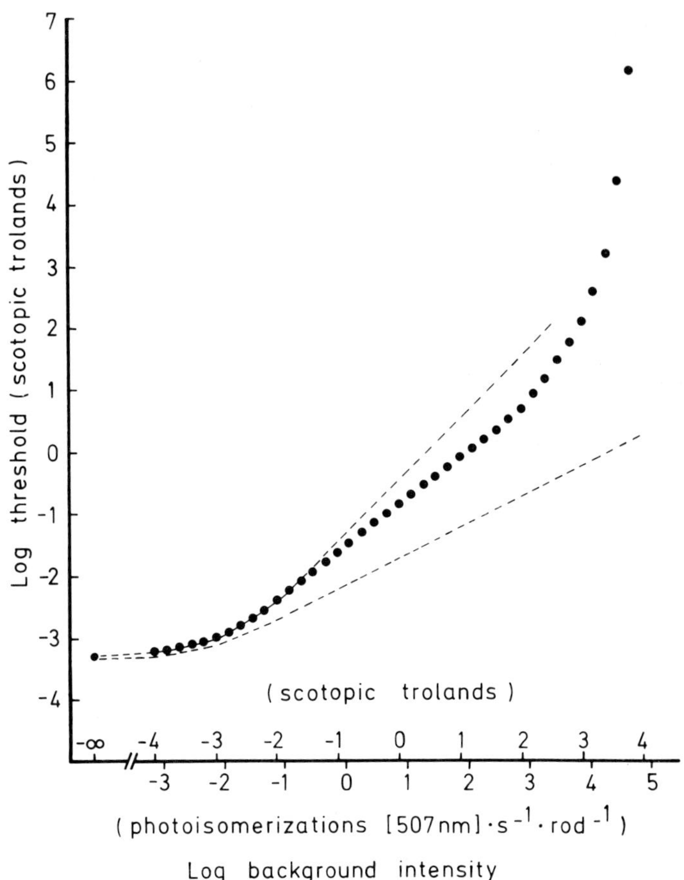

Fig. 2.19. The increment threshold curve of achromat K.N. from Fig. 2.1 (filled circles) plotted along with the theoretical upper and lower limits to his incremental sensitivity (dashed lines). The lower limit, calculated from Barlow's Fluctuation Theory (from Fig. 2.9), follows the de Vries–Rose square-root law and is determined by physical noise and dark noise in the photoreceptors. The upper limit follows Weber's law and indicates the additional influence of neural mechanisms upon increment threshold in the normal observer.

Aguilar & Stiles average function). It is also true when the target is brief and small (see Table 2.5*b*; Scholtes & Bouman, 1977). Interestingly, the background intensity at which Weber's law starts to govern threshold behaviour all over the retina is approximately $-10.0 \log_{10}$ W deg^{-2} or 2.75 $\log_{10}$ scotopic td. This corresponds to between 2000 and 3000 quanta arriving per second at the entrance aperture of each photoreceptor (Scholtes & Bouman, 1977; I estimate a value between 3400 and 4100 quanta from my conversion factors); almost exactly the level at which the

Table 2.8. *Variation of achromat K.N.'s increment threshold (ΔI), for a 200 ms, 6 deg diameter target, as a function of background intensity (I)*

I^a	ΔI^a	$\Delta I/I$	I^a	ΔI^a	$\Delta I/I$
−4.0	−3.24	5.75	0.0	−0.86	0.14
−3.8	−3.20	3.98	0.2	−0.72	0.12
−3.6	−3.16	2.75	0.4	−0.56	0.11
−3.4	−3.12	1.91	0.6	−0.40	0.10
−3.2	−3.08	1.32	0.8	−0.26	0.09
−3.0	−3.00	1.00	1.0	−0.10	0.08
−2.8	−2.92	0.76	1.2	0.05	0.07
−2.6	−2.80	0.63	1.4	0.20	0.06
−2.4	−2.70	0.50	1.6	0.36	0.06
−2.2	−2.54	0.46	1.8	0.52	0.05
−2.0	−2.40	0.40	2.0	0.68	0.05
−1.8	−2.24	0.36	2.2	0.92	0.05
−1.6	−2.10	0.32	2.4	1.16	0.06
−1.4	−1.94	0.29	2.6	1.44	0.07
−1.2	−1.80	0.25	2.8	1.76	0.09
−1.0	−1.64	0.23	3.0	2.10	0.13
−0.8	−1.48	0.21	3.2	2.60	0.25
−0.6	−1.32	0.19	3.4	3.20	0.63
−0.4	−1.16	0.17	3.6	4.40	6.31
−0.2	−1.02	0.15	3.8	6.20	251.20

[a] Values are given in $\log_{10}$ scotopic trolands.

rod visual system is assumed to be saturating (see below). Thus the rod-driven visual system of the achromat may only achieve Weber's law when it is too late, when the rods are already saturating.

There is some support for this speculation in Table 2.8, which gives the variation of K.N.'s increment threshold for the long, large target as a function of background intensity. His Weber–Fechner fraction reaches a constant value of 0.05 to 0.06 only in the background range from 1.4 to 2.4 $\log_{10}$ scotopic td. This is the value reached by the normal observer on the long-wavelength background at a much lower level (−2.0 $\log_{10}$ scotopic td). And it suggests that the total flux of signals required for Weber's law behaviour may be reached at a much lower level in the normal observer because his cone signals are summing with his rod signals to raise the level of the adaptation pool (see also Chapter 1 for an alternative explanation).

2.5 The saturation of the rods

2.5.1 Psychophysically estimating saturation

Aguilar & Stiles (1954) were the first to observe the precipitous rise in rod increment threshold that occurs above 2.0 $\log_{10}$ scotopic td. To quantify this sudden loss of sensitivity, they took as their criterion the background intensity causing the Weber–Fechner fraction to increase to 100 times its minimum value in the region of constant slope. They found the increase occurred at backgrounds between 3.59 and 3.77 $\log_{10}$ scotopic td – on average, 3.65 $\log_{10}$ scotopic – for their four observers.

A very similar value is found for achromat K.N., whose change in the Weber–Fechner fraction, as a function of background intensity, is quantified in Table 2.8 and shown in Fig. 2.6. K.N.'s minimum Weber–Fechner fraction for the 200 ms, 6 deg flash is 0.05; and the background causing it to increase 100-fold is near 3.65 $\log_{10}$ scotopic td. (The values for the two normal observers are 3.50 and 3.60 $\log_{10}$ scotopic td, respectively.) This corresponds to more than 32 500 quanta (507 nm) s^{-1} being absorbed by each rod (see also Figs. 11.1–11.3).

Unlike the value of the absolute sensitivity asymptote and the slope of the Weber–Fechner region, K.N.'s saturation constant does not change with target parameters. This is apparent in Fig. 2.5 (see also Figs. 11.1 and 11.2), where it can be seen that achromat K.N.'s curves measured with different target diameters converge at high intensities. For the 1 deg diameter, 100 ms flash, K.N.'s saturation constant is about 3.5 $\log_{10}$ scotopic td; and for the 10 min, 10 ms flash it is about 3.6 $\log_{10}$ scotopic td. The small difference is well within the error of extrapolation.

The Aguilar & Stiles criterion for rod saturation is very stringent. It is difficult, especially in the normal observer whose upper thresholds are obscured by the cones, to extrapolate to the background that drives the rod threshold so high. A more convenient measure is to find the background intensity that specifies the onset of saturation. This can be done by assuming that the Weber–Fechner relation holds in the absence of saturation and by determining the background causing its fraction to double (Hayhoe, MacLeod & Bruch, 1976; Lennie, Hertz & Enroth-Cugell, 1976; Adelson, 1982). On this assumption, the onset of saturation occurs for achromat K.N. at a background near 2.6 $\log_{10}$ scotopic td or about 2900 isomerizations (507 nm) s^{-1} rod $^{-1}$, regardless of target size. The value for the normal observer in Fig. 2.2 is 2.15 $\log_{10}$ scotopic td (1000 isomerizations (507 nm) s^{-1} rod^{-1}); and the value derived from the Aguilar & Stiles average curve is 2.5 $\log_{10}$ scotopic td (2300 isomerizations (507 nm) s^{-1} rod^{-1}).

2.5.2 The site of rod saturation

Saturation is a breakdown of the regular Weber–Fechner relation, which is believed to be regulated by the sensitivity control mechanisms. So it might be argued that the frequent quantal absorptions at high backgrounds drive the sensitivity regulatory network to its response ceiling, resulting in a neural response compression. Indeed, this may be what happens under some special conditions; when say the background is flashed simultaneously with the onset of the test flash (see below). But it cannot strictly be the case for typical, steady background conditions; because the rods and cones share the same sensitivity pathways to the brain and there is no impairment or response compression in the cone visual system at levels where the rod visual system saturates.

Saturation also cannot be due to photopigment bleaching; for it occurs well before even a significant fraction of visual pigment has been inactivated by bleaching (see Fig. 2.7). At the adapting level corresponding to K.N.'s onset of saturation (2.6 $\log_{10}$ scotopic td) less than 1% of the rhodopsin is bleached; and at the level corresponding to his complete saturation (3.65 $\log_{10}$ scotopic td) more than 85% still remains. In fact, photopigment depletion, by decreasing the number of molecules available to absorb quanta, would actually forestall saturation; as it seems to do in the cone visual system. Moreover, bleaching a little pigment may cause the receptors to get noisy (Lamb, 1987) and increase threshold in a way consistent with Weber–Fechner behaviour, but not with saturation.

Nor can saturation be strictly due to the suppression of rod signals by the cones (see Whitten & Brown, 1973); for it sets in at the same level in K.N. as in the normal trichromat, even though the former has only rod vision (this has also been remarked in other achromats by Blakemore & Rushton, 1965 and Sakitt, 1976; Sharpe & Nordby, The photoreceptors in the achromat, Chapter 10). To be sure, suppression by the cones is consistent with the fact that rod saturation is unique to species with mixed (i.e. rod and cone) retinae (see Green *et al.*, 1975). But there is no need in the duplex retina for the cones to suppress rod signals at higher intensities. The rods largely do it themselves (Baylor *et al.*, 1984). This can be deduced by referring back to Fig. 2.8, which plots the relative desensitization by steady backgrounds of individual macaque rod outer segments and of K.N.'s rod vision. The single rod and the rod visual system curves differ in shape, save in one respect: the photoreceptor function is driven to its maximum response and starts to saturate in a manner analogous to that exhibited by the psychophysical increment threshold function. Thus rod saturation, as measured psychophysically, would seem to directly reflect signal compression at the rod outer segment.

Or, at least this is how it appears at first glance. Upon closer inspection, however, we find that the correspondence is not exact. In fact, in macaque photoreceptors the sensitivity to a test flash is reduced to half the value found in the dark (comparable to saturation onset) by a background that gives about 100 isomerizations (507 nm) s^{-1} rod^{-1} (1.15 $\log_{10}$ scotopic td; the psychophysical estimate for K.N. is 2.6 $\log_{10}$ scotopic td); and is reduced 100-fold (comparable to Aguilar & Stiles's estimate of the upper limit of saturation) by a background that gives about 700 isomerizations (507 nm) s^{-1} rod^{-1} (1.98 $\log_{10}$ scotopic td; the psychophysical estimate for K.N. is 3.65 $\log_{10}$ scotopic td). In short, individual rods become unresponsive at backgrounds more than one order of magnitude lower than those causing rod vision to saturate.

2.5.3 *Subtractive filtering*

One could reasonably argue that the disparity between the physiological and psychophysical estimates of saturation is due to the problem of not knowing exactly how to compute the limits of saturation from an increment threshold curve; or to erroneous assumptions about how to relate photons incident on the cornea to isomerizations per rod; or to slight differences between monkey and human rods; or to the fact that the responses of the monkey rods were measured in an artificial medium; or to the different flash conditions used in the electrophysiological (11 ms flash duration) and psychophysical (200 ms flash duration) measurements. Indeed, with reference to stimulus parameters, it has been shown that when the target is flickered at temporal frequencies near 4 Hz the onset of saturation in the human occurs at lower background levels, between 20 and 50 scotopic td or between 150 and 370 photoisomerizations (507 nm) s^{-1} rod^{-1} (see Conner, 1982; D'Zmura & Lennie, 1986).

Nevertheless, these arguments – valid as they may be – do not dispose of the problem; because, as has been shown in the previous sections (see Figs 2.13 and 2.17), the intensity required for psychophysical saturation depends upon background exposure and size. In particular, when the background is flashed simultaneously with the target onset, saturation begins at levels as low as 3 scotopic td or 23 photoisomerizations (507 nm) s^{-1} rod^{-1} (Hallett, 1969; Adelson, 1982; see also Geisler, 1979; Alexander & Kelly, 1984); and when the background is small (2 deg) and exposed for more than 5 min, saturation begins near 40 scotopic td or about 290 photoisomerizations (507 nm) s^{-1} rod^{-1} (Alexander *et al.*, 1986).

For flashed backgrounds, the quantal absorptions yielding saturation are much fewer than those driving individual rod photoreceptors into response compression (see Fig. 2.13). This must be contrasted with steady backgrounds, where the onset of saturation occurs at many more quantal absorptions. It suggests that flashed backgrounds are more effective in penetrating to and overloading the neuronal sites controlling adaptation, which are proximal to the photoreceptors. For steady backgrounds, on the other hand, it may be that, even as the outer segment is saturating, the receptors may still be responding, and the visual system may still be able to extract information if it is given enough time to make compensatory sensitivity adjustments.

Adelson (1982) has argued that the earlier onset of saturation with flashed backgrounds is rod-specific. But at least three other studies have found that rod system saturation with flashed backgrounds is strongly influenced by cones at higher backgrounds; evidence, once again, that cones have access to the neuronal sites regulating the sensitivity of the rods (Alexander & Kelly, 1984; Fach, Sharpe & Stockman, 1989; Sharpe *et al.*, 1989; Schneck, Volbrecht & Adams, 1989). Alexander & Kelly (1984), for instance, have shown that when the background flash is made less effective for cones, through the Stiles–Crawford effect, the onset of rod saturation occurs at a higher luminance of background flash than normal; and, further, that protanopes – who lack the long-wave sensitive cones – do not show the characteristic of rod saturation until a much higher-than-normal luminance of the background flash. (Preliminary measurements suggest that this is also true for the achromat K.N.)

Not only the exposure of the background, but also its size, alters markedly the quantum catch per receptor required for saturation to appear in increment-threshold curves. Saturation for a small target (10 ms, 24 min) occurs earlier on a small background (2 deg in diameter) than on an equiluminous large one (8 deg in diameter); though the influence is only manifest when the background exposure is prolonged for more than 5 min (Alexander *et al.*, 1986). Since changing background diameter has no effect upon the quantum catch per receptor – it only increases the number of receptors having the same quantum catch – this would seem to provide solid support for the role of spatial high-pass filtering in rod system desensitization. Otherwise, why should smaller backgrounds have a greater effect than larger ones? If anything, one would expect larger fields to drive the system closer to its response ceiling, through the pooling of more rod signals.

Indeed, this is what is found in electrophysiological recordings from cat ganglion cells (Lennie *et al.*, 1976). Large (15 deg diameter) backgrounds, covering the entire receptive field, provoke an earlier onset of rod saturation (a doubling of the Weber–Fechner fraction) for a small test flash (0.2 deg, 125 ms on, 125 off) than small backgrounds (0.4–0.6 deg): 420 as compared to more than 20000 quanta s^{-1} rod^{-1}. And, what is more, varying the target size from 0.2 to 1.0 deg does not markedly alter the quantum catch (per receptor) required for saturation to appear against either background; even though the larger test flash has more than six times the area of the small background. Over the whole range of the increment-threshold curve (including saturation), thresholds for the different flashes are in the ratio of their areas. Thus receptors in the region neighbouring the small background are desensitized even though unilluminated.

A possible basis for the discrepant human and cat results may be the background sizes used. The small backgrounds used to test rod saturation in the cat (0.4–0.6 deg) were much smaller than those used in the human (2 deg). It could be, then, that spatial sensitization effects of the Crawford–Westheimer type were occurring with the larger field. That is, when the background was small, there may have been no lateral inhibitory signal from the light-adapted surround of ganglion cell receptive fields to prevent overloading of the centre mechanism's response to the adapting light (Buss *et al.*, 1982). But this argument does not really help out because the two backgrounds (2 and 8 deg) used in the Alexander *et al.* experiments were very much larger than backgrounds producing the optimal rod Crawford–Westheimer effect (Alexander, 1974) and psychophysical estimates of the adaptation pool size (see above). Regardless of the differences between the cat and the human results, however, the point remains that if rod saturation occurs solely within the photoreceptor outer segments, then the background diameter – as well as the background exposure – should have no effect whatsoever.

2.6 Conclusions

Macaque rods and presumably human ones as well do not light-adapt, though events within them define, to a large extent, the lower and upper limits of the rod light-adaptation process. Absolute sensitivity is determined mainly by intrinsic dark noise in the photoreceptor; saturation, by the overloading of the transduction process in the outer segment. Between these limits, the regulation of sensitivity is determined by neuronal network processes that sum the signals of many rods. Photopigment bleaching and the speeding up of the photoresponse – individual photoreceptor events which in principle could underlie human rod light-adaptation – do not contribute importantly to it.

The function of the network processes is to prevent the rod signals from exceeding the very limited dynamic range (about 2.0–2.5 $\log_{10}$ units) of the visual neurones; to escape saturation and to continuously use the steepest part of their neuronal stimulus–response function for detection of increments and decrements. Their means of doing so can be likened to automatic gain controlling and subtractive filtering. But the physiological substrates subserving these means have yet to be identified. Although some evidence suggests that automatic gain control arises in the bipolar cells and that subtractive filtering occurs in the outer plexiform layer, this is undoubtedly an oversimplication and may well be erroneous, especially since subtractive filtering is generally assumed to be antecedent to multiplicative gain control. It is more likely that there are parallel series of sensitivity regulation processes involved in rod desensitization (cf. Green, 1986); and that every stage of the retinal processing 'machinery' participates in some way (see Werblin & Copenhagen, 1974; Hood & Finkelstein, 1986). And, it may be that the visual system takes advantage of different pathways through the interneuron circuitry to optimalize its performance at different ambient levels of illumination. An example from each the cat and the macaque serves to underscore this point.

In the cat – the mammal about whose visual system we have the most anatomical and physiological information – at least 22 different morphological varieties of amacrine cell can be recognised (Kolb, Nelson & Mariani, 1981). Two of these conduct signals directly to ganglion cells. They are the wide-field A17 cell, without antagonistic surround, and the narrow-field AII cell, with antagonistic surround, which also connects to cone bipolars. The A17 cell may be an example of a sustained rod–amacrine integrating signals over a large area and improving detection at absolute threshold; whereas the AII amacrine cells may serve to concentrate and quicken the slower signals of the rods; thereby providing a significant improvement in the speed of perception for small luminous objects on scotopic backgrounds (Nelson, 1982).

In the Rhesus monkey, approximately two per cent of all ganglion cells have a long dendritic process that bypasses bipolar cells and directly contacts rods (Mariani, 1982; Zrenner, Nelson & Mariani, 1983). These cells could transmit scotopic signals to the brain more rapidly than the other types of retinal ganglion cells since they circumvent the usual interneuronal circuitry of the retina. In seemingly good analogy, two different pathways for conducting rod flicker signals – one sluggish, the other fast – have been demonstrated psychophysically (Conner & MacLeod, 1977; Conner, 1982; Stockman & MacLeod, 1989b; Stockman *et al.*, 1990). At 15 Hz the rod signals transmitted through the two pathways emerge out-of-phase, so that destructive interference produces a nulling of the apparent flicker.

The question arises as to whether or not these distinct pathways are unique to rods or whether they are shared with the cones. But, given the wealth of synaptic interconnections in the retina, it is more than likely that the same pathways summing and regulating the rod signals are probably involved in summing and regulating the cone signals as well. In fact, adaptive independence is inconsistent with the morphology, physiology and psychophysics of the visual system. True, at low adapting levels, the rods function autonomously because they are the only photoreceptors sensitive enough to respond to the gentle rain of photons. And, at high adapting levels, the cones function alone because the heavy rain of photons forces the collapse of the rods. But, in between at mesopic levels where both rods and cones are active, the sensitivity of the visual system must be being regulated by the flux of their combined signals to some extent, as is made clear by comparisons between the increment thresholds of the normal and achromat observer.

Acknowledgements

The preparation of this manuscript was supported by the Deutsche Forschungsgemeinschaft, Bonn (SFB 325, B4) and the Alexander von Humboldt-Stiftung, Bonn–Bad Godesberg. I am grateful to Clemens Fach, Dr Knut Nordby and Dr Andrew Stockman for providing some of the data described here. I thank Drs Horace Barlow (Cambridge), Friedrich Heitger (Zürich), David Pepperberg (Chicago), Tom Reuter

(Helsinki), Lothar Spillmann (Freiburg im Breisgau), Andrew Stockman (La Jolla), Paul Whittle (Cambridge), Henk van der Tweel (Amsterdam) and Eberhart Zrenner (Tübingen) for critically commenting on the manuscript.

3

Physiological mechanisms of visual adaptation at low light levels

Maureen K. Powers and Daniel G. Green

3.1 Introduction

We are largely unaware of the large variations in ambient illumination that exist between one location and another and those that slowly occur over a period of time. Thus one of the truly amazing aspects of vision is generally ignored, until one tries to photograph a scene. Through our photographs we discover that even with the aid of a variety of apertures and shutter speeds and films it is next to impossible to get the camera to register precisely what we see. *Visual adaptation* is the process through which retinal sensitivity is adjusted so that even when the environmental intensity changes by orders of magnitude our visual world remains relatively constant.

One of the reasons adaptation is possible is that the natural world is composed of objects illuminated by a distant source. To the extent that objects are diffuse reflectors, the point to point variations in luminance of a scene are given by

$$L = p(x)E$$

where E is the intensity of illumination from the source and $p(x)$ is the spatial variation in the reflectivity of the objects in the scene. The information extracted by the visual system from the image on the retina is an impression of $p(x)$ which is relatively independent of E. The system does this by performing a logarithmic transform and suppressing the steady component. Thus, in terms of the classical adaptation paradigm in which an increment is added to steady background, the just detectable increment varies with background according to Weber's relation. That is,

$$\mathrm{d}I/I = \text{constant}.$$

The above description of the behavior of the visual system during adaptation says little about the activity of individual system components, and how their responses might be causally related to the phenomena of adaptation. In Selig Hecht's early model (Hecht, 1924), the reduced sensitivity to incremental stimuli observed during light adaptation was thought to be directly related to the reduced concentration of photopigment in the photoreceptors in light adapted eyes. But in the early 1950s Campbell & Rushton developed the means of testing Hecht's ideas directly by using a new instrument, the retinal densitometer (Campbell & Rushton, 1955), to measure the actual concentration of visual pigment in the living human eye. Subsequent work showed that pigment concentration and visual threshold were indeed related, but not as directly as Hecht had thought: reducing the pigment concentration by only a small amount had a devastating effect on the ability to detect dim stimuli (Rushton, 1961). The subsequent work of Rushton and others (e.g. Lipetz, 1961; Rushton, 1965*a*, *b*; and Cleland & Enroth-Cugell, 1968; Easter, 1968) was consistent with the notion that all aspects of light adaptation originated beyond the photoreceptors. This notion also turned out to be incorrect. We now know that significant adaptation can occur in photoreceptors in some species and for some photoreceptor types (bufo, snapping turtle, frog, and gekko, but not primate rods) especially at higher light levels (Green *et al.*, 1975; Green & Powers, 1982).

The first direct demonstration of adaptational phenomena within rod photoreceptors was by Grabowski, Pinto and Pak (1972), who showed that a steady background could desensitize axolotl rods. Naka & Rushton's (1968) and Dowling & Ripps's (1970, 1971, 1972) recordings from horizontal cells showed that rod-mediated adaptation occurred at an early stage of retinal processing. Experiments in a variety of cold blooded vertebrates using sodium aspartate to isolate receptor potentials subsequently provided evidence that photoreceptors can display a wide range of adaptive phenomena (Dowling & Ripps, 1972; Witkovsky, Nelson & Ripps, 1973). Intracellular recordings from single photoreceptors showed directly that receptors can significantly regulate their own sensitivity (Grabowski *et al.*, 1972; Baylor & Hodgkin, 1974; Normann & Werblin, 1974; Kleinschmidt & Dowling, 1975; Fain, 1976). Thus light adaptation can begin at the very first stage of visual processing and, as we will see, is manifest at all subsequent levels of retinal processing as well as in the brain.

In this chapter we review the basic phenomena of visual adaptation at low luminance, with an emphasis on the physiological mechanisms that may be responsible. In its broadest sense the term 'adaptation' would include all aspects of light and dark adaptation as well as contrast adaptation (e.g. Ohzawa, Sclar & Freeman, 1982, 1985) grating adaptation (e.g. Movshon & Lennie, 1979), and probably other topics as well. However, in keeping with the theme of the book, we have limited our review to material that is relevant to rod-mediated vision, focusing on the effects of dim, steady, spatially uniform backgrounds on the ability to detect spots or gratings. We leave to a later chapter (Chapter 5) by Lamb the exposition of principles of dark adaptation and to the preceding ones (Chapter 2) by Sharpe and (Chapter 1) by Hess a discussion of the psychophysical effects of adaptation. Other relevant reviews include Shapley & Enroth-Cugell (1984), Green (1986), part 3.2.6 in Hood & Finkelstein (1986) and Chapter 7 in Dowling (1987).

3.2 Effects of background light on luminance detection

Two experimental procedures have been used extensively in the study of luminance adaptation as it affects detection of incremental, spatially uniform stimuli: intensity–response functions and increment thresholds. The bulk of knowledge about the physiological mechanisms of adaptation has come from such work. In both paradigms the dependent measure is usually response amplitude. It is important to note, however, that luminance adaptation almost always affects the kinetics of cellular response as well. While some have attempted to link changes in speed with changes in sensitivity (e.g. Fuortes & Hodgkin, 1964) this aspect of adaptation is generally ignored, perhaps because the kinetic changes during adaptation are very much smaller in magnitude than the reduction in response amplitude.

3.2.1 Description of the phenomenon

Typical intensity–response functions recorded at several levels of retinal processing are illustrated in Fig. 3.1. The data are from rat retina (Green & Powers, 1982). Circles show functions under full dark adaptation, with no background present. Under these conditions, the ganglion cell appears most sensitive because its response is relatively greater in amplitude than that of the receptor potential and b-wave to comparable intensities. In the example shown here the ganglion cell has reached saturation (Fig. 3.1*c*) before any response is seen at the level of the

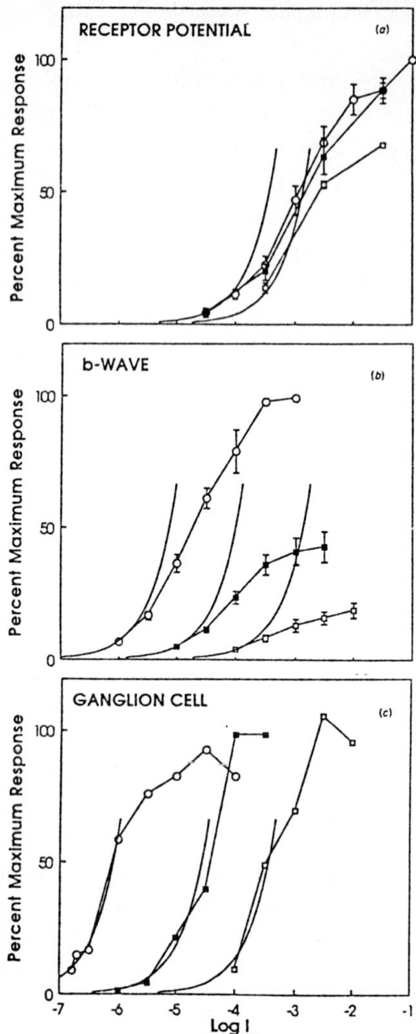

Fig. 3.1. Intensity–response functions at different levels of background illumination and different levels of retinal processing in mammalian (rat) retina. Percent maximum amplitude is shown for the aspartate-isolated 'receptor potential', and for the b-wave in normal preparations. Percent maximum spike discharge (number per second) is shown for an individual ganglion cell. Circles are data obtained after dark adaptation with no background present. With backgrounds that raised the b-wave absolute threshold by 1 log unit (squares) or 2 log units (open squares), little adaptation of the receptor potential was observed. The b-wave was compressed in amplitude and shifted toward higher thresholds; the ganglion cell was merely shifted and displayed no response compression. Figure adapted from Green & Powers (1982). Full-field, monochromatic stimuli. To give an idea of the quantal sensitivities involved, at log $I_T=0$, the 200 ms stimulus was equivalent to 12×10^4 quanta absorbed in each rod per second. Absolute threshold for the ganglion cell (circles in *c*, measured at 50% response) was about 0.08 quanta per second per rod or 1 photon absorbed per 13 rods. The background that raised threshold to about 1.2 quanta per second per rod (solid squares in *c*) was itself equavalent to 9.5 quanta per second per rod.

receptors (Fig. 3.1*a*). It is of course important to note that the inability to observe a response may be due to limitations of the experimental approach; individual receptors must be responding, or more distal responses could not occur.. The receptor potential does not reflect the sensitivity of individual receptors.

The effect of background illumination depends upon the level of processing within the retina (Fig. 3.1). Backgrounds that depress b-wave responsivity by 1 log unit (solid squares) or 2 log units (open squares) have practically no effect on the intensity–response function of the receptor potential. The same backgrounds cause a lateral shift in the intensity–response functions of the ganglion cell, and a lateral shift plus response compression in the b-wave.

Examination of the increment threshold functions demonstrates that sensitivity is regulated at different levels of retinal processing as background luminance increases (Fig. 3.2). The data (from the rat) in Fig. 3.2 are plotted relative to threshold in darkness for each of the retinal responses. This transformation is justified because we know that individual rods respond to the absorption of individual photons (Hecht, Shlaer & Pirenne, 1942; Fain, 1975; Baylor, Nunn & Schnapf, 1984; also see Chapters 4 and 6); as implied above, the low absolute sensitivity of the receptor potential is presumed to be due to problems of measuring a mass potential far from its site of origin. The same argument holds for the b-wave, which is also less sensitive in absolute terms than the ganglion cell. Fig. 3.2 shows that the amplitude of the receptor response is not influenced by backgrounds of relatively low luminance – the incremental stimulus required to elicit a threshold response is no higher than that required in darkness until the background intensity reaches 1–2 log units above threshold for the b-wave and ganglion cell. Thus, the absorption of individual photons by rods, and the amplification of the signal produced by these absorptions is proximal retina, is responsible for determining increment threshold at low background luminances.

At higher luminances the situation is different. At backgrounds that are 2.5 to 3.5 log units above absolute threshold for the rat receptor potential, b-wave and ganglion cell (Fig. 3.1), the increment threshold curves are parallel. That is, the imposition of mesopic backgrounds causes equivalent increases in threshold for all three response types. At these background levels, however, the rods are probably no longer the exclusive mediators of visual response because the backgrounds are at the high end of the intensity–response function for the receptor potential, which is close to its level of saturation (Fig. 3.1; Kleinschmidt

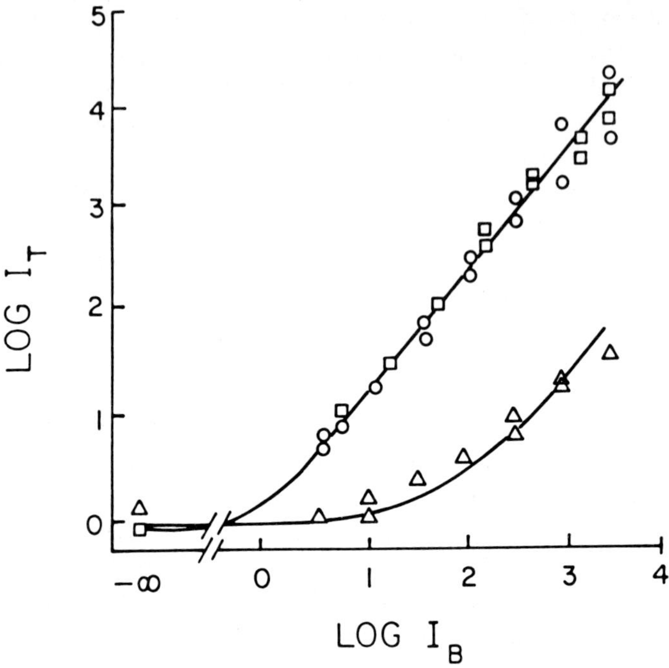

Fig. 3.2. Increment threshold curves for receptor potential, b-wave and ganglion cell from dark adapted rate retina. Triangles show receptor potential thresholds (log I_T) as a function of background intensity (log I_B). Circles and squares show thresholds for b-wave (circles) and ganglion cell (squares) in the presence of the same tungsten backgrounds. Redrawn from Green & Powers (1982). Test stimuli were monochromatic (500 or 600 or 625 nm; see Green & Powers, 1982, for details).

& Dowling, 1975). At and above these background luminances, then, the rod receptor response cannot contribute much to the regulation of threshold, and cones or elements beyond them must be responsible for determining threshold (see Green & Powers, 1982).

For the b-wave there is also a shift in operating range toward higher intensities, but the intensity–response function also changes shape. Comparison of Figs. 3.1*b* and *c* shows that the b-wave generally saturates at intensities where the ganglion cell has reached its asymptote as well, indicating stimulus intensities beyond the ganglion cell's operating range. In the scotopic range, it is only when the intensity of the test stimulus begins to approach that of the background that its presence or absence will produce a significant change in the total response. The result is that threshold for the test is related to background luminance by a ratio scale: if the background is increased in intensity by some factor then the test must also be increased by about the same amount before its effects will be significant (Fig. 3.2). This is Weber's law.

These illustrations show that, in general, background lights in the scotopic range reduce sensitivity. For the ganglion cells, the sensitivity reduction is reflected in a wholesale shift of the intensity–response function, so that stimuli that are saturating with no background present now produce smaller responses (Fig. 3.1*c*). The important effect of this is, of course, that the message received by the brain reflects *relative* changes in stimulation, independent of the background luminance.

3.2.2 *Mechanisms and models*

Recent physiological recordings of photoreceptor currents in primate rods (Baylor *et al.*, 1984) have confirmed the classical psychophysical evidence that quantum fluctuations can place limits on dark adapted rod sensitivity. Thus, one way that a background could affect detection of a test stimulus is through the increased *quantum noise* from the background (see Aho *et al.*, 1988). That is, for a Poisson random process the fluctuations from a background of intensity I_B are proportional to $(I_B)^{1/2}$: increasing background intensity would correspondingly increase the quantum noise. If reliable transmission of information required a fixed signal/noise ratio, then sensitivity (see also Chapters 1, 4 and 6) expressed in terms of the increment required to maintain a set level of performance would decrease inversely with the square root of background intensity (the De Vries–Rose Law). In this context, three points can be made about recordings from ganglion cells: (1) light-included increases in the variability of the maintained spike discharge have not been clearly demonstrated; (2) in a species where the rod ganglion cell ratio continually increases during normal growth, the variability of the maintained discharge of ganglion cells does not change (Falzett, Nussdorf & Powers, 1988); and (3) the effect of a background on ganglion cell sensitivity is not described by the de Vries–Rose Law over any range of background intensities. Thus, it appears that noise from quantum fluctuations contributes little to the process of light adaptation.

One of the simplest mechanisms one can imagine is one where the effect of adaptation is to decrease the potency of the test probe. MacLeod (1978) has called this the *dark glasses model* of adaptation. That is, desensitization produces an effect that is equivalent to reducing the intensity of the stimulus. Pigment depletion would have such an effect but this might also occur if (for example) adaptation depleted the store of chemical synaptic transmitter. In both instances a stimulus presented against a background light would have less effect than in the dark. The amplitude of the response, however, could be restored to its original size by simply increasing stimulus intensity. In other words, the effect of an adapting stimulus in the dark glasses model is to cause a shift of the intensity–response function rightward along the log intensity axis. A dark glasses model could account for the behavior of ganglion cells (Fig. 3.1), but such a model is clearly too simplistic to account for adaptation of the receptor potential or of the b-wave (Fig. 3.1).

An alternative to the dark glasses model is *response scaling*. Visual response can be described by a function which is the product of two functions, one depending on I_D and the other on I_B.

$$R = g(I_D)\, f(I_B)$$

where I_D = threshold intensity with no background present and I_B = intensity of background. In this model adaptation attenuates the size of the response without affecting the form of the light dependency. Probably the best known model of this kind of adaptation was proposed by Alpern, Rushton & Torii (1970).

In *physiological* terms, we know the following about the mechanisms of adaptation at the various retinal locations. The rods do not change in sensitivity (if they change at all) until they approach the limit of their response range in darkness. Until then they rely on internal amplification of photon events (see Fung, Hurley & Stryer, 1981; Fesenko, Kolenikov & Lyuborsky, 1985) to relay signals to other cells, and the inner retina then further amplifies these signals (Ashmore & Falk, 1980). Adaptation within mammalian rods normally only occurs at higher background levels, after the cones have become the functional receptors. At these levels adaptation involves complex ionic events related to Ca^{2+} flow during sustained hyperpolarization (see Kleinschmidt & Dowling, 1975; Yau & Kakatani, 1985). Recent work suggests that Ca^{2+} is in fact the feedback messenger that is responsible for adaptation in rods (Matthews *et al.*, 1988; Nakatani & Yau, 1988; Koch & Stryer, 1988; see Pugh & Altman, 1988), even in mammalian rods (Koch & Stryer, 1988).

Beyond the photoreceptors, at the low background levels where photoreceptors themselves are not affected but where rods are responsible for vision, again control mechanism operates to effect adaptation (see Enroth-Cugell & Shapley, 1973). This mechanism must be synaptically stimulated by transmission of small signals from the photoreceptors, and probably also involves response compression (see b-wave data,

Fig. 3.1). This type of adaptation has been called 'network' adaptation (Green *et al.*, 1975). Response compression can not account for changes in sensitivity at low luminances, because the ganglion cell maximum response is unattenuated by backgrounds (see Fig. 3.1*c* and Sackman & Creutzfeld, 1969).

3.2.3 Adaptation pools

Many investigators have addressed the question of whether or not an adapting stimulus falling in one place can affect the sensitivity at other points in the retina (Rushton & Westheimer, 1962; Rushton, 1965*a*, *b*; Barlow & Andrews, 1973; Cleland & Enroth-Cugell, 1968; Easter, 1968; Green, Tong & Cicerone, 1977). The impetus for these experiments concerned the sites of visual adaptation (See Green, 1986). We will use the term 'adaptation pool', suggested by Rushton (1965*b*), to denote the collection of receptors that combine their signals to control the sensitivity in an area of retina.

There is good reason to have an adaptation pool. Returning to the photographic process to illustrate our point, as anyone with a camera knows, natural scenes frequently have highlights and shadows wherein the ambient illumination greatly exceeds the dynamic range of film. Varying the aperture allows one to register either light or dark areas, but not both. Living things solve this problem in a way that, as far as we are aware of, no human-made image processing device does (see also Chapter 13). In the eye there is local control of sensitivity over restricted areas of the retina: the adaptation pool. The adaptation pool needs to be small enough to be able to regulate independently sensitivity in the dark and light areas of a scene, but not too small. If the size of the pool begins to approach the size of the detail in the image, the adjustments of gain will not improve the neural image. Turning down the gain in the brighter areas and turning it up in the darker areas will reduce contrast and degrade the image. Exactly what the optimum size is for the pool will depend on the nature of the scene (Chapter 1 gives an account of this from the psychophysical point of view.). What is clear is that the pool should be considerably larger than a photoreceptor and considerably smaller than the scene as a whole.

Do such pools exist in the retina? For cells other than rod photoreceptors, the answer in general has been affirmative – pooling does occur – and consequently these experiments again provide compelling evidence that the photoreceptor outer segment is not the major place where sensitivity is regulated.

3.2.4 Adaptation and speed response

One of the fascinating aspects of adaptation is the change in speed of response that is almost always associated with changes in sensitivity. A system in which speed of response and sensitivity are inversely related makes biological sense. The only way that a photon-limited system can gain in absolute sensitivity is to sum light over time. This is a direct analog of using long exposures to take low level photographs. The price one pays for the increase in sensitivity so gained is a loss in the ability to react rapidly to changing conditions. Quickness of response is of such great survival value that it has to be advantageous to trade off sensitivity for greater speed at higher levels of illumination.

There is ample evidence for such changes from human psychophysics (e.g. Barlow, 1958), but the biochemical/synaptic mechanisms behind these changes are uncertain. Recordings from turtle, frog, and toad rods (Schwartz, 1975; Baylor & Hodgkin, 1974; Hood & Grover, 1974; Fain, 1976) show that the incremental response is significantly shortened in duration by backgrounds. A simple gain control or response compression model of visual adaptation cannot give an account of these changes. What is required is a process where the rate constants are functions of light intensity. One of the best known of these is the scheme that Fuortes & Hodgkin (1964) proposed to fit visual responses in *Limulus*. Their model, which consists of a cascade of ten first-order processes with the rate constant of each depending on light adaptation, does an admirable job of reproducing the light-induced changes in both sensitivity and speed.

The above might seem to suggest that the phototransduction apparatus is the primary source of changes in temporal integration. More recent work, however, indicates primate rods are different in this regard (Baylor *et al.*, 1984): light adaptation has little effect on the response kinetics of photocurrents in monkey rods (see also Figs 1.11–1.15). Thus in spite of tremendous theoretical progress in recent years, we are still a long way from being able to explain the mechanisms that are responsible for changes in sensitivity and speed of response that characterize human rod adaptation.

3.2.5 Rod saturation

There are lower and upper limits on the magnitude of the neural signals. The lower limit is determined by factors such as the size of the quantized input variable (i.e. the photon nature of light or the contents of a synaptic vesicle) or the magnitude of the intrinsic noise. On the other end of the scale, intensity–response curves of cells always plateau at higher stimulus intensities (see Fig. 3.1). The upper limit in response is reached in a cell giving graded potentials when all the active channels are closed (or open) or in a spiking neuron when it is firing at its maximum rate. When a cell is driven to its limit no greater response can be elicited. It is saturated, in the sense that it cannot signal further increases in light intensity.

Aquilar & Stiles (1954) were the first to infer saturation of rod signals in humans using psychophysical methods (also see their results discussed in Chapters 1, 2 and 11). They calculated that saturation begins to occur when each rod is absorbing several hundred photons per second. Because rods contain on the order of 10^8 molecules of rhodopsin such a background bleaches only a small fraction of the pigment and thus has a negligible effect on the pigment content of the rods. Consequently, Aquilar & Stiles suggested that 'rod saturation' might represent *neural* over-load of the photoreceptors.

Electrophysiological recording of rod signals in a variety of animals (e.g. skate, goldfish, toads, lizards, rats and primates) have shown that a bright steady light that causes about 400 photoisomerizations per second evokes a response of nearly maximum amplitude. After exposure to steady backgrounds brighter than this, the ability to respond to incremental stimuli is suppressed. With continuous illumination, in cold-blooded vertebrates but not in mammals, the incremental response returns (the 'silent period' ends; see Powers & Easter, 1978). Receptor recordings show that responsivity returns because the cell membrane potential can recover from saturation (Dowling & Ripps, 1970; Kleinschmidt & Dowling, 1975; Fain, 1976; Matthews, 1983). Associated with return toward resting membrane potential is a decrease in flash sensitivity. Photoreceptor adaptational mechanisms can thus play an important role in reducing both sensitivity and steady membrane potential in some vertebrate species, allowing recovery from saturation and permitting rods to continue to respond in the presence of brighter backgrounds.

3.2.6 *Impact of receptor coupling*

We have implicitly assumed so far that a photoreceptor's response is dependent only on the light it absorbs in its own outer segment. This is clearly not so, especially in non-mammalian retinas (Baylor, Fuortes & O'Bryan, 1971; Baylor & Hodgkin, 1973; Fain, 1975, 1976; Schwartz,

1975; Copenhagen & Owen, 1976). In toad, for example, up to 60% of the hyperpolarization observed in a rod originates from its illuminated neighbors (Fain, 1975). Photoreceptors in some retinas are synaptically coupled to their near neighbors through sign-conserving synapses, and to their more distant neighbors through sign-inverting synapses. The basis for the synergistic effects is electrical in some species (Detwiler & Hodgkin, 1979; Copenhagen & Owen, 1980) and possibly chemical in others (Normann *et al.*, 1984); in either case the effects are mediated through direct photoreceptor-to-photoreceptor contacts. The basis for the antagonistic effects is feedback from horizontal cells onto photoreceptors (Baylor *et al.*, 1971). Thus, rather than functioning independently each photoreceptor is an integral part of an elaborate synaptic network.

How does photoreceptor coupling affect adaptation? Copenhagen & Green (1985) have recently answered this question for the rods of the snapping turtle. Their first experiments were stimulated by Rushton's finding that it took very few photons to elevate threshold in human subjects (Rushton, 1965*b*). From this Rushton argued that the rods that saw the background must somehow raise the threshold of the ones that did not. Copenhagen & Green (1985) found that a background so dim that each rod absorbed a photon only once every ten seconds could halve the flash sensitivity of the rod response (note that this seems inconsistent with mammalian results as depicted in Fig. 3.1). This seemed much like the Rushton result and initially suggested pooling of adaptation early in retinal processing. However, detailed measurements of the spatial spread of adaptation failed to show pooling over distances greater than could be accounted for by stray light. Fig. 3.3 shows sample records from these experiments. An adapting slit superimposed on a small test spot had a much larger desensitizing effect than when it was moved 20 m away. This was true in spite of the fact that the hyperpolarizing responses evoked in the central rod by the slit alone under the two conditions (central and displaced stimulation) were virtually identical.

These results caused Copenhagen & Green to rethink their original conclusion. What they had neglected to consider is that the logic of inferring pooling involves an implicit assumption about how long the effect of each photoisomerization persists. If the absorption of 0.1 photon per rod per second can adapt, as Copenhagen & Green found, then before one can conclude that there is pooling, the possibility that a single photoisomerization produces a massive desensitizing effect which persists for 10 seconds or more must be excluded. Rather than eliminat-

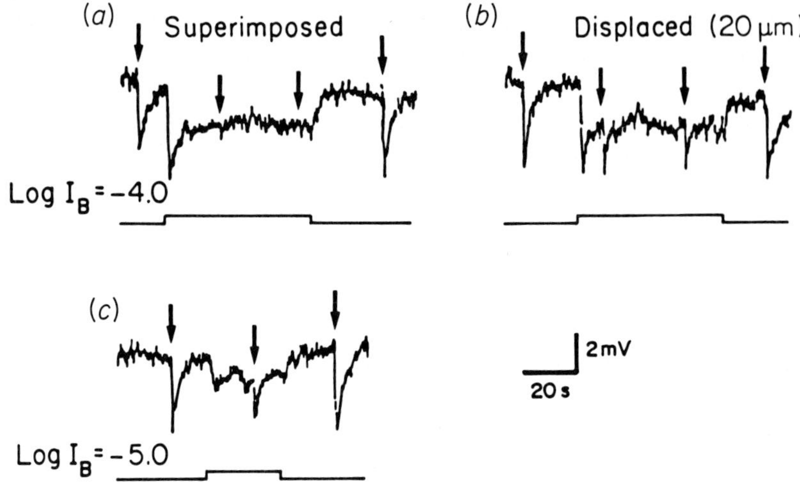

Fig. 3.3. Failure to find spread of adaptation through coupled rod network in snapping turtle retina. Effects of superimposed and displaced slits on intracellular responses from rod photoreceptors. All flash responses (arrows) are to a 25 μm diameter spot centred on the impaled rod. (*a*) An initial control flash response (arrow) was followed by presentation of a background, during which greatly reduced responses to two test flashes were observed (arrows). After removal of the background, flash response returned to its original amplitude. (*b*) Same as in (*a*), except the adapting background was displaced 20 μm relative to the center of the rod's receptive field. (*c*) Same as in (*a*) except the intensity of the adapting background was reduced by 1 log unit, to give the same effect on flash sensitivity as in (*b*). Redrawn from Copenhagen & Green (1985), who concluded that the effect of the background in (*b*) could parsimoniously be due to stray light (hence the effect in (*c*)), and therefore that adaptation did not spread laterally through the photoreceptor sheet.

ing this possibility, Copenhagen & Green's experiments suggested that this is exactly what happens: the results imply that the effect of a single photon absorption spreads longitudinally along the length of the outer segment and desensitizes the whole photoreceptor. The lack of spread to other rods implies that receptor coupling does not play a major role in light adaptation, even in cold-blooded species.

3.2.7 Adaptation beyond the retina

Adaptation of the visual system to uniform background fields originates in the retina, and its effects are generally weaker in the brain. In the lateral geniculate nucleus, responses are relatively more sustained at lower luminances (Virsu, Lee & Creutzfeldt, 1977) but this effect is not nearly as striking as in retinal ganglion cells (Jakeila, Enroth-Cugell &

Shapley, 1976; see Fig. 3.5). When measured with spot-like stimuli, receptive field surrounds of geniculate cells have somewhat greater inhibitory effects on their centers than do those of retinal ganglion cells (Hubel and Wiesel, 1961), and at lower luminances this still seems to be the case because surround inhibition is decreased during dark adaptation, but not to the extent that it is in retina (Maffei & Fiorentini, 1972; Virsu *et al.*, 1977; but see Kaplan, Marcus & So, 1979, discussed below).

3.3 Effects of background light on spatial vision

There are very few studies on this topic, which is clearly an important one for practical applications. In their 1966 paper, Enroth-Cugell & Robson observed that the spatial contrast sensitivity of cat retinal ganglion cells seemed to depend on background luminance level. Daitch & Green (1969) and a variety of others (e.g. van Meeteren & Vos, 1972; DeValois & Morgan, 1974; Pasternak & Merigan, 1981; see also Koenderink *et al.*, 1978, and Hess & Howell, 1988) have subsequently demonstrated a clear dependence of psychophysical spatial sensitivity of luminance level in humans and animals. In this section we discuss the evidence for neural mechanisms that underlie these changes, first within the retina and then within the brain. A recent discussion of the analysis of spatial pattern by the visual system at higher luminances may be found in Shapley & Lennie (1985).

3.3.1 Retinal ganglion cells

Barlow, FitzHugh & Kuffler (1957) noted, before the use of grating stimuli became widespread, that the spatial organization of cat retinal ganglion cells changed during dark adaptation. Specifically, they observed a diminished inhibitory influence of the surround near absolute threshold, so that the receptive field center size appeared to increase when background luminance was low. Subsequent work (Fig. 3.4) has shown that the actual sizes of the center and surround components of ganglion cell receptive fields change very little with adaptation (Cleland & Enroth-Cugell, 1968; Derrington & Lennie, 1982), but has confirmed that the surround becomes relatively less effective at very low levels of illumination (Enroth-Cugell & Lennie, 1975; Barlow & Levick, 1976; Derrington & Lennie, 1982). Enroth-Cugell & Lennie (1975) concluded that the apparent 'dropping out' of the surround response observed by Barlow *et al.* (1957) was due to the differences in sensitivity of surround

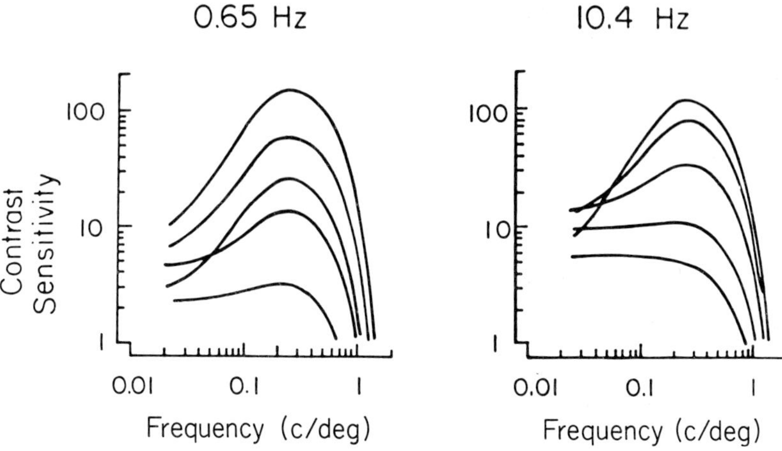

Fig. 3.4. Spatial contrast sensitivity functions for an X-on cell in cat retina, measured at different levels of background illumination. Left set of curves shows data for sine wave gratings modulated in time at 0.65 Hz; right set for gratings modulated at 10.4 Hz. From lower to upper curves in both sets, background illumination (mean luminance of the gratings) increased as follows: 3.8×10^{-5} cd/m^2, 4.9×10^{-4} cd/m^2, 0.087 cd/m^2, 15 cd/m^2, 200 cd/m^2. Contrast sensitivity (the height of the curve) improved by more than a log unit with background illumination over this range of background intensities. Spatial resolution (cutoff frequency) also improved, but only by about a factor of 2. Redrawn from curves given in Derrington & Lennie (1982).

and center mechanisms, so that at very low luminances the surround was too insensitive to exert an inhibitory influence on the center, while the more sensitive center was still quite capable of responding. Thus one effect of background illumination on retinal ganglion cells is to increase contrast sensitivity by increasing the lateral inhibitory effect of the surround (Kuffler, 1953). Precisely how this occurs, by changes at the level of the synapse or some other mechanism, is not known.

A consideration that becomes important in any discussion of retinal mechanisms and spatial vision is the response type of the ganglion cell in question. There is clear evidence that X and Y cells differ in response properties (Enroth-Cugell & Robson, 1966), and some evidence that ON and OFF cells within these classes differ in spatial properties as well (Bilotta & Abramov, 1987). Given that X and Y cells (Linsenmeier & Jakeila, 1979) and ON and OFF cells (Falzett *et al.*, 1988) can still be characterized near absolute threshold, we can ask whether their response properties remain invariant over the various cell types at scotopic levels of adaptation. Jakeila *et al.* (1976) addressed this question in cat retina,

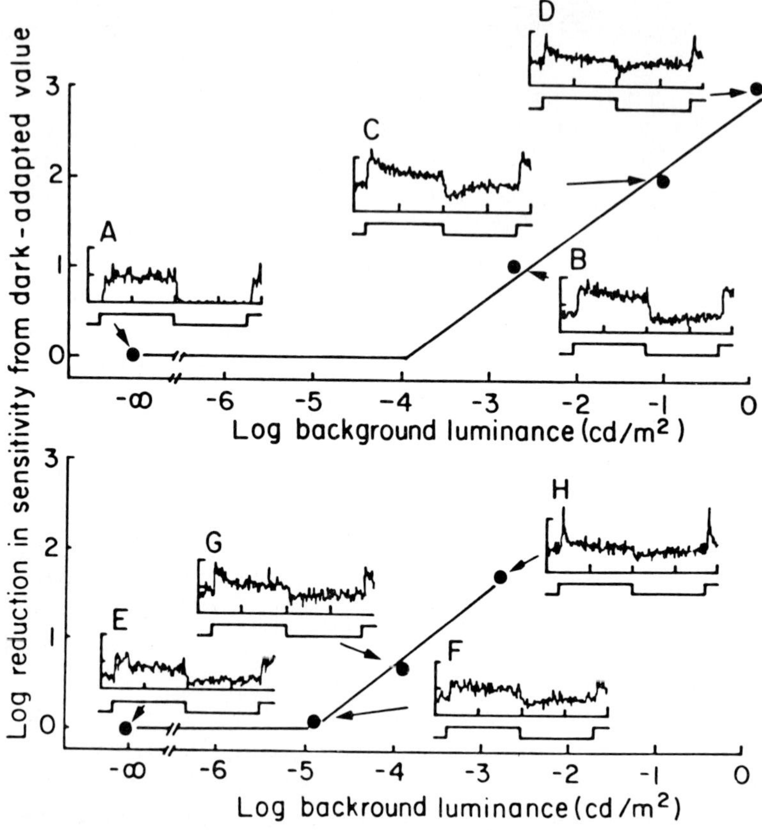

Fig. 3.5. Another effect of background illumination on ganglion cell response is to introduce transients. This shows response time courses for a cat X-on cell (top) and a Y-on-cell (bottom) at several different background levels. In A and E, no background was present and the cells' responses are sustained. In B and F, the responses were still sustained in the presence of a dim background. At higher levels (C, D, G, and H) transient components appear in the responses of both X and Y cells. Unit on histograms are 1 s and 50 spikes/s (20 ms bin width, 30 repetitions). From Jakeila *et al.* (1976).

and found that both X and Y cells became fully sustained under full dark adaptation (Fig. 3.5). Most ganglion cells in goldfish retina are also sustained at absolute threshold (Falzett *et al.*, 1988). In cat, adaptation to a background within the scotopic range (that is, a dim background that does not render the retina 'light adapted') resulted in the emergence of transient responses from both cell types (Jakeila *et al.*, 1976). This result suggests again that background illumination may enhance cellular response.

Interestingly, spatial summation and linearity are not obviously affected by background levels, at least when these are very low (Linsenmeier & Jakeila, 1979), nor are there any obvious differences between X and Y cells in the changes brought about in receptive field organization by low background levels (Derrington & Lennie, 1982). Derrington & Lennie (1982) also showed that the optimum spatial frequency of both X and Y cells is invariant with adaptation level (Fig. 3.4).

A classification that has recently revealed clear differences in the effect of adaptation level on physiological response is based on the projections of retinal ganglion cells to the LGN. The primate LGN contains discrete cellular layers that are characterized by relatively large (magnocellular) or small (parvocellular) cell bodies. By recording synaptic potentials from ganglion cells within the LGN simultaneously with action potentials from intrinsic LGN cells, and using the eye of origin to determine which layer and thus which LGN cell type is being recorded, it is possible to determine whether a particular ganglion cell is presynaptic to an M type LGN cell or to a P type LGN cell. Kaplan & Shapley (1986) have recently used this technique to show that these two types of retinal ganglion cell have distinctly different properties when light adapted: cells presynaptic to LGN M cells are high in contrast sensitivity, while those presynaptic to LGN P cells are low.

It is the effect of adaptation to different luminance levels that concerns us here, and in very recent work Purpura, Kaplan & Shapley (1986, 1987) have examined the effect of mean luminance on the contrast gain and gain control of P and M cells in macaque monkey. They find that the gain of M cells while dark adapted is on average 100 times that of P cells, and that the amount of light needed to turn on the gain control mechanism was 10 times lower in M cells than in P cells. It would thus seem that M cells in monkey might be primarily responsible for vision at low luminances, because they amplify receptor signals more and they are more sensitive to light adaptation.

Much less is known about the effect of adaptation on temporal response, so the mechanisms of the effects that have been observed remain obscure. In cat retinal ganglion cells, increasing background luminance preferentially increases contrast sensitivity when temporal frequency is high; stimuli of constant spatial frequency but lower temporal frequency were less affected by changes in background luminance (Derrington & Lennie, 1982; Fig. 3.4). This selective effect was attributed to the improvement in temporal resolution of photoreceptors at relatively high luminances, as noted by Baylor & Hodgkin (1974).

Hopefully more physiological studies will be designed in future to address the important and interesting topic of spatiotemporal interactions during adaptation.

3.3.2 Lateral geniculate nucleus neurons

No full contrast sensitiviity functions exist at this writing for lateral geniculate neurons at different levels of adaptation. Bisti *et al.* (1977) measured response amplitude (number of spikes) as a function of spatial frequency for stimuli of constant contrast approximately 3 times threshold. They reported a reduction of contrast sensitivity and spatial resolution with decreasing background luminance, but their results are difficult to compare with later work because of their stimulus conditions.

One of the conclusions Bisti *et al.* (1977) drew was that the surround of geniculate cells was still present under dark adapted conditions, as Maffei & Fiorentini (1972) had concluded before them. Kaplan *et al.* (1979), using sinusoidal stimuli and measuring full contrast–response functions, showed that although the surrounds of LGN cells are certainly still present, they are 4–10 times less sensitive under dark adaptation. This value approached that of retinal ganglion cells measured in the same way (Kaplan *et al.*, 1979). The diminished influence of the surround under dark adaptation results, as it does in retinal ganglion cells, in an increase in the apparent size of the receptive field center. Kaplan *et al.* (1979) could not account quantitatively for the change in center size by either (*a*) a change in center–surround balance, which is probably the mechanism used by ganglion cells, or (*b*) phase differences between the responses of center and surround brought about by dark adaptation. They postulated that the apparent increase in center size that occurs in LGN cells is not apparent at all, but real, and they speculated that it may be related to an actual difference in anatomical pathways feeding LGN cells in light and dark. This possibility remains to be tested.

As in the retina, there are several different cell classifications in LGN (X, Y; ON, OFF; etc.), but any changes observed in LGN responses under dark adaptation seem to be independent of these classifications. They are not independent along the magnocellular–parvocellular dimension, but the differences observed are due to changes that occur at the retinal level (Kaplan & Shapley, 1986).

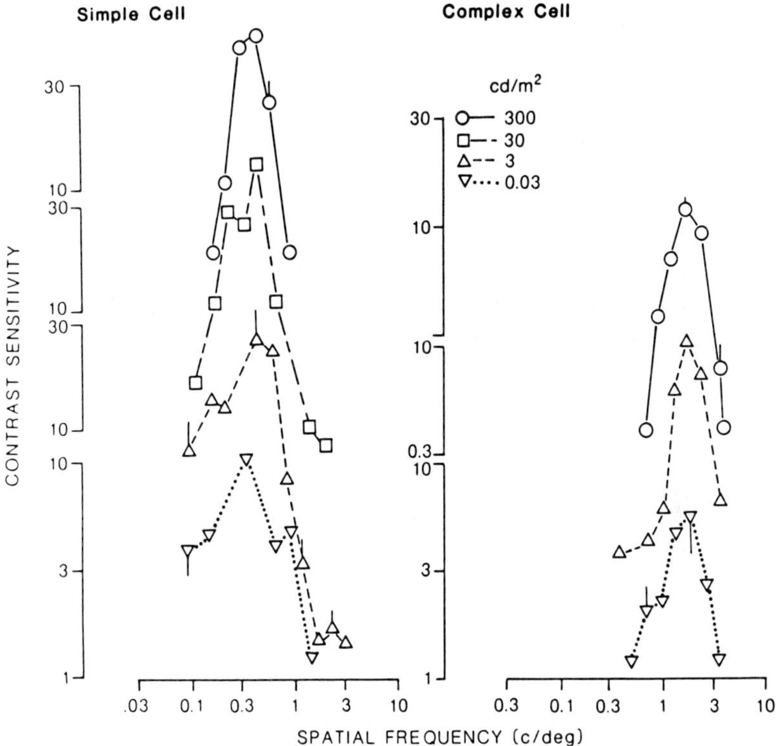

Fig. 3.6. Contrast sensitivity of a simple and a complex cell in cat retina shows that peak sensitivity declines with dimmer backgrounds, but there is no change in the overall shape of the functions or on their placement along the spatial frequency axis. Bisti *et al.* (1977) have shown that contrast response functions peak at lower spatial frequencies when backgrounds are dimmer than those used here. Unpublished data from a study by Hess & Lillywhite (1980).

3.3.3 Cortical neurons

Background illumination affects cortical neurons somewhat differently than LGN neurons. As is the case for LGN, no full contrast sensitivity functions have been published where mean luminance was a parameter, so the conclusions reached here must be tentative. Nonetheless the data that do exist suggest that cortical neurons, which are more narrowly tuned to spatial frequency than cells earlier in the visual pathway (Cooper & Robson, 1968; Campbell, Cooper & Enroth-Cugell, 1969; Tolhurst & Movshon, 1975; Movshon, Thompson & Tolhurst, 1978; DeValois, Albrecht & Thorell, 1982), have reduced contrast response and slight shifts in spatial frequency peaks but no overall change in the shape of spatial tuning curves (Bisti *et al.*, 1977) or contrast sensitivity functions (Hess & Lillywhite, 1980; Fig. 3.6, also see Figs 1.5, 1.6 and 1.19 in Chapter 1) as background illumination is decreased. The range of background luminances tested was larger in Bisti *et al.* (1977) than in Hess & Lillywhite (1980), and the peak shift toward lower spatial frequencies was consequently more obvious at the lower luminances than in Fig. 3.6. Simple and complex cells seem to respond similarly as background levels change, with the exception that complex cells are generally still responding to grating stimuli at mean luminances that are a log unit or more below threshold for simple cells (Bisti *et al.*, 1977). This finding is consistent with the idea that larger cells determine threshold at low luminances, and that as background luminance is increased more smaller cells are recruited (see Figs 1.3–1.5 for further evidence).

Although there are some changes in spatial tuning of cortical neurons as background level is changed, they are very small (see Fig. 1.19 for comparable temporal effects). The cortex thus seems to maintain its tuning properties over a wide range of mean luminances. This behavior probably serves to mediate findings like those of Graham (1972) and those displayed in Fig. 1.18, which show that spatial frequency channels are relatively invariant even in dim light.

3.4 Summary

In darkness the visual system is most sensitive to luminance as a stimulus dimension and much less sensitive to spatial variables. Background lights serve to desensitize the system to luminance but to increase its sensitivity to space, even within the scotopic range. The physiological mechanisms that underlie the changes in sensitivity in both domains reside in the retina. Within the luminance domain, high amplification of the signal by the post-receptoral network renders adaptation by the photoreceptors themselves unnecessary in the presence of dim backgrounds, but the network's sensitivity is decreased. The ability to maintain responding even when a background is present is due to a gain control mechanism beyond the receptors. At higher background levels, the receptors in non-primates also adapt.

The physiological mechanisms underlying changes in sensitivity to grating stimuli have been most extensively studied in ganglion cells, but they probably have their origins earlier in retinal processing. As background level changes, the relative sensitivities of the center and surround mechanisms of the ganglion cell change, resulting in apparent increases or decreases in receptive field center size, spatial frequency peak and cutoff, and contrast response. How the change in balance is itself mediated is not clear; one interesting possibility is that synaptic changes at the horizontal cell level may be responsible (Raynauld, LaViolette & Wagner, 1979).

Cells beyond the retina benefit from the adaptation mechanisms in retina but appear to have few of their own, at least in the stimulus realms considered here. Although the data base is small, we can conclude that LGN and cortical neurons do not change their response properties very much as light levels change, and the changes that are observed (such as cells with larger receptive fields showing higher sensitivity) can generally be attributed to processes that occur in the retina.

Acknowledgments

Work was supported by grants from the National Eye Institute (M. K. P. and D. G. G). We thank Dr A. B. Bonds for useful discussion, Dr Joseph Bilotta for reading an earlier version of the chapter, and Dr Robert Hess for providing Fig. 3.6.

4

Absolute sensitivity

Walter Makous

The direct observation of events within dark adapted primate rods, by Baylor, Nunn & Schnapf (1984), now offers data in place of conjecture and indirect inferences about processes that limit the absolute sensitivity of the human eye. New psychophysical data on influences over absolute sensitivity point in directions previously unexplored, and some of the less new data have never been fully exploited. Hence, it seems timely to revisit the classic question of absolute visual sensitivity. This effort leads to an improved estimate of the amount and sources of the noise that limits absolute sensitivity.

4.1 Basic concepts

Absolute sensitivity refers here to the ability of an observer to detect the presence of small amounts of light. This essay emphasizes the limits to that ability and skirts, as much as possible, related problems. It represents an attempt to go as far as possible with a minimum of assumptions, eschewing even those assumptions that may be *reasonable* if they are not *necessary*. The result is simple enough that mathematical notation can be avoided without loss of rigor.

Much is said here of noise, and yet most psychophysical work with noise during the past decade receives scant attention. Partly this results from the stricture on assumptions and partly from the fact that such work applies primarily to the photopic system, whereas the focus here is on the scotopic system.

One may be primarily interested in understanding visual function under ordinary conditions, and even so find that such understanding is fostered by use of a formal system that may be applicable only under artificial conditions. Such a formalism, adopted here, is information theory as introduced by Shannon (Shannon & Weaver, 1949); the artificial conditions to which it applies are the controlled conditions of an experiment. Presumably, the understanding so derived generalizes beyond the laboratory.

As the concept of noise is central to the ensuing discussion, and as its use is often ambiguous or misunderstood, a few words are devoted to it here. The concept is used here strictly in the context of an information system. Stripping the classic information system (Shannon & Weaver, 1949) of all but its essentials, it is defined here simply as a transmitter and a receiver with a channel of communication connecting the two. The state of the transmitter is defined by the experimenter's manipulation of the stimulus apparatus, and the state of the receiver is defined by the observer's response. Performance, i.e. transmission of information, is perfect if the receiver assumes a unique state for each state of the transmitter. If the state of the receiver (the observer's response) does not depend uniquely on the state of the transmitter (manipulation of the apparatus), the lack of perfect correlation is attributed to addition of noise, as originally defined by Shannon & Weaver (1949, p. 34). Insofar as noise is, by definition, unpredictable (if it were, the signal could be decoded), it is a chance variable, and it is often represented by stochastic processes. However, the word carries no necessary implications except that the response contains variability not inherent in the experimental manipulations, such as opening and closing the shutter. Specific sources of such noise, with particular properties, are considered separately below.

4.2 Light as a noisy carrier

Owing to the stochastic nature of light, a channel of communication that depends on the intensity of light is inherently noisy. For example, if the mean number of quanta passing through an aperture every time it is uncovered is 2, on 13.5% of the trials no quanta pass at all. As an ideal receiver might or might not detect light when the shutter is opened, the system contains noise.

4.3 Quantum detector with light loss

Turning now to the human scotopic system, we begin with the experiment of Hecht, Shlaer & Pirenne (1942) on the absolute sensitivity of the human eye, for it is prototypical. (It is so well known that it will not be summarized; see Chapter 2.) Barlow showed long ago (1956) that their data necessarily imply a source of noise within the observer. As Barlow defined noise more narrowly than here, and as his purpose was to characterize the noise and to make other points as well, not all readers have appreciated the robustness of this conclusion; that is, its independence of many of the assumptions and particular estimates made in that and subsequent papers on this topic.

The criterion for threshold used by Hecht *et al.* is detection of a stimulus on 60% of its presentations. If no noise arose within the observer, a response would be elicited from the observer on 60% of the trials by a stimulus that delivered a mean of 0.9 quanta per trial. This is below the 54–148 quanta delivered to the observers' corneas, and also below the 5–14 quanta that the authors estimated activated the observers' rods. More important, it is well outside the probable range of error in that estimate. Any noiseless system would yield a substantially higher correlation between stimuli (shutter openings) and responses, given any estimate of the mean number of effective quanta that is within established limits on the ratio of incident to effective light. Hence, by Shannon's definition, the system must be subject to noise other than that attributable to the quantum fluctuations of light.

It is worth mentioning parenthetically that if absolute sensitivity were limited by quantum noise, image intensifiers, which amplify the noise as much as the signal, would not improve vision. As they do dramatically improve vision (van Meeteren, 1978; also see Chapter 13 for more detail), they must fail to amplify part of the noise that limits performance, namely, the noise arising within the visual system.

4.4 Poisson noise

As Barlow (1956) pointed out, observers sometimes report a stimulus when none was presented; that is, they make false positive responses. This is attributable to noise. Barlow (1956) and others have suggested that one source of such noise might be quantum-like events that occur spontaneously. It is now established that primate rods are subject to such random spontaneous events that are indistinguishable from those caused by photons. Baylor *et al.* (1985) report that in monkey rods they occur in the dark at a mean rate of once every 160 s. As the frequency distribution of the number of such events within intervals of fixed duration follows a Poisson distribution, such noise is often referred to as Poisson noise, as it will be here (see also Chapter 6 for neurophysiology).

It is of interest to compare human light detection to an ideal quantum detector that is subject to such Poisson noise. One can then determine how much Poisson noise must be delivered to an ideal detector to degrade its performance to a level equivalent to that of the human. That amount of noise, sometimes called dark noise, will be denoted here as the *equivalent Poisson noise*, to emphasize its descriptive as opposed to theoretical origin.

4.4.1 Equivalent Poisson noise

Barlow estimated that the equivalent Poisson noise (as it is denoted here) in the experiment of Hecht *et al.* lay between 3.1 and 66 such events per trial. More recently, Prucnal & Teich (1982) reported estimates for four observers ranging from 8 to 36, with standard errors of the estimates ranging from 13 to 88. Estimates of equivalent Poisson noise based on psychometric functions, such as these are, depend on involved computations and evidently are not tightly constrained by the data. ROC (receiver operating characteristic) curves based on rating scales, such as those of Sakitt (1972), more tightly constrain inferences about both the distribution of noise and the estimates of its parameters. However, Sakitt's original paper did not make use of ROC curves, and a later analysis that did (Sakitt, 1974) was based on a fit of Gaussian functions instead of Poisson functions to the data. This is inappropriate, as Sakitt acknowledged, for both the quanta in the stimulus and the spontaneous quantum-like events must follow a Poisson distribution. Therefore, it has been necessary to analyze her data a third time, this time comparing the observed ROC curves with theoretical ROC curves derived on the basis of the Poisson processes that we know affected her observations. That analysis is presented below.

4.4.2 Estimate of noise in Sakitt's experiment

Description of experiment

The recent measurements of Baylor *et al.* (1984) allow a better estimate of the effective capture area of a primate rod, 1.2 μm^2, than has been available before. This value includes the optical aperture of the rod, its optical density, and the proportion of absorbed quanta that produce activations. Assume in addition: about 4% of the light is lost to reflection at interfaces; the density of the lenses of her observers at the wavelengths she used (470–520 nm) was about 0.15; there are 120 000 rods mm^{-2} at an

(a)

p(hit)

0.0 0.2 0.4 0.6 0.8 1.0

p(false positive)

0.0 0.2 0.4 0.6 0.8 1.0

(b)

p(hit)

0.0 0.2 0.4 0.6 0.8 1.C

p(false positive)

0.0 0.2 0.4 0.6 0.8 1.0

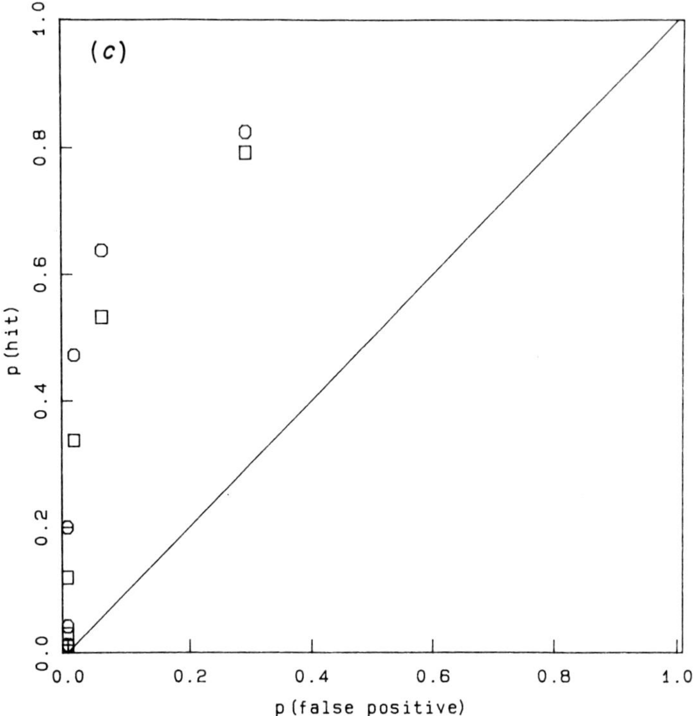

Fig. 4.1. ROC curves for Sakitt's (1972) three observers. Octagons represent the results with the stronger stimulus; squares, those with the weaker stimulus. Part (*a*), K.D.; part (*b*), L.F.; and part (*c*) B.S.

eccentricity of 7 deg in the temporal retina, where the test flash fell (a 29′ disk presented for 16 ms). According to these assumptions, stimuli containing a mean of 55 and 66 quanta (the stimulus intensities Sakitt used) would cause a mean of 5.3 and 6.4 physiological activations, respectively. Blank trials, of course, cause no activations.

Sakitt allowed her observers to grade their responses on each trial according to a seven step rating scale, where '0 meant that we did not see anything,' and '6 meant a very bright light.' As the observers made 7 different responses to the identical stimulus, noise (as defined above) clearly enters into their performance.

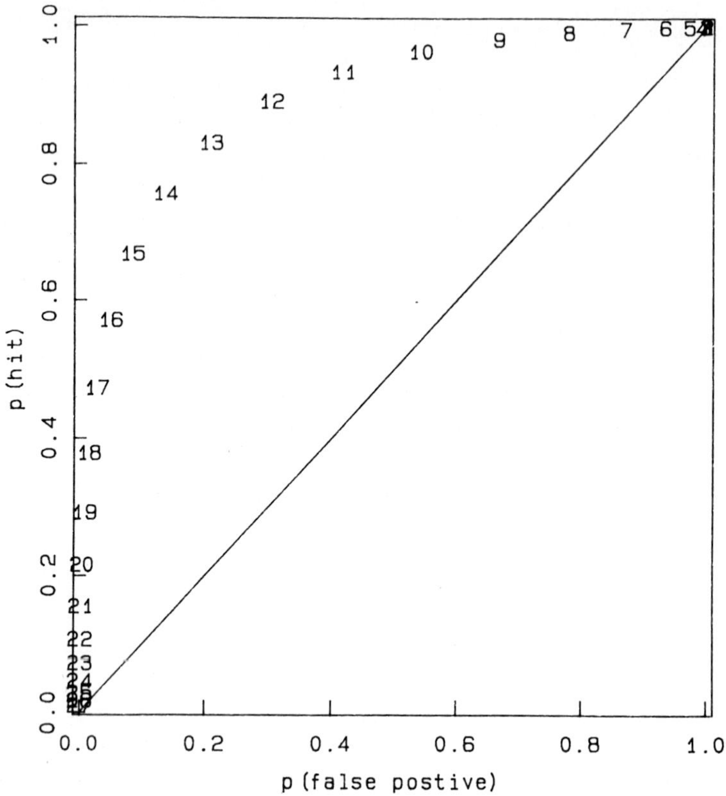

Fig. 4.2. Theoretical ROC curve for Poisson distributed signal and noise. The mean of the noise distribution is 10 events per trial, and the mean of the signal plus noise, 16.3 events per trial. The location of each numeral represents the hits and false positives corresponding to a criterion set at the number of events indicated by the numeral.

The data

Following conventional signal-detection theory, blank trials are assumed to reflect noise only, and trials in which the shutter was opened, signal plus noise. The data obtained by this seven-category rating scale are shown in Fig. 4.1 as conventional ROC curves, each point representing the proportion of responses of rating i or greater made on trials containing a signal (hits), versus those made on blank trials (false positives). Octagons represent results with the stronger stimulus; squares, those with the weaker stimulus.

Correspondence between theory and data

Fig. 4.2 is a theoretical ROC curve generated by a Poisson distribution of noise, with a mean of 10 events per trial, and a signal that is also Poisson distributed, adding a mean of 6.3 events per trial to the noise. Each symbol shows the probabilities of hits and false positives when the criterion corresponds to the numeral forming the symbol. For example, suppose the observer signaled a detection if and only if 14 or more events occurred on any given trial; then the probability of hits would be about 0.75, and the probability of false positives would be about 0.15. Juxtaposition of this curve with the data for the stronger stimulus in Fig. 4.1 would show that the two fit reasonably well. However, the viewer's evaluation of the fit is complicated by crowding of the points near the origin, and by unequal confidence intervals in different regions of the figure. Consequently, in Fig. 4.3, the probabilities, p, shown in Fig. 4.1 and 4.2, have been transformed into values, p', such that the 0.95 fiducial limits (according to X^2) are uniformly equal to 1 unit. (The transformation is:

$$p' = 0.51n^{0.5}\cos^{-1}(1 - 2p),$$

where n is the number of observations.)

The data presented in Fig. 4.3 (denoted by closed symbols) are from Fig. 4.1, and the upper set of numerals in Fig. 4.3*a* are from Fig. 4.2. So, a data point and a theoretical point separated by more than one unit differ from one another significantly. To assist the eye, lines corresponding to plus or minus the 0.95 fiducial limits are drawn about the data points. This transformation preserves the aspects of the ROC curve that are important here but eases evaluation of the correspondence between data and theory.

The theoretical ROC curves were derived according to the following assumptions.

(1) There is a source of Poisson noise not associated with light that generates a mean of n photon-*like* events per trial, i.e. an equivalent Poisson noise equal to n.

(2) The number of such events during the weaker stimulus follows a Poisson distribution with a mean of $n + 5.3$ events per trial.

(3) The number of such events during the stronger stimulus follows a Poisson distribution with a mean of $n + 6.4$ events per trial.

If these assumptions were true, then, except for statistical errors, each of the 32 points in the 6 curves of Fig. 4.3 would tend to lie within one

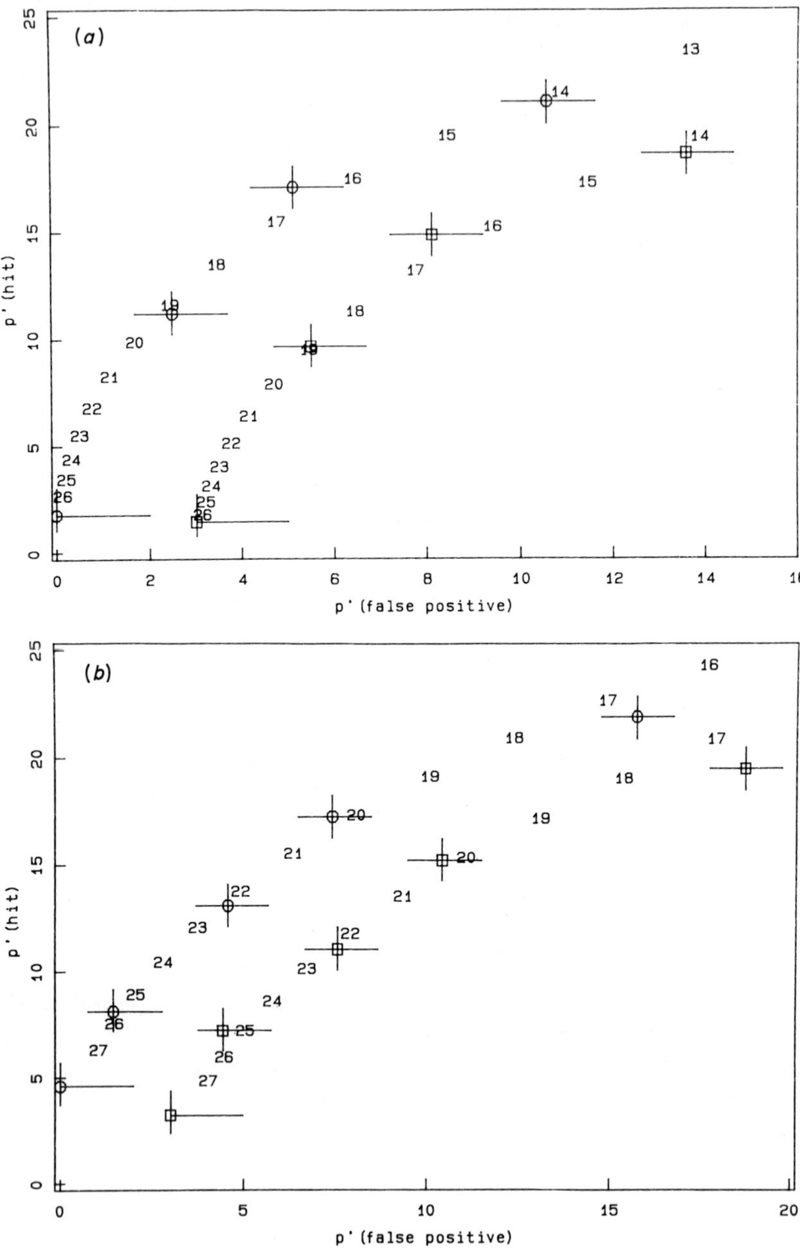

Fig. 4.3. Transformed ROC curves of Sakitt's (1972) three subjects and the best fitting theoretical ROC curves. The probabilities of a hit and a false positive have been transformed (see text) so that the fiducial limits span the same distance everywhere in the figure. The symbols follow the same conventions as

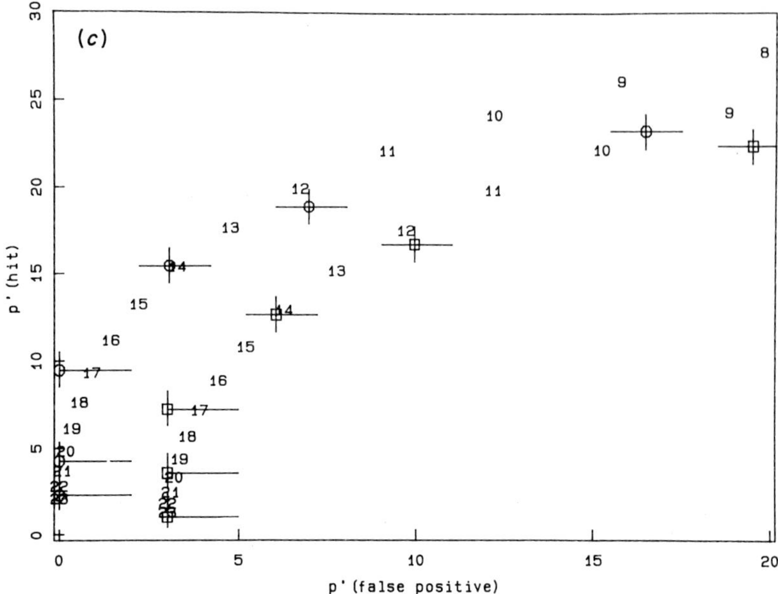

fiducial interval (half the length of the horizontal and vertical lines spanning the closed symbols) of a theoretical point, and corresponding points for the weaker and stronger stimulus would have to lie near corresponding points of the theoretical curve. That is, the criteria the observers use for the stronger stimuli must be the same as those they use for the weaker stimuli. As the assumptions above lead to discrete estimates, the constraints on the fit of data to theory are greater than they would be if the data were being fit to continuous curves. Note that there is but a single free parameter: n, the equivalent Poisson noise.

Table 4.1 shows the best-fitting theoretical values derived from the assumptions above for the three observers. 'Best n' is the best estimate of the equivalent Poisson noise; 'Range n' is the range of values that the equivalent Poisson noise can assume without significantly (0.05 level) increasing X^2; and 'Estimated criteria' is the estimated number of events corresponding to each observer's criterion at each of the 6 levels of detection (ratings 1–6).

Fig. 4.3 (*cont.*)

for Figs. 4.1 and 4.2. The squares and lower theoretical curve in each section have been displaced to the right by 3 units for clarity. The upper theoretical curve is based on the assumption that the noise follows a Poisson distribution with a mean of n events per trial, and signal plus noise is a Poisson distribution with a mean of $6.3 + n$ events per trial; and the lower theoretical curve is based on the assumption that the mean of the signal plus noise is $5.4 + n$ events per trial. The values of n are: part (*a*), 10; part (*b*) 14; part (*c*) 7. The lines spanning the data symbols represent the 0.95 fiducial limits.

Table 4.1

Obs.	Best *n*	Range *n*	Estimated criteria for ratings					
			1	2	3	4	5	6
K.D.	10	8–13	14	16	19	27	n.a.	n.a.
L.F.	14	9–17	17	20	22	25	28	—
B.S.	7	4–9	9	12	14	17	20	23

To illustrate the findings, the best interpretation of K.D.'s performance (Fig. 4.3*a*), according to the assumptions above, is that he was subject to an equivalent Poisson noise of 10 events per trial, and he responded according to the following criteria: '0' when 13 or fewer events occurred; '1' when 14 or 15 events occurred; '2' when 16–18 events occurred; '3' when 20–25 events occurred; and '4' when 26 or more events occurred. The other two responses were never used by this observer. Evidently, there are slightly too few false positives associated with a response of '1' to be consistent with a criterion of 16 events (and slightly too many hits to be consistent with a criterion of 17 events), but the deviation is not great.

In Fig. 4.3*b*, the theoretical point for a criterion of 28 events is not shown because of computational limitations; consequently, the estimate of a criterion of 28 events is made by extrapolation. For this observer the hit rate for category '1' with the weaker stimulus (squares) is slightly too low, but one such deviation is expected among 10 observations, each of which can deviate in either of two orthogonal directions.

The data of observer B.S. (Fig. 4.3*c*) show the greatest inconsistency with the assumptions: responses of '1' to both intensities of stimulation involved too few hits for a criterion of 9 events (and too many false positives for a criterion of 10 events).

Noise and signal-plus-noise distributions

Although evaluation of correspondence between theory and data may be best done with ROC curves such as are shown in Fig. 4.1 and 4.2, they do not always foster intuitive understanding. Fig. 4.4 presents the same results in a form that may be easier to appreciate. The histogram on the left represents the distribution of non-photon (noise) events per trial when the mean is 7. The two histograms on the right represent the distribution of events per trial when a mean of 5.3 (middle distribution)

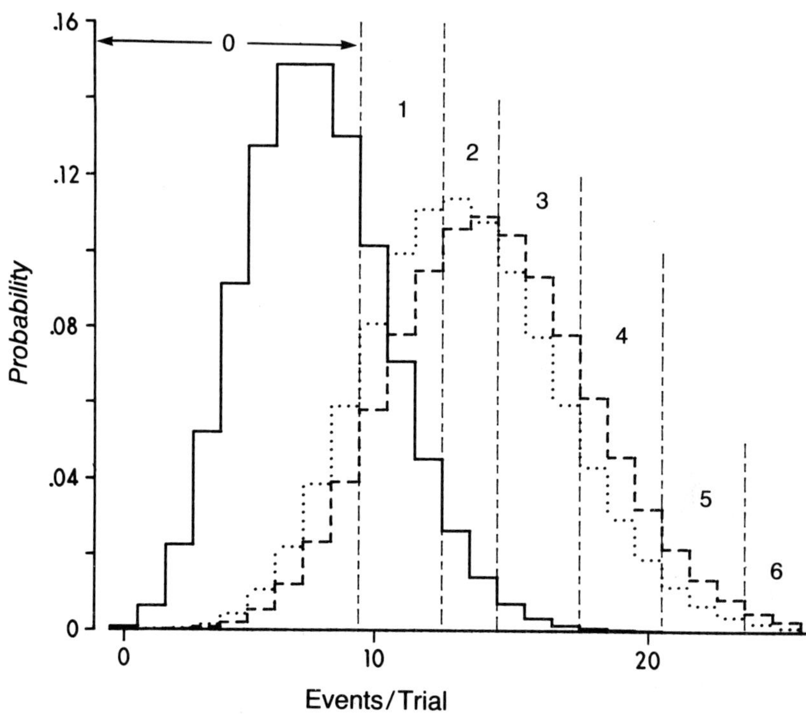

Fig. 4.4. Best fitting distribution of noise and signal plus noise for the two stimulus intensities of Sakitt (1972). Observer B.S. The vertical lines of dashes represent the best estimates of the criteria used by this observer. The mean of the noise distribution is 7 events per trial, the signal was 5.4 and 6.3 for the two distributions of signal plus noise.

or 6.4 (right distribution) effective quanta are added to the noise. Thus, the left distribution represents noise alone, and the other two represent the summed effects of signal and noise.

The dashed vertical lines represent the criteria of Table 4.1 for observer B.S. For example, if the number of events on a given trial (including both noise and any events elicited by the stimulus) were 8 or less, it is supposed that the observer gave a 0 rating; and if the number of events were more than 8, it is supposed the observer gave a rating greater than 0. The areas of the three distributions separated by the lines correspond to the observed response frequencies of observer B.S.; as the number of events per trial are discrete, the criteria separating response categories coincide with boundaries between integers, e.g. betweeen 8 and 9 events.

Comparison with other findings

The estimate of an equivalent Poisson noise of 7–14 events per trial falls in the lower range of Barlow's (1956) estimate of 3–66 events per trial, and overlaps with the lower end of Prucnal and Teich's estimate of 8–36 events per trial. However, the confidence limits here, 5–8 events per trial, are smaller than the standard errors of 13–88 events per trial in the latter study. The improvement is attributed to use of ROC curves based on rating scales as opposed to psychometric functions based on single-criterion thresholds.

Sakitt's first analysis (1972) of her own data yielded estimates of 0.36–1.2 events per trial, with unknown error (the fits were 'only fair'). However, these estimates depend on the unsupported assumption that the numeral the subject chose for a response was arithmetically equal to the number of rod activations on that trial. In her second analysis (Sakitt, 1974), based on the inappropriate assumption that both signal and noise have Gaussian distributions, the estimates of the number of noise events ranged from −0.677, significantly below zero in the statistical sense, to 0.41 events per trial.

Conclusions

To summarize this section, a model observer with a single free parameter, the equivalent Poisson noise, provides an approximate description of the performance of Sakitt's three observers. The best estimate of the equivalent Poisson noise for these observers varies from 7 to 14 quantum-like events per trial. However, the data cannot be entirely attributed to a noise of this kind, owing to a few observations that deviate reliably from the requirements of the model. Of course, even if the fit were perfect, it would not necessarily mean that an average of 7–14 quantum-like events per trial actually occurred in Sakitt's observers, for other models, more complex but perhaps more plausible, might also fit the data. Nevertheless, this is an economical and reasonably good description of the observers' performance, and the equivalent Poisson noise serves at least as an index of merit for the observers' performance.

4.4.3 Noise coincident with the stimulus

Let us minimize, for the present, the misfits of the model, and emphasize instead the degree to which the model describes human performance. It is worth considering the implications of a conclusion that the performance of Sakitt's observers is like an ideal quantum detector that is subject to a mean of 7–14 spontaneous, quantum-like events on each trial.

Any such events occurring within the image of the stimulus during its presentation would, by definition, be indistinguishable from those caused by the stimulus itself. The stimulus in Sakitt's experiment covered 0.83 deg^2, about 22000 rods. If these 22000 rods generated 7–14 spontaneous events in 16 ms, each would have to generate such events at the rate of once every 25–50 s. This interval is much shorter (that is, they occur at a faster rate) than the once every 160 s reported by Baylor *et al.* (1984) for monkey rods (the lower 0.95 fiducial limit of their estimate is once every 111 s). According to the physiological evidence, only 2 or 3 such events should have occurred per trial, not 7–14. Data from monkey rods, *in vitro*, may not apply to Sakitt's observers, but, supposing they did, to what could one attribute the extra noise in the human observer?

4.4.4 Spatio-temporal summation of noise

If noise in rods near the image of the stimulus or the effects of noise just before or just after the stimulus cannot be distinguished from events caused by the stimulus itself, then such events might contribute to the unassigned noise being sought. The data on the amount of noise attributable to such events are scarce. This is because the issue turns on *discriminating* events separated in time or space, not *summing* events over time and space. That is, an observer that is *able* to integrate information over a large area or time to detect a stimulus is not necessarily *forced* to do so. So use of data on Ricco's law or Block's law to infer the area and time over which noise must be summed is inappropriate, for the observer may be able to reject the noise if necessary. Zuidema *et al.* (1984) have shown that observers can *discriminate* a time separation of only 4 ms under conditions, similar to those of Sakitt's experiment, where quanta can be *summed* over hundreds of milliseconds to reach a threshold. Zacks (1970) has reported such paradoxical discrimination and summation under identical conditions.

By analogy in the spatial domain, Sakitt (1971) showed that observers can *discriminate* stimuli separated by 3.4′ at absolute threshold, even though the quanta can be *summed* over more than 30′ to bring a stimulus to threshold.

So, much of the signal that can be summed to reach threshold can also be discriminated. Therefore, much of the noise arising within these spatio-temporal boundaries presumably can also be discriminated from a more confined signal. Spatio-temporal discriminations at threshold seem to be so good that the undiscriminated noise that seeps over the spatio-temporal boundaries of the stimulus is probably too little to account for much of the extra noise implicated above.

4.4.5 Conclusion

Of the 32 data from Sakitt's experiment, 5 are inconsistent with the assumption that only spontaneous quantum-like events in the rods limit absolute sensitivity. This is supported by comparison of psychophysical evidence with the best physiological evidence available.

This is not new, having been examined many times since the classic study of Hecht *et al.* Barlow (1977) estimated that about half what is called noise here arises centrally, that is, in the brain. The evidence that has accumulated since then strengthens this conclusion.

4.5 Non-Poisson noise

Having concluded that there are other sources of noise, we turn next to the properties of this noise and the identity of its sources.

An initially attractive hypothesis is that some of this noise follows a Gaussian distribution: all practical communication systems are subject to a finite Gaussian noise, a consequence that follows from application of the central limit theorem to the manifold, independent sources of noise that exist within any such system; such noise has been observed in primate rods (Baylor *et al.*, 1984); and Sakitt (1974) concluded that Gaussian distributions fit her data even better than Poisson distributions. Computations confirm Sakitt's conclusion, but fit depends on use of four free parameters, the means and standard deviations of both noise and signal-plus-noise distributions; and it requires use of impossible results, such as a negative number of noise events. When Gaussian noise is added to Poisson noise, and the free parameters of the Gaussian distribution are restricted to the two related directly to the hypothesis, namely, the mean and standard deviation of the Gaussian noise, then any combination of Gaussian and Poisson noise fit worse than Poisson noise alone. Gaussian noise tends to flex the ROC curves toward symmetry, away from the direction of the deviations shown in Fig. 4.3.

It should perhaps be stated, parenthetically, that all computations were done by APL programs written by the author, that fit the data directly, without transformation, and weigh each deviation in proportion to the inverse of the standard error of the estimate. The programs use an iterative, 'hill-climbing' approach to find the set of parameters that fit best. Naturally, care was taken to avoid entrapment in local minima, and so forth.

So addition of Gaussian noise to Poisson noise can be excluded here as the principal cause of the deviations of theory from data, for it only increases the deviations. To fit the data, the distribution of added noise must be more skewed, not less skewed, than the hypothesized Poisson noise. That the Gaussian noise we know is present does not predominate may be attributed to its suppression by a process, proposed by Baylor *et al.*, that acts like a threshold, and to other mechansisms discussed below.

No plausible source of such noise exists at the periphery of the visual system. Suppose, however, that the signal (and associated noise) undergoes a logarithmic or other compressive transformation, like a saturating function. Symmetrically distributed noise (e.g. Gaussian noise) added *after* the transformation has the same effect as noise skewed in the appropriate direction added *before* the transformation.

Several authors have discussed evidence of a multiplicative noise in the visual system (Teich *et al.*, 1982; Lillywhite & Laughlin, 1979; Lillywhite, 1981; Massof, 1987; see also Chapter 6). Multiplicative noise, in itself, would fail to produce the required skew (Lillywhite, 1981). However, additive noise entering the system after a logarithmic or similar transformation has the same effect as multiplicative noise entering before the transformation. So a symmetrically distributed noise added to the signal after a compressive transformation can explain both the evidence of multiplicative noise and the failures of the Poisson model.

Of course, it is difficult to infer the effect of complex central or cognitive processes on the shapes of ROC curves. Such processes might cause the observed discrepancies with or without the assistance of a compressive transformation. In any case, noisc must certainly enter the system as the signal propagates from the rods and through the brain.

4.5.1 Noise entering proximal to the rods

Many things raise thresholds, but few demonstrably affect estimates of absolute threshold. There are, however, new lines of evidence that thresholds can be lowered below what would otherwise be considered an absolute threshold, by operations that cannot easily affect the rods directly. Therefore, these threshold-lowering operations remove a

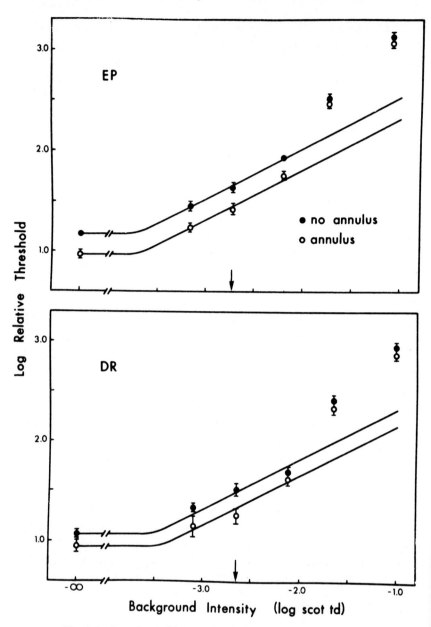

Fig. 4.5. Log threshold versus log background intensity. Test flashes were presented either in the absence of annuli (filled symbols) or 200 ms after session of a 300 ms (observer D.R.) or 500 ms (observer E.P.) annulus surrounding and contiguous to the location of the test stimulus. Theoretical curves (from Barlow, 1957) fitted by least squares to the four points furthest to the left. Brackets span plus and minus one standard error of the mean thresholds. The annulus lowered absolute thresholds by 0.2 log unit. (From Pulos & Makous, 1982.)

source of noise (according to the present definition) that acts proximal to the rods to raise the absolute threshold.

Let it be stated at the outset that none of these has been demonstrated under optimal conditions, such as those of Hecht *et al.* or even those of Sakitt. So it is not certain that any of these sources contribute to the unassigned noise discussed above. They remain, however, as interesting candidates especially because they have not been tested.

4.5.2 *A monoptic effect*

The upper curve of Fig. 4.5, from Pulos & Makous (1982), shows a typical threshold-versus-intensity curve. The test stimulus was a 2.5 deg disk of 530 nm light, presented for 20 ms, 7 deg temporal to fixation.

The lower curve shows the threshold under the same conditions, except that the test flash followed (by 200 ms) the removal of an annulus (2.5 deg inside and 9 deg outside diameter) surrounding the location of the test flash. The pairs of points on the extreme left show that removal of the annulus reduces the absolute threshold below its value when tested conventionally, with no annulus at all. As light in the annulus does not fall on the rods hit by light from the test flash, and with no plausible pathway for these effects to reach to those rods, the sensitizing effect of removing the annulus reduces *desensitizing* effects (noise) that act proximal to the rods themselves. Control experiments showed that the effect cannot be attributed to stray light or to reduction of uncertainty about the test flash.

4.5.3 *Binoptic effects*

Although the sensitization shown in the experiment of Pulos & Makous (1982) does not occur when the annulus is presented to the opposite eye, interocular interactions are not ruled out in that experiment. It is possible, for example, that the contralateral eye exerts a threshold elevating effect on signals from the test eye, and that the annulus temporarily reduces this effect. Several recent experiments mitigate the implausibility of this idea.

Fig. 4.6 shows a pair of dark adaptation curves from Makous, Teller & Boothe (1976). The test stimulus was a 1 deg disk presented for 20 ms, 5 deg temporal from fixation. The upper dark adaptation curve was obtained in the conventional way, with the fellow eye patched and in the dark, as in most experiments on dark adaptation and absolute threshold.

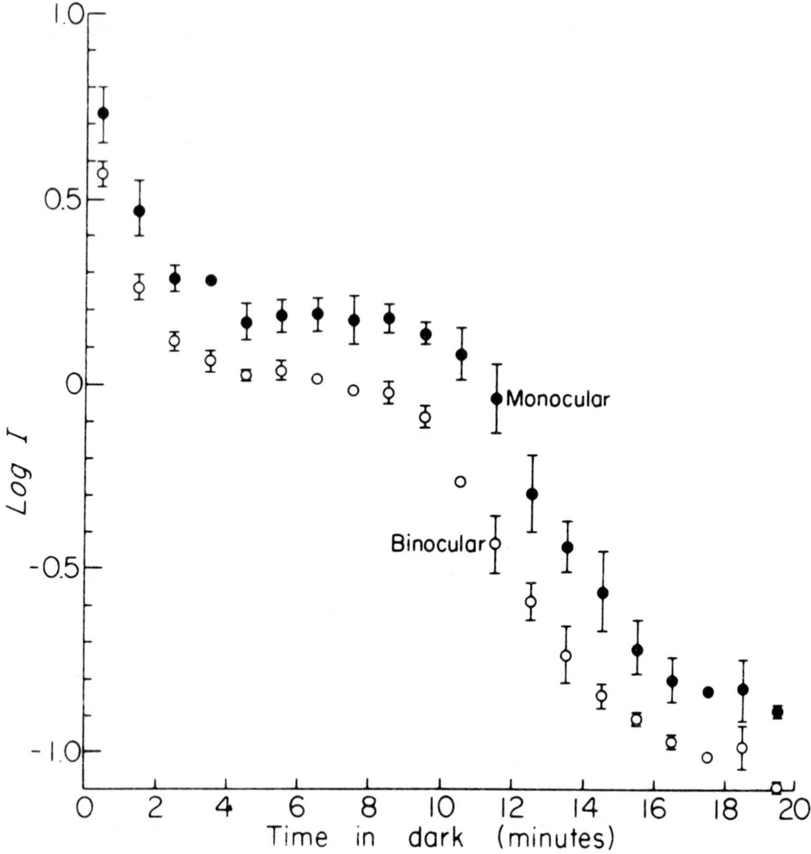

Fig. 4.6. Monocular dark adaptation following monocular (filled symbols) and binocular (unfilled symbols) light adaptation. (From Makous *et al.*, 1976.)

The lower curve was obtained following light adaptation of both eyes. This shows that light adapting one eye increases sensitivity (lowers threshold) to light entering the other eye.

Fig. 4.7 shows an example of the results of a similar experiment during which the fellow eye was briefly pressure-blinded. The dip in the upper dark adaptation curve illustrates the finding that pressure-blinding the fellow eye has the same effect as light adapting it. A dark adapted eye, then, qualifies as a source of noise that interferes with detection of signals elicited from the other eye. Evidently, both pressure blinding and light adaptation reduce that noise.

These experiments did not proceed to absolute threshold, for eventually the effect of light adapting the fellow eye must dwindle away. However, extrapolation of the dark adaptation curves in Figs 4.6 and 4.7

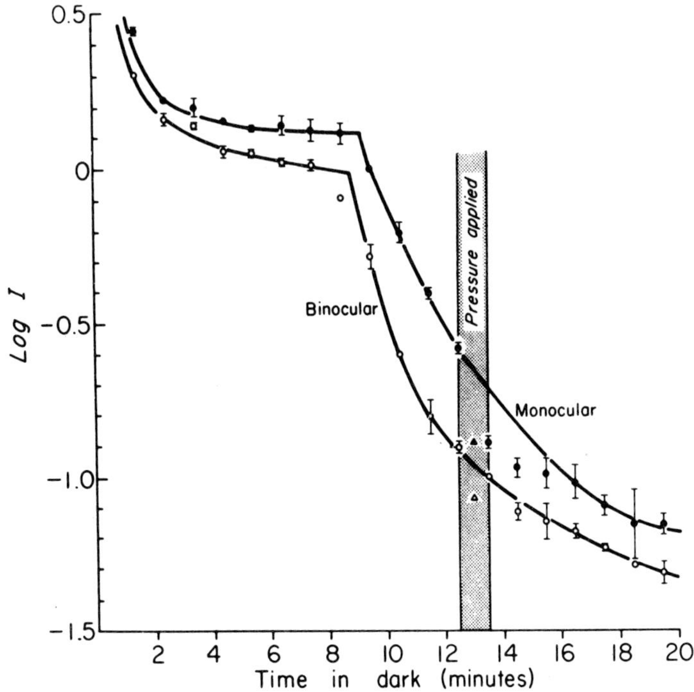

Fig. 4.7. Pressure blinding during dark adaptation after monocular (filled symbols) and binocular (unfilled symbols) light adaptation. The eye tested was light adapted in both conditions, and pressure was applied, during the shaded interval, to the eye not tested. Brackets span plus and minus one standard error of the thresholds when they were larger than the symbols themselves. (From Makous *et al.*, 1976.)

might lead one to speculate that the pair of curves in each of these figures do not approach the same asymptote. Fig. 4.8 shows the result of an unpublished test of that possibility. It shows the thresholds of the same observer under the same conditions. However, all thresholds were obtained after both eyes had been in the dark for more than an hour. Each point represents the mean of the thresholds obtained by the method of adjustment over a period of 5 min, and the bars represent plus or minus one standard error of the mean. Evidently light adaptation of the fellow eye temporarily lowers the threshold (increases the sensitivity) of the test eye. The white and black symbols represent two different runs, in which 5 min rest periods occurred at different times, establishing that the process of measuring the thresholds did not affect the thresholds. (In the run represented by the black symbols, the observer rested during the periods from 10 to 15 min after the beginning of light adaptation, and

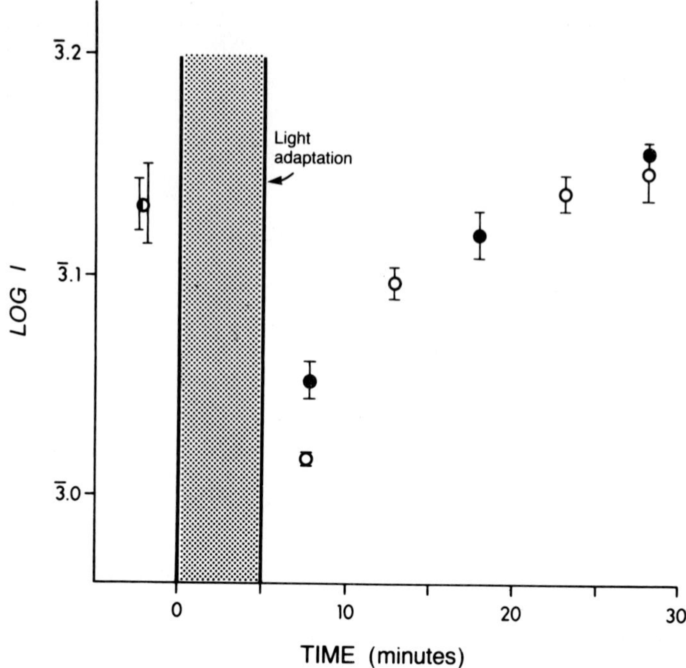

Fig. 4.8. Absolute threshold after contralateral light adaptation. The filled and unfilled symbols represent mean thresholds during intervals of 5 min, with different periods of rest. The brackets indicate plus and minus one standard error of the mean threshold.

from 20 to 25 min after light adaptation. In the other run, the observer rested during the period from 15 to 20 min after the beginning of light adaptation.)

These results are not wholly convincing in themselves, but they have been independently observed by Auerbach & Peachey (1984), and by Reeves, Peachey & Auerbach (1986). Fig. 4.9, from Auerback & Peachey, shows thresholds for both eyes of an observer before and after light adapting one eye. The panel at the extreme left shows the thresholds after both eyes have been dark adapted. While light adapting the right eye raises thresholds, as expected, the thresholds in the contralateral eye simultaneously decrease (next panel). The following panel shows the same effects with conditions reversed for the two eyes. Finally, the last panel traces dark adaptation under the original conditions until it returns to the preadapted state in both eyes.

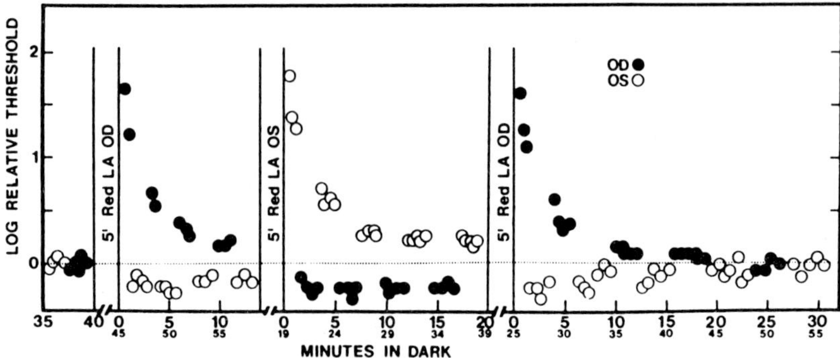

Fig. 4.9. Thresholds of both eyes, in absolute darkness, after monocular light adaptation. (From Auerbach & Peachey, 1984.)

4.6 The nature of the centrally acting noise

This is evidence, then, that not all the noise that limits absolute thresholds comes from the immediate neighborhood of the test flash. In the cases summarized in the last section, it comes from the other eye altogether. As stated above, this possibility cannot be excluded even in the monoptic example (from Pulos & Makous, 1982), for the annulus could leave a brief after-effect that interferes with the noise originating from the contralateral eye.

The most plausible explanation of these interocular effects is that noise arising from the contralateral eye is mixed with that from the test eye. As noise originating from opposite eyes presumably is uncorrelated, according to the simplest assumption it should raise the threshold in proportion to the square root of 2. This seems not enough to account for the entire unexplained noise.

However, the visual system may not mix noise in the way that linear systems do. When two uncorrelated signals enter opposite eyes, observers usually report the phenomenon of binocular rivalry, and, at the same time, the threshold for test flashes presented to the suppressed eye rises about 300%, i.e. half a log unit (Wales & Fox, 1970), not merely by the 40% dictated by addition of uncorrelated noise. Whether the mechanism of rivalry is disabled in the dark is not known. Makous *et al.* (1976) speculated that it might not be. Evidently a dark adapted eye can enter rivalry with a stimulated eye (Makous *et al.*, 1976; Rozhkova, Nickolayev & Shchadrin, 1982; Bolanowski & Doty, 1987). When neither eye is externally stimulated, experimental test of the idea is complicated by the difficulty of determining which is dominant and which suppressed at any given instant. Nevertheless, an indirect test for this idea is possible by examining the shape of the psychometric function.

4.6.1 Psychometric functions

If an eye fluctuates between a dominant and suppressed state, its sensitivity also fluctuates between two states differing by about a factor of three. If test flashes are presented willy nilly during both states, as they generally must be, the psychometric function is the sum of two psychometric functions separated by about half a log unit, each being associated with separate states of rivalry. The sum of two such curves might be expected to show three inflections instead of one: a negative inflection associated with each of the underlying curves, and a positive inflection between the two. Differentiation of the psychometric function should show two modes separated by about half a log unit.

That such curves are rare may be taken as evidence against the present hypothesis, except for two things: (1) few psychometric functions contain enough points and enough precision to show all the inflections; and (2) changes of sensitivity during the experiment would tend to smooth out the curves and obscure the inflections.

Exceptions to (1) above are contained by the paper of Teich *et al.* (1982), who reported 7 psychometric functions of 10 points each, under the conditions of Hecht *et al.* (1942). The octagonal points connected by a solid line in Fig. 4.10 show the means of the points in these psychometric functions after the curves have been aligned with respect to the threshold parameter, *t*, of the authors' model. As the curve consists of discrete points, it cannot be differentiated, but the corresponding difference function is shown in Fig. 4.11 by the octagonal points.

The reliability of the result is marginal, but it is not inconsistent with a bimodal curve with peaks separated by half a log unit. Confidence in this interpretation is strengthened by the fact that the data fall reliability below the theoretical curve, a curve with 4 free parameters, at lower intensities, and consistently above the curve at higher intensities, as it would if the curve were a composite of the two psychometric functions hypothesized here. These deviations of data from theory, with their standard errors, are shown in Fig. 4.12.

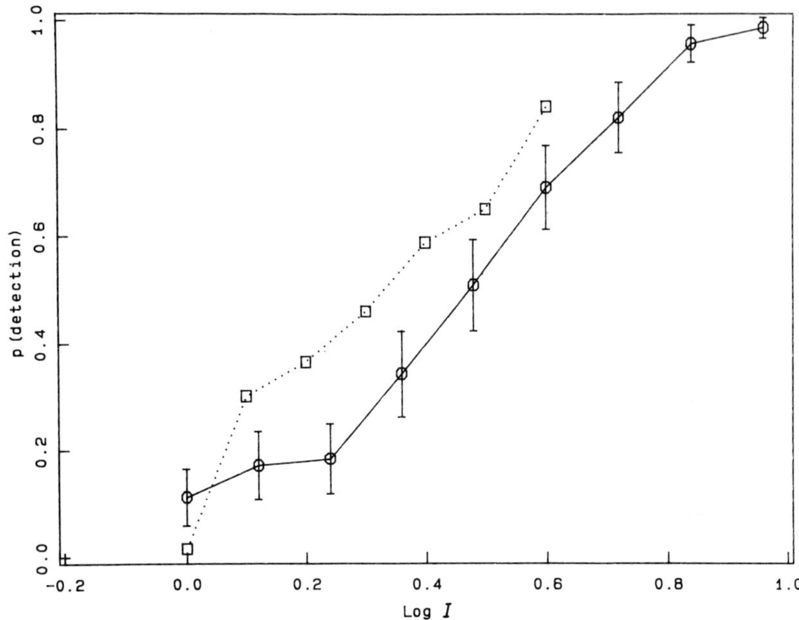

Fig. 4.10. Psychometric functions. The data represented by octagons are from Teich *et al.* (1982), and data represented by squares are from unpublished observations of the author. The brackets span plus and minus one standard error of the mean of the seven observers, after adjustment on the abscissa to align the observers' thresholds. The standard errors of the other data, which are approximately 0.07, are omitted to avoid clutter. The ordinates of the squares are adjusted so that chance performance (25% correct) corresponds to zero. The abscissae for both curves are arbitrary.

Even if the bimodality of this curve be accepted, the interpretation offered here might be questioned, for an average of the data from two sessions each from seven observers, could produce spurious results resembling these if there were substantial differences of sensitivity between sessions or between observers (although the adjustment of the curves with respect to the threshold parameter should minimize danger of the latter). To obviate such problems, the psychometric function shown in Fig. 4.10 by the squares were obtained (unpublished). The observer and conditions are the same as those of Fig. 4.8. The task was four-alternative forced choice, in which the 7 intensities of test flash were randomly distributed within 7 blocks of 42 trials each. Thus, each point represents 42 trials. All observations were made in a single session, and performance during the individual blocks showed that sensitivity was stable among blocks of trials. To ease comparison of the data with those

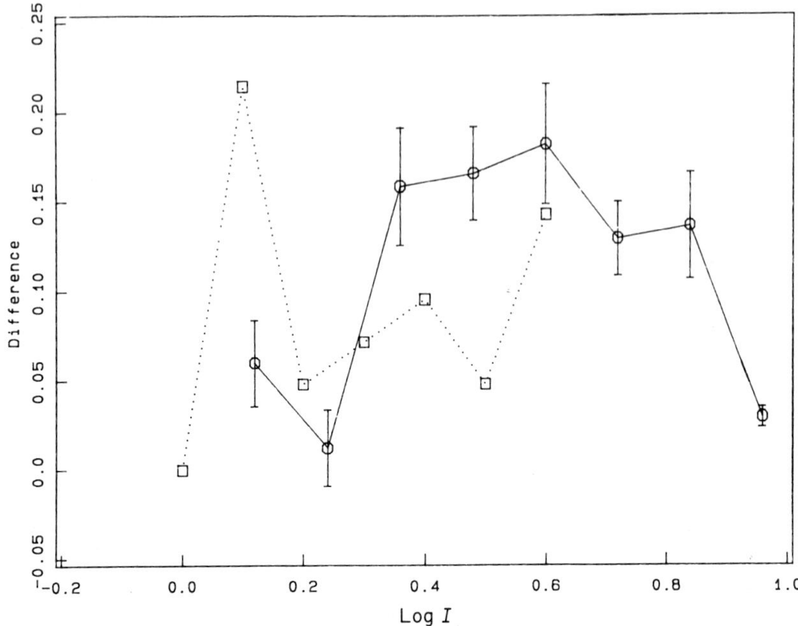

Fig. 4.11. Differenced psychometric functions. The ordinate of each point represents the difference between adjacent pairs of points in Fig. 4.10. The brackets represent the standard errors of the means of the corresponding differences for each of the seven observers of Teich *et al.* (1982). The standard errors of the means represented by the squares, which are omitted, are about 0.10.

of Teich *et al.*, they are plotted so that zero on the ordinate corresponds to chance performance (25% correct). (The position on the abscissa is arbitrary.) In Fig. 4.11 the squares connected by lines of dots is the differenced curve. Although an F test of these differences is significant ($p < 0.01$), the reliability of the individual features of the curves is marginal. The point at the extreme right represents a true maximum, for the psychometric function at this intensity is so close to the upper asymptote that differences represented by any points to its right must quickly approach zero. The two maxima of this curve, if they be accepted as reliable, do differ by about half a log unit.

In conclusion, although the data of Figs. 4.10 and 4.11 are not strong support of the possibility that absolute thresholds fluctuate between two states differing by half a log unit or so, neither are they inconsistent with it. The mechanism of binocular rivalry deserves to be considered a possible source of noise in monocular tests of absolute threshold.

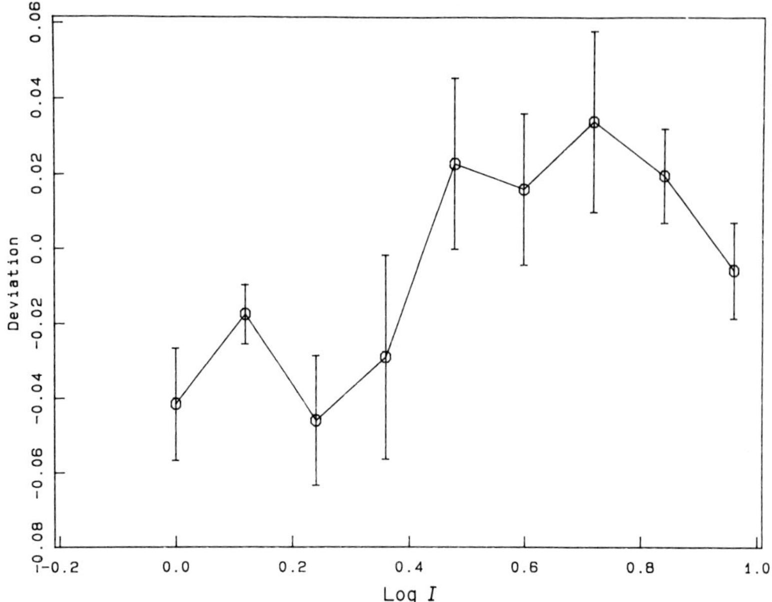

Fig. 4.12. Mean differences between the data of the seven observers of Teich *et al.* (1982) and the corresponding theoretical curves. Brackets represent plus and minus the standard error of the differences.

4.6.2 Direct tests of rivalry

If the sensitivities of opposite eyes alternate during tests of absolute threshold, it might be thought that a direct test of such alternation would be possible. If the sensitivity of one eye is depressed at any given instant by rivalry, the opposite eye must be at its most sensitive. Binocular presentation of test flashes should always find one or the other eye at its most sensitive, and comparison of binocular detections with monocular detections should show differences reflecting any underlying alternations of sensitivity. Such experiments are considered tests of binocular summation. Any such summation must be compared to the effects of probability summation, which requires no physiological interpretation and would occur even if the two eyes belonged to different observers (Pirenne, 1943).

Most treatments of probability summation assume that the eyes are mutually independent. If more binocular summation is observed than can be attributed to probability summation between independent detectors, then direct neural summation or facilitation of the signals from the two eyes is inferred. However, no such neural interaction between signals is required if the sensitivities of the two eyes is not independent but is *negatively* correlated, as is hypothesized here. Thus, the typical finding (Blake & Fox, 1973; de Weert, 1984), of super-summation, i.e. summation exceeding probability summation between independent detectors, is ambiguous, allowing either or both of two interpretations: negative correlation between the sensitivities of the two eyes, or neural summation of signals elicited from the two eyes by the test flash.

Perhaps a more complex experiment might unconfound these interepretations. Makous & Sanders (1978) attempted to by presenting simultaneous, spatially separate pairs of flashes, sometimes both in the same eye, and sometimes one to each eye. The rationale is that detection of a subthreshold flash (approximately 0.3 probability of seeing when presented monocularly), means that the eye to which it was presented is likely to be in its more sensitive state; consequently, presentation of a second flash to the same eye, close enough to be in the same state of rivalry but far enough to be distinguished, allows a test of the sensitivity of an eye that is likely to be in the dominant state of rivalry. Conversely, if the second flash is presented to the opposite eye instead of the same eye, it is likely to fall on a suppressed retina. So the frequency of reports of single as opposed to double flashes in the two instances provide a basis for estimating the correlation of sensitivities between the two eyes. Quantitative evaluation of the results is complicated by fluctuations of sensitivity common to both flashes, by other fluctuations that might be specific to a given retinal location, and by false positive responses. Although these complications are involved, they are tractable. What proved *not* to be tractable in this experiment is the very problem encountered with binocular summation experiments, namely, neural interactions between signals from the two test flashes. Test flashes presented close enough together to fall within the same domain of dominance also seem to interact neurally. If enough degrees of freedom were introduced in the experiment to evaluate all the probable interactions, either the propagation of error in the resulting computations obliterates the required precision, or the number of observations required vitiates the necessary assumption of ergodicity.

Another problem with such experiments must be mentioned. Unless eye position is monitored, fixation targets must be presented to both eyes to enable presentation of stimuli to corresponding locations on opposite retinas, and in a position that minimizes the observer's uncertainty.

Whether such fixation stimuli affect the mechanism of rivalry being investigated is not known.

So a direct test of the hypothesis of rivalry in the dark poses a challenge for future investigators.

4.6.3 Other candidates

No doubt undue emphasis has been placed here on binocular rivalry to the exclusion of other, perhaps more probable sources of noise, such as the observer's uncertainty about the stimulus (cf. especially Pelli, 1985), variability of the observer's criterion, and other limits imposed by the observer's decision processes. However, these other sources of noise are already receiving attention, but the influence of the patched eye in putatively monocular experiments has received less attention than it may deserve. Perhaps a moral may be permitted: covering an eye does not block its noise.

4.7 Neural noise

The data discussed above, on what has been called the unassigned noise, are entirely psychophysical. Attempts are sometimes made to evaluate such noise by observing the variability of discharge of individual neurons while environmental conditions are held as nearly constant as possible. Relating the results of such observations to performance of the psychophysical observer is complicated by two problems: (1) ignorance of the code used by the communication system (i.e. the nervous system); and (2) ignorance of the correlations of discharge among the neurons affecting the behavior.

4.7.1 Neural filters

Most analyses of signal and noise in spiking neurons depend on the assumption that the signal is encoded by the rate of discharge by the neurons. However, at and near absolute threshold, responses of ganglion cells to individual quantum-like events consist of bursts of 2 or 3 impulses (Barlow, Levick & Yoon, 1971; Mastronarde, 1983*b*). If the pattern of impulses is put through a filter, or decoder, that responds only to bursts of impulses, then the state of the receiver of the communication system is unaffected by individual impulses, and the variability of such impulses does not qualify as noise. Insofar as behaviour is concerned, then, noise in neurons cannot be evaluated without knowing the filters or coding scheme applicable to the neurons.

4.7.2 Correlations among neurons

The signal encoded by the discharge of an individual neuron, and the associated noise, are relevant for performance of the psychophysical observer only if that performance depends on the cell observed, or on one like it. If performance depends on signals and noise in more than one cell, it depends on the relative correlation of signal and noise in all the cells affecting the behavior, and on how the discharge of these cells combines to determine behavior.

If the correlation between the activities in two cells is different, i.e. either greater or less, during the response to a stimulus than it is in the absence of a stimulus, then more signal can be extracted from the noise in the pair of cells than appears possible from observation of either cell alone.

In the simplest case, imagine that in the absence of any stimulus, an increase in the activity of one cell is accompanied by an equal decrease in that of the other cell and vice versa, whether through a sign inverting synapse between a source of noise and one of the cells, reciprocal inhibition, or any other mechanism. Then, if a third cell sums the activity of the first two, its activity must be constant in the face of any amount of variability in the other two cells. And if, for any reason, the correlation between the responses of the two cells *to a stimulus* is anything other than the perfect negative correlation existing in the absence of a stimulus, then the activity of the summating cell contains a finite signal and no noise: that is, the signal-to-noise ratio is not limited by the noise in the individual cells. The signal-to-noise of a cell that sums the activity of two other cells is greater than that of either cell whenever the correlation between the responses of the two cells to a stimulus is greater than the correlation of their spontaneous activity.

Conversely, if the correlation between the responses of two cells to a stimulus is *less* than that of their spontaneous activity, a cell that is post-synaptic to both cells has a greater signal-to-noise ratio than that of either cell if it takes the difference of the activities in those two cells, i.e. if one cell is excitatory and the other inhibitory. Only if the correlations between the activities of two cells is identical in the stimulated and unstimulated state is it impossible to increase the signal-to-noise ratio by subsequent processing.

All combinations of correlations during responses and spontaneous activity of ganglion cells have been reported (Mastronarde, 1983*a*, *b*, *c*; Ginsburg, Johnsen & Levine, 1984). Evidently, this is due to differing amounts of common, as opposed to private, sources of signal and noise for different pairs of cells (Ginsburg *et al.*, 1984); to differing sign inverting networks between such sources and the individual cells; and to electrical coupling between ganglion cells that communicates noise between all types of cells but enhances responses between pairs of on-cells to quantum-like events in the rods (Mastronarde, 1983*c*).

Ginsburg *et al.* (1984) attribute less than 20% of the noise in light adapted goldfish ganglion cells to a common source, but the proportion is likely to be greater in the activity of dark adapted mammalian ganglion cells (Mastronarde, 1983*a*, *b*), which is dominated by the spontaneous, quantum-like events in rods (Mastronarde, 1983*b*). In these preparations, the overlap of receptive fields causes a high correlation among responses to rod activations in neighboring cells, and most of the other noise tends to be uncorrelated. Since it has not been possible to record activity in dark adapted ganglion cells in the absence of spontaneous rod activations, it has not been possible to correlate quantitatively ganglion cell activity not elicited by rod activations, i.e. what has been called here the unassigned noise.

So, the neurophysiological observations of greatest relevance to behavioral manifestations of noise entail simultaneous observations of at least two neurons both in the presence of stimuli (to evaluate correlations between signals) and in the absence of stimuli (to evaluate correlations of the noise). Obvious as it may seem, it is worth noting that the conditions and species used for physiological observations should be at least similar, if not identical, to those of the psychophysical observations that the physiology is used to explain.

4.8 Summary

This essay begins with an exploration of the conclusions about the sensitivity of the human scotopic system enabled by a minimum of assumptions. Whatever raises threshold above that of an ideal detector is defined as noise. Comparison of Sakitt's classic data (1972) to ROC curves in which both signal and noise are Poisson distributed shows that the variance in the performance of 3 observers can be reasonably described by a single quantity, defined as the equivalent Poisson noise. Estimates of this noise for these observers are 7, 10, and 14 events per trial, with 0.95 fiducial limits of 4–9, 8–13, and 9–17. The number of spontaneous quantum-like events observed in monkey rods are consistent with no more than 3 such events within the temporal and spatial boundaries of the stimulus. Psychophysical data on the ability to discriminate (not sum) signals outside these limits from those within them excludes spatial and temporal integration of noise as the explanation of the difference. Gaussian distributed noise is rejected as a large component of the unassigned noise. Evidence that absolute thresholds can be lowered by manipulations of distant rods, and by manipulations affecting only the fellow eye, implicate noise distant from the site of the stimulated receptors. However, simple addition of noise from candidate sources also cannot account for the unexplained noise. Binocular rivalry in the dark is examined, through the shape of psychometric functions, as a possible source of some of this noise and remains a possible candidate. The essay ends with discussions of impediments to a test of this hypothesis, and of limitations that neural filters and correlated activity in ensembles of cells impose on efforts to draw inferences about behaviorally significant noise from the activity of individual neurons.

Acknowledgements

I thank Denis Pelli for many helpful comments on an early draft, and Lewis O. Harvey for pointing out an embarrassing error. This work was supported by NIH grants EY-04885 and EY-1913.

5

Dark adaptation: a re-examination

T. D. Lamb

5.1 Introduction

The visual system, both in the human and in other vertebrates, functions effectiveiy over an enormously wide range of intensities, from starlight to bright sunlight, a range of about 10 log units. Obviously there must exist mechanisms which permit the visual system to attain extreme sensitivity at the dimmest levels of lighting, yet which avoid saturation and work effectively at very high light levels. This ability to 'adapt' to the ambient level of illumination is of fundamental importance to vision.

One mechanism permitting the wide range of operating levels is the use of a duplex receptor system, with rod photoreceptors specialized for operation at extremely low light levels and cone photoreceptors designed for operation at much higher levels. In this way each system need only function over the more restricted range of about 5 log units of intensity. Nevertheless, even this operating range of 100000:1 in each system is impressively wide, and indicates that both the scotopic (rod) and photopic (cone) systems have a very powerful ability to adapt to the ambient lighting level.

To bring about these adaptational changes the degree of amplification in the overall visual system must be altered, and the retina apparently possesses an *automatic gain control* to achieve this. In the photopic system, much of the gain control occurs within the cone photoreceptors themselves. In contrast, although considerable gain changes occur within the rod photoreceptors, the scotopic system appears to achieve its automatic gain control mainly through post-receptoral mechanisms.

5.1.1 Light adaptation versus dark adaptation

From the outset it is convenient to distinguish two rather different phenomena which are both referred to as adaptation, and which may be confused.

Light adaptation (synonymous with *background adaptation* or *field adaptation*) refers to the ability of the visual system quickly to establish a new steady state of visual performance when the incident level of illumination changes. Such intensity changes may either be *increases* or *decreases* in illumination; in both cases a new operating point is reached within seconds, provided the intensity change is restricted to a few log units (e.g. Crawford, 1947).

The term *dark adaptation*, as used here, is synonymous with *bleaching adaptation*. It refers not simply to the behaviour observed after a reduction in light level, but is instead reserved for the special case of recovery following the cessation of extremely intense illumination, which has 'bleached' a substantial fraction (say more than 0.1%) of the photopigment in the receptors. This recovery may be extremely slow. For example, following exposure to a very intense light bleaching 90% of the rhodopsin, one's visual sensitivity is initially enormously depressed and only recovers to its final dark-adapted level after some 40 minutes.

5.1.2 Analogies of visual adaptation

As an analogy of visual adaptation it is helpful to consider the operation of a television receiver. In a television set an *automatic gain control* (AGC) circuit automatically adjusts the receiver's sensitivity very rapidly in approximately inverse proportion to the signal strength, so that a picture of similar contrast is obtained for stations of very different signal strengths. In this way the output of the television set, the picture, is given by the *modulation* of the transmitted signal rather than by the absolute strength of the signal received. For a weak station the gain of the amplifiers in the television set is high and the picture may appear noisy, while for a strong station the gain is greatly reduced and relatively noise-free reception is obtained.

In much the same way, background adaptation acts automatically and fairly rapidly to adjust visual sensitivity approximately in inverse proportion to the mean light intensity. This has the consequence that early stages in visual processing detect *contrast* (or modulation) in the visual scene. As has been pointed out by Shapley & Enroth-Cugell (1984), such contrast coding may be of immense importance to the visual system. Most of the visual scenes which we normally encounter involve *reflecting* objects. In a scene composed of reflecting objects and illuminated by a single source, the contrast in the scene is independent of the intensity of illumination. Extraction of information about contrast in the retinal image means that, for such scenes, the signals sent from the retina to the brain will not depend on the ambient level of illumination. In this way the brain may be presented primarily with information about the scene, rather than with information about the light level.

In terms of the television receiver analogy, dark adaptation would correspond to the situation of tuning from an extremely powerful local station to a very weak distant station and finding (to one's surprise) that it was necessary to wait a long time for the receiver to resensitize so that a picture could be obtained. Obviously, the manufacturer of a television receiver with this kind of performance would be likely to have some trouble selling it, and one is left wondering why such an undesirable property should be built into the visual system. One attractive possibility is to suppose that the slowness of dark adaptation represents an unavoidable consequence of some other important property of visual transduction; perhaps it is a consequence of the particular biochemistry needed to obtain the enormously high sensitivity of the rod photoreceptors.

An alternative analogy of visual adaptation is represented by the television *camera*. Such a camera has an *automatic light control* (ALC) which rapidly compensates for changes in the scene illumination in order to provide an output signal which represents contrast in the scene rather than the absolute level of illumination. The television camera, however, differs from the visual system in a major respect, in the mechanism whereby this automatic light control is achieved. In the case of a conventional television camera, control is achieved primarily by means of varying the aperture of the lens, i.e. the size of the iris. In this way the amount of illumination falling on the light-sensitive image tube is held reasonably constant over a wide range of scene illumination levels. Our visual system, on the other hand, has available only a quite restricted range of pupil size (from 2 to 8 mm dia.) and most of the gain control is exercised at the level of the retina itself, as will be explained later. (A similar approach has recently been implemented in modern CCD cameras, where the image summation time can be regulated.)

In terms of the television camera analogy, dark adaptation would correspond to the situation of exposing the camera to intense illumination (such as an electronic flash or a focused image of the sun), and finding subsequently that the camera only very slowly recovered its ability to generate signals under dim lighting conditions. Such behaviour is in fact quite characteristic of certain television camera tubes. Some may be permanently damaged by extremes of illumination, while most exhibit a transient after-image. The presence of this after-image indicates that for a period of time the camera experiences a phenomenon rather similar to the effect of real light. Such a situation is surprisingly similar to that which occurs during dark adaptation in our own visual system.

5.2 Psychophysics

For excellent reviews of the psychophysics of visual adaptation the reader is referred to Barlow (1972), MacLeod (1978), Shapley & Enroth-Cugell (1984) and Pugh (1988).

5.2.1 Psychophysics of light adaptation

The steady-state performance of the scotopic visual system, when light-adapted to a wide range of illumination levels, was studied in a classic paper by Aguilar & Stiles (1954), and their results are replotted in Fig. 5.1 (also see Fig. 1.2 for further analysis). In their investigation the conditions were chosen to provide stimulation selectively of the *rod* system, by making the test stimulus: (i) blue-green (*c.* 520 nm), (ii) of large area (9° dia.), (iii) of relatively long duration (200 ms), and (iv) positioned in the parafovea. The unit of retinal illuminance, the scotopic troland, may be converted to isomerizations s^{-1} in each rod using the conversion factor given by Baylor, Nunn & Schnapf (1984, p. 603) that 1 scotopic troland $\simeq 4.2$ isomerizations s^{-1} rod^{-1}.

The continuous curve in Fig. 5.1 (left-hand ordinate) plots the stimulus luminance required for a subject just to be able to detect the incremental stimulus on the background; this is called the 'increment threshold'. As the background luminance (plotted on the abscissa) was increased from extremely low levels up to quite high levels, three regions of behaviour could be distinguished. At the lowest background levels (below 10^{-3} trolands) the increment threshold was approximately constant, and its value (about 5×10^{-4} trolands) is referred to as the 'absolute threshold'. Next, over a range of background intensities of about 4 log units, from 0.01 to 100 trolands, the increment threshold rose steadily. On these double logarithmic coordinates the curve in this region approximated a straight line with a slope, n, of about 0.93.

Hence, for intensities up to 100 trolands the increment threshold, ΔI, could be related to the background, I, by

$$\frac{\Delta I}{\Delta I_0} = \left(1 + \frac{I}{I_D}\right)^n \quad \text{with } n \simeq 0.93, \tag{5.1}$$

where ΔI_0 is the absolute threshold and I_D is a constant termed the 'dark

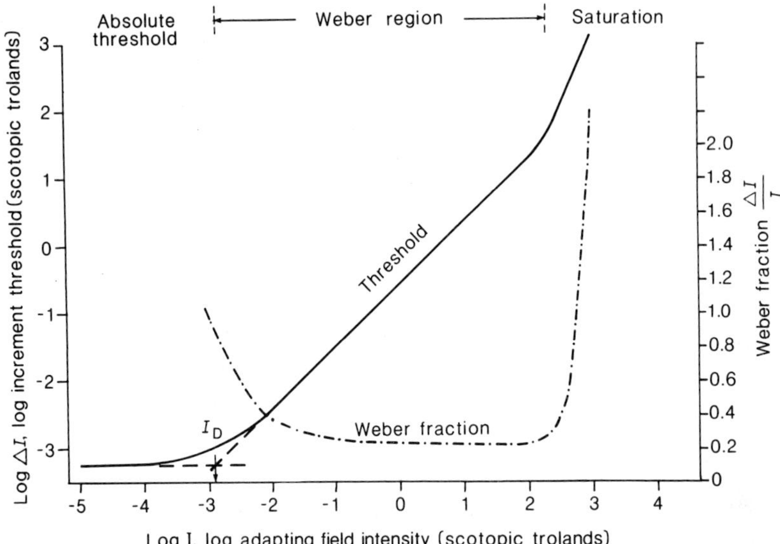

Fig. 5.1. Human scotopic increment threshold curve, showing desensitization by adapting light; averaged results for normal observers redrawn from Aguilar & Stiles (1954). The continuous curve (left-hand ordinate) is a double logarithmic plot of the threshold intensity, ΔI, for the detection of a test field presented on a steady background field of intensity, I. The interrupted curve (right-hand ordinate, linear scale) plots the contrast $\Delta I/I$ of the test field at threshold. The test and adapting fields were chosen so as to favour detection by the rod system; test flash: 520 nm, 200 ms duration, 9° dia., parafoveal; adapting field: 650 nm, steady, 20° dia.; the test and adapting fields were concentric, centred 9° from the fovea in the temporal field. ΔI and I are measured as retinal illuminance (light flux at cornea) in trolands. The intersection of the horizontal and sloping regions of the threshold curve gives the absolute dark light, I_D (see equation (5.1)).

light'. Above a background level of about 300 trolands the increment threshold increased steeply for further increases in background, and this third region is referred to as 'saturation' of the rod system increment sensitivity.

In (5.1) the value of the exponent n required to fit the threshold data under these conditions was fairly close to unity. The value obtained, however, varies markedly with stimulus conditions, and generally lies within the range 0.5 to 1 (see Chapter 1). A value of unity provides what is referred to as *Weber law* behaviour, where, over quite a wide range of background intensities, the increment threshold is simply directly proportional to the background intensity. Hence, in considering the Weber region, where $I \gg I_D$ and $n \sim 1$, (5.1) reduces to

$$\frac{\Delta I}{I} \simeq \frac{\Delta I_0}{I_D}, \text{ a constant.} \tag{5.2}$$

The parameter $\Delta I/I$ on the left side of (5.2) is the *contrast* of the stimulus, and (5.2) indicates that in the Weber region of the experimental curve the threshold for detection of the stimulus occurs at approximately a fixed level of contrast (see Fig. 1.2). This value of the contrast at threshold, given by the right side of (5.2), is termed the *Weber fraction* or *Fechner fraction* and, under the conditions of Fig. 5.1, had a value of about 0.2 (see right-hand ordinate scale).

In analysing psychophysical results (for example the dark-adaptation experiments in Sections 5.2.2 and 5.4.1), it is particularly convenient to employ conditions which give Weber law behaviour, since the occurrence of direct proportionality ($n = 1$) in (5.1) represents a major simplification in the analysis. Generally speaking, the conditions which lead to n approaching unity are that the test stimulus should subtend as large an area as possible and be as long in duration as possible. Recently, Sharpe *et al.* (1989) have found that Weber's law is most closely approximated when the adapting background is *red* (and therfore stimulates the cones), as in the experiment of Aguilar & Stiles (1954). With a green background the slope is roughly $n = 0.8$.

The interpretation of the remaining two parameters ΔI_0 and I_D in (5.1) and (5.2) is as follows. The absolute threshold, ΔI_0, represents the minimum intensity of the test flash which can be detected in the absence of background illumination. When multiplied by the duration of the stimulus it gives the minimum quantity of light, ΔQ_0, detectable by the visual system; under fully dark-adapted conditions this corresponds to perhaps 10–15 photon absorptions in rods in the retina. For the conditions above, with a 9° dia. test stimulus, these few photon hits would be distributed over perhaps 10000 rods, so that the probability of any single rod receiving two or more photons would be negligibly small. In their far-sighted paper, Hecht, Shlaer & Pirenne (1942) interpreted this and other results to indicate that rod photoreceptors must be able to respond reliably to single photon hits (see also Chapter 6). It was not, however, until the late 1970s that advances in methods enabled this prediction of psychophysics to be verified electrophysiologically, first in rods of lower vertebrates (Baylor, Lamb & Yau, 1979*b*) and subsequently in primate rods (Baylor *et al.*, 1984), as will be discussed in Section 5.3.1.

The meaning of the parameter I_D in (5.1) is shown graphically in Fig. 5.1 as the intensity at the intersection of the horizontal and sloping regions of the curve. As the intensity of the background illumination is reduced, the observed threshold intensity decreases, until the background reaches I_D (i.e. until $I = I_D$). With further decreases in background intensity there is essentially no further decrease in threshold intensity, and the visual system in darkness may be considered to be behaving as if it were experiencing a real background of intensity I_D. Thus, the term $(I + I_D)$ in (5.1) represents the total of the real and apparent light being experienced by the eye, and it is for this reason that I_D has been referred to as the 'dark light' of the scotopic visual system. Since, as will be shown later, there are conditions under which the visual system may experience a greatly elevated dark light, the parameter I_D determined from Fig. 5.1 should preferably be referred to as the 'absolute dark light'; that is, the dark light under fully dark-adapted conditions. It has a value of *c.* 2×10^{-3} scotopic trolands, or about 0.008 isomerizations s^{-1} rod^{-1}.

5.2.2 *Psychophysics of dark adaptation: Rushton's classical description of sensitivity recovery*

It has been known for a very long time that, following exposure to very intense illumination, recovery of visual sensitivity in the human is composed of two components, a rapid cone-dominated phase followed by a slower rod-dominated phase. The original results of Hecht, Haig & Chase (1937) are presented in Fig. 5.2*a*, and illustrate the recovery of sensitivity following bleaching exposures of different magnitude. Subsequently, a more thorough study of dark adaptation in a normal observer was made by Pugh (1975*b*), and sample results for both a small (2%) and a large (98%) bleach are plotted in Fig. 5.2*b*. An unfortunate complication with experiments on normal subjects relates to the difficulty in studying the rod-phase at early times when the cone system dominates. At any given time the more sensitive of the two systems will detect the stimulus, so that it is not easy to investigate the less sensitive system.

In order to overcome this problem Rushton was able to investigate an achromat (or rod monochromat), an observer apparently lacking any functional cone system (Rushton, 1961*b*; Blakemore & Rushton, 1965*a*, *b*). His results are illustrated in Fig. 5.3*a* for a bleach of approximately 50%. Subsequently, in studying normal observers, Alpern, Rushton & Torii (1970) developed a technique (which they called the contrast flash technique) designed to favour detection by the rod system even in the presence of a functioning cone system. In this way they were able to follow the behaviour of the rod system of the normal observer to early times, and they obtained results similar to those in the achromat. More

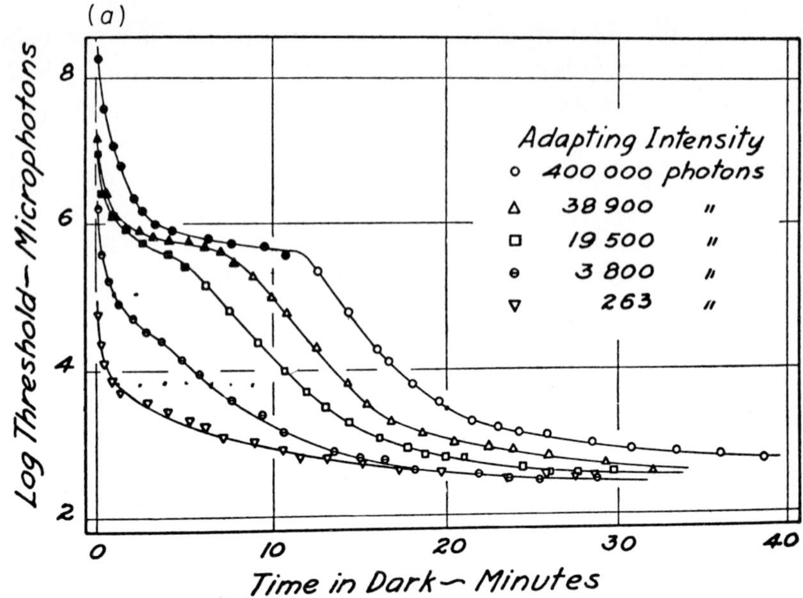

Fig. 5.2. Dark-adaptation curves for normal observer. (*a*) Classical results obtained for a series of bleaching intensities by Hecht *et al.* (1937), showing distinct cone- and rod-dominated regions. (Note: the unit of retinal illuminance, the troland, was then called the 'photon'.) (*b*) More recent results obtained by Pugh (1975*b*), redrawn by Lamb (1981), illustrating recovery after bleaches of 2% and 98% on different scales. Reproduced with permission from Hecht *et al.* (1937) and Lamb (1981).

recently a thorough study has been made of dark adaptation in an achromat by Nordby, Stabell & Stabell (1984) (also see Chapter 10) whose results for a range of bleaching intensities are plotted in Fig. 5.3*b*.

Rushton and his colleagues also investigated the time course of regeneration of visual pigment following a bleaching exposure (Campbell & Rushton, 1955; Rushton, 1961*a*, *b*; Alpern, 1971; Alpern *et al.* 1970; Pugh, 1975*a*). They concluded that for the human retina the fraction, B, of pigment remaining bleached decayed exponentially with time following the return to darkness. Thus:

$$B = B_0 \, e^{-t/T} \tag{5.3}$$

where B_0 is the initial fraction of pigment bleached and where for the rod system the time constant, T, was reported to vary from 4.5 to 7.5 min.

In combining the threshold elevation results and the pigment regeneration results, use was made of the observation by Dowling (1960) that for the rat electroretinogram (ERG) the logarithm of sensitivity reduction was proportional to the fraction of pigment remaining unregenerated

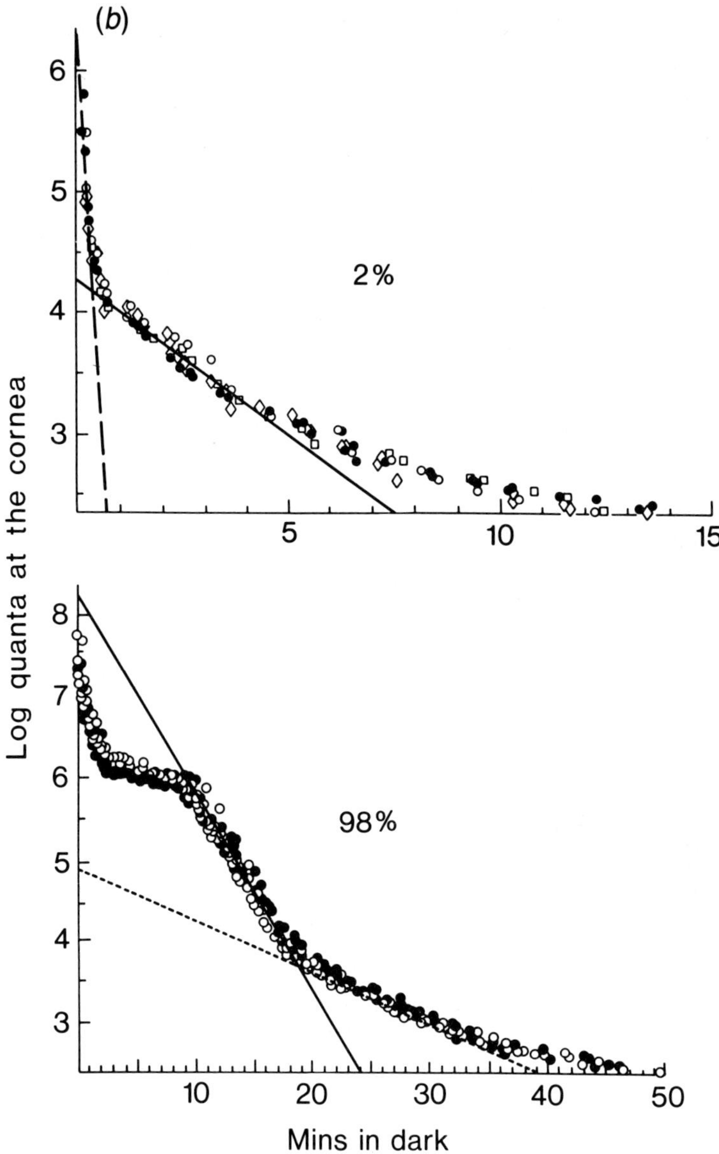
(b)
6
5
4
3
2%
5
10
15
Log quanta at the cornea
8
7
6
5
4
3
98%
10
20
30
40
50
Mins in dark

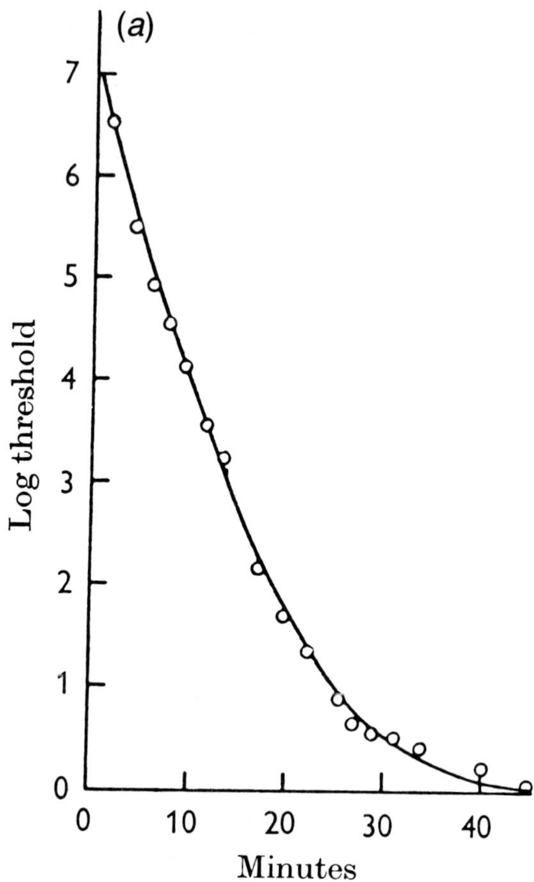

Fig. 5.3. Dark adaptation curves measured for achromats (rod monochromats). (*a*) From Blakemore & Rushton (1965*a*, Fig. 2*a*) for an exposure thought to have bleached around 50% of the rhodopsin; test field 6° dia. (*b*) From Nordby *et al.* (1984) for bleaches of 12%, 21%, 49%, 83% and 98%; test field 1° by 2°. For the achromat, desensitization of the rod system can be followed far above the level corresponding to cone threshold in the normal. Note the close similarity between the curve in (*a*) and the middle curve in (*b*) (49% bleach). Reproduced with permission from Blakemore & Rushton (1965*a*) and Nordby *et al.* (1984).

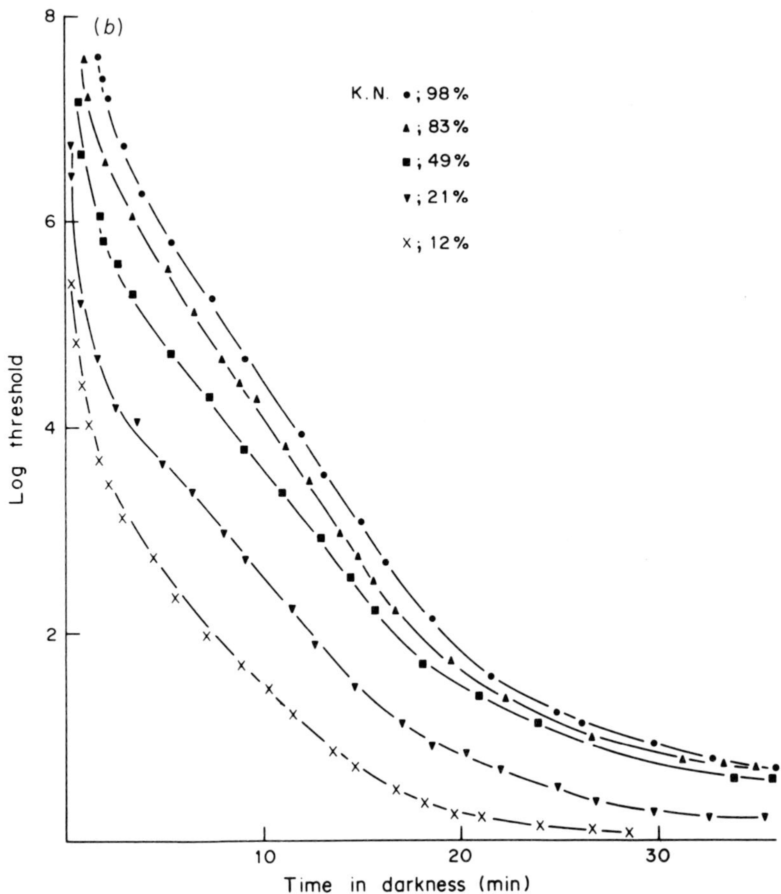

Rushton and his colleagues then reported that in humans the log sensitivity recovery and the pigment regeneration similarly followed a common time course, which was roughly exponential, as shown in Fig. 5.4 (from Rushton, 1961*b*, 1965*b*). Hence, both for the rat ERG (Dowling, 1960) and for human perception (Rushton, 1961*b*, 1965*b*), the threshold elevation following bleaching was given by what has been termed the Dowling–Rushton relation

$$\frac{\Delta I}{\Delta I_0} = 10^{aB}. \tag{5.4}$$

The constant, a, for the human rod system was reported to be $a = 20$ (Rushton, 1961*b*, 1965*b*), subsequently modified to $a = 12$ (Alpern *et al.*, 1970).

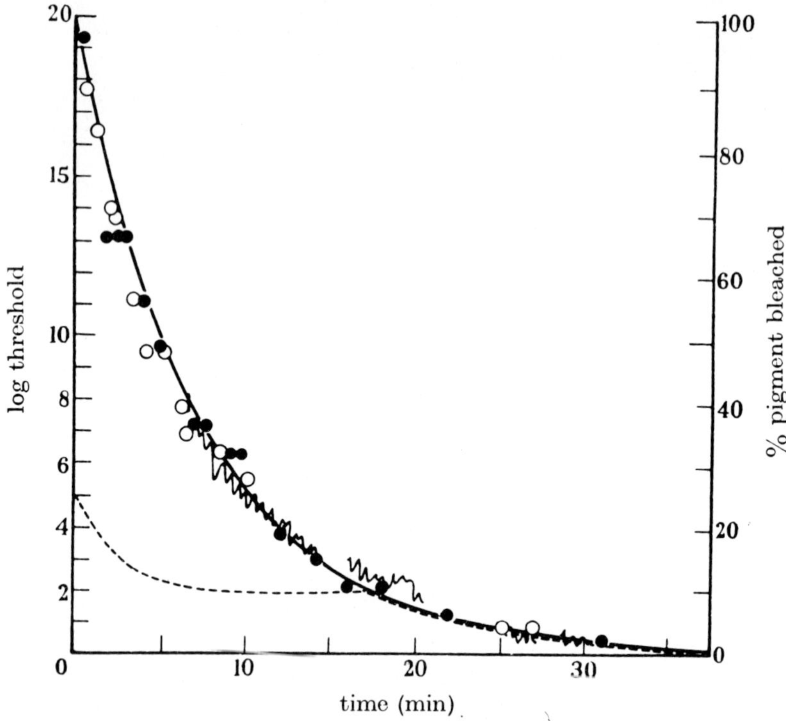

Fig. 5.4. Comparison of recovery of threshold and regeneration of visual pigment following an almost total bleach (from Rushton, 1965*b*, Fig. 3, modified in turn from Rushton, 1961*b*). Irregular line, threshold recovery measured for achromat (ordinate at left). ●, ○, pigment regeneration measured by retinal densitometry for normal observer and achromat, respectively. Continuous curve is equation (5.3), exponential decay, with $T = 7.5$ min. Interrupted curve shows approximate cone and rod branches of normal observer. Reproduced with permission from Rushton (1965*b*).

Equations (5.3) and (5.4) form the cornerstone of Rushton's description, which was most fully developed in his Ferrier Lecture (Rushton, 1965*b*), and which has been widely accepted as an adequate model of dark adaptation since the mid-1960s.

Barlow's hypothesis

An alternative description of dark adaptation was put forward by Barlow (1956, 1964) who proposed that, both in fully dark-adapted conditions and during recovery from bleaches, the visual system is limited by *noise* internal to the photoreceptors. He proposed that, by some unknown mechanism, the photoreceptors become noisier during the after-effect of a bleach, thereby raising the visual threshold, as a result of the same signal-to-noise considerations which apply during steady illumination (Barlow, 1957). This idea was was not developed further, and appears to have received relatively little support over the years. However, it will be returned to in Section 5.4.

5.2.3 Problems with the Rushton description

Upon close inspection it turns out that there are serious problems with both the experimental and theoretical bases of Rushton's description. The equations do not, in fact, provide a reasonable fit to the psychophysical results, and (5.4) is without theoretical foundation. As was stated by Alpern *et. al* (1970), in relation to a slightly more complicated form of (5.4) used to describe the additional effects of backgrounds, 'the formula is not easy to interpret and can only be regarded as a compact parcel of trouble'.

In the first place the model provides a reasonable description for the recovery of sensitivity only under a restricted set of conditions; namely in the late stages of recovery from a large bleach. With small bleaches the theory greatly underestimates the threshold elevation (Rushton & Powell, 1972; Pugh, 1975*b*). For example, with a bleach of only 2% ($B = 0.02$), (5.4) predicts an initial threshold elevation of 0.4 log units if $a = 20$, or 0.22 log units if $a = 12$. Experimentally, however, it is found that the initial threshold elevation exceeds 3 log units, but falls within 1 min to about 1.6 log units and declines slowly from there; see Fig. 5.2*b* (from Pugh, 1975*b*). Hence for small bleaches the Rushton description can be in error by more than a factor of 10.

With large bleaches the errors at early times may be even greater. For a 90% bleach ($B = 0.9$) the Rushton (1965*b*) description with $a = 20$ predicts an initial desensitization of 18 log units, declining within 2 min to perhaps 15 log units. Recent psychophysical measurements on a rod monochromat (one of the editors of this volume; Nordby *et al.* 1984) have shown that 2 min after such a bleach the measured threshold elevation is about 7 log units, indicating an error in the model of perhaps 8 log units, this time in the opposite direction. With $a = 12$ the prediction is considerably closer at early times, but the late behaviour is worse.

A third problem involves the time course of the recovery of sensitivity, described in (5.3) and (5.4) by the single time constant, T. In his comprehensive examination of dark adaptation kinetics, Pugh (1975*b*) measured the time constant of the best-fitting exponential at a series of bleaching intensities and found a monotonic increase from $T = 3.5$ min at a 0.5% bleach to $T = 11.5$ min at a 98% bleach. Hence at best the constant T in (5.3) is not actually a constant, but varies with B_0. However, closer examination of the experimental results would seem to indicate that the individual dark adaptation curves are in any case not very well fitted by an exponential decay. Instead, both in Rushton's results (Fig. 5.3*a*) and in more recent results (Figs 5.2*b* and 5.3*b*) the decay of log threshold elevation appears to be well-described over a substantial range by a straight line. This point will be taken up in detail later.

Although not directly relevant to human results, it is of some interest to note that in the cat retina the pigment regeneration results obtained with retinal densitometry measurements fail to fit a simple exponential. Both Bonds & MacLeod (1974) and Ripps, Mehaffey & Siegel (1981) have shown that regeneration of rhodopsin, rather than fitting an exponential time course, is essentially linear with time until at least 75% has been resynthesized. This nearly-linear relationship suggests that in the cat retina rhodopsin regeneration involves a rate-limited reaction; i.e. one which proceeds at essentially a constant rate when the concentration of reactant is high.

A quite substantial difficulty with Rushton's description would seem to relate to the degree of lateral spread across the retina of the signal for desensitization. A necessary part of his model is the 'pooling', at a site proximal to the receptors, of 'desensitizing' signals from rods; according to Rushton this pooling needed to cover a vast area of the retina. Hence, one of the main experiments taken as supporting Rushton's theory was the uniform desensitizing effect obtained upon bleaching either with a pattern of bars, as reported by Rushton & Westheimer (1962) or with a pattern of dots (Rushton, 1965*a*). However, in repeating this experiment Barlow & Andrews (1973) found the opposite result, that the sensitivity in retinal regions where the dark bars had been was not reduced to the same extent as in regions where the bleaching bars had been. The difference at times exceeded 1 log unit, indicating a substantial problem with the model as formulated by Rushton. The more recent experiments of MacLeod, Chen & Crognale (1989) indicate that pooling of post-bleach adaptational signals is restricted to about 10 min arc of visual angle.

A final pair of objections arise on aesthetic grounds. Rushton's model of dark adaptation requires (for reasons that will not be elaborated here) that the rod photoreceptors independently signal two parameters, on the one hand the incident light intensity and quite separately the fraction of pigment bleached; it is difficult to conceive of a mechanism whereby this could be achieved. Additionally Rushton's scheme requires that the reduction in sensitivity be related *exponentially* to the fraction of pigment remaining unregenerated (Equation (5.4)), and such a relationship appears inelegant and perhaps unphysical.

5.2.4 Equivalent background intensity

In considering any alternative description of dark adaptation behaviour, it seems important to take full account of the classical observations of Stiles & Crawford (1932) and Crawford (1937). They showed that during the course of dark adaptation the elevation of threshold could accurately be described in terms of an 'equivalent background intensity'. That is, following an intense bleaching exposure the visual system behaves as if it is viewing the world through a veiling light and, during the course of dark adaptation, the intensity of this equivalent background slowly fades away.

This equivalent background hypothesis has the great attraction that it removes the need to invoke special mechanisms of desensitization in explaining dark adaptation. All that it is necessary to postulate is that by some unknown mechanisms the after-effects of a bleach give rise to events which the visual system is unable to distinguish from real photon hits. Thus, dark adaptation simply becomes a special case of light adaptation, in which the adapting field is stabilized on the retina. Equally, it is not essential to have an explanation of light adaptation itself; all that is required is the experimental measurement of the effects of stabilized adapting lights. What is necessary, of course, is first to test whether the equivalent background hypothesis fits the experimental results, and then ideally to seek some explanation for the origin of the equivalent light.

The adapting effects which occur during recovery from a bleaching light consist not only of an elevated threshold, but also comprise improved spatial and temporal resolution and changes in pupil size. Additionally, at early times after the bleach a pronounced after-image is apparent, but normally this fairly rapidly becomes unnoticed. According to the equivalent background hypothesis above, each of these phenomena during dark adaptation should be exactly equivalent to the effects produced by a real light of appropriate intensity stabilized on the retina. There is a substantial body of experimental evidence in support of this assertion with respect to threshold elevation and after-image appearance, but only a qualitative equivalence has been established for the other cases (pupil size, etc.).

In the case of threshold elevation it is well known that the threshold for detection, ΔI, depends greatly upon the stimulus parameters, in particular upon the size and duration of the test field. Consequently the form of the relationship between threshold and background intensity varies according to the stimulus parameters. But at any given time during dark adaptation a *single* value of equivalent background intensity correctly describes the threshold elevation for all stimulus configurations which have been tested (Crawford, 1937, 1947; Blakemore & Rushton 1965*a*, *b*).

Similarly, the brightness of an after-image determined by matching it to a stabilized field of real light is found to correspond exactly to the equivalent background required to describe the threshold elevation at a corresponding time (Barlow & Sparrock, 1964). And in the case of pupil size it has been shown that during dark adaptation constriction occurs which is qualitatively similar to that produced by an adapting field (Alpern & Campbell, 1963).

On the other hand the equivalence has been reported to break down with respect to the sensitizing effect obtained when the background diameter is enlarged (Westheimer, 1968), and for the improved flicker fusion frequency obtained with brighter backgrounds (Ernst, 1968). Unfortunately, however, both of these studies were performed with backgrounds which were not stabilized and, as discussed by Barlow & Sakitt (1973), it seems likely that the visibility of the real background may have influenced thresholds. What now seems fairly clear is that, in order to test whether the effect of bleaching is identical with the effect of an 'equivalent background', it is essential to employ a precisely stabilized retinal image (Geisler, 1980).

A natural criticism of the equivalent background hypothesis would seem to be that during dark adaptation (following exposure to a bleaching light) we experience a sense of darkness rather than of light. However, this apparent difficulty is again related to the perfect retinal stability of any effects of bleaching, and the observation that a properly stabilized retinal image rapidly disappears from our perception. But also important is the surprising observation that the presence of a real veiling light on the retina leads to a sense of *greater darkness* in the relatively dark areas of the scene. This may be demonstrated readily by viewing a scene in bright sunshine. Provided that the observers' eyes are shaded from direct sunlight then a high-contrast percept will be obtained. However, if the sunlight is allowed to fall directly upon the observer's eyes (a simple means of producing a veiling light) then the relatively dark parts of the scene will immediately appear still darker, rather than lighter. It is as if our eye has 'automatic black level compensation' whereby the lowest intensity level over the entire scene is 'defined' as black, and our sense of darkness or brightness is mapped onto the remaining intensity range.

The point of this complicated diversion is simply that our lack of awareness of the presence of a long-lasting after-image of bleaching, and our subjective sense of darkness during this recovery, are in no way incompatible with the equivalent background hypothesis of Stiles & Crawford (1932) and Crawford (1937).

5.2.5 *Additional points*

An important observation, made originally by Crawford (1946) and recently confirmed in exhaustive experiments by Pugh (1975*b*), is that the time course of human dark adaptation is identical for adapting exposures of different duration which bleach the same amount of visual pigment. This intensity × time trade-off was shown to hold for bleaches ranging from 0.01% to 99%, at least for exposure durations less than 30 s. It has been pointed out by Pugh (1988) that it would seem extremely unlikely that any mechanism beyond the rod synapse could integrate the effects of bleaching exposures of different durations to give such perfect intensity × time trade-off, especially since all the exposures cause saturation of the rod's electrical response. Pugh has therefore concluded that it is reasonable to believe that it is indeed the amount of pigment bleached, or something functionally related to it, which determines the state of dark adaptation.

It is important to emphasize that the slowness of recovery of visual sensitivity after exposure to bright lights must be disadvantageous to the owner of the eye (Barlow, 1972). As in the case of the television camera and receiver analogies the slow recovery cannot in any way be beneficial to the system. Hence, perhaps the most productive approach would be to view dark adaptation as an unavoidable consequence of some presumably very important feature of visual transduction.

5.3 Receptor physiology

To the extent that the equivalent background hypothesis can be accepted as an adequate description of dark adaptation, the need for investigating the detailed physiology of the photoreceptors is reduced. In this section a brief description will be given of the rod's electrical response to illumination and of its desensitization by steady backgrounds. This will be followed by a short account of the changes in the electrical response induced by bleaching, and a description of recent results which show a phenomenon in the rod outer segment resembling an equivalent background. Reviews of the rod's electrical response and the nature of the transduction process may be found in Lamb (1984*a*, 1986*b*), Pugh & Cobbs (1986), Stryer (1986) and Baylor (1987), while various aspects of light adaptation in photoreceptors are discussed by Shapley & Enroth-Cugell (1984), Lamb (1986*a*), Pugh (1988), and Pugh & Altman (1988).

5.3.1 Rod responses to light

Perhaps surprisingly, the rod response to illumination comprises a *reduction* in the magnitude of a current which flows into the rod outer segment in darkness (Hagins, Penn & Yoshikami, 1970). Although this can at times be confusing and may seem at variance with the operation of other sensory receptors, it is clearly established as the mode of operation of all vertebrate photoreceptors.

As discussed in Section 5.2.1, Hecht *et al.* (1942) predicted, from their measurement of human absolute threshold, that rod photoreceptors must be able reliably to signal the absorption of individual photons (see Chapter 4). However, even after the advent of intracellular voltage recordings (see Chapter 6) from photoreceptors in the late 1960s, experimental verification of this prediction did not prove possible (Fain, 1975). It turned out that, because of the extensive electrical coupling which exists between neighbouring photoreceptors, the electrical responses were spread out over many cells (Gold, 1981). Hence, instead of there being a large single-photon voltage response in one rod, there is in fact a much smaller voltage response distributed over many rods, and this smaller response could not be resolved in the presence of other sources of noise.

With the development of the suction pipette technique for recording the outer segment current of individual photoreceptors (Baylor, Lamb & Yau, 1979*a*, *b*) it became possible to measure the activity of single rods and to show conclusively that rods do indeed respond reliably to each photon hit (at least at low intensities). This work was first performed on the very large rods of amphibia, but was later extended to primate rods (Baylor *et al.*, 1984). In both toad and monkey rods in fully dark-adapted conditions the average response to a single photon was around 1 pA in amplitude, representing about 2–5% of the maximal response obtainable

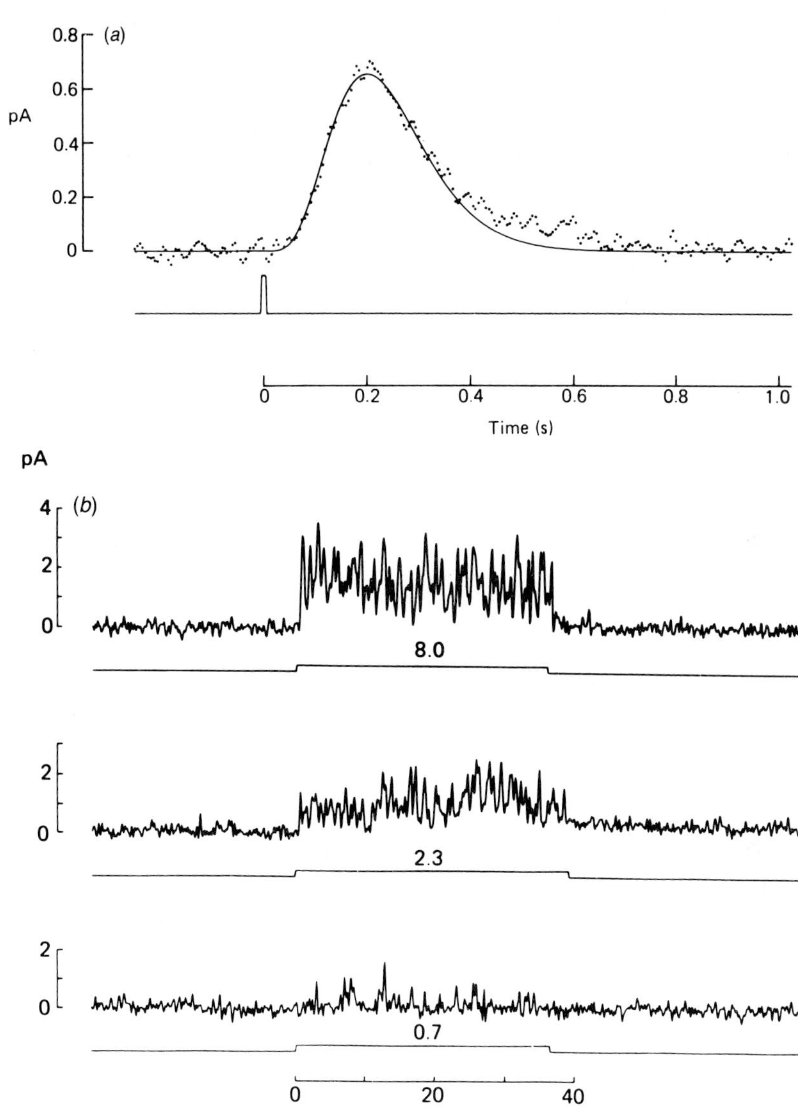

Fig. 5.5. Responses of a monkey rod photoreceptor to brief flashes and to steady lights. (*a*) Average photocurrent response to brief dim flashes, delivering approx. 1 isomerization per trial, on a relatively fast time base. (*b*) Individual responses in a different rod to steady dim lights of three intensities, delivering approx. 18, 5, and 1.5 isomerizations s^{-1}; the figures near the traces indicate the light flux in photons μm^{-2} s^{-1}. Note the slower time-base and lower gain. Reproduced with permission from Baylor *et al.* (1984).

with a bright flash. The average time course of this quantal response in a monkey rod is illustrated in Fig. 5.5*a*; consistent with earlier psychophysical predictions it has a time to peak of around 200 ms.

In response to steady dim illumination, rods from amphibia and primates display pronounced fluctuations, as illustrated in Fig. 5.5*b* for monkey (Baylor *et al.*, 1984). At the lowest intensity in Fig. 5.5*b* it is just about possible to resolve individual events a little under 1 pA in amplitude, elicited by the low rate of random bombardment of photons with this very dim light. At the slightly higher intensities in the upper two traces, individual photon hits cannot be resolved, and a wildly fluctuating trace is observed, similar to that obtained from a photomultiplier tube. It is possible to show from noise analysis that these fluctuations are entirely consistent with the notion that the rod's electrical response to dim illumination is composed of the superposition of random occurrences of the single photon events.

5.3.2 *Receptor desensitization by background illumination*

The flash sensitivity, S, of the overall phototransduction process may conveniently be defined as the size of the incremental response, ΔR, divided by the size of the increment in illumination, ΔQ, which induced it, so that

$$S = \Delta R / \Delta Q. \qquad (5.5)$$

Electrophysiological recordings from cones and from the large rods of lower vertebrates have shown that the transduction process in these photoreceptors becomes desensitized in the presence of background illumination, as illustrated in Fig. 5.6 for a toad rod (Lamb, 1984*b*). The upper-most trace was obtained for flashes presented in darkness, and the height of the trace represents the dark-adapted flash sensitivity, S_D, in this cell; the lower traces were obtained with test flashes presented on steady backgrounds of progressively greater intensity. These responses show that in the toad rod the effect of background illumination is to desensitize the rod and to accelerate its response; that is, the peak of the response both decreases in size and moves to earlier times as the background intensity increases.

The relationship between sensitivity and background intensity for toad rods is plotted in Fig. 5.6*b* (Fain, 1976). In order to aid comparison with psychophysical measurements the ordinate plots $1/S$, the reciprocal of the sensitivity defined in (5.5) above. This parameter represents the

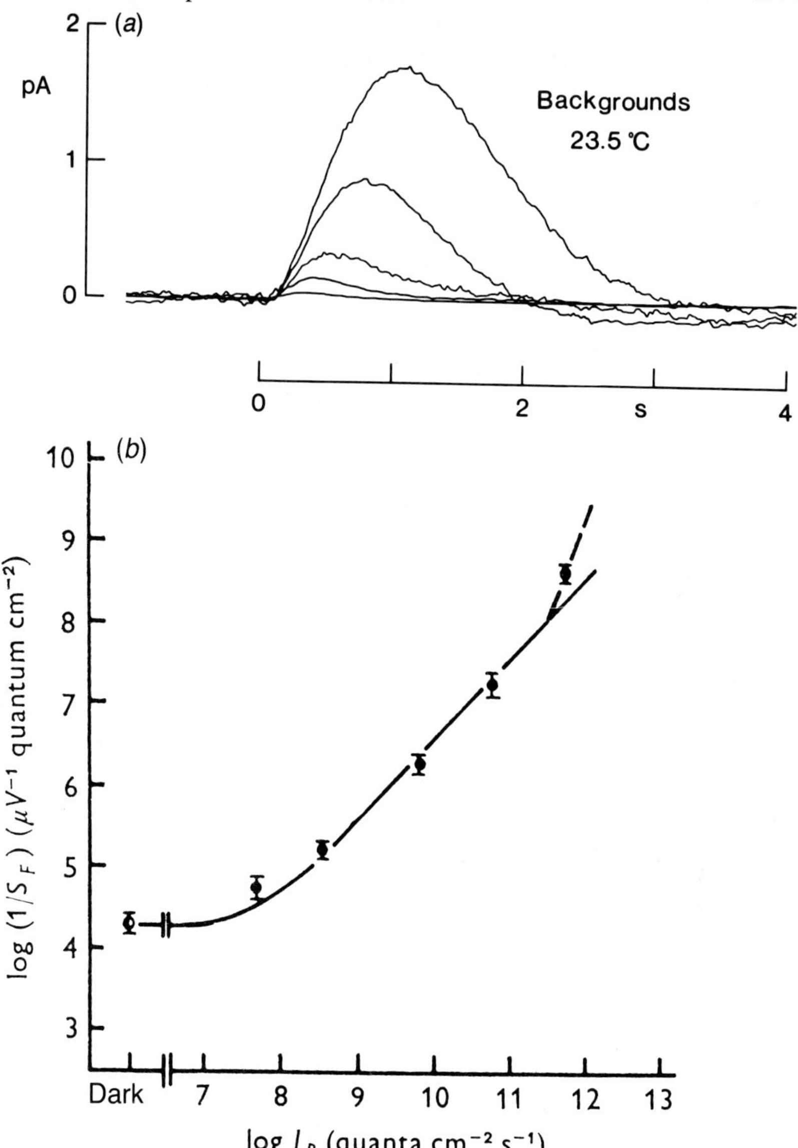

Fig. 5.6. Desensitization of a toad rod by background illumination. (*a*) Photocurrent in response to dim flashes. Uppermost curve was obtained for flashes presented in darkness, while the remaining curves were for flashes presented on backgrounds of progressively greater intensity. With the brighter backgrounds the test flash intensity was increased, and the plotted responses have been scaled down accordingly; i.e. the curves are equivalent to sensitivity, $S = \Delta R/\Delta Q$. Reproduced with permission from Lamb (1984*b*). (*b*) Desensitization plotted as a function of background intensity, for voltage responses from a toad rod. Log reciprocal sensitivity ($1/S$) is plotted against log background intensity, and over a considerable range the results are fitted by a straight line with unit slope (Weber law behaviour). Reproduced with permission from Fain (1976).

quantity of light required to elicit a criterion response amplitude, and is therefore comparable to the threshold, ΔI, in (5.1) and (5.2). The straight-line behaviour (with slope of unity) in the double logarithmic coordinates of Fig. 5.6*b* indicates that, over a considerable range of backgrounds, $1/S$ is directly proportional to background intensity I. Hence

$$\frac{S_D}{S} = 1 + \frac{I}{I_0}, \tag{5.6}$$

indicating Weber law behaviour at the level of the photoreceptor, analogous to (5.1) with $n = 1$ in the psychophysical case.

Photoreceptor desensitization of this kind is observed over a wide range of intensities in cones (Baylor & Hodgkin, 1974; Normann & Perlman, 1979) and in the large rods of lower vertebrates (Fain, 1976). Recently it has been shown that mammalian rods also desensitize according to Weber's law (Tamura, Nakatani & Yau, 1989), but this desensitization does not set in until a relatively high intensity. Although it had previously been reported that in primate rods the main effects of backgrounds were explained simply by saturation without desensitization (Baylor *et al.*, 1984), the results of Tamura *et al.* (1989) indicate that some adaptation does occur. H. R. Matthews (personal communication) has, however, now shown that in guinea pig rods the Weber-law region occupies only about 2 log units of intensity immediately prior to saturation.

The desensitization has been shown to occur primarily in the light-sensitive outer segment, and is intimately associated with the biochemical cascade of transduction (see, for example Pugh & Cobbs, 1986). From consideration of the very low intensities at which rod desensitization occurs, Donner & Hemilä (1978) and Bastian & Fain (1979) concluded that the desensitization resulting from absorption of a single photon spreads to affect many disks, and therefore that it involves a diffusible messenger substance. The degree of spread of desensitization was investigated by Lamb, McNaughton & Yau (1981), who concluded that the diffusion of a small molecule could account for the observed results.

It has now been shown that the major part of the desensitization is caused by a light-induced decline in cytoplasmic free calcium concentration (Torre, Matthews & Lamb, 1986; Matthews *et al.* 1988; Nakatani & Yau, 1988; Fain *et al.*, 1989; Matthews *et al.*, 1990). There is general agreement that calcium's internal action is mediated by an effect on the

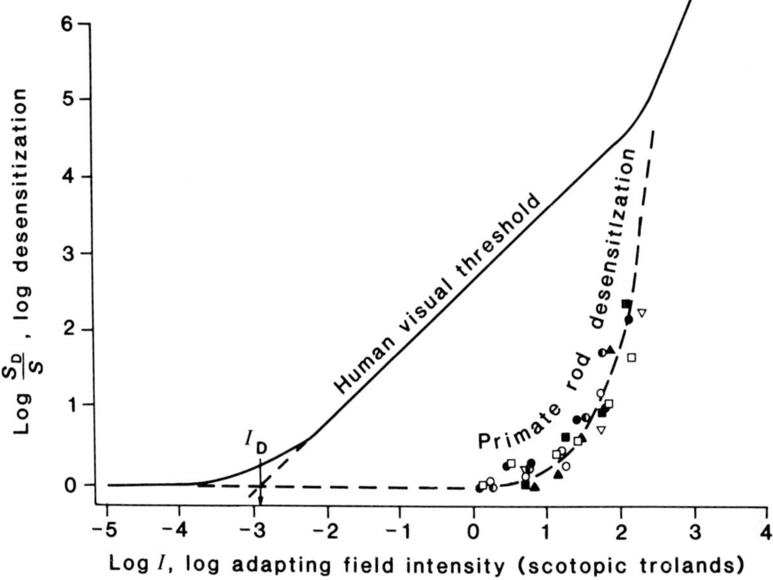

Fig. 5.7. Desensitization of primate rods by background illumination, plotted on the same coordinates as Fig. 5.1. The symbols are derived from Fig. 9 of Baylor *et al.* (1984) using the conversion factors given in their paper to convert to trolands. (Specifically, t_i is taken as 282 ms and k_f as 0.0563 μm^2 (their Table 4), so that $k_s = k_f t_i = 0.0158$ μm^2 s; also, 100 tolrand = 365 photons μm^{-2} s^{-1} (their p. 603); hence $k_s I_s = 1$ in their Fig. 9 corresponds to 17.3 trolands.) Solid curve, human increment sensitivity, redrawn from Fig. 5.5.1; interrupted curve drawn by eye. It is clear that, for most of the intensity range over which the human visual system displays Weber law behaviour, the rod photoreceptors remain fully sensitive. Also it appears that saturation in the psychophysical case may result from saturation of the rod response.

cyclic nucleotide cascade (Pugh & Cobbs, 1986; Stryer, 1986), and a powerful effect on the enzyme guanylate cyclase has been demonstrated (Hodgkin & Nunn, 1988, 1988; Koch & Stryer, 1988). An important test of any model of phototransduction will be to see whether it correctly predicts the invariant rising phase of the receptor response at the earliest times, as shown in Fig. 5.6*a*.

The monkey rod measurements of Baylor *et al.* (1984) have been replotted in Fig. 5.7 (on co-ordinates similar to Fig. 5.1) for comparison with the behaviour of the overall scotopic system. Over much of the psychophysical Weber law region the electrophysiological results show that individual rods continue to operate with essentially full sensitivity. This indicates that the desensitization observed for the overall system is contributed by post-receptoral mechanisms; see Chapters 1 and 3. For the purposes of consideration of the equivalent background hypothesis of dark adaptation, however, the site of such desensitization, although interesting, is not of any critical importance.

An intriging question then, is why it is that the rods of lower vertebrates should desensitize in a Weber law manner, over a wide range of intensities, whereas primate rods show little desensitization and instead retain most of their flash sensitivity until saturation. The answer may lie simply in the prevention of saturation in the larger and slower rods of the lower vertebrates (Fain, 1976; Shapley & Enroth-Cugell, 1984; Lamb, 1986*a*). Because of the much larger rhodopsin content (*c*. 20×) of the larger rod, a given light intensity will activate many more rhodopsin molecules than in a mammalian rod. And because of the much slower response (*c*. 10×, due to the lower temperature of *c*. 20 °C, cf. 37 °C), the effects of each activated rhodopsin will last much longer in the lower rod. (Additionally, account should be taken of differences in the numerical aperture of the ocular lens in the different species, but such differences are likely to be small.) From these combined factors we would expect that, at some arbitrary intensity of ambient illumination, the number of simultaneous 'photon effects' will be vastly greater in a toad rod than in a monkey rod. But apparently, in order to permit visual detection at extremely low light levels, all rods have evolved a large single-photon response amplitude, of several percent of the standing dark current. Therefore, at a moderate scotopic intensity, where a primate rod would still be able to register single-photon hits as in Fig. 5.5*b*, a large rod of a lower vertebrate would, in the *absence* of desensitization, be totally saturated and unable to respond. Hence in this way, the automatic gain control (AGC) in cones and in large rods serves to prevent saturation, and thereby to improve the sensitivity of the visual system. At the higher absolute intensities at which primate rods saturate, the cone photoreceptors are able to respond adequately, so that the small extent of adaptation in these rods represents no disadvantage.

5.3.3 Photochemistry of rhodopsin

Before considering the experimental work on bleaching recovery of rod photoresponses it is necessary to mention briefly some properties of the photochemistry of rhodopsin.

The rhodopsin molecule consists of a large protein, opsin, with attached to it a small hydrocarbon, retinal (the chromophore). Retinal can exist in a variety of isomeric forms, of which the two important to vision are termed 11-*cis* and all-*trans*; the native form of rhodopsin consists exclusively of the opsin bound to the 11-*cis* isomer.

Upon absorption of a photon of light the rhodopsin molecule is converted to an active form, often indicated as Rh*. The initial event in this activation is the photoisomerization of the 11-*cis* chromophore to its all-*trans* form. Subsequent steps in the rapid activation of rhodopsin appear to be thermal reactions which proceed without the involvement of enzymes. Although it had previously been thought that the inactivation steps similarly proceeded spontaneously, this now seems not to be the case and enzymes appear to be involved. In the rhodopsin activation/inactivation cycle a number of intermediate forms exist (termed photo-intermediates), which traditionally were identified because of their different absorption spectra (i.e. because they had different colours), and a considerable body of information exists on the nature of these photochemical changes (see, for example, Langer, 1973).

Recently it has been realized that part of the inactivation of Rh* involves multiple phosphorylation of the opsin, followed by binding to a specific protein ('48 kDa protein' or retinal S-antigen), as discussed in Sections 5.4.4. Such reactions appear not to alter the absorption spectrum of the photointermediates, and are therefore not spectroscopically observable. Consequently, the changes in concentration of the various intermediate forms through which Rh* progresses are not known, and are certainly not simply obtainable from the total fraction of pigment, B, remaining spectrophometrically unregenerated.

Furthermore, since these reactions require the intervention of at least one enzyme (rhodopsin kinase) they are most unlikely to proceed by simple first order kinetics. Perhaps related to this point, Donner & Hemilä (1975) have shown that the relative proportions of the long-lasting spectrophotometric intermediates (metarhodopsins II and III) depend greatly on the magnitude of the initial bleach.

Hence, in summary, although it is known that 11-*cis* retinal is required for the eventual regeneration of native rhodopsin, the detailed kinetics of the photointermediates are complicated, and incompletely understood.

Finally, in the normal retina all-*trans* retinal is re-isomerized to 11-*cis* retinal by a pathway involving transport from the rod outer segment to the pigment epithelium and back again. Hence, in experiments involving isolated retinae (where the retina is detached from the pigment epithelium), the normal source of 11-*cis* retinal is interrupted and the normal regeneration of native rhodopsin will not occur. Nevertheless rods in the isolated retina contain small amounts of 11-*cis* retinol, and the regeneration of about 3% of the pigment is possible (Donner & Hemilä, 1975; Cocozza & Ostroy, 1987; in frog and toad).

5.3.4 *Receptor sensitivity during dark adaptation, and effects of 11-*cis *retinal*

It has been shown in many studies of lower vertebrates that the sensitivity of the rod photoreceptors themselves is greatly reduced following a bleach, and that the sensitivity gradually recovers over a period of tens of minutes (see for example, Grabowski, Pinto & Pak, 1972; Green *et al.*, 1975). Experiments measuring intracellular voltage changes have usually been performed on isolated retina preparations, and the interpretation is complicated by the fact that regeneration of visual pigment does not then occur (in significant amounts) because of the absence of the pigment epithelium. In these cases bleaching leads initially to a very large desensitization of the rods followed by partial recovery to a permanently desensitized level. The level of this permanent desensitization is graded with the magnitude of the bleach, and is far greater than expected for the reduced quantal catch resulting from absent pigment (Donner & Hemilä, 1978; Pepperberg *et al.*, 1978).

In the isolated retina preparation it has been shown that substantial recovery of rod sensitivity, even to the fully dark-adapted level, can be obtained by addition of the chromophore 11-*cis* retinal to the bathing medium (e.g. Pepperberg *et al.*, 1978; Perlman, Nodes & Pepperberg, 1982). As shown in Fig. 5.8, from Pepperberg *et al.* (1978), addition of 11-*cis* retinal during the plateau level of permanent desensitization following a bleach of 40% led to rapid recovery of sensitivity to almost the original dark-adapted value. Subsequently a further bleach of 80% led to a continual recovery of sensitivity without a permanent desensitization.

Similar results have recently been obtained by Jones *et al.* (1989), who showed that 11-*cis* retinal (but not retinol) leads to steady recovery when incorporated by means either of liposomes or interphotoreceptor retinoid-binding protein. In cones, 11-*cis* retinal causes very rapid recovery, while 11-*cis* retinol causes somewhat slower (but nevertheless complete) recovery.

Such experiments indicate that in these retinae the normal recovery of rod sensitivity requires the regeneration of rhodopsin. However, since the quantities of the different intermediates of bleaching are not known,

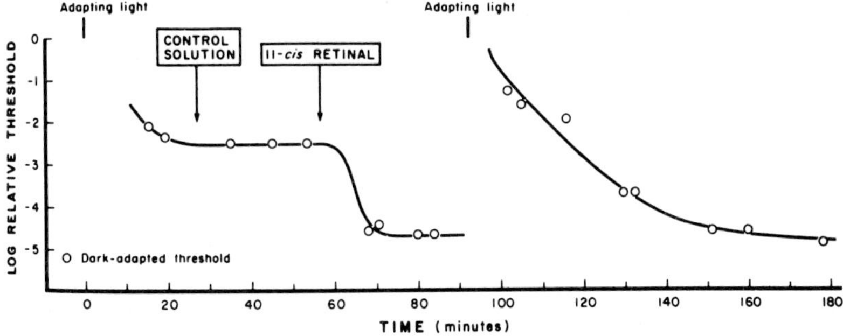

Fig. 5.8. Recovery of sensitivity in photoreceptors in the isolated skate retina following bleaches. The dark-adapted sensitivity is indicated by the symbol prior to time zero, and then two bleaching exposures were presented: 40% at time zero, and 80% after 90 min. Following the first bleach the photoreceptor sensitivity recovered only to a plateau level about 3 log units above the dark-adapted value. Application of 11-*cis* retinal then caused the threshold to recover to near its original value. Following the second bleaching exposure full recovery occurred, presumably because of the continued presence of 11-*cis* retinal. Reproduced with permission from Pepperberg *et al.* (1978).

it is difficult to make quantitative statements about the influence of such intermediates on rod sensitivity. Furthermore, it is also difficult to know what relation to expect between desensitization of the rods themselves in these experiments and desensitization of the overall visual system since, as shown in Fig. 5.7, these need not be closely related.

5.3.5 Bleach-induced fluctuations in rod photoreceptors

Events in dark-adapted conditions

In Section 5.3.1 the responses of rod photoreceptors to individual quanta of light were examined. Not only do rods show quantal events during illumination, but in addition they exhibit exactly similar events even in total darkness. This phenomenon, illustrated in Fig. 5.9*a*, was first demonstrated in toad rods by Baylor, Matthews & Yau (1980) and the observation was subsequently extended to primate rods by Baylor *et al.* (1984). In dark-adapted monkey rods they found spontaneous events, indistinguishable from the photon-induced events, occurring on average about once every 160 s. Thus, even in darkness, there is a low rate of quantal events, and Baylor *et al.* (1980) provided evidence that these events probably represent *thermal* isomerizations of rhodopsin. The rate

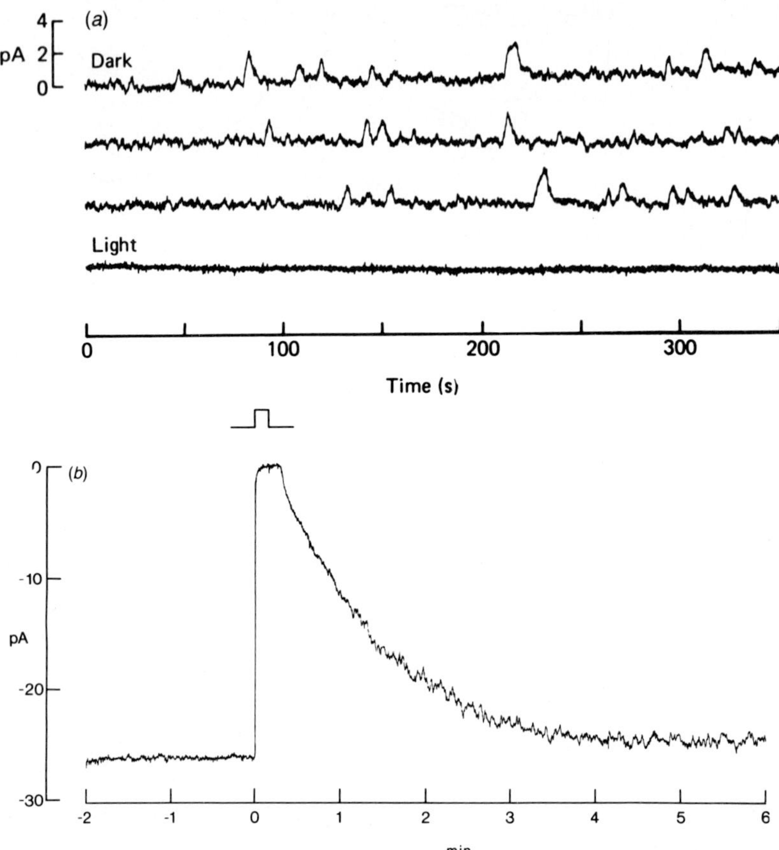

Fig. 5.9. Spontaneous photon-like events in toad rod photoreceptors, in dark-adapted conditions and following a bleaching exposure. (*a*) Events recorded at high gain and on a slow time-base under dark-adapted conditions (upper three traces) and in the presence of steady saturating light (lowest trace); this last case represents the instrumental noise in the recording system. The discrete events in the upper traces have approximately the same amplitude and time course as the average response to a single photoisomerization in the same rod. Reproduced with permission from Baylor *et al.* (1980). (*b*) Fluctuations occurring during the recovery phase following exposure of the rod to an intense light bleaching about 0.7% of the pigment. Initially the circulating dark current was completely suppressed, but as the current recovered it was accompanied by pronounced fluctuations. Power spectral analysis showed these fluctuations to be indistinguishable from the noise produced by the random bombardment of photons during illumination with dim light. Reproduced with permission from Lamb (1980).

of occurrence of these events (1/160 s $\simeq$ 0.006 events s^{-1}) coincides remarkably closely with the rate of equivalent isomerizations corresponding to the psychophysical 'absolute dark light' (see Section 5.2.1), of approximately 0.008 isomerizations s^{-1} in each rod. The close similarity of these values suggests that the scotopic absolute dark light may be determined by the spontaneous occurrence of these discrete events in the rod outer segment. This would indicate the thermal events to be of great importance, setting the absolute limit for detectibility of dim stimuli.

Bleach-induced events

Rather more unexpectedly, rod photoreceptors also display photon-like noise following intense bleaching exposures. A recording of toad rod current following a bleach of about 0.7% of the rhodopsin is shown in Fig. 5.9*b*, from Lamb (1980). Prior to the bleach, in the fully dark-adapted state, the baseline was relatively quiet. When the bleaching light was delivered the photocurrent was at first totally suppressed, and then as it slowly recovered it was accompanied by greatly increased noise. This noise gradually faded away (after the end of the illustrated record) over a period of 10–20 min.

It was possible to show from power spectral analysis that the bleach-induced fluctuations were indistinguishable from the effects of background light (Lamb, 1980). In other words, the rod was behaving as if it was experiencing an enormously increased rate of spontaneous photon-like events, and during the course of dark adaptation the intensity of this 'equivalent background illumination' gradually declined.

The same phenomenon is illustrated in another cell in Fig. 5.10, this time with a continuous record lasting 60 min. The timing of an intense exposure, bleaching about 0.5% of the pigment, is marked by the arrow in trace B.

In the fully dark-adapted state (trace A and beginning of trace B) occasional spontaneous quantal events are apparent on an otherwise quiet baseline. Towards the end of trace A the sensitivity of the rod was measured with a series of 20 dim flashes, marked by open circles (○). Note the considerable fluctuation in the size of these responses, due to the quantal nature of light. Further test flashes, similarly marked by circles, were presented in each of the subsequent traces in order to monitor recovery of the rod's sensitivity. (The bright test flash towards the end of trace E was presented in order to check that the cell's dark current had not declined.)

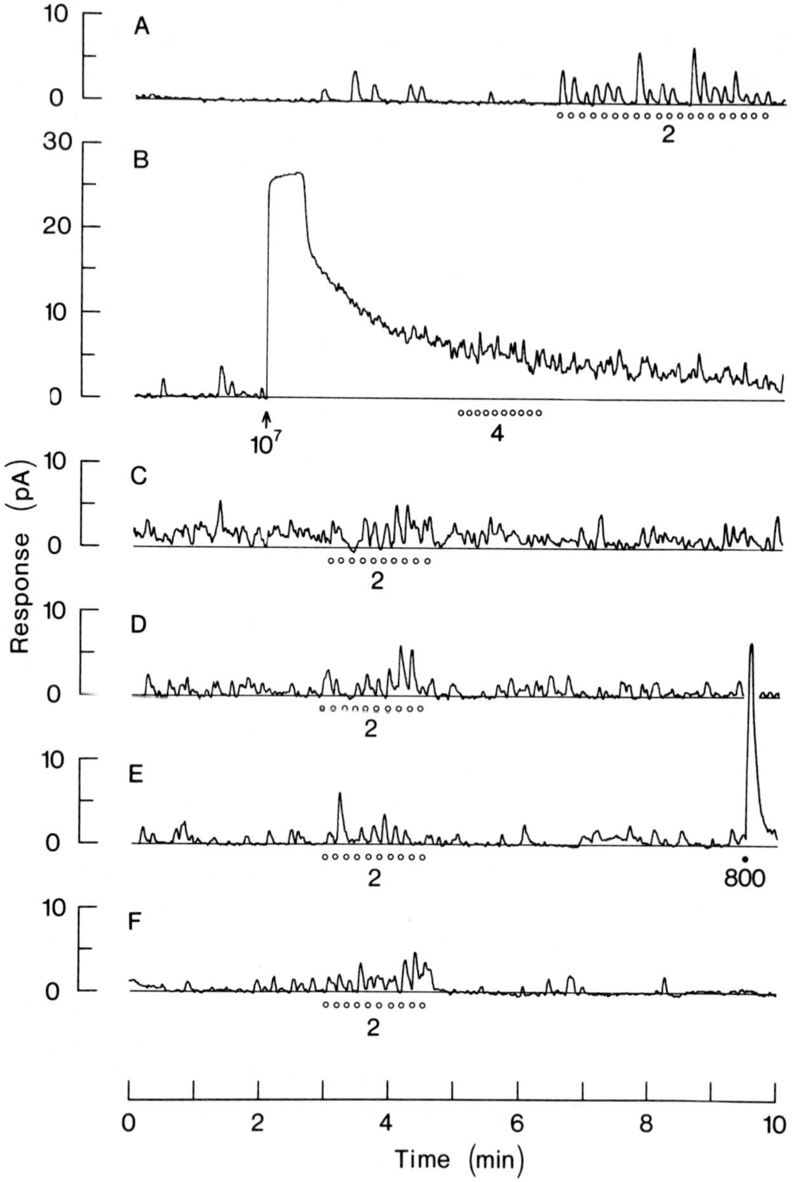

Fig. 5.10. Bleach-induced fluctuations, together with flash sensitivity measurements, during a continuous recording lasting 60 min. Timing of dim test flashes is marked by open circles (○), and numbers nearby indicate approximate mean number of isomerizations elicited per flash; the brighter flash (●) near the end of trace E was presented in order to check that the circulating current had not deteriorated. At 2 min into trace B an intense flash was presented delivering *c.* 10^7 isomerizations (approx. 0.5% bleach). The photocurrent remained saturated for roughly 45 s, and the recovery phase was accompanied by pronounced current fluctuations. In the earliest stages of recovery the fluctuations are not at all prominent, presumably because of the reduced sensitivity of the cell.

In this experiment it is again clear that the recovery phase of the response to the bleach is accompanied by prominent fluctuations. During the latter part of trace B these fluctuations contribute (or are superimposed on) a decaying d.c. component, while in trace C it appears that the steady current has settled back essentially to its original level. In the later traces (D, E and F) the fluctuations appear gradually to become resolvable into discrete events having approximately the form of the original spontaneous events in the dark-adapted state. Hence this figure is again qualitatively consistent with the idea that following a bleach the rod response is accompanied by a greatly elevated rate of occurrence of photon-like events, and that slowly this rate declines.

The dim test flashes presented in trace B, just a few minutes after the bleach, show that at this time the rod was desensitized by a factor of roughly 4 (note that these flashes were double the intensity of those in trace A). It is presumably because of this desensitization that fluctuations are not very prominent at early times since, as indicated in (5.7) below, the power spectral density in the fluctuations is proportional to the square of the flash sensitivity. Consistent with this notion, a similar phenomenon is seen when real lights are presented. At moderate to high intensities of real light the cell becomes desensitized and the fluctuations are then less pronounced than at dimmer steady intensities, as shown for example in Fig. 1 of Baylor *et al.* (1979*b*). In the present figure (Fig. 5.10), by the time the next set of test flashes was delivered (approximately 12 min after the bleach, trace C), the rod's sensitivity had recovered quite substantially, and pronounced spontaneous fluctuations were occurring.

In the case of fluctuations arising as a result of steady illumination, classical methods of power spectral analysis are applicable, and have for example been used by Baylor *et al.* (1979*b*). For the case of a series of identical events with shape $r(t)$ occurring randomly in time at rate $\nu\ \mathrm{s}^{-1}$, and adding linearly, the zero frequency asymptote $S(0)$ of the power spectral density of the noise is given by

$$S(0) = 2\nu\left[\int_0^\infty r(t)\,\mathrm{d}t\right]^2. \qquad (5.7)$$

For $r(t)$ corresponding to the rod's single-photon response, (5.7) becomes

$$S(0) = 2\nu\left[f\, r_{\mathrm{peak}}\, t_{\mathrm{peak}}\right]^2, \qquad (5.8)$$

where r_{peak} and t_{peak} are the amplitude and time-to-peak respectively of the single-photon response, and f is a 'shape factor' typically having a value of 1.5–1.7 for the rod response. Hence, in order to estimate the event rate v, it is necessary to determine $S(0)$ from the spectrum of the fluctuations, and r_{peak} and t_{peak} from the flash sensitivity. Because of the random nature of the occurrence of quantal events, quite long records are needed to obtain reliable estimates for the power spectra, and in practice durations of at least 2–3 min are required. And similarly, to determine flash sensitivity it is in practice necessary to present at least 10–20 dim flashes, at intervals of 10 s or so. Hence it may take 5 min or more to obtain a single reliable estimate of the event rate in steady illumination, for the time-course of responses obtained at room temperature from toad rods.

Analysis of such results is further complicated by non-stationarity; that is, the cell's sensitivity (r_{peak}), kinetics (t_{peak}), and equivalent event rate (v) are all changing with time. Strictly speaking this invalidates (5.7) and (5.8) but, provided the parameters are changing relatively slowly, it is probably reasonable to use these equations to provide an approximate value for v. Since it is not possible simultaneously to measure the flash sensitivity and the fluctuations, it is in practice necessary to present dim flashes before and after each section of noise and to estimate an average sensitivity.

Such a method was applied to the bleach-induced fluctuations in another cell, using a protocol similar to that in Fig. 5.10, to give the results illustrated in Fig. 5.11. The open symbols plot the raw estimates of event rate v, while for the filled symbols the dark-adapted event rate (approx. 0.03 s^{-1}) has been subtracted to give an estimate of the bleach-induced event rate. After the first 10 min it appears that the equivalent event rate decays with a time constant of approx. 15 min (in a toad rod at 25 °C). The first point, at 6 min, is well above the solid line, indicating either the existence of a component with a faster decay or perhaps that the method is not very accurate during the early rapidly-changing phase. In this cell a bleach of *c*. 10^7 isomerizations induced an initial event rate extrapolated as 1–2 events s^{-1}.

Hence these results are consistent with the idea that, following a small bleach, the toad rod outer segment experiences a greatly elevated rate of events indistinguishable from photon-events, and that slowly this event rate declines. Similar results to these have been observed in all rods in the toad retina which have been tested with bleaches in the range 0.1–2.5%. At higher bleach intensities the rod is, unfortunately, permanently desensitized (presumably as a result of the absence of 11-*cis* retinal) and the lowered sensitivity renders the fluctuations much smaller. This latter

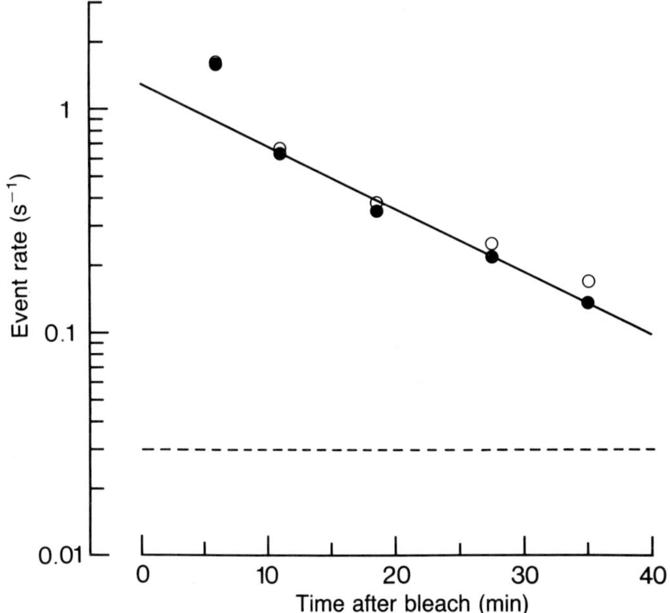

Fig. 5.11. Calculated rate of equivalent photon events in a toad rod exposed to a bleach of 0.5%. Protocol was similar to that in Fig. 5.10, with dim test flashes given periodically. Open circles (○) are calculated event rates for power spectra obtained over periods of approx. 3 min centred at the indicated times; flash sensitivities were averaged before and after these periods. Event rate was calculated from equation (5.7). Filled circles (●) give the bleach-induced rate, obtained by subtracting the mean dark-adapted spontaneous event rate of 0.03 s^{-1} (shown by broken line) from the open circles. Dark-adapted single photon response was 1.1 pA in amplitude; 25 °C.

result seems consistent with the recent report that in this species (*Bufo marinus*) not more than 3% of the pigment can be regenerated in the isolated retina (Cocozza & Ostroy, 1987).

Primate

At very small bleaches, of around 0.003% or about 3000 isomerizations, monkey rods have been reported to exhibit step-like transitions in the recovery phase (Baylor *et al.*, 1984), but it is not known how these events might affect the overall behaviour of the scotopic system. More recently it has been reported that, at higher bleaches of around a few percent, monkey rods exhibit photon-like fluctuations similar to those in toad (Schnapf *et al.*, 1987). Such events are certainly predicted on the basis of the model of dark adaptation developed by Lamb (1981), and presented in the following section. It will be of great interest in the future to examine quantitatively how these recently found fluctuations compare with predictions.

5.4 A model of dark adaptation

This section describes a model of dark adaptation developed as an alternative to Rushton's formulation, in which the observed threshold elevation in the overall visual system originates from photon-like events within the rod transduction machinery (Lamb, 1981). In certain respects it may be seen as an extension of the hypothesis of Barlow (1964) that the elevated dark light following a bleach arises from increased noise in the rod photoreceptors.

5.4.1 Origins of the model

Components of psychophysical threshold recovery

In the course of analysis of Pugh's (1975*b*) dark adaptation results, it was noted that the recovery of log threshold elevation could accurately be described in terms of several straight-line sections, rather than the convential exponential form. Examples of such straight-line behaviour are illustrated in Fig. 5.2*b* for 2% and 98% bleaches. Although the changes in scale between the two parts in Fig. 5.2*b* complicates comparison, the solid lines in the two parts actually have the same slope, of approximately 0.24 log units min^{-1}. Indeed, for all bleaches in the range 0.5–98% the recovery over a substantial region could be fitted with a line of this slope. Similar behaviour may be seen in Fig. 5.3 for the case of two rod monochromats, where the threshold elevation may be followed to higher values; see also Stabell, Stabell & Nordby (1986). The results of Nordby *et al.* (1984) in Fig. 5.3*b* and those of Stabell *et al.* (1986) were, however, not available when the original analysis described here was performed (see Chapter 10 for more detail).

The significance of a straight-line decline in semi-logarithmic coordinates is that it indicates exponential decay of the quantity with time; that is, decay according to exp $(-t/\tau)$ where τ is a time constant. Hence the threshold elevation (rather than the *log* threshold elevation in Rushton's formulation) appeared to decline exponentialy with time.

As may be seen in Fig. 5.2*b*, two other regions of the decay were also well-fitted by straight lines, and again this was a general feature seen over a wide range of bleaching strengths. From these observations it was concluded that recovery of threshold elevation following any bleaching exposure could be described in terms of three components of exponential decay, and it was found that the time constants were roughly 5 s, 100s and 400 s.

Furthermore, in analyzing the magnitude of the separate components of recovery, it was shown that the first two components increased in size in direct proportion to the bleach, at least for small bleaches. Thus, in going from a 0.5% bleach to a 5% bleach the magnitudes of both these components increased by approximately 1 log unit. This appeared to indicate an underlying linearity in the threshold elevation induced by bleaching.

Basic hypotheses

To interpret these psychophysical observations two basic hypotheses were made, one fundamental and the other for simplicity.

(1) Fundamental hypothesis The fundamental hypothesis was that the 'equivalent background' of Stiles & Crawford (1932) and Crawford (1937) arises from the generation, within the rod transduction machinery (and as a direct consequence of the presence of the bleaching products), of events indistinguishable from photoisomerizations.

(2) Supplementary hypothesis For convenience of analysis it was further assumed that the dark adaptation data of Pugh (1975*b*) were obtained under conditions that gave very nearly Weber law behaviour. (The exponent n in (5.1) would actually have been $n \simeq 0.8$–0.9 for Pugh's conditions, but this was approximated as unity.)

From the second hypothesis the equivalent background intensity for Pugh's experiments was simply directly proportional to the measured threshold elevation, and from the first hypothesis this equivalent background intensity was in turn directly proportional to photoproduct concentration. Together these hypotheses indicated that, to a good approximation, the photoproduct concentration should have been directly proportional to the measured threshold elevation. In other words, the dark adaptation curves could be considered in a simplistic way as plots of the concentration of photoproducts.

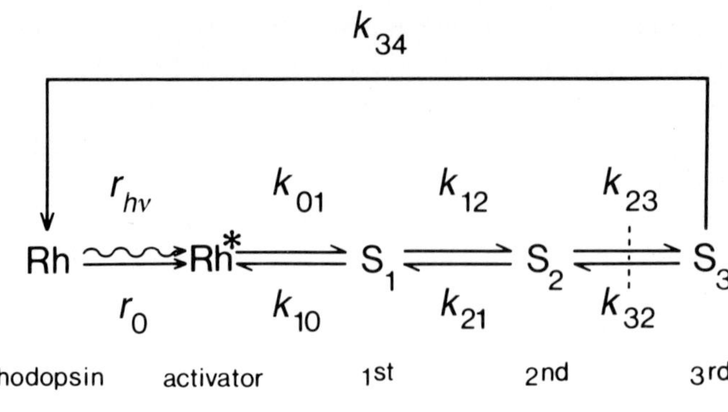

Fig. 5.12. Scheme to account for the kinetics of the three components in the recovery of the elevated 'equivalent background intensity'. Rh is isomerized to Rh* either by light (hv) or thermally (at rate r_0). Rh* is inactivated to S_1, which is converted to S_2, and in turn to S_3, before being resynthesized to native rhodopsin. S_1, S_2 and S_3 give rise to the three distinct components of recovery, through the reverse reactions with rate constants k_{10}, k_{21} and k_{32}. The time constants of the three components of decay are given by the reciprocals of the rate constants of removal, k_{12}, k_{23} and k_{34}. The broken vertical line represents rate-limiting of the interconversion of S_2 and S_3 (see text). Reproduced with permission from Lamb (1981).

5.4.2 Reverse reactions from photoproducts

On the basis of these hypotheses, the presence of three separate components in the bleaching recovery was taken as evidence for the existence of three separate photochemical intermediates, each producing photon-like events in the rod and each decaying with a separate time constant. The details of the specific model chosen, incorporating these three separate photoproducts and giving rise to photon-like events, will now be described.

The model is shown in Fig. 5.12, beginning and ending with rhodopsin, Rh, and with a series of intermediates labelled Rh* and S_1 to S_3, Rh* is the substance which activates the light response, and apparently corresponds to an early form of metarhodopsin II. S_1, S_2 and S_3 represent the substances which cause the three components of elevation of equivalent background.

The absolute dark light (or rate of thermal isomerizations, is represented by the rate r_0, real light by the rate r_{hv}, and the elevated background light during recovery from bleaching by the reverse reaction from S_1 to Rh*, with rate constant k_{10}. Hence, according to this model the formation of Rh*, whether by photoisomerization, thermal isomerization or reverse action from S_1, is assumed to trigger the transduction process in the same way. This means that, as far as the electrical response is concerned, the rod cannot distinguish whether Rh* was generated by photoisomerization, thermal isomerizaiton or reverse reaction. Accordingly the total rate of 'photon-like events' in the rod will be the sum of the real light, the thermal events, and the events produced as a result of the presence of the bleaching products.

The second and third components of recovery are assumed to arise in a similar way from reverse reactions in the chain of removal reactions. S_1, S_2 and S_3 are removed with rate constants k_{12}, k_{23} and k_{34} respectively, set to give the observed time constants of 5 s, 100 s and 400 s. The influence of S_2 and S_3 is exerted through the weak reverse reactions with rate constants k_{21} and k_{32} respectively. Hence at a late time in recovery, when most of the bleached rhodopsin has been converted through to S_3, this third substance will decay with a time constant of around 400 s. It will produce a small amount of S_2 and a smaller amount of S_1, which will in turn produce a tiny rate of activation of Rh*, equivalent to real light.

Although the details will not be given here, it was straightforward to determine all the parameters of the model from Pugh's psychophysical data. The only complication was the necessity to assume rate-limiting of the interconversion of S_2 and S_3 (indicated by the dotted line in Fig. 5.12). This arose because the non-linear behaviour of the second component at large bleaches, together with the delayed onset of the third component, suggested a bottleneck at this point (see Lamb, 1981, Fig. 4). This rate-limiting turns out to be an important feature of the model.

5.4.3 *Predictions of the model*

Electrophysiology

A clear prediction of this model is the presence of an elevated rate of occurrence of photon-like events in rods following bleaches. Such events are now well-documented (Section 5.3.5), but at the time that the model was formulated they had not been observed. (The experiments of Lamb, 1980, were in fact performed as a direct test of this hypothesis but, regrettably, the theoretical paper forecasting the existence of the fluctuations, Lamb, 1981, was not actually published until after the experimental work had been published.)

Section 5.3.5 showed that the increased fluctuations found in rods

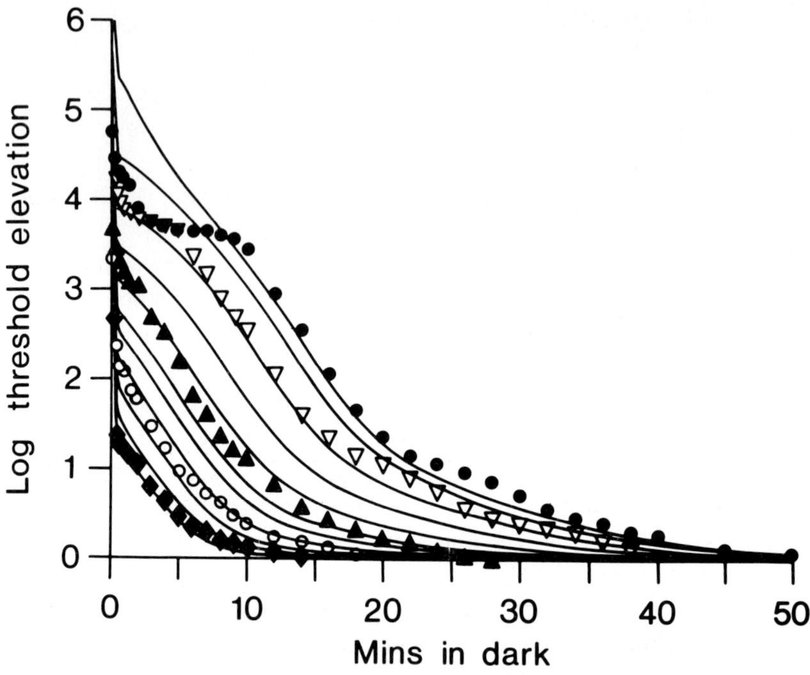

Fig. 5.13. Reconstructed behaviour of the model for a family of dark adaptations. Curves are predictions of the model for the eleven bleaching intensity-time products used by Pugh (1975*b*), while the symbols are averaged points measured from his data for five of the bleaches (◆, 0.5%, ○, 3.9%, ▲, 22.2%; ▽, 86.4%; ●, 98.1%). Reproduced with permission from Lamb (1981).

following a bleach are broadly consistent with the expectations of the theory, but a rigorous test is not feasible because of the differences between the human and toad systems. The situation is further complicated by the non-stationary nature of the system under analysis and by the requirement for very long and stable recordings. Hence, although it is not possible to say that the toad rod recordings precisely confirm the theory, they are qualitatively consistent with it and provide no reason to doubt the theory.

Psychophysics

The reconstructed behaviour of the model for human dark-adaptation behaviour is shown in Figs 5.13 and 5.14, for superimposed and separate traces respectively. In each case the solid curves are predictions of the model, while the symbols are measured threshold elevations redrawn from Pugh (1975*b*).

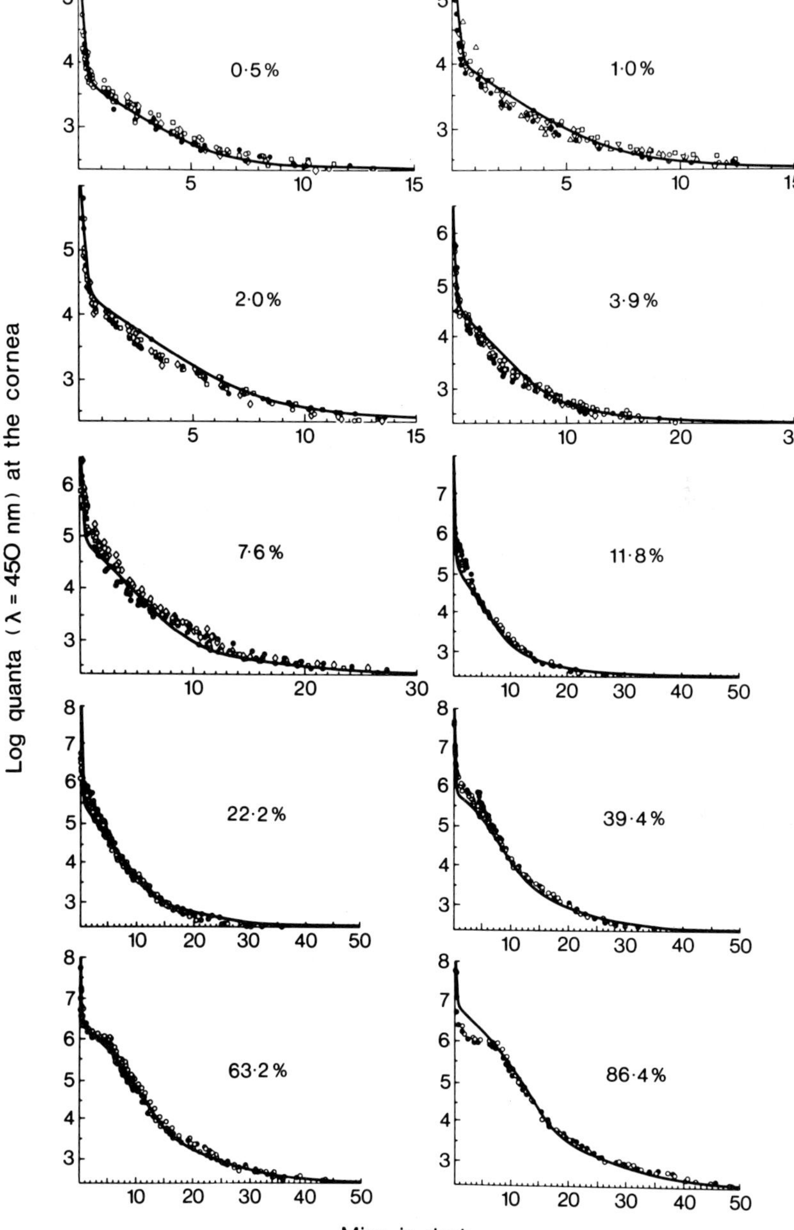

Fig. 5.14. Observed recovery and predicted behaviour of model for dark adaptation following bleaches of ten different magnitudes. Data redrawn from Pugh (1975*b*, Fig. 5.13), with individual reconstructed curves from superimposed. Values on each panel show percent bleached. Reproduced with permission from Lamb (1981).

It may be seen that below the region of cone domination the predicted behaviour is very similar to the observed behaviour, throughout the tested range of 3 log units of intensity corresponding to bleaches from 0.5% to 98%. Comparison with Fig. 5.3*b* for a rod monochromat suggests that the form of the predicted behaviour above cone threshold is also qualitatively correct.

However, in comparing the psychophysical results of Pugh (1975*b*) with those of Nordby *et al.* (1984) there appears to be a minor difference in vertical scaling between the two studies, whereby the latter results for the rod monochromat show log thresholds some 30% greater than Pugh's. Whether this represents a relative difference in calibration attenuations between the two studies, or whether perhaps the data of Stabell *et al.* corresponds to more-nearly Weber law behaviour (i.e. n closer to unity), is not clear. In either case fairly minor changes to the parameters could be made, as discussed by Lamb (1981, p. 1781), which would provide an equivalent fit to the more recent results. Ideally, of course, the full analysis should be applied to dark adaptation data from a rod monochromat, where the increment-threshold function has been measured under identical conditions. Unfortunately, such increment-threshold data do not appear to be available at present.

Even without such additional data, the accuracy of the prediction of Pugh's results (upon which the model was based) over a very wide range of bleaches, and the qualitative comparison with the monochromat results, would appear to provide considerable support for the ideas underlying the model.

An essential feature of the model is the rate-limited removal of the second product, S_2, which is needed to account for the form of the recovery curves with large bleaches. This assumption does not accord with earlier ideas that the photochemical bleaching reactions are thermal, but there is in any case evidence now against those ideas. For example, Donner & Hemilä (1975) showed that in frog retina the rate constants of removal of metarhodopsins II and III appeared to be much higher (i.e. there was faster removal) with small bleaches than with large bleaches. And in cat retina, Bonds & MacLeod (1974) and Ripps *et al.* (1981) have shown that the regeneration of rhodopsin is essentially linear with time until at least 75% has been resynthesized. These results are strongly indicative of rate-limited reactions in frog and cat photoreceptors, and they suggest that a similar limit in the human would not be unreasonable. Indeed, the regeneration of visual pigment in the achromat shown in Fig. 2 of Sharpe, van Norren & Nordby (1988) (see also Chapter 10) appears consistent with this idea.

Magnitudes of the reverse reaction rates

It is interesting to consider the approximate magnitude of the reverse reaction rates. From the parameters chosen to fit the psychophysical data the time constant, $k_{10}{}^{-1}$, of the reverse reaction from S_1 to Rh^* is approx. 20000 s, and the equilibrium constants of the following two reactions (conversion of S_1 to S_2, and S_2 to S_3) are approximately 100 (i.e. the reactions proceed well to the right). The first of these figures indicates that in the early stages of a 1% bleach, with about 10^6 Rh molecules (in a human rod) converted through to S_1, there will be a rate of reactivation of Rh^* of approx. 50 molecules s^{-1}. Similarly, in the late stages of a 100% bleach, when most of the 10^8 Rh have been converted through to S_3, there will remain of the order of 10^6 S_2 molecules, 10^4 S_1 molecules, and a rate of reactivation of Rh^* of approx. 0.5 molecules s^{-1}. These figures give an indication of the very small degree of overall reversibility in the removal reactions required to account for the psychophysical results.

5.4.4 *Possible molecular basis for the model*

In order to consider the possible molecular basis for the model it would be highly desirable to identify the three substances S_1, S_2 and S_3 with physical intermediates in the photobleaching sequence. However, none of the *spectrophotometrically* identified intermediates have appropriate kinetics, and it seems likely that the differences between the substances involve more subtle changes in the rhodopsin molecule than the known spectrophotometric transitions.

Of the classical photochemical intermediates, metarhodopsin II is produced within a few milliseconds of photoisomerization (at 37 °C), but decays only very slowly, with a time constant of more than 80 s (in isolated human retina; Baumann & Bender, 1973). The later product metarhodopsin III builds up to a peak in about 180 s and decays thereafter with a time constant of around 250 s.

It had often been thought difficult to explain the role of metarhodopsin II, since it is produced much faster than the electrical response of the rod, yet it remains in the cell for much longer than the duration of the electrical response. However, it now seems likely that the single spectral species metarhodopsin II actually encompasses a variety of chemically different forms. Chemical modification at a region of the rhodopsin protein molecule remote from the chromophore site could alter the chemical properties of the protein (converting it into a different 'species') without altering its absorption spectrum. Such an 'isochromic' change could not, by definition, be detected spectrophotometrically; a similar change has been reported for metarhodopsin I (Williams, 1970).

At present it is widely thought that Rh*, the form of rhodopsin which activates the light response, corresponds to an early form (perhaps the first form) of metarhodopsin II produced following photoisomerization. There is evidence that the transition from metarhodopsin I to metarhodopsin II represents a substantial rearrangement of the molecule, perhaps involving an opening-up of the protein. In this way a key enzymatically-active site presumably becomes exposed, and it is this opening-up step which represents the formation of Rh*.

The most likely physical candidates for the step(s) corresponding to the removal of Rh* are firstly phosphorylation of the protein and secondly the capping action of another protein. It has been known for some years that the biochemical transduction cascade is 'quenched' by ATP (Liebman & Pugh, 1980), and that photo-activated rhodopsin is phosphorylated at multiple locations as the result of the catalytic action of rhodopsin kinase, a 65 kDa peripheral protein (Bownds *et al.*, 1972; Kühn & Dreyer, 1972). More recently it has been shown that this reaction is sufficiently fast to participate in the quenching of activated rhodopsin (Sitaramayya & Liebman, 1983; Sitaramayya, 1986). Once rhodopsin has been phosphorylated it is able to bind a soluble protein, variously referred to as 48 kDa protein, arrestin and retinal S-antigen (Kühn, Hall & Wilden, 1984). It has now been shown that, with the 48 kDa protein bound, the phosphorylated rhodopsin is inhibited in its ability to trigger the later stages of the transduction cascade (Wilden, Hall & Kühn, 1986). Hence on this scheme Rh* is removed by multiple phosphorylation followed by binding of the 48 kDa protein.

Hence a number of biochemical transformations are known to affect activated rhodopsin, and other reactions probably remain to be discovered, but regrettably it cannot at present be said whether any of these reaction products are the substances represented by S_1, S_2 and S_3 in the model.

Phosphorylation and reverse reactions

A theoretical consideration has been made by Lisman (1985) of the energetics which may be involved in the phosphorylation of rhodopsin, and the effects that such phosphorylation might have on the rate of reverse reactions. Although his arguments relate to invertebrate metarhodopsin they are equally applicable to the vertebrate case. Lisman postulated that the non-phosphorylated form of metarhodopsin II is active, and that the attachment of one or more phosphates leads to inactivation. The existence of multiple phosphorylation sites on a single rhodopsin protein molecule is explained as a way of ensuring that the probability of subsequently returning to the completely unphosphorylated form is very small.

Phosphorylation reactions are generally quite reversible under physiological conditions. Lisman suggests that with a typical ATP/ADP ratio in the cytoplasm the equilibrium ratio, R, of the singly phosphorylated to the unphosphorylated form might only be about 100:1, corresponding to a free energy change of about 2 kcal. On this basis m similar phosphorylation reactions occurring on the same molecule would lead to an equilibrium ratio of final to initial product of R^m, or about 10^{10}:1, corresponding to a free energy change of *c.* 10 kcal, for $m = 5$. In this way the multiple phosphorylation steps would drastically reduce the overall rate of reverse reactions.

In Lisman's scheme a single phosphorylation is sufficient to inactivate Rh*, and additional phosphorylations serve primarily to decrease the probability that inactive metarhodopsin will revert to its active state. (They may also contribute to the stereotypical smooth waveform of the single photon response.) In considering the probability of reversal it is interesting that seven to nine phosphates have been observed to be added to activated rhodopsin (Wilden *et al.*, 1986). This would suggest that such reactions could easily provide the required low degree of overall reversibility shown in the previous section to be necessary.

Hence, it seems that the appropriate kinds of chemistry and intermediates exist in the transduction chain, in order for the model to be correct. But the tantalizing link between physics and psychophysics remains to be established firmly.

5.5 Summary

A variety of problems with the Dowling–Rushton model of dark adaptation have led to a re-examination of the subject, and an alternative description has been advanced.

This formulation is based on the equivalent background hypothesis of Stiles & Crawford (1932) and Crawford (1937), which states that during dark adaptation the visual system behaves as if the world is being viewed through a veiling light that slowly fades. Although this hypothesis has never been given an absolutely rigorous test, it appears to provide a very good description of most of the observed psychophysical behaviour. Extending the ideas of Barlow (1964), the present formulation proposes that during dark adaptation the equivalent background hypothesis is literally correct, in that the rod phototransduction process experiences events indistinguishable from photon hits, but caused by the presence of bleaching photoproducts in the rod outer segment.

A model based on this hypothesis is capable of providing a very good description of the kinetics of the recovery of visual threshold following bleaches ranging from 0.5% to 98%. The model predicts the occurrence of photon-like fluctuations in recordings from rods following bleaches, and such fluctuations are indeed observed, with qualitatively the correct form. While it has not been possible to subject the model to any particularly strong test, there are no obvious suggestions of any serious failures on its part. This is not, however, to claim that the model is correct in all its details, but rather to suggest that it represents a more satisfactory description than the Dowling–Rushton formulation.

Three attractive features of the model are as follows. Firstly, it is capable of explaining the observed desensitization reasonably accurately over a wide range of bleaches. Secondly, it removes an exponential dependence of sensitivity on fraction bleached (the Dowling–Rushton equation), and replaces it with a *linear* dependence on photoproducts, thereby avoiding some of the difficulties which arise with non-uniform bleaches. And, thirdly, it presents a fairly simple physical basis for the origin of the equivalent background (or noise), namely reverse reactions from photoproducts.

An interesting consequence of acceptance of the equivalent background hypothesis is that it then becomes unnecessary to provide any special description of the mechanisms of desensitization which occur in the overall visual system. Whatever changes occur during *light adaptation* with a steady stabilized light, whether at the receptor or subsequently, will automatically apply during dark adaptation also. Obviously it would be desirable to provide a description of such changes eventually, but it is by no means necessary to consider dark adaptation as entirely separate from light adaptation.

An obvious question of interest is why the transduction machinery should experience such events following bleaches; that is, why is it not possible to design a system where reverse reactions do not occur? It seems likely that the answer involves the energetics of the reactions involved, and the extremely high sensitivity of the rod photoreceptor. In order to trigger the light response reliably the activated rhodopsin Rh* needs to be present for an adequate length of time; thus the removal reactions cannot be too rapid or sensitivity would be thrown away. But any chemical reaction, such as the removal of Rh*, is bound to exhibit some degree of reversibility determined by the free energy change of the reaction. Given the biological constraints within which the living cell has to operate, it would seem that the photoreceptor performs exceedingly well. In many ways it appears that our visual system outperforms most electronic devices operating at low light levels and at the same temperature.

It is worth remembering that the slowness of dark adaptation can in no way be beneficial to the owner of the eye. Rather it is a distinct disadvantage, and we would presumably be better off with a visual system that could rapidly adapt to dim light after very intense light. (In just the same way the designer of a television camera or of a photomultiplier tube would prefer to use materials which did not phosphoresce and which could rapidly attain full sensitivity after intense exposures but, until the recent arrival of CCD cameras, this goal seemed extremely difficult to attain.) In this context dark adaptation may be considered as an unfortunate consequence of some kind of trade-off which has had to be made in order to attain the exquisite sensitivity of the rod photoreceptor.

As a final point we might consider some evolutionary aspects of the time-course of dark adaptation: that is, just how serious a problem for the survival of an animal is the slowness of dark adaptation? It would seem that in normal life the rod system needs to be brought to its full sensitivity only relatively slowly, at a rate comparable to the fading light at dusk, and of this the rods are readily capable. In fact, if the rate-limiting step in the model is correct, the resensitization is actually slower than it might otherwise have been. Such rate-limiting may then conceivably be advantageous to an animal, since the rods spend much of their time completely incapacitated in daylight conditions. Accordingly it would seem undesirable continually to expend large amounts of energy on rhodopsin resynthesis when the light level seldom drops precipitously.

On the argument above, that the fading light at dusk represents the norm, it might be expected that in the evolution of vertebrates a sudden decrease in the ambient lighting level over a range of 6 or more log units would be a relatively infrequent and unimportant occurrence. However, for cave-dwelling and burrowing animals travelling between bright daylight and the subterranean world, a more rapid adaptation to darkness might be advantageous. It would be interesting to know whether this has evolved in such animals.

Acknowledgements

I am most grateful to Professors D. A. Baylor and E. N. Pugh Jr for helpful comments on the manuscript. This work was supported by grants from the M.R.C., the N.I.H. (EY-06154), and the Wellcome Trust.

6

Invertebrate vision at low luminances

Simon B. Laughlin

6.1 Introduction

The problem of seeing at low luminances is one of extracting information from an unreliable signal. Unreliability stems from the lack of available light. The process of photon absorption is stochastic and, as recognised by De Vries and Rose (rev. Rose, 1977), quantum fluctuations set an upper limit to the signal to noise ratio of the visual system. The more photons one has, the better the signal-to-noise ratio and the more one sees. It follows that the efficiency of vision at low luminances depends upon three sets of factors, each of which must be optimised to maximise the signal and minimise the noise. The three sets of factors correspond to three levels of visual processing, the collection and imaging of light, the transduction of light energy into a signal and the transmission and processing of this signal. One must collect and image light with an optical system of high sensitivity. The photoreceptors must collect and register photons efficiently by mechanisms that introduce little extra noise. Finally the nervous system must use efficient means for transmitting and processing the receptor signals. Neural networks must be designed to minimise added noise and their properties must be tailored to the statistics of the incoming signal to enable them to extract the maximum amount of information.

The compound eyes of insects, crustaceans and arthropods such as the familiar horseshoe crab, *Limulus*, are bound by these same constraints. In addition, their eyes are often amenable to a rigorous quantitative analysis that provides an opportunity to study the efficiency of vision and visual processing at several levels. This facility enables us to identify the fundamental optical and neural problems associated with vision at low intensities, and to investigate their solutions. For this reason the study of compound eyes offers far more than the satisfaction of zoological curiosity. I will attempt to demonstrate some of the principles that promote efficiency by reviewing the fundamentals of phototransduction, sampling and neural processing. This broad overview is intended to demonstrate the range and subtlety of the mechanisms that arthropods employ to ensure reasonable night vision, and to emphasise that performance is improved by matching the form of sampling and processing to the available light and by minimising the effects of intrinsic noise. We will start by examining the efficiency with which photoreceptors transduce signals at low intensities and the efficiency with which single photon signals are transmitted in the brain. We will then turn to the question of adjusting sampling and neural processing to the optical quality of incoming signals.

6.2 Responses of invertebrate photoreceptors at low luminances

To attain maximum sensitivity the retina must register the absorption of single photons efficiently. The maximum efficiency would pertain if the signal-to-noise ratio of the photoreceptor responses equalled the limit imposed by the corneal photon flux. To obtain this maximum the photoreceptors have to transduce the energy of every available photon into a brief response of constant energy (e.g. an electrical response of fixed amplitude and duration). In this case the retina would be an ideal device with a unit quantum efficiency, i.e. the signal-to-noise ratios at the input and the output would be equal (e.g. Rose, 1977). In invertebrates the comparative ease with which recordings can be made from intact photoreceptors, viewing the world through undisturbed optics, offers an excellent opportunity to study the factors that prevent a retina from attaining perfect quantum efficiency. Because many of these limitations can be directly related to biological materials and biological processes that are analagous to those found in the retinas of vertebrates, the findings are of general significance. For example, invertebrates offered the first insights into the nature of a biological photoreceptor's response to single photons. Indeed, the statistical techniques used to establish the relationship between discrete photoreceptor responses and photon absorptions were forged on invertebrates, particularly by Yeandle and his associates (for a concise summary see Yeandle, 1977).

In 1958, Yeandle reported that the dark-adapted photoreceptors of the lateral eye of the horseshoe crab, *Limulus*, generated discrete depolarising waves (bumps) at random intervals (e.g. Fig. 6.2). These 'bumps' occurred in total darkness but their frequency increased in proportion to light intensity. Yeandle repeated Hecht, Shlaer & Pirenne's (1942) classical 'frequency of seeing' experiment on *Limulus* photoreceptors and found that the probability of observing a bump after a brief flash increased with stimulus intensity in a manner that was consistent with a bump being triggered by a single photon. This analysis was extended to show that the numbers of bumps elicited by each flash followed a Poisson distribution, as did the intervals between the bumps generated during prolonged periods of dim illumination. In both cases the means of the appropriate Poisson distribution increased in proportion to stimulus intensity (Fuortes & Yeandle, 1964). This statistical evidence was consistent with each absorbed photon triggering a quantum bump, but it was impossible to gauge the efficiency of bump generation. As Fuortes & Yeandle pointed out, the bumps followed a flash of light with a variable latency, indicative of a stochastic process connecting photon absorption to the generation of membrane potential. As an example, they suggested that transduction could involve the generation of droplets of 'internal transmitter substance' and that the action of these droplets might follow Poisson statistics. In this case, a photon absorption could generate large numbers of drops, each with a low probability of generating a bump. Such a wasteful process introduces multiplicative noise (e.g. Cohn, 1983) that would lower the quantum efficiency by introducing extra uncertainty but bump statistics would remain Poisson. In Fuortes & Yeandle's preparations the ratio between bumps and incident photons was usually less than 1 in 100 and the attenuation by the optics was uncertain. Thus there were plenty of photons available to allow for the possibility that a highly inefficient transduction process generated the Poisson statistics. Indeed, statistical theory shows that when the probability that an absorbed photon triggers a bump is low one cannot distinguish between mechanisms that trigger just one bump per effective photon, and mechanisms that trigger a daughter Poisson process which generates, on average, more than one bump. Unless the ratio between bumps and available photons is greater than about 0.2, the statistics of adaptation and transduction cannot be disentangled (Weiss & Yeandle, 1975).

The compound eye of the locust provides the high quantum efficiency required to analyse the statistics of transduction. In eye slice preparations, locust photoreceptors produce quantum bumps, with properties similar to *Limulus* (Scholes, 1964). By using an intact preparation (Wilson, 1975), in which the natural optics and the retinal air and blood supply is undisturbed, one is able to record larger bumps (Fig. 6.2). The number of bumps produced in darkness is routinely as low as 6 per receptor per hour and with stimuli of the optimum wavelength and direction, 60% of incident photons produce a quantum bump. This high ratio enables one to distinguish between mechanisms that produce one bump per photon and mechanisms that produce, on average, more than one bump (Lillywhite, 1977). For example, if more than one bump is produced per photon, the bumps will tend to occur in clusters, each group being generated by a single photon absorption. When the mean interval between photon absorptions greatly exceeds the duration of a cluster, these clusters will manifest themselves as an unexpectedly large number of short intervals between bumps. By analysing bump intervals it was concluded that a single photon absorption produces just one bump. Thus the locust photoreceptor is an extremely efficient photon counter that produces a single bump for each effective photon. High ratios between incident photons and bumps have been measured in flies (0.5), and crabs (0.45) (Dubs, Laughlin & Srinivasan, 1981; Doujak, 1985). For the case of the fly the value of 50% of incident corneal photons absorbed fits well with data on the optics (de Ruyter, 1986); 80% of the energy is transferred from the diffraction pattern of the lens to the modal pattern of the photoreceptive waveguide (van Hateren, 1984). The density of pigment and length of the photoreceptive waveguide suggests that 85% of this light will be absorbed. The remaining loss can be explained by reflection at the corneal surface of 10% and a quantum efficiency of the photopigment of 80%.

6.3 Photoreceptor intrinsic noise

Although the locust photoreceptors are, by vertebrate standards (e.g. H. B. Barlow, 1977), extremely effective at trapping and registering incident photons, the biochemical processes of transduction introduce intrinsic noise. Two types of noise have been observed. The first is dark noise – spontaneous fluctuations in membrane potential produced in darkness. The second is transducer noise – fluctuations in response amplitude generated during the phototransduction of photon signals.

6.3.1 Dark noise

As in vertebrate rods, photoreceptor dark noise has two components: a continuous fluctuation in membrane potential and larger discrete events that resemble photon bumps. The continuous dark noise has not been analysed in invertebrate photoreceptors but the published records suggest that it poses little threat to the resolution of single photon events in fully dark adapted cells (Fig. 6.2). It will be interesting to see if this dark noise can be associated with intermediate stages in the transduction process, as in rods (Baylor, Matthews & Yau, 1980). In insect and crab photoreceptors the rates of dark bumps reach low levels, in the order of 10 per hour at 25 °C (Lillywhite & Laughlin, 1979; Dubs *et al.*, 1981; Doujak, 1985). In fully dark adapted photoreceptors of the intact *Limulus* lateral eye, dark bump rates drop to practically zero (R. B. Barlow *et al.*, 1987). These levels compare with rates of 360 per hour in toad rods at 20 °C (Baylor *et al.*, 1980). However, a toad rod contains 3×10^9 rhodopsin molecules while a single locust or fly photoreceptor contains approximately 10^8 rhodopsin molecules. The higher rates in rods can be attributed to the larger number of rhodopsin molecules. Thus there is no evidence at present that the invertebrate transducer is inherently superior to the vertebrate with respect to dark noise.

Several explanations have been advanced for dark bumps. Because the dark bumps have properties that are similar to, but not necessarily identical to (e.g. Lisman, 1985) light induced bumps, they can be attributed to the spurious activation of photopigment. In the invertebrates a photon absorption isomerises rhodopsin to an active metarhodopsin (Fig. 6.1) and this triggers the enzymatic cascade responsible for producing a bump. The active form is then converted to a stable but inactive form of metarhodopsin, probably by phosphorylation (Paulsen & Bentrop, 1984; Lisman, 1985). This inactive metarhodopsin is then isomerised back to rhodopsin by the absorption of a second photon, and reactivated by dephosphorylation. This general scheme suggests two origins for dark bumps. The first is the spontaneous generation of active metarhodopsin from rhodopsin, either by thermal isomerisation or by activation of the enzymatic site to produce an anomalous active rhodopsin. The second is the production of an active meta- by a back reaction from inactive meta-. All schemes are compatible with the observation that in *Limulus*, as in rods, the dark bump rates increase markedly with temperature. All components of the transduction process will be temperature sensitive (R. B. Barlow *et al.*, 1987).

There is compelling evidence for the production of dark bumps by metarhodopsin. In many arthropod photoreceptors, a bright brief flash of light produces a saturated response which is followed by an after-potential that can take up to an hour to decay. This after-potential is a prolongation of the light response, for it has the same electrical prop-

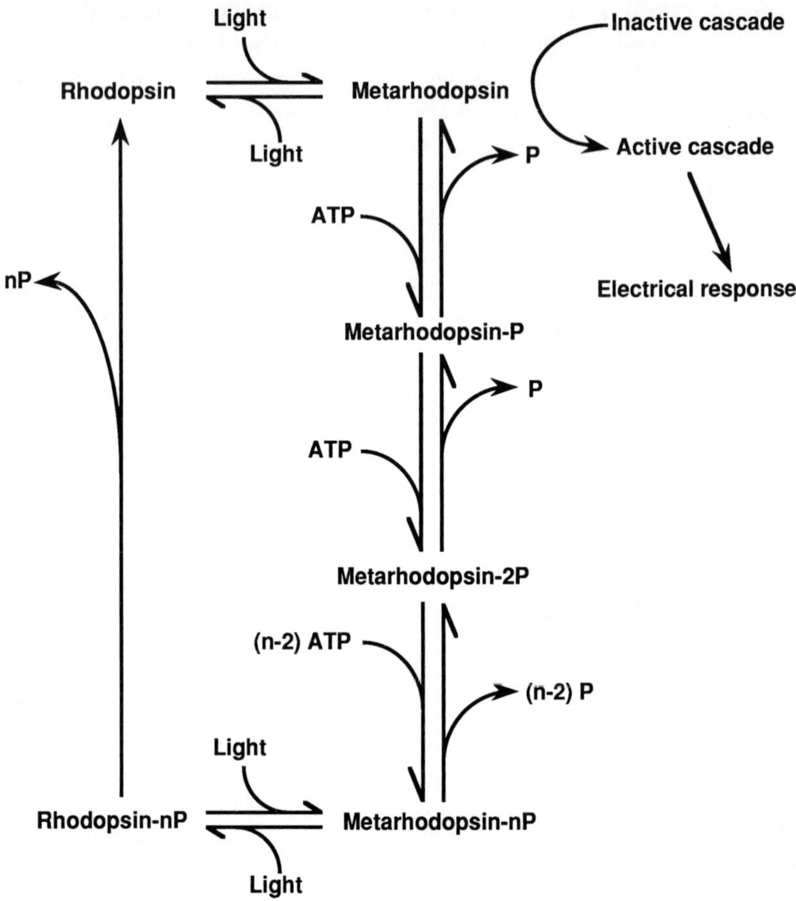

Fig. 6.1. An outline of the photopigment cycle in an invertebrate photoreceptor showing how metarhodopsin is thought to activate the electrical response before being inactivated by successive phosphorylations. These phosphorylated metarhodopsins could spontaneously hydrolyse to regenerate the active metarhodopsin, so producing electrical dark noise (after Paulsen & Bentrop, 1984, and Lisman, 1986).

erties and decays to a train of bumps. A large body of work, performed throughout the 1970s (rev. Hamdorf, 1979) showed that the after-potential depended upon the presence in the photoreceptor of a photoproduct of the initial flash. Light which reisomerised metarhodopsin back to rhodopsin truncated the after-potential. Recent experiments suggest that the after-potential bumps are generated by a large pool of inactivated metarhodopsin (Lisman, 1985). The dark bump rate increases with the amount of metarhodopsin formed in the photoreceptor by the initial bright flash (e.g. Lisman, 1985). Furthermore, the dark bump rate is increased by depleting cells of ATP (Stern *et al.*, 1985). This suggests that the dark bumps are generated by phosphorylated metarhodopsin reverting to its active form. A successive multiple phosphorylation of individual metarhodopsin molecules could be responsible for the decay of the after-potential if each additional phosphorylation decreased the probability of the molecule reverting to the active form. Thus, as suggested for rods by Lamb (1981), relatively stable photoproducts generate a strong signal that is equivalent to light, and the decay of these photoproducts is an important component of the recovery of full sensitivity during dark adaptation.

There are insufficient data to conclude that stable photoproducts invariably impose a lower limit to photoreceptor dark noise. The after-potential is generated by an unusual stimulus, namely a brief and intense illumination of a dark adapted photoreceptor which overloads the cell with newly formed metarhodopsin (Hamdorf, 1979). Furthermore, the inactive forms of metarhodopsin are extremely stable and would generate little noise in smaller quantities. The probability of inactive metarhodopsin reverting to the active state is of the order of 10^{-9} (Lisman, 1985). The after-potential is generated because there is a pool of several hundred million inactivated metarhodopsins in a system that is sensitive enough to respond to the activation of just one molecule. The more natural situation is the slow dark adaptation of a cell that has been illuminated constantly for several hours. To my knowledge, the role of metarhodopsin in generating dark noise has not been investigated under these conditions.

Not all dark bumps are produced by metarhodopsin. Dark bumps persist at rates of over 100 per hour in *Limulus* ventral photoreceptors where all metarhodopsin has been converted to rhodopsin (Lisman, 1985). Similar bump rates are observed in the photoreceptors of *Limulus* lateral eye but these rates are modulated by a circadian rhythm (R. B. Barlow *et al.*, 1987), an observation which lessens the likelihood that thermal isomerisations of the chromophore are responsible. If a lateral eye photoreceptor is kept in darkness, the bump rate increases during the day to over 2000 per hour, and decreases at night to rates approaching zero. The decrease in dark bump rates is associated with an increase in bump amplitude. Thus an increase in sensitivity (size of response to single photon) is associated with a decrease in dark noise. To those familiar with photoelectric devices, this finding seems counterintuitive. However, an increase in the sensitivity of photoreceptors is generally associated with an increase in response latency and duration. If the decreased speed of response were associated with reductions in the rate constants of transduction intermediates, and these reductions were brought about by raising energy barriers, this would explain the lower dark noise. In this case the speed of response is being sacrificed for both sensitivity and for lower dark noise.

The clock controlling the circadian rhythm is located in the brain, and efferent activity in the optic nerve is responsible for setting the retina into the night state. Consequently the high dark bumps rates encountered in the original experiments on excised eyes (e.g. Yeandle, 1958; Fuortes & Yeandle, 1964) result in part from the denervated retina reverting to its day state. In summary, dark noise in the form of spontaneous bumps originates from stable photoproducts and from other intermediates. The effects of dark noise on behavioural or neural thresholds has not been investigated, but the stable metarhodopsins of invertebrate photoreceptors offer the possibility of manipulating dark noise in predictable ways.

6.3.2 Transducer noise

Quantum bumps vary greatly in their latency, duration and amplitude. These variations originate in the chemical reactions responsible for signal amplification, and they must contribute noise (Laughlin, 1976; Yeandle, 1977). The extent to which this *transducer noise* reduces quantum efficiency depends critically upon both the light intensity and the criteria used to define efficiency. At low light levels the signal will be carried by discrete bumps and efficiency can be maintained by converting each bump into an action potential (i.e. a unit pulse) (Lillywhite & Laughlin, 1979), as in *Limulus* lateral eye (see below). In this case only latency variations will contribute noise. The influence of latency variations has not been assessed, but given that a low rate of photon capture precludes fine temporal discrimination, latency variations will usually be of small effect.

At higher intensities the quantum bumps fuse to generate a continuous but noisy receptor potential. This noise results in part from variations in the rate of photon absorptions (photon noise) and in part from variations in bump waveform (transducer noise). If one takes the amplitude of the receptor potential as a measure of the signal, then transducer noise adds to photon noise. This effect of transducer noise was investigated by Lillywhite & Laughlin (1979) using locust photoreceptors as a model system. Lillywhite's earlier paper on bumps (1977) established that the intact locust retina is an ideal preparation for examining the effects of intrinsic noise on the statistical efficiency of vision at low luminances. With a very low dark bump rate in the photoreceptors, and each light induced bump corresponding to an effective photon, one can precisely calibrate the quantum catch. An exact calibration is essential because any measure of the efficiency of transduction and neural processing is only as accurate as the estimation of photon catch (e.g. H. B. Barlow, 1977). In other words, to be confident that the signal-to-noise ratio has been reduced by intrinsic noise, one must be certain that the reduction is not an artefact due to an overestimation of photon catch.

The effects of transducer noise on the efficiency of locust photoreceptors were estimated using a simple procedure (Fig. 6.2). The effective quantal content of the stimulus was calibrated for each cell by making bump counts. The dark adapted photoreceptors were then presented with flashes of known mean quantal content. The cells responded with a receptor potential whose amplitude increased with quantal content, and it was assumed that all information about the effective intensity of the stimulus was coded as this peak response amplitude. The relationship between effective quantal content and amplitude was established by measuring the average response amplitudes to calibrated stimuli. A train of 100 or more flashes of constant known mean quantal content was then delivered and the response amplitudes recorded. Photon and transducer noise generated considerable variability among the amplitudes of these responses and their absolute contributions were measured as follows. Each response amplitude was converted to an equivalent effective quantal catch using the curve relating mean response to mean quantal content. The mean and variance of this set of apparent catches were calculated and compared to the mean and variance expected from the known effective quantal content of the flash. As expected, the mean equivalent catch equalled mean quantal content of the flash, but there was considerable excess variance. In a photon noise limited system the variance among catches should equal the mean catch, but for our measure of the locust's response, the variance always exceeded the mean by a significant factor (Fig. 6.2*d*). This excess variance represents transducer noise. This experiment was repeated at a number of different intensities to examine the relationship between transducer noise and effective quantal content. For low intensities (1–60 effective photons per flash) the variance added by transducer noise approximately equalled the photon noise and, like the photon noise, increased in proportion to the mean (Fig. 6.2*d*). Thus transducer noise is multiplicative, in the sense

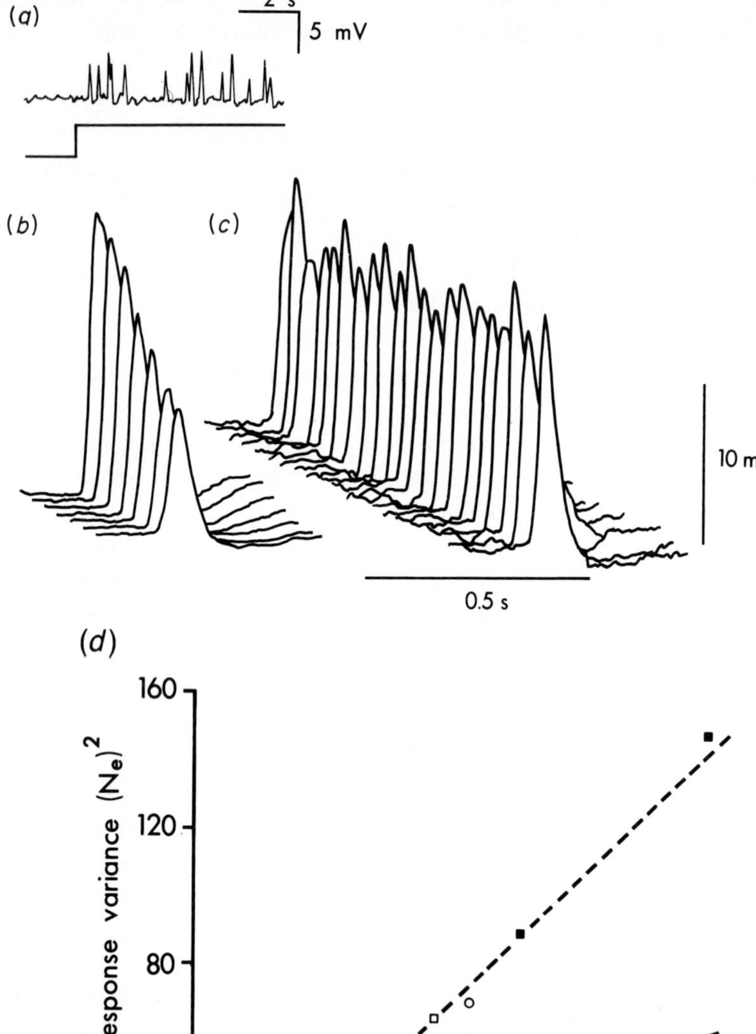
(a)
2 s
5 mV
(b)
(c)
10 mV
0.5 s
(d)
160
120
80
40
total response variance $(N_e)^2$
20
40
60
effective photons flash^{-1}(N_e)

that it contributes a variance proportional to the mean. Monte Carlo simulation established that the observed variations in bump amplitude and latency were capable of generating this type of multiplicative noise. This analysis of locust photoreceptors provided the first experimental measurement of multiplicative noise in a visual system.

Multiplicative noise has important implications for the interpretation of response thresholds at low intensities (Lillywhite, 1981). For example, it is often assumed that when threshold (and by inference the masking noise) is proportional to the square root of intensity, the system is limited by photon fluctuations. In this case the statistical distribution of responses can be used to determine the mean number of photons absorbed at threshold. In locust photoreceptors this assumption would produce consistent but erroneous results. Although noise is proportional to the square root of intensity, transducer noise and photon noise contribute equal amounts. If one uses noise analysis methods (e.g. Kirschfeld, 1965; Katz & Miledi, 1972) to derive the effective photon catch it is underestimated by a factor of 2 (Lillywhite & Laughlin, 1979; Lillywhite, 1981). In addition, when the results of noise analysis were used to assign equivalent quantum catches to the responses recorded at one mean intensity, the apparent distribution of catches was Poisson, with a mean equal to the erroneously lower quantal catch. Not only did multiplicative noise lower the apparent quantal content of the stimulus, it generated the Poisson distribution of response amplitudes that corresponded to the apparent and lower mean. This experimental finding was corroborated by a computer simulation (Lillywhite, 1981). Clearly, if one had performed a noise analysis on this locust data, and were unaware of the true quantum efficiency and the multiplicative nature of the noise, one would have been tempted to conclude that the locust photoreceptor was a purely photon noise limited system. In this case the quantum catch would be seriously underestimated but there would be nothing in the

Fig. 6.2. Quantum bumps and transducer noise in the locust photoreceptor. (*a*) Intracellular records of photon bumps at the low intensity used to determine the effective quantal content of the stimuli – lower trace shows stimulus onset. (*b*) The averaged responses to flashes of different effective quantal content, as used to determine the relationship between response amplitude and quantum catch. (*c*) Part of a train of responses elicited by constant intensity flashes of mean effective intensity 12.5 photons per flash, showing the variations in response amplitude resulting from photon noise and transducer noise. (*d*) The total variance among responses, expressed in (effective photons)^2, increases with the effective quantal content of the stimulus, but exceeds the variance expected from photon noise. This excess variance constitutes transducer noise. Figures reproduced from Laughlin & Lillywhite (1981) with the permission of The Physiological Society.

statistics of the noise to indicate that efficiency had been lowered by intrinsic noise. Because rods also produce responses to single photons that vary in amplitude, duration and latency, this type of multiplicative noise could be a significant factor in accounting for the low statistical efficiency of human vision (Lillywhite, 1981).

The suitability of locust photoreceptors for studies of the factors limiting coding efficiency at low intensities has been exploited by Cohn (1983). He points out that multiplicative noise arises because each event in a Poisson process (in this case photon absorption) generates a second process that is itself Poissonian, and that these types of process are likely to be widespread in early visual processing. Examples include the release of synaptic vesicles at chemical synapses and the mechanism of action potential generation (H. B. Barlow, Levick & Yoon, 1971). This latter effect has recently been modelled by Teich *et al.* (1982) but these effects have not been incorporated into a receiver operating characteristic (ROC) analysis (Cohn, 1983). Cohn suggests that the form of coding can reduce the effects of intrinsic noise by exploiting its structure. For example, in his recordings from locust photoreceptors he finds that there is a negative correlation between response amplitude and response duration. Thus the total area of the response shows much less variance than the peak amplitude. This result contradicts an extensive analysis of quantum bumps in locust (Howard, 1983) which finds that bump amplitudes, latencies and durations are uncorrelated. Nonetheless, when Cohn uses the area as a measure of response, his ROC analysis indicates that the noise results from a Poisson process with a mean that nearly equals the true photon catch, as calculated from counts of quantum bumps. Thus for certain measures of response the efficiency approaches 100%. As Cohn points out, this study emphasises that the way in which information is processed critically determines the quantum efficiency. This observation is as true for the way that the nervous system processes photoreceptor responses as it is for the way in which physiologists analyse them.

These investigations of the efficiency of locust photoreceptors at low light levels resemble a psychophysical task in which observers are presented with a flash, and are asked to judge its intensity (see Chapter 4 for specific details). Judgements are made on the assumption that the stimulus will always be a flash that punctuates a much longer period of darkness. The world is far less predictable than this and this uncertainty must lower efficiency. For the case of total uncertainty about the world, the effects of intrinsic noise on efficiency can be quantified by measuring the response of a photoreceptor to a random stimulus of known quantal content. This approach has been undertaken by de Ruyter and H. van Hateren (see de Ruyter, 1986). A pseudorandom stimulus of several seconds duration (in this case a moving pseudorandom grating of moderate contrast) is repeatedly delivered to a photoreceptor and the responses recorded. The average response is taken and this is subtracted from each individual response to give the noise. Analysis of the signal and noise shows that the noise was essentially unaffected by the signal, so confirming that the photoreceptor was operating in its linear range. In this case the signal-to-noise ratio, and hence the efficiency, is given by the ratio between the spectral densities of signal and noise. Their data suggest that fly photoreceptors are extremely efficient at low frequencies, but efficiency declines for frequencies above 10 Hz, perhaps due to random variations in bump latency. It appears that this type of analysis has the potential both to define efficiency in the most general terms, and to indicate, through changes in efficiency with signal frequency, the source of intrinsic noise.

6.4 The efficiency of transmission of single photon signals

Efficiency requires that quantum bumps are reliably transmitted to higher order neurons. Bump transmission has been investigated in flies and in *Limulus*. In flies the second order neurons produce discrete potentials, corresponding to the bumps in photoreceptors (Fig. 6.3), but the degree to which these interneuron bumps have been contaminated by the intrinsic noise generated at the photoreceptor synapses has not been analysed. The second order neuron of the *Limulus* lateral eye, the eccentric cell, is connected to the 10 or more receptors in an ommatidium by electrical synapses. Intracellular recordings demonstrate that, in the dark adapted intact eye, the quantum bumps trigger regenerative potentials of up to 80 mV amplitude in the photoreceptors (R. B. Barlow & Kaplan, 1977). These large amplitude events can trigger an action potential in the eccentric cell. The coupling of bumps to regenerative events provides an extremely efficient means of coding single photons because thresholding could remove the continuous component of receptor dark noise, while the regenerative event converts quantum bumps of variable amplitude into unit pulses.

The efficiency with which single photon signals are coded by the eccentric cell has been examined by measuring the intensity dependence of action potentials close to the absolute threshold of the light response

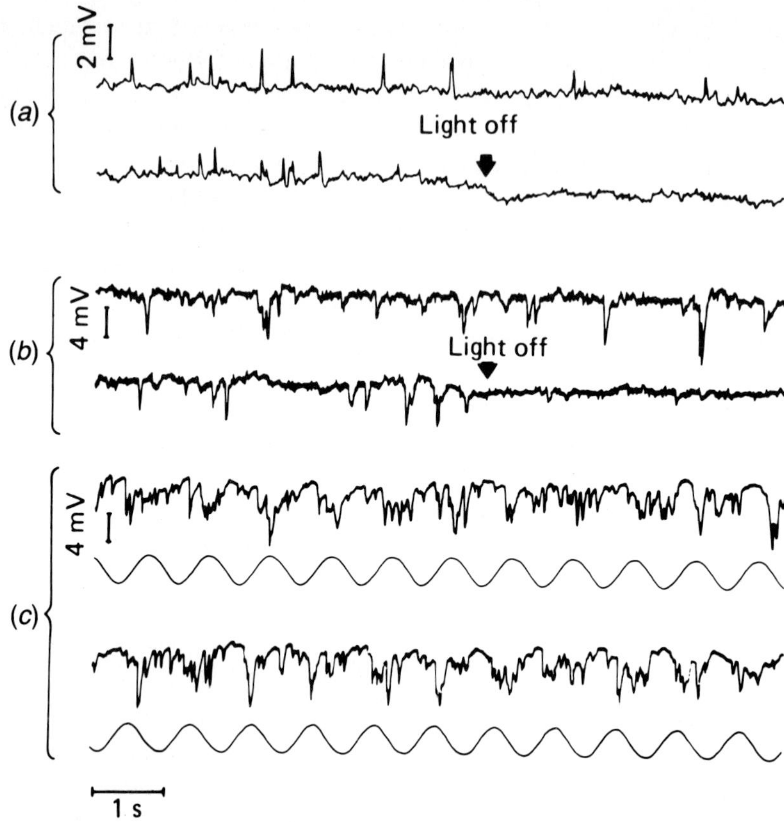

Fig. 6.3. Intracellular responses recorded from a photoreceptor and a second order large monopolar cell of a fly when the animal is viewing stimuli that are close to the absolute threshold of the fly's optomotor response. (*a*) The response of a photoreceptor to a uniform screen with a luminance equal to the mean luminance of the grating at absolute threshold. (*b*) Response of a large monopolar cell to a mean luminance that is 1.2 log units below absolute threshold. (*c*) Response of a large monopolar cell to the threshold grating. The lower trace shows that modulation in intensity that is generated by the grating stimulus passing through the centre of the cell's field of view. All recordings are from the dorsal frontal eye region of *Musca domestica*. The figure is reproduced from Dubs *et al.* (1981), with the permission of The Physiological Society.

(Kaplan & R. B. Barlow, 1976). Frequency of response curves (equivalent to frequency of seeing curves) were determined for observations of the numbers of spikes following brief dim flashes of different intensity. The curve for observing a single spike corresponded to a threshold of one photon. Interestingly, the curves for seeing 2 spikes and for seeing 3 spikes followed the curves for thresholds of 2 and 3 photons respectively. In addition, the curve relating spike frequency to intensity was linear over this range and the distribution of responses was Poissonian. These statistics support the physiological data that spikes are triggered by quantum bumps. However, the eccentric cell seems to be extremely inefficient under the conditions of these experiments. The stimulus was a light guide cemented to a single facet and, given uncertainties in light guide alignment and in the optical coupling of the light guide to the graded refractive index optic system of the *Limulus* ommatidium (Land, 1981), it is virtually impossible to derive an accurate estimate of the number of available photons. The best estimate of quantum efficiency was less than 0.1%. Kaplan & R. B. Barlow (1976) showed that intrinsic noise, in the form of a varying threshold of response, would flatten the frequency of seeing curves. Such variations in threshold could be generated by spontaneous bumps driving the lateral inhibitory network of the *Limulus* lateral eye. The flattening of the frequency of response curve would allow a process that depended on the coincidence of several photons to masquerade as a single photon process. A similar argument has been advanced by H. B. Barlow (1977) in an attempt to reconcile the low quantum efficiency of human vision with the frequency of seeing curves. However, given the subsequent physiological data on regenerative potentials in *Limulus* photoreceptors it seems more probable that the stimulus configuration is primarily responsible for the low efficiency. Transducer noise may also lower efficiency (Lillywhite & Dvorak, 1981). Because of the spread in quantum bump amplitudes, some of these single photon signals may be too small to trigger a regenerative event in the receptor, and hence a spike in the eccentric cell.

The approach taken by Kaplan & R. B. Barlow (1976), and by H. B. Barlow and colleagues (1972) on cat retinal ganglion cells, has been extended to an identified fourth order cell in the fly visual system, the giant movement detector cell, H1. This cell is part of a small set of neurons coding patterns of motion in the visual field (rev. Hausen, 1984). At higher luminances, H1 responds selectively to horizontal movement in one direction. When dark adapted it responds to weak stationary flashes by generating a small burst of action potentials. H1 provides an excellent opportunity to investigate the efficiency with which single photon signals are transmitted through neural networks. Because the level of dark discharge is less than 1 spike per second, and weak flashes generate spikes in proportion to intensity, one can test the hypothesis that single photons are capable of generating an action potential, and compare the efficiency of H1 with the accurate data for the quantum catch of fly photoreceptors (e.g. Dubs *et al.*, 1981). Lillywhite & Dvorak (1981) found that the frequency of response curves, and the distributions of response amplitudes, were in accord with a single photon generating a spike. They also used the powerful reciprocity test (e.g. Reichardt, 1970) to dismiss the requirement for photon coincidences. A given number of photons is delivered over a variable time interval (i.e. intensity is the reciprocal of duration). For stimulus durations that exceed the integration time of the system, the probability of coincidences decreases as duration increases. By comparison, the probability of observing responses to single photons remains constant. When this test was performed on H1, the quantum/spike ratio did not change with stimulus duration.

The quantum/spike ratio varied greatly from cell to cell. Using a precise determination of H1's receptive field, optical data on the angular spacing photoreceptors and the point spread function and measurements of the ratio between quantum bumps and incident photons, one can express the quantum/spike ratio in terms of effective quanta (i.e. those that are likely to generate a bump). The best H1 cells had an efficiency of 1 spike per 4 effective photons while the worst scored 1 in 40. Lillywhite & Dvorak emphasised that for fly, as for man, detection efficiency depended critically on the physical condition of the subject. Some of the less efficient individuals were raised at sub-optimal temperatures. However, there was no indication that the rate of spontaneous discharges was higher in the less efficient individuals. The spontaneous activity in H1 was low enough to be attributed to photoreceptor dark bumps. However, there was an anomalous excess of short intervals in the spike interval distribution that could represent intrinsic noise generated in neural networks.

Lillywhite & Dvorak's study exploits the opportunity offered by compound eyes for defining the efficiency of biological image processing. The precise characterisation of the optics of the ommatidial array is combined with a knowledge of the neuroanatomy and with measurements of photoreceptor signals in intact preparations to determine the quality of the retinal image and hence the efficiency of neural processing. A second example of this approach is provided by the motion sensitive cell, H1. De Ruyter (1986) has used a reverse correlation technique to determine the amount of information coded by H1 as it responds to random movements of a white noise grating. The responses of photoreceptors to the same stimulus were measured and the photoreceptor signal-to-noise ratio was combined with measurement of H1's receptive field and experimentally derived parameters of correlation model of movement detection (Reichardt, 1970), to define the amount of information on movement available to the H1 neuron. The available information on movement was approximately twice that coded by H1, indicating that the post-receptoral efficiency of the movement detection system is around 50%. Such direct measures of efficiency should enable one to relate the properties of higher order processes to their function because efficiency is likely to be a critical parameter that determines the ways in which neural receptive fields and response properties are organised, and adjusted during dark adaptation. An example of this efficiency approach is provided in the next section, which reviews the relationship between photon noise level, sampling and information content with respect to optical sampling at low luminances.

6.5 Sampling and processing

The goal of the sampling and processing of images is to generate a representation of the available optical information that is suitable for controlling behaviour. For invertebrate vision at low luminances the optics, sampling and processing are related by a common principle – the trade-off between spatial resolution and sensitivity. To obtain reliable data at low intensities, sampling and processing must integrate signals over space and time to obtain sufficient photons. Thus in invertebrates, as in humans (e.g. H. B. Barlow, 1972) and as for night-viewing instruments (see Chapter 13), spatial summation and temporal integration continually adjust the grain and timescale of vision to match the available light. In invertebrates this trade-off is performed both optically and neurally.

6.6 Optical trade-offs

The majority of insects and crustacea use compound eyes. These are arrays of optical sub-units, the ommatidia. In general, an ommatidium consists of a lens, a cone, a set of photoreceptors and pigment cells (Fig. 6.4). The lens is a comparatively rigid and immovable acellular structure of high refractive index, crafted from the animal's integument. The cone is usually cellular and it separates the lens from the receptors. There are commonly 8 photoreceptors arranged in a column. At the centre of the column the photoreceptors form dense arrays of microvilli. Each microvillus is a tube of membrane, filled with a narrow core of cytoplasm and densely studded with visual pigment molecules. Thus the densely packed microvilli are equivalent to the lamellae of vertebrate cone cells, forming a cylinder of high refractive index which acts as a waveguide (rev. Snyder, 1979). The pigment cells are important optical structures in a compound eye (e.g. Stavenga, 1979). Their position determines the field of view, and hence the absolute and angular sensitivities of the photoreceptors. The basic ommatidial structure is modified and combined in a number of ways to produce a wide range of compound eyes. The simplified account presented here introduces a number of sensitivity–resolution trade-offs, relating to image formation and sampling at low intensities. For a definitive account of the many variations and subtleties of compound eye design, consult the review by Land (1981).

There are two basic types of compound eye, apposition and superposition (Fig. 6.4). Structurally and optically the apposition eye is the simpler. In each ommatidium the receptors lie at the focus of the lens, and receive light from a small acceptance angle. This angle is determined by the angular diameter of the photoreceptor, the point spread function of the facet lens and, where appropriate, the interaction of the lens diffraction pattern with the waveguide modes of the photoreceptor (van Hateren, 1984). Light is prevented from passing between ommatidia by dense screening pigment around the cone and the photoreceptors. Thus each ommatidium samples a small area of space through the restricted aperture of one facet. A composite image is built up by assigning each ommatidium a unique line of sight. From the viewpoint of a photoreceptor, this system is functionally equivalent to a vertebrate eye. Light is mapped in an orderly fashion from the object to the photoreceptor array via a lens system (e.g. Kirschfeld, 1976).

The optical properties of apposition compound eyes are subject to a familiar set of design trade-offs. At low intensities spatial resolution is sacrificed for sensitivity (Walcott, 1975). Fourier Optics has been combined with Information Theory to quantify his trade-off in a manner that is applicable to visual sampling in general (Snyder, Stavenga & Laughlin, 1977; Snyder, Laughlin & Stavenga, 1977). This approach is summarised by a simplified account of the ways in which apposition eyes are designed for vision for low luminances. The array of ommatidia is analogous to the matrix of pixels in a digital image. The number of different signals that can be reliably discriminated in each ommatidium is equivalent to the range of grey-levels that can be assigned to a pixel. The information content of the image is determined by two factors, the spatial density of ommatidia and the number of discriminable signal levels that each ommatidium can generate. The sensitivity–resolution trade-off boils

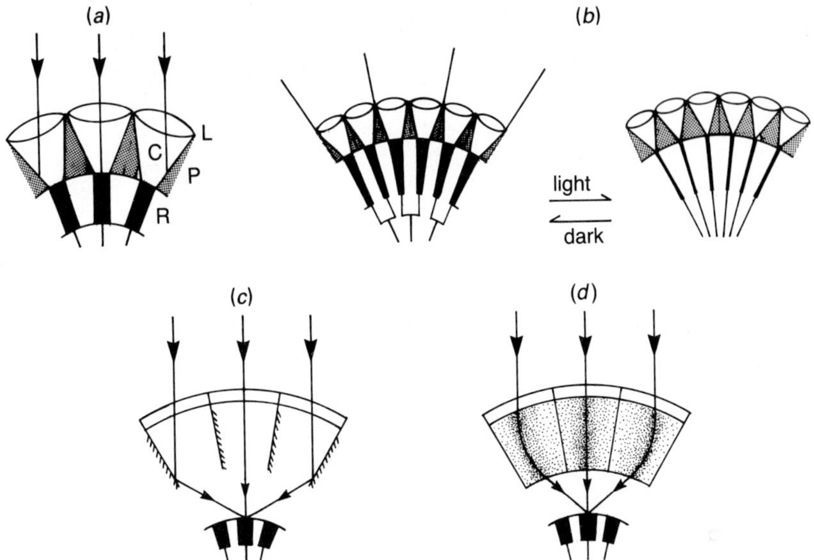

Fig. 6.4. Sampling at different intensities and the design of apposition and superposition eyes. (*a*) An apposition compound eye that is designed for vision at low luminances sacrifices sampling density for sensitivity by using a small number of large ommatidia, with fat photoreceptors subtending a large visual angle. (*b*) An apposition eye designed for work at day and night has many smaller ommatidia with narrow photoreceptors, to obtain maximum spatial resolving power at high light levels. When this eye dark adapts the photoreceptors increase their effective diameter. This change is combined with pooling of receptor outputs to produce a system that is equivalent to the ommatidia of the low luminance eye (*a*). (*c*) The reflecting superposition eye collects light over an aperture of several ommatidia and uses mirrored cones to direct parallel rays to a single photoreceptor. The large aperture improves sensitivity. (*d*) The refracting superposition eye uses lens cylinders with a parabolic refractive index gradient to achieve the same superposition of parallel rays. L = lens; C = cone; P = screening pigment; R = photoreceptor.

down to exchanging spatial sampling density (i.e. the number of ommatidia) for signal levels.

The number of signal levels is determined by detail available from the object, the mean quantal catch of an ommatidium, and the demodulation of the signal by the ommatidial optics. For the purpose of analysing trade-offs we assume that the object is random and has a mean contrast of 0.3. The signal amplitude is proportional to the number of photons received and the stimulus contrast. The photon catch increases with lens diameter and photoreceptor diameter, but the available contrast decreases with receptor diameter and increases with lens diameter. If we restrict our attention to optical constraints, the only source of noise is the

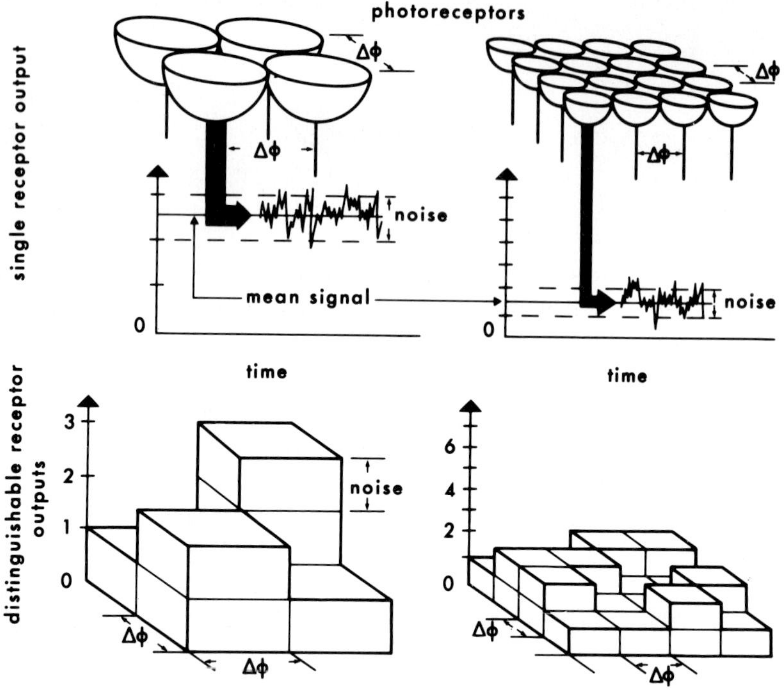

Fig. 6.5. Sampling density, noise and information capacity. Two sets of ommatidia (or retinal ganglion cells) view the same area of a scene at the same luminance. The 4 large ommatidia each absorb enough light to receive several resolvable signal levels. The 16 smaller ommatidia only receive enough light to resolve 2. Nonetheless, the smaller ommatidia have a higher information capacity at this light level because they can generate a larger number of discriminably different patterns of response.

random process of quantal absorption. Thus the noise has a variance equal to the mean photon catch and for an ommatidium of fixed dimensions the number of discriminable signals increases with intensity according to the square root law. Given a compound eye of fixed radius, how should it be divided into ommatidia to obtain the best image? The choice is between a larger number of smaller ommatidia or a smaller number of larger ommatidia (Fig. 6.5). By going for larger ommatidia one sacrifices signal levels (SNR) for sampling density. The larger lens receives more light and has better resolving power and this boosts the SNR, but fewer ommatidia are accommodated in an eye of fixed radius. The efficiency of a particular eye design can be assessed by calculating the maximum number of different pictures that it can form. This is simply the number of combinations that can be generated by the O ommatidia producing S signal levels.

$$P = S^O$$

The number of ommatidia is dictated by eye radius and lens diameter, while the number of signal levels is determined by signal strength and photon noise. Signal strength is calculated by assuming a fixed mean object contrast and a flat spatial frequency spectrum, and then analysing the modulation transfer from object to image using Fourier optics. The noise is determined by the photon catch of the ommatidia, as dictated by the intensity of incident light and the optics.

This analysis shows that for every given combination of intensity, eye radius and object contrast there is one ommatidial geometry that is most effective at receiving pictures. As intensity falls the lens of this optimum ommatidium increases in size to collect more light and, as a result, sampling density decreases. Thus the analysis of image quality in terms of available pictures (i.e. information capacity) predicts precisely how spatial acuity should be traded off against sensitivity. The treatment predicts that the apposition compound eyes of insects active at low light levels can be expected to have larger facets and larger angles between facets than strictly diurnal relatives. Such trends are seen in dragonflies, bees, wasps and butterflies (Horridge, 1978; Wehner, 1981). In addition the treatment accounts for the increase in area summation in the human retina that accompanies dark adaptation (Snyder *et al.*, 1977).

Many apposition eyes are designed to cope with a range of intensities. In this case an excellent strategy is to arrange the ommatidia for vision at high luminance (many small facets). When intensity falls the ommatidial optics is adjusted to sacrifice spatial resolving power for photon catch. Because photon noise precludes high spatial resolution at low intensities this makes a great deal of sense (Laughlin, 1975). The quantitative analysis of these effects shows that optical adjustment is very effective when it is combined with the neural summation or pooling of ommatidial signals (Snyder, 1979). Neural summation effectively creates larger ommatidia with a lower sampling density (e.g. Fig. 6.4). In this case neural summation is the most significant blurring factor and the optics can be readjusted to sacrifice spatial resolving power for increased photon catch. One can think of the human pupil operating in a similar manner. In apposition compound eyes the optics are adjusted by a number of mechanisms, all of which depend on the precise and coordinated control of cellular processes within single ommatidia. For example, locusts enlarge the cross-sectional area of their photoreceptors by growing longer microvilli at dusk. This requires that light controls the cycle of membrane turnover and control is augmented by an endogenous diurnal rhythm (Williams, 1987). In many eyes the receptors are moved closer to the lens to increase their angular subtense (rev. Walcott, 1975) or the screening pigment around the cone withdraws to increase the entrance aperture of the system. The lateral eye of *Limulus* provides a fine example of these mechanisms: combining photoreceptive membrane synthesis, receptor movement and pigment movement under the control of a circadian clock (e.g. R. B. Barlow *et al.*, 1987). At a microscopic level, the intracellular movement of pigment granules and membrane cisternae generate refractive index changes around the photoreceptor waveguide and this increases the number of modes propagating down the waveguide (e.g. Snyder, 1979). This variety of ingenious mechanisms demonstrates how important it is to match the sampling strategy to incident illumination in the pursuit of efficiency, but such subtlety and diversity do obscure a sad fact for animals with apposition eyes – they have optimised a sub-optimal structure.

The apposition eye is badly suited for vision at low luminances. Most of the light entering the eye is wasted by striking the screening pigment at the sides of the cone. Not surprisingly, many types of nocturnal insects and crustacea have evolved a second type of eye, the superposition. In the superposition eye, the light entering many facets is brought to a focus on one set of receptors. Thus the compound optical system acts as if it is a simple lens, bringing parallel light falling over a wide aperture to focus at one point (Fig. 6.4). This remarkable optical feat is accomplished by reflecting or refracting light in the cone, and then projecting it across a clear zone to the underlying receptors (Fig. 6.4). The reflecting mechanism is exemplified by crayfish and shrimps (rev. Land, 1981). The cone has flat sides which are mirrored by a dense layer of guanine crystals and it is comparatively simple to see how this works for a single strip of ommatidia (Fig. 6.4). For the realistic case of parallel rays falling on a two-dimensional surface, the cones must be right-angled prisms, as is observed in these reflecting eyes (Vogt, 1977). The second type of superposition eye, the refracting, occupies a place in the history of optics. It was here that Sigmund Exner discovered the lens cylinder and, together with another student of physiological optics, Matthiesen, founded the field of graded refractive index optics. Exner (1891) deduced that the firefly eye formed a superposition image and showed that this was achieved by virtue of a refractive index gradient in each cone

(Fig. 6.4). Each cone is a lens cylinder of length sufficient to act as a pair of confocal lenses. This arrangement directs a parallel beam back towards the centre of the eye. Exner demonstrated that a lens cylinder must have a parabolic refractive index gradient to form an image (e.g. Wood, 1911). Although the superposition eye is clearly more sensitive than the apposition (Kirschfeld, 1974), and typifies nocturnal insects and crustacea, there is no systematic comparison of behavioural acuity and sensitivity in the two eye types.

6.7 Neural sampling and processing

Optics and transduction generate a neural image of a scene in the form of a mosaic of photoreceptor responses. The degree to which information is extracted from this depends critically upon the mechanisms used by the nervous system. Although relatively little is known about this aspect of invertebrate vision at low luminances, there is every indication of extensive parallels with vertebrate systems. Before discussing these findings it is necessary to establish that animals with compound eyes can respond to stimuli of low intensity.

Some of the best data on invertebrate vision come from the study of the compound eyes of the housefly *Musca*. A classical behavioural assay of acuity is to place a fly on a miniature torque meter, present a large field of moving stripes and measure the torque generated by flies as they turn with the stripes so as to stabilise themselves with respect to their surroundings. In the 1960s, optomotor experiments of this type formed the basis of an extensive systems analysis of fly movement detection, using sinusoidally modulated stimuli of controlled contrast, spatial wavelength, intensity and velocity (rev. Reichardt, 1970). A part of this programme addressed the question of sensitivity at low luminances. Two lines of evidence suggested that the housefly visual system detected a moving pattern from a pattern of discrete single photon triggered events in photoreceptors. First, close to absolute threshold the relationship between threshold contrast and mean intensity or threshold spatial wavelength and mean intensity followed the classical square root law for a photon noise limited system (Fermi & Reichardt, 1963). Second, calibrations of the stimuli combined with electrophysiological measurements of the acceptance angle and spectral sensitivity of single photoreceptors showed that at absolute threshold each receptor received, on average, 2–3 photons per second (Scholes & Reichardt, 1969). The fact that the fly is obtaining information about movement from isolated single photon events was confirmed by recording the responses of photoreceptors to stimuli that were known to lie at the optomotor threshold (Fig. 6.3). At the absolute threshold, the photoreceptors are generating quantum bumps at the mean rate of 1.7 s^{-1} (Dubs *et al.*, 1981).

From the point of view of a single photoreceptor, this threshold flux is moderately low but, in comparison with the other animals, flies do not have good night vision. The absolute threshold is at the lower end of the human mesopic range, at approximately 10^{-3} cd m^{-2} (Fermi & Reichardt, 1963). Since the optical systems of fly and man have similar F-ratios, their retinal images are of equal brightness, and optical factors alone cannot explain the fly's comparative insensitivity. In all probability the fly, a diurnal animal, has not evolved the area summation mechanisms required to increase sensitivity at low intensities (see Fig 1.3 for human). The shore crab, *Leptograpsis*, does better than a fly. It is able to detect the movement of point source which has the brightness of a 0.5 magnitude star (Doujak, 1985). Intracellular recordings show that this threshold corresponds to a quantum bump every three seconds in each of the receptors looking directly at the point source. If one takes into account the fact that, with a finite acceptance angle, a number of other receptors view the point source obliquely, with a lower efficiency, one derives an estimate of a total retinal signal of 18 bumps per second (Doujak, 1985). Nonetheless, the point source is 900 times brighter than the minimum intensity required for detection by humans. A remarkably exhaustive review of insect vision (Wehner, 1981) suggests that there are no other quantitative studies of night vision in arthropods where one can relate absolute thresholds to receptor quantum catch. Given the information available on optics and transduction, this is an area of research that would repay further study.

Returning to the optomotor response of flies, the analysis of thresholds suggests that dark adaptation is accompanied by changes in the pattern of neural processing. There is a great deal of evidence that the optomotor response is driven by large arrays of elementary movement detectors (revs. Reichardt, 1970; Buchner, 1984). Each detector compares signals from two separate areas of the retina. Before comparison the signals are filtered, both spatially and temporally, and the temporal filtering introduces a delay into the signal arriving from one of the areas. This delay allows the elementary movement detector to correlate the filtered signal received from one area of the retina with the filtered signal received in another area a brief time before. Correlation of the two signals is taken to be an indication of movement. At high intensities the response is dominated by the elementary movement detectors that pick out correlations in the signals from neighbouring ommatidia. However, at lower intensities the sampling base widens. Responses are dominated by elementary detectors that compare points that are separated by 2, 3 or 4 ommatidia (Pick & Buchner, 1979). This increase in separation is accompanied by a decrease in temporal resolution that can be largely attributed to changes in the photoreceptor frequency response (Zettler, 1969; Pick & Buchner, 1979). There are also changes in the spatial filtering of signals that preceded movement detection. As intensity falls the high frequency roll off of the contrast sensitivity function moves to lower frequencies and the low frequency roll off disappears. These changes suggest that dark adaptation of the movement detection system is accompanied by an increase in area summation and a decrease in lateral inhibition (Srinivasan & Dvorak, 1980). Pick & Buchner point out that the movement detector system is trading sensitivity for resolution in a manner that typifies vision at low luminances.

It is possible to model this sensitivity/acuity trade-off and the results suggest that both the filtering and the sampling are matched to the characteristics of the stimulus so as to maximise sensitivity to movement (Srinivasan & Dvorak, 1980). According to their model, the task of the movement detection system is to stabilise the retinal image during flight. Measurements of pattern fixation during flight show that the fly stabilises the image imperfectly, wandering off target according to a Gaussian distribution of error angles. In the model these conditions are approximated by a Gaussian distribution of instantaneous angular displacements of the image, and the image is assumed to be random (i.e. equal power at all spatial frequencies). Under these conditions the motion signal varies in strength with spatial frequency. Low spatial frequencies generate weak signals because, when displaced by small angles they produce small changes in intensity at any given point on the retina. The strength of motion signal increases with spatial frequency up to the point where two limitations come into play. The first is the attenuation of high spatial frequencies by the optics. The second is the loss of signal that occurs when the angular displacement of the image shifts a spatial frequency by more than half a wavelength. Thus there is a band of intermediate spatial frequencies in which the motion signal is strongest. It is suggested that lateral inhibition attenuates low frequencies to keep the movement detector inputs tuned to the most favourable spatial frequencies. The position of this band depends upon the size of the step displacements. When steps are large, the high spatial frequencies are less effective and the band of most effective frequencies is shifted downwards. Srinivasan & Dvorak (1980) noted that at low intensities a fly's ability to stabilise its surroundings diminishes. The mean step size of movement increases and this necessitates a retuning of the elementary movement detector inputs to lower frequencies. Thus the loss of lateral inhibition and the increased area summation match the input filters of the movement detection system to the most favourable band of frequencies. A related argument accounts for the increase in sampling base at low intensities. If the sampling bases are too far apart then higher frequencies will be undersampled and will appear to move in the wrong direction (e.g. Gotz, 1964), while when they are too close together the point spread functions of the input filters will overlap more and this will introduce correlations that are independent of movement. The optimum sampling distance is two thirds the half-width of the input filter. Thus as these filters widen at low intensities the sampling base must increase. The theoretical analysis of Srinivasan & Dvorak (1980) demonstrates an important principle, namely that the performance of the movement detection system can be enhanced by matching sampling and prefiltering to the quality of the input signal. A number of its conclusions should engage anyone with an interest in motion detection. Furthermore its original findings and its approach might profitably be extended to embrace other movement detection systems, both in those insects such as locusts which fly at night, and to vertebrates such as ourselves, which are active by day and by night. Nonetheless, one aspect of their approach should be questioned. They suggest that the changes in sampling and prefiltering are required because photon noise generates larger errors in stabilisation. These errors feed back onto the input as larger movements. Thus the system modifies the way in which it filters and samples its input to take account of inaccuracies in the motor response. But these inaccuracies ultimately derive from the light intensity of the input. Might not area summation reduce these errors by improving the signal-to-noise ratio in the elementary movement detectors? Nonetheless, the analysis of motion sensitivity in flies suggests that the photon noise necessitates a reorganisation of the mechanisms undertaking movement detection and this is a consideration that may help account for changes that take place in retinal filtering during light adaptation.

The best documented changes in neural filtering concern the second order neurons. The most familiar second order neuron from a compound eye is the eccentric cell of *Limulus*. Two neural processes operate at the level of the eccentric cell – namely the lateral inhibition and the self-inhibition described by Hartline and his colleagues. Lateral inhibition gives the eccentric cell high pass filter characteristics principally in the spatial domain, and self-inhibition generates high pass filter characteristics in the time domain. The strength of lateral inhibition decreases with discharge rate and hence light intensity (rev. Laughlin, 1981). The strength of inhibitory interactions is also reduced when the retina passes from the day state to the night state, and measurements of 'Mach bands' suggest that the spatial extent of antagonism is unchanged (Batra & R. B. Barlow, 1982). This reduction in the strength of inhibition must be of functional significance because it is directly controlled by the circadian clock mechanism discussed above. Indeed, it appears to be a common principle of visual processing that inhibitory interactions decline during dark adaptation (but see Figs 1.9 and 1.11 for opposing view). For example, the low frequency roll off in human contrast sensitivity corresponds to lateral inhibition and disappears with dark adaptation (rev. H. B. Barlow, 1972). A similar effect is seen in the flicker response (Kelly, 1972). The fact that inhibition declines with intensity in both invertebrate and vertebrate visual systems, suggest that inhibitory interactions are either unnecessary or impede efficiency, at low intensities.

One possible explanation for the intensity dependence of inhibition is provided by a study of second order neurons in the fly visual system (Srinivasan, Laughlin & Dubs, 1982). The large monopolar cells show both lateral and self-inhibition when light adapted. As the background intensity falls, inhibition declines in amplitude and increases in space constant or time constant. This behaviour can be explained in terms of a predictive coding model. It is suggested that the function of inhibition is to remove correlated components from the incoming retinal signal. Spatial correlation has been introduced by the optics and is an inherent property of natural scenes (Srinivasan *et al.*, 1982). Temporal correlation is introduced by the finite duration of phototransduction. The lateral inhibitory mechanism derives a weighted mean of the signals in a small area of retinal image and subtracts this from the output of the second order neuron. This weighted mean is a statistical 'best-estimate' of the correlated components. Self-inhibition performs the equivalent function in the time domain. Note that predictive coding is basically a mechanism for deriving the local mean intensity and subtracting this from the incoming signal to reduce its amplitude by suppressing the background component. At low intensities photon noise reduces the accuracy of signals and simple statistics shows that the local means must be estimated over larger areas or longer periods to derive an accurate measure. Hence the need to reduce the strength and increase the extent of inhibition. Measurements of signal-to-noise ratio have been combined with measurements of contrast sensitivity functions and temporal impulse responses to show that inhibition is well regulated to perform this function. Note that predictive coding demands a reliable (i.e. relatively noise free) estimate, so ensuring that efficiency is not severely curtailed by subtracting one independently noisy signal from another. Thus the predictive coding argument substantiates a more general observation, namely that retinal inhibition is being regulated to minimise the effects of photon noise. Because photon noise is uncorrelated in both space and time its components will add in inhibitory networks where the signals are subtracting from each other. This problem is avoided by decreasing inhibition and by averaging out the photon noise in the inhibitory components. Inhibition may well disappear entirely from second order neurons at absolute threshold because, under these conditions, the background signal is so close to zero as to be negligible. However, antagonistic spatio-temporal interactions are likely to occur at a higher level of processing, if only to confirm that one area is brighter than another, and the extent to which these higher order interactions are regulated to suppress photon noise is an open question.

In conclusion, we see that invertebrate visual systems allow for the precise definition of optical, receptoral, neural and behavioural performance in the intact animal. This experimental facility allows us to quantify that key parameter in vision at low luminances, efficiency. We have seen that the recordings of receptor responses to stimuli of known quantal content allow us to measure the ways in which the inherently stochastic processes of transduction degrade the signal-to-noise ratio. Such measurements of signal-to-noise at the visual systems inputs have been combined with the precise knowledge of the receptor sampling mosaic, the neural connectivity and recordings of interneuronal responses to analyse the efficiency of neural processing. Finally, the effects of the determined constraints, both optical and neural, can be assessed theoretically, and this enables us to understand the relationship between factors such as sampling density and photon noise at low light levels. These analyses confirm that efficiency dictates that the aperture of the optics, the grain of sampling and the receptive fields of interneurones are matched to the signal to noise ratio of the image and the many subtle mechanisms employed by arthropods to achieve this matching attests to the importance of this principle.

PART II

Achromatopsia

7

Total colour-blindness: an introduction

Lindsay T. Sharpe and Knut Nordby

'Color est pluribus unis.' (Vergil, *Moretum*, l. 104)

'Among the several kinds of beauty the eye takes most delight in colours. We nowhere meet with a more glorious or pleasing show in nature than what appears in the heavens at the rising and setting of the sun' (Joseph Addison, *The Spectator*, 3 June 1712). Indeed, the ability to see colours is such a compelling and vivid part of visual experience that one may be forgiven for, occasionally, regarding it, instead of object recognition – which it merely subserves – as the fundamental aspect of visual perception. But so it often seems: for though a blind man can perceive the size and surface properties of objects from his sense of touch, he is at a loss to determine their colour. Hence, the signification of the medieval proverb: 'A blind man can not juggen [judge] wel in hewis [hues]' (G. Chaucer, *Troilus und Criseyde*, *c.* 1380, Bk ii, l. 21).

Chaucer and his contemporaries – and even Addison and his – were surely unaware that not only the completely blind, but also the colour-blind, 'deemeth' wrong of colours and are unable to discriminate between hues that are easily distinguished by the colour-normal. In fact, the most severely afflicted of them, the completely colour-blind, are unable to experience any hue differences at all. Their visual world, a world without colour, is at odds with the world of the colour-normal. To be sure, the two worlds are not equally exclusive; for the colour-normal have access to the world of the totally colour-blind. They can witness, as night falls, how the many colours blend into one, and how, in the moonlight, colours take on darker and lighter shades of pale. But the totally colour-blind have no obverse means of entering the world of the colour-normal. For them, there is no 'sweet approach of even or morn'

(Milton, 1667, *Paradise Lost*, III); the day dawns, as it ends, in all-pervasive black and white.

Given the stark contrast between the vision of the totally colour-blind and the colour-normal, it is surprising that the earliest reports of colour-blindness appear relatively late in the history of science. After all, 'The nature of sight and the structure of the organ of vision rank among the foremost subjects with which the minds of thinking men have been preoccupied since the dawn of recorded history' (Polyak, 1941, p. 95). Did no medieval artist or dyer ever employ a colour-blind apprentice? Did no ancient Egyptian, Mesapotamian, Indian, Greek or Chinese physician ever encounter a colour-blind or day-blind patient? This seems more than doubtful. Thousands of sufferers flocked to the ancient Aesclepeia, alone, to benefit from the highly developed ophthalmological services offered there (Lascaratos, 1980). And an oblique reference to the pathology of eyesight and colour vision appears in the classical Chinese medical textbook, *The Yellow Emperor's Canon of Internal Medicine*, which summarizes the traditional Chinese literature from 722 to 221 B.C. (Dong & Jin, 1989).

But, it must not be forgotten that recognition of a colour-anomaly is a subtle one, complicated by our use of language. For the colour-blind, it is not clear whether the confusion about colour lies within, in themselves, or without, in the language of others:

> It is to be remembered that a person in whom colour vision is defective may go through life quite unconscious of his inferiority and without making any incriminating mistakes, differentiating objects by their size, shape and luminosity, using all the time a complete colour vocabulary based on his experience which teaches him that colour terms are applied with great consistency to certain objects and to certain achromatic shades, until circumstances are arranged to eliminate these accessory aids and he realizes that his sensations differ in some way from the normal. (Duke-Elder, 1964, pp. 661–2)

For the colour-normal, on the other hand, it is all too easy to impute the colour confusions of others to ignorance, carelessness or idiosyncrasy. It seems quite possible, therefore, that the perceptual confusion is so confounded by the linguistic one that only the introduction of the scientific approach, with its emphasis upon careful observation and attention to particulars, allowed for the discovery of colour-blindness (see Sherman, 1981).

Indeed, the lateness of historical recognition parallels three relevant facts. First, many colour-deficient individuals, especially deuteranopes (those missing the green or middle-wave sensitive cone pigment) and anomalous trichromats (those having a deviant cone pigment), are unaware of their deficiency until they are tested in the course of military or occupational screening. In this regard, it is significant that the earliest reports of colour-blindness originated among Quakers (cf. the Harris and Dalton families below); a group who counted 'the fine arts as worldly snares' and 'whose most conspicuous practice was to dress in drabs'. Flagrant errors in dress, caused by colour confusions, attracted more notice amongst them.

Second, the frequency of colour-blindness 'rises in proportion to man's distance from his primitive state, with the lowest rate in the aborigines of Australia, Brazil, Fiji and North America, and the highest rate in Europe and the East, including the Brahmins of India' (Trevor-Roper, 1960, p. 153). A possible explanation of this is that defective colour vision is a less life-endangering handicap in a more developed society; for even the partially colour-blind are disadvantaged relative to the colour normal at identifying objects in the wild, having 'especial difficulty in detecting coloured fruit against dappled foliage that varies randomly in luminosity' (Mollon, 1989, p. 21). If so, it follows that the prevalence of the disorder – and the likelihood of discovering it – increases with the advancement of technology and worldly comforts.

Third, the most profoundly afflicted of the colour-blind, the complete achromats – for whom colour errors are most incriminating and endangering – are legally classified as blind in many countries because of the severity of their accompanying symptoms. Given their greatly reduced visual acuity, which is frequently attended by large refractive errors, it seems highly likely that in ancient and medieval times (when refractive errors went uncorrected) complete achromats were dismissed as completely or functionally blind. Thus the greater fact – their poor sight – may have eclipsed the lesser – their colour-blindness. Pertinently, the first reading glasses were only invented late in the thirteenth century (cf. Polyak, 1941); probably in what, today, we call Yugoslavia (Dugacki, 1977; cited in Weale, 1988).

In this chapter we consider first the early anecdotal accounts of colour-blindness, which confound partial with total colour-blindness; for, even in the late seventeenth century, colour-blindness was thought to be a 'strange and singular' phenomenon. The recognition that the complete inability to distinguish colours is merely the most uncompromising form of colour-blindness came only later. After considering the early accounts, we briefly review the theories that have been offered to explain congenital, total colour-blindness, or *achromatopsia* as it is better described. The proliferation of theories may have arisen, in part, from the failure, in the past, to differentiate between the major types of total colour-blindness. We, therefore, end the chapter, aided by hindsight, with a short taxonomy of achromatopsias.

7.1 Early observations about colour-blindness

Whatever the reasons for the historical delay, colour-blindness was probably not generally recognized in Europe until the end of the eighteenth century. There was, apparently, little or no recognition of any form of colour-blindness in the ancient classical world, as far as we can ascertain from a close reading of the Aristotelian, Galenic, Ptolemaic, Alhazennian, Avicennian, and other theories of vision, though Hippocrates (460?–377? B.C.) may have been aware of it. In the *Corpus Hippocraticum*, he provides a description of *hemeralopia*, or 'day-blindness' (Hirschberg, 1982), and he makes the remarkable observation that: 'Colours do not look the same at all times, nor when north or south winds blow, nor do they seem the same to all ages' (*Corpus Hippocraticum* V, l. 500, quoted from Lascaratos & Marketos, 1988, p. 37).

Indeed, the conceptual framework for the discovery of colour-blindness seems to have been largely lacking. The ancient Greeks and Arabs (except for Alhazen) considered the crystalline lens of the eye to be the chief organ of sight and, with notable exceptions (including Democritos, Aristotle, Alhazen, Avicenna and Averroes), conceived vision as arising from rays, or emanations, *emerging* from the eyes (see Polyak, 1941, 1957). These errors were set right by Felix Platter (1583), who succinctly described the correct arrangement and function of the eye:

> Light enters the eye from outside, passing through the opening of the pupil and into the dark chamber of the eye, where its rays are collected by the crystalline lens and distributed over the whole expanse of the retina. This membrane is, then, the true photoreceptor, while the lens is no more than its 'spectacle'.
>
> (Platter, quoted in Polyak, 1941, p. 134)

Nevertheless, the theories of the Ancients continued to influence thinking as late as the eighteenth century (see the observations of Turbervile below). Moreover, before the publication of Newton's *Opticks* in 1704, most scientists and natural philosophers accepted unquestioningly Aristotle's vague assessment in the *De Coloribus* that colour vision derives from 'the intermingling of the elements of light and darkness'. Perhaps then, we seek without hope in the literature of classical antiquity for an analogy to the modern sense of total colour-blindness.

Like the Ancients, the greatest writers on geometric optics and dioptrics during the seventeenth century, Johannes Kepler (1604, 1611), René Descartes (1638), Christian Huygens (1690) and Isaac Newton (1704), make no conspicuous references to colour-deficient or colour-anomalous vision. Even in the eighteenth century, Joseph Priestly, in his *The History and Present State of Discoveries Relating to Vision, Light and Colours* of 1772, gives no mention of people who see colours abnormally. In fact, colour-blindness, as a deviation from normal vision, was hardly recognized before the remarkable self-analysis of John Dalton (1798), who summed up the anomalous characteristics of himself and others in the celebrated report *Extraordinary Facts Relating to the Vision of Colours; With Observations*, which he presented to the Manchester Literary and Philosophical Society on 31 October 1794. His address, tellingly, begins by declaring how unthinkable it is, even in the late eighteenth century, for such an anomaly to be manifest among men:

> *it will scarcely be supposed*, that any two objects, which are every day before us, should appear hardly distinguishable to one person, and very different to another, without the circumstance immediately suggesting a difference in their faculties of vision; yet such is the fact, not only with regard to myself, but to many others also . . .
>
> (Dalton, 1798, p. 28; our emphasis).

Yet, more than a hundred years earlier, in the late seventeenth century, the first scattered references to colour-blindness had begun to appear in the English literature.

7.1.1 *The Maid from Banbury*

The earliest Western observations about a totally colour-blind person were published in 1684 in *The Philosophical Transactions of the Royal Society*. A letter, written by the 'great, and experienced Oculist' Dr Dawbenry Turbervile of Salisbury, briefly describes the 'supernatural' vision (as it was then called) of:

> A maid, two or three and twenty years old, . . . from *Banbury*, who could see very well, but no colour beside *Black and White*. She had such Scintillations by night, (with the appearances of Bulls, Bears, &c.) as terrified her very much; she could see to read sometimes in the greatest darkness for almost a quarter of an hour. (p. 736)

Note that Turbervile held to the erroneous belief that the Maid was capable of emanating 'Scintillations' or *phosphenes* by which she could read at night; suggesting that the true nature of light rays and the function of the eye was not known in the late seventeenth century, even by 'a great and experienced Oculist'.

The same Maid was, very probably, the subject of a similar, but more detailed, account given by Robert Boyle in: *Some Uncommon Observations about Vitiated Sight* of 1688 (see Mollon *et al.*, 1980; Mollon, 1989). From Boyle's account we learn that the Maid's colour-blindness was acquired by illness, 'having been upon a certain Occasion immoderately tormented with Blisters, applied to her Neck and other Parts, she was quit deprived of her sight' (p. 265). (The 'Blisters' here presumably refer to the therapeutic use of *cupping*, then generally practised.) We further learn that her acuity was better than normal even in bright sunlight (see below). Boyle also remarked upon the poor Maid's phosphenes, though he did not believe she saw by them: 'she is not unfrequently troubled with flashes of Lightning, that seem to issue out like Flames about the External Angle of her Eye, which often make her start, and put her into Frights and Melancholy Thoughts'. But he thought such issuances less 'Strange and Singular' than the relevations that: 'she can distinguish some Colours, as Black and White, but is not able to distinguish others, especially Red and Green' (p. 256); and 'when she looks upon a Turk[e]y Carpet, she cannot distinguish the Colours, unless of those parts that are White or Black' (p. 268).

Boyle added observations from a more trustworthy source whose vision, 'tho' not so odd' as the Maid's, had an 'Affinity' with it and 'so may make it more Credible' (p. 268). The individual, 'a Mathematician, Eminent for his skill in Opticks, and therefore a very competent Relator of Phaenomena belonging to the Science' (p. 268), confided to Boyle that:

> there are some colours, that he constantly sees amiss, and particularly instanced in one, which in a clear day (for so it was when we discoursed together of this matter) seemed to him to be the same with that of a darkish sort of cloth, that he then wore, whilst to me and other men it appeared of quite differing colour. (p. 269)

Nothing further, however, was made of these observations, though they very well may constitute the first recorded description of a genuine case of congenital, as opposed to acquired, colour-blindness; at least in the Western literature. In the Eastern literature, they may be antedated by some observations recorded in Ming dynasty China. The Chinese opthalmologist Wang-Ken-Tang (1549–1613) provides a description of a syndrome, whose ancient Chinese term was 'sees red like white' (Dong & Jin, 1989). In the *Standard of Diagnosis and Treatment of Six Categories of Diseases* (1602), he writes:

> The viewed objective colour is not like its original one. Due to individual differences, some see the sun like an ice-wheel, some see flame like white, or some see white like red or green, or see yellow like blue or green. (quoted from Dong & Jin, 1989)

7.1.2 The Harris brothers

The next European account of 'Persons who could not distinguish Colours' appeared nearly a hundred years later, also in the *Philosophical Transactions of the Royal Society*. In a letter addressed to the Rev. Joseph Priestly (the acknowledged authority on geometric and physiological optics), Mr Joseph Huddart (1777) describes the vision of two brothers, living in Mary-port in Cumberland: Thomas Harris, a shoemaker, and Jonathan Harris, a master of a trading vessel (the exact identification of the brothers was later established by Crerar & Ross, 1953). The brothers were Quakers. This is significant for two reasons. First, among the Quakers, as Huddart noted, 'a general uniformity of colour is known to prevail' and (erroneous) departures from uniformity would be remarkable. Second, the proportion of colour-defectives among Quakers was later found to be nearly twice the normal percentage (Trevor-Roper, 1960, p. 153); presumably because of their interbreeding within small communities.

Huddart first investigated Thomas Harris, who he '*had often heard from others* could discern the form and magnitude of all objects very distinctly, but could not distinguish colours' (p. 261). The italics are ours to emphasize that by the late eighteenth century the idea of colour vision anomalies seems, at last, to have breached the threshold of public consciousness.

The discovery had been made by Thomas Harris himself; wholly from introspection, he had come to believe that:

> other persons saw something in objects which he could not see; that their language seemed to mark qualities with confidence and precision, which he could only guess at with hesitation, and frequently with error. His first suspicion of this arose when he was about four years old. Having by accident found in the street a child's stocking, he carried it to a neighbouring house to inquire for the owner: he observed the people called it a red stocking, though he did not understand why they gave it that denomination, as he himself thought it completely described by

> being called a stocking. The circumstances, however, remained in his memory, and together with subsequent observations led him to the knowledge of his defect. (p. 261)

Unlike Turbervile and Boyle, Huddart did not rely solely on the statements of his subject, he also tested Thomas Harris's vision with coloured objects. On the basis of what now would be considered far too rudimentary tests, he concluded that Harris:

> could never do more than guess the name of any colour; yet he could distinguish white from black, or black from any light or bright colour . . . In general, colours of equal degree of brightness, however they might otherwise differ, he frequently confounded together . . . though he could see other objects at as great a distance as [other persons] . . . where the sight was not assisted by the colour. (p. 262)

Thus, like Boyle's Maid, Harris the shoe-maker appears appears to have had normal photopic acuity. This suggests either that he had a form of achromatopsia without concomitant amblyopia (see the Taxonomy below) or, more likely, that he was not totally colour-blind – despite Huddart's remarks to the contrary (see Dalton's interpretation below).

Huddart then tested Thomas's brother, Jonathan the mariner, in Dublin in December 1776. The tests were performed with a 'striped ribbon . . . in the day-time, and in good light' (p. 265). Huddart found that:

> the several stripes of white he [Jonathan Harris] uniformly, and without hesitation, called white: the four black stripes he was deceived in, for three of them he thought brown, though they were exactly of the same shade with the other, which he properly called black. He spoke, however, with diffidence as to all those stripes; and it must be owned, the black was not very distinct: the light green he called yellow; but he was not very positive: he said, 'I think this is what you call yellow.' The middle stripe, which had a slight tinge of red, he called a sort of blue. But he was most of all deceived by the orange colour; of this he spoke very confidently, saying, 'This is the colour of grass; this is green.' I also shewed him a great variety of ribbons, the colour of which he sometimes named rightly, and sometimes as differently as possible from the true colours. I asked him, Whether he imagined it possible for all the various colours he saw, to be mere difference of light and shade; whether he thought they could be various degrees between white and black; and that all colours could be composed of these two mixtures only? With some hesitation he replied, No, he did imagine there was some other difference. (pp. 263–4)

Jonathan Harris's remarks and test results are open to interpretation. However, given that he was a master mariner, it seems likely that he must have had normal photopic acuity, like his brother Thomas, and been able to distinguish some colours (see below). Huddart also mentions a third colour-blind brother, but he did not interview him.

7.1.3 Scott and Colardeau

Huddart's communication attracted little general attention, but it prompted the publication of two more observations about colour-anomalous vision; one in England (Whisson, 1778); the other in France (L'Abbé François Rozier, 1779). The first, also appearing in *The Philosophical Transactions of the Royal Society*, contained a letter from a retired textile merchant named J. Scott. The letter was transmitted to Whisson, a fellow of the Royal Society, by the Reverend Michael Lort. In the letter, Scott describes his colour defect in enough detail to establish *incontrovertibly* that he, unlike the Maid from Banbury, Thomas Harris the shoe-maker and Jonathan Harris the sea-captain, could see some colours:

> I do not know any green in the world. A pink colour and a pale blue are alike, I do not know one from the other. A full red and a full green are the same, I have often thought them a good match; but yellows (light, dark and middle) and all degrees of blue, except those very pale, commonly called sky, I know perfectly well . . . A full purple and deep blue sometimes baffle me. (p. 611)

Scott then went on to describe the prevalence of the confusions among three generations of his family. His father and maternal uncle had the defect, as did one of his two sisters and her two sons (the pedigree of the Scott family has been published by Cole, 1919). The letter is remarkable for two reasons. It contains the first reference to congenital (as opposed to acquired) colour-blindness in a female; and it includes the first speculation in print that the defect might be inheritable. Although his own son and daughter did not have the defect, Scott was, nevertheless, troubled by the question of descent to his grandchildren.

Huddart's letter about the two Harris brothers prompted L'Abbé François Rozier (1779) to translate it into French and to publish it in his journal *Observations sur la Physique, sur l'Histoire Naturelle et sur les Arts*, along with several anecdotes about the French poet Charles-Pierre Colardeau (sometimes referred to as Collardeau). Colardeau, who died in 1776, had been fond of pencil sketching and, according to Rozier, painting. Painting, however, posed problems; Colardeau made amusing mistakes, unless his friends selected the colours for him. Left to his own devices, he confused bright red and deep blue, yellow and blue, and red and green. Rozier, noting the similarity between the confusions of Colardeau and the Harris brothers, suggested that perhaps defective colour vision was more widespread than previously believed.

Rozier's anecdotes and Huddart's letter were referred to in an article by J. H. Voigt that appeared in 1781 in J. C. Lichtenberg's *Gothaisches Magazin für das Neuste aus der Physik und Naturgeschichte*. The article was entitled 'Des Herrn Giros von Gentilly Muthmassungen über die Gesichtsfehler bey Untersuchung der Farben' or 'The speculations of Giros von Gentilly (a pseudonym for George Palmer; see below) about the visual field in investigations of colour'. After commenting upon the colour-blindness of (Thomas) Harris the shoe-maker and Collardeau [*sic*] the poet, Voigt added that von Gentilly (read Palmer) had encountered several similar persons, a particularly severe case being that of 'einem Apotheker in Strassburg' (an apothecary in Strasbourg), referred to as M**.

The Huddart and Whisson letters were cited in 1792 in the third edition of the *Encyclopedia Britannica* under the headings of 'Colour' and 'Vision', respectively (see Sherman, 1981, p. 120). But little was made of the scattered material – even though enough information was now available to make broad inferences about the prevalence and inheritability of the visual defect – until attention was dramatically focused on the subject by John Dalton.

7.1.4 Dalton's epochal analysis

Dalton's investigations into colour-blindness were kindled by his own discovery of his *protanopic* defect (see below). His first self-doubts, like those of Thomas Harris, were awakened by an incident with a red stocking, which he mistook for blue. (Dalton, like the Harris brothers was a Quaker. He once shocked a Quaker meeting by wearing scarlet stockings instead of blue ones (Synder, 1967).) But the doubts lay dormant, until they were vexed into conviction in the autumn of 1792, by his accidental observation that the colour of the flower of the *Geranium zonale* appeared blue by daylight, though red by candlelight (1798, p. 29). The perceptual change was confirmed by his brother, but not by other observers (including another brother and a sister, who were colour-normal); which thus proved to Dalton beyond a doubt that his and his brother's vision deviated from the normal.

At first, Dalton assumed that his own defect and that of his brother were singular occurrences (1798, pp. 37–8). But upon reading Huddart's report about the Harris brothers, he sensed that something more was amiss and decided to have the Harris family investigated more thoroughly. (He was evidently unaware of Whisson's report about the Scott family.) He, therefore, solicited a friend, Joseph Dickinson, living near the Harrises, to seek them out and to elicit their responses to a set of coloured ribbons. Both Thomas and Jonathan Harris were long dead. But Dickinson was able to test and interview the two surviving brothers, Joseph and John, who also had the defect (Crerar & Ross, 1953); and apparently with symptoms similar to Dalton's.

Huddart had mistakenly noted that Thomas Harris: 'had two [actually three] brothers in the same circumstances as to sight; and two other brothers and sisters who, as well as their parents, had nothing of this defect' (p. 263). And Dalton (1798) seems to have thought that there was only one surviving colour-blind brother. This is all put right by Crerar & Ross (1953). There seems to have been some confusion about the colour vision of the brother John, but genealogic analysis of the descendants of the Harris family (which include Joseph, first Baron Lister, the founder of antiseptic medicine) convincingly establishes that John Harris was colour-deficient as well (Bell, 1926; Crerar & Ross, 1953). Incidentally, the interviewer, Joseph Dickinson, married Mary, the sole daughter of Thomas Harris the shoe-maker; their only son, Isaac, was colour-blind (Crerar & Ross, 1953).

The results of Dickinson's interview led Dalton to speculate that: 'a considerable number of individuals might be found whose vision differed from that of the generality, but at the same time agreed with my own' (1798, pp. 38–9). He then conducted a further search, finding some 20 other persons whose vision was like his own. None of his colour-blind individuals were female; and he thought it remarkable that he had not heard of one female subject to the peculiarity – though evidence to the contrary was already available from Scott's account in the *Philosophical Transactions*.

7.1.5 Dalton's theory

Dalton thought that *all* colour-blind individuals had the same defect as himself, a loss of sensitivity to red (i.e. long wavelengths), which we nowadays call *protanopia* or *red-blindness*. When observing a spectrum, for instance, he found: 'that part of the image which others call red, appears to me little more than a shade, or defect of light' (Dalton, 1798).

He hypothesized that the loss of red sensitivity was caused by one of the humours of his eye being tinted with blue, thus absorbing the red:

> one of the humours of my eye must be a transparent but coloured, medium, so constituted as to absorb red and green rays principally, because I obtain no proper ideas of these in the solar spectrum; and to transmit blue and other colours more perfectly. (Dalton, 1798, p. 43)

Dalton's contemporaries, Thomas Young, and Sir John Herschel, were unsatisfied with this hypothesis. Young (1807), invoking his own trichromatic theory, reasoned that the deficit could be more parsimoniously attributed to the 'absence or paralysis of those fibres of the retina, which are calculated to perceive red' (Young, 1807, vol. 11, pp. 315–6; cf. Sherman, 1981, p. 17); and Herschel (1833), echoing these sentiments somewhat, opined that 'we [the normal] have three primary sensations when you [Dalton] have only two' (in a letter from Sir John Herschel to Dalton, 20 May 1833; quoted in Bell, 1926, pp. 24–5). This is more or less how we explain protanopia today.

But Dalton rejected these explanations, preferring his own hypothesis as the more scientific (see Sherman, 1981, p. 126). To prove it, he directed that his eye should be examined upon his death (or at least he was not adverse to the idea, see Miles, 1957). A post-mortem examination was conducted on the day following his death (27 July 1844) by his physician, Joseph A. Ransome, in the presence of George Wilson, Regius Professor of Technology at the University of Edinburgh and an authority on colour-blindness. It revealed that the two humours and the lens of one eye were clear and transparent:

> the *aqueous* was collected in a watch-glass from a careful puncture of the cornea, and viewed both by reflected and transmitted light, [and] was found to be perfectly pellucid and free from colour. The *vitreous humour and its envelope* (the hyaloid membrane) *were also perfectly colourless*. The *crystalline lens* was slightly amber-coloured, as usual in persons of advanced age. (Ransome, in a letter to William Henry, Dalton's biographer, quoted in Duveen & Klickstein, 1954, p. 361)

The posteriormost part of the other eye was removed by a vertical section 'with as little disturbance as possible to the humours' and thereafter observations of coloured objects were made through it by Ransome. He judged the contrast of scarlet and green to be undiminished when viewed through the eye, which was contrary to Dalton's prediction; since Dalton 'was unable to discover any difference between the colour of the scarlet geranium flower and its leaves' (Ransome, quoted in Duveen & Klickstein, 1954, p. 362). Thus, Dalton's theory of colour-blindness could be rejected outright at its *fons et origo*. Ransome concluded, and Sir David Brewster later concurred, that 'the imperfection of Dalton's vision arose from some deficient sensorial or perceptive power rather than from any peculiarity of the eye itself [*sic*]' (Ransome, quoted in Duveen & Klicksten, 1954, p. 362). Alternative versions of the *modus operandi* of the examination of John Dalton's eye exist (Playfair, 1899; Miles, 1957), but the essential facts remain the same.

7.1.6 *After Dalton*

Dalton and his predecessors assumed that colour-blindness was a singular phenomenon; an idea that Dalton stubbornly held to until his death. But, even before Dalton's post-mortem examination, evidence was available for questioning the unity of expression of colour-blindness and for elementarily distinguishing between its different types. In 1837, Seebeck had introduced a systematic and objective approach for diagnosis and classification of colour-blind persons, and had demonstrated that there were at least two classes of them, corresponding roughly to the distinction we now make between protanopes and deuteranopes. Seebeck's classification system was followed by others, including those of Wartmann (1843), George Wilson (1855) and Holmgren (1878). Wilson, who was in attendance at Dalton's post-mortem examination, screened 1154 soldiers, policemen and students in Scotland; identifying three types of the colour-blind, depending on whether they confounded red, brown or blue with green (see Sherman, 1981, Table 7.2). And Holmgren, who screened a population of many thousands in Sweden, noted (seemingly for the first time) that, within an affected family, both the type and degree of the colour defect were usually the same.

Seebeck, Wartmann, Wilson and Holmgren all made use of simple, though often elaborate, colour tests, usually involving naming of spectral or interference colours or sorting of coloured glass, wool skeins or papers. With the introduction of the first series of pseudo-isochromatic plates, published by Stilling (1878*a*, *b*), and with Lord Rayleigh's introduction of the red–green colour-matching equation in 1881, and Nagel's anomaloscope for measuring it in 1898 (1907), more exact and quantitative analysis became available. (For a history and description of the early colour tests, see Linksz, 1964.)

7.1.7 *The first case?*

Prior to the advent of the spectroscopic test and the anomaloscope, it is difficult to say who described the first *bona fide* case of total colour-blindness. In the century-and-half following Huddart's report, 119 cases were recorded according to Bell (1926); only one of which originated from America (Colburn, 1897; Bell seems to have missed the earliest report from America; Earle, 1845). In the same time span, Shindo (1932) reported 78 and Hohki (1938) reported 89 cases in Japan; some of which are included in Bell's (1926) survey.

Although the disorder is sometimes referred to as the *Daubeney–Huddart anomaly*, the attribution is incorrect. First of all, Daubeney is a misnomer for Dawbenry Turbervile, which originates from Polack (1939). Polack, writing in French, apparently had trouble reading English; among other things, he refers to the age of the Maid of Banbury as 32–32 instead of 22–23. Moreover, Daubenry Turbervile's case was one of colour-blindness acquired by sickness or mental distress rather than heredity; and Huddart's cases were probably ones of congenital, partial (protanopic) colour deficiency rather than cases of congenital, total colour-blindness Dickinson and Dalton's diagnosis being more credible than Huddart's (see Bell, 1926; Crerar & Ross, 1953). Of course, these objections are largely beside the point; for, as Walls & Heath (1954) put it: 'total colour blindness was believed in for so long before it was actually seen, that the first genuine case [may have] attracted so little attention to its describer that we cannot now determine who he was' (p. 257). Rather than having to set total colour-blindness apart from the incomplete colour-blindness; it had to be disentangled from them.

The first adequately documented cases of congenital, total colour-blindness are probably those of Donders (1871), Nettleship (1880) and Landolt (1881), (see François, Verriest & De Rouck, 1955*a*, *b*, Table I). The earlier reports, including those of D'Hombres Firmas (see below), Galezowski (see below), Schopenhauer (1812), Spurzheim (1825), Böhm (1857) and Niemetschek (1868) – like those of Turbervile, Huddart and Rozier – provide too few observations to ascertain the exact nature of the colour vision defects described (see François *et al.*, 1955*a*, *b*, Table V). For a review of the early cases of total colour-blindness, one can refer to the genetic study by Julia Bell (1926) for the *Francis Galton Laboratory for National Eugenics* in London – listing 199 cases of achromatopsia, 39 of which have genealogies – or to the survey of

François *et al.*, (1955*a*, *b*) – listing 316 cases in Europe and America, 215 of which are probably cases of typical, complete achromatopsia with amblyopia (see their Table I.) Important genealogical evidence from the Japanese literature is listed in Waardenburg (1953); and Okuzawa (1987) provides a list of reports of colour-blindness in the Japanese and Western literatures, dating from 1602.

7.1.8 The island of Fur

The single most important study of an interrelated group of total colour-blind people is that of Holm & Lodberg (1940; see also Franceschetti *et al.*, 1958, 1959; Jaeger & Krastel, 1981). They investigated the accumulation of cases found on Fur (earlier spelled Fuur); a small island situated in the Limfjord in the northern part of Jutland, Denmark. Conditions on the island 'were very propitious for the manifestation of a recessive disease'. In fact, total colour-blindness was so well known there that the mothers in the most heavily afflicted families, could decide whether the child had the anomaly when it was only a couple of months old (Holm & Lodberg, 1940, p. 236).

In a population of about 1600 inhabitants, Holm & Lodberg gathered reports of 23 cases of total colour-blindness; 18 of which they examined themselves. Nineteen of their cases were registered in one pedigree comprising about 300 individuals; the remaining four were recorded in a pedigree comprising 57 individuals. (The rate of frequency, 1:70, is 4000 times higher than that reported for normal populations, see below.)

One of the cases referred to, but not examined, by Holm & Lodberg, was Mikkeline Nielsen, born 15 January 1892. She had a dizygotic twin sister, Christiane, a younger sister, Ane, and two younger brothers, Mikkel and Anthon, who had the same condition; while her parents, four other brothers and three other sisters had normal colour vision (Larsen, 1918, p. 1130; Holm & Lodberg, 1940, pp. 241–4). Lodberg and Holm themselves investigated Christiane, Ane and Mikkel. Mikkeline Nielsen had first been diagnosed in 1914 at the eye department of the *Rigshospitalet* (The National Hospital) in Copenhagen, where she was later employed as a 'gangpige' (domestic), and was extensively tested by Harald Larsen (Larsen, 1918). In 1921, when she suddenly died from pneumonia, she became the first achromat to be subjected to a histological investigation (Larsen, 1921*a*, *b*; see below).

7.2 Theories of total colour-blindness

7.2.1 The receptor loss theory

Dalton's theory, referred to above, was not strictly speaking a theory of total colour-blindness – nor was it the first such theory. More than a decade before Dalton's speculations, the first physiological theory of achromatopsia appeared in the English and French literature. It was, apparently, the brainchild of the mysterious Englishman, Mr George Palmer (1777, 1786; see also Voigt, 1781), whose identity, long and unsuccessfully sought by Walls (1956), was finally revealed by Mollon (1985*a*, *b*). Assuming that all light was constituted of only red, yellow and blue primary rays, Palmer hypothesized that:

> 'la rétine doit être composée de trois sortes de fibres, ou membranes analogues chacune à un des trois rayons primitifs, et susceptibles d'être mues par lui seul' (Palmer, 1786, p. 52; 'the retina must be composed of three kinds of fibers, or membranes, each analogous to one of the three primary rays, and susceptible to being stimulated by it').

Whiteness he attributed to stimulation of all three kinds of fibres in unison; darkness to lack of stimulation; and 'false vision' (read, colour-blindness or colour-anomaly) to an absence or deficiency in one or more of the fibres. Palmer was either personally acquainted with the colour-blind poet Charles-Pierre Colardeau or had heard about Colardeau's defect second-hand from mutual acquaintances, for he adds:

> 'Il existe des personnes qui, quoique voyant très-clair, ne distinguent pas de couleurs, et n'ont sensation que de plus ou moins de lumière, c'est-à-dire, de clair et d'ombre, parce que chaque classe des fibres peut être mue distinctement par chacun des trois rayons: de ce nombe étoit la poëte Colardeau' (Palmer, 1781, p. 52; 'There exist persons who, although they see very clearly, cannot distinguish colours, and have only the sensation of more or less of light, that is to say, of light and dark, perhaps because each class of fibres is not differentially stimulated by each of the three rays: to these individuals belongs the poet Colardeau').

Thus, Palmer speculated that Colardeau must have been deficient in all three colour sensitive fibres, or, more precisely, that Colardeau's three fibres failed to respond differentially throughout the spectrum. Since their response was always in unison, *ipso facto*, only a sensation of whiteness could result. In modern terms: if we read *short-wave*, *middle-*

wave and *long-wave* sensitive cones for the three kinds of fibres, this hypothesis anticipates the receptor loss theory of colour-blindness proposed by Leber (1873) and Fick (1874) a hundred years later. (Palmer was evidentally unaware of Turbervile's and Huddart's reports in the *Philosophical Transactions*; and he believed that Colardeau saw only black, white and grey, though it seems more likely that the poet was only insensitive to red.)

Thomas Young, who knew of Palmer's writings (see Mollon, 1985*a*), put forward a similar – indeed correct – hypothesis to explain Dalton's (protanopic) reduced sensitivity to the red end of the spectrum. Palmer's version, however, fails to explain total colour-blindness because of an unfortunate anatomical/physiological shortcoming: Palmer did not know, nor was it logical for him to deduce – the necessary knowledge did not exist – that a fourth process, or fibre, in the retina was responsible for night vision. Its discovery would have to await Schultze's (1866) functional and morphological distinction between rods and cones, which was possible only after extensive anatomical researches.

7.2.2. The rod only theory

Two years after Schultze's (1866) great discovery, the French opthalmologist X. Galezowski (1868) proposed a physiological theory of the origins of total colour-blindness. (He was almost certainly unaware of Palmer's works.) Galezowski first carefully considered the different varieties of congenital colour-blindness, dividing the cases known to him into three groups: 'ceux qui ne reconnaissent point de couleurs' ('those who do not recognize colours at all'); 'ceux qui ne distinguent pas une des couleurs principales' ('those who do not distinguish one of the principal colours [blue, yellow and red]') and 'ceux qui ne peuvent distinguer des teintes et des nuances secondaires ainsi que des tons' ('those who cannot distinguish the tints and secondary shades as well as the tones'). In the first group he placed: Thomas Harris the shoe-maker (Huddart, 1777), Collardeau [*sic*] the poet (Rozier, 1779), an individual (*De.*, a melancholic from Anduze) investigated by D'Hombres-Firmas (1849), and another (*M.E.*, a distinguished man of letters) investigated by Galezowski himself (M.E., it should be pointed out, had nystagmus, but normal visual acuity after optical correction for myopia!). Dalton was placed in the second group. Galezowski reasoned that, for the cases in the first group, the cones: '... devraient être ou incomplétement dévelоppés, ou peut-être même ils seraient complétement absent ...' ('... are deviant or incompletely developed, or perhaps even completely absent . . .'; p. 146). Accordingly, he concluded that the visual functions of the totally colour-blind: '. . . se passeraient toutes dans les bâtonnets' ('. . . take place wholly in the rods'; p. 147).

This speculation, which is still valid (see Chapter 10), has since become known as the *pure rod* theory. However, it would be much better termed the *rod only* theory because almost all of those who have supported it have been careful not to rule out the possibility that total colour-blindness is due to an abeyance or disorder in the cones' function, rather than strictly to their absence. Thus von Kries (1897) wrote: '. . . lediglich Mangel oder Functionsunfähigkeit des Zapfenapparates vorliegt, während die sonstigen Verhältnisse, insbesondere die räumliche Vertheilung der Stäbchen, mit der Norm übereinstimmen, . . . [und dass also der Monochromat nur] . . . mit Stäbchen sieht' ('. . . merely a defect or malfunction of the cone system exists; while the other features, particularly the spatial distribution of the rods, agrees with the normal standard, . . . [and thus the totally colour-blind only] . . . sees with his rods'). König (1894) likewise reasoned, as recorded by Nagel (1911), that: 'in the case of eyes that are totally colour-blind, vision is performed entirely by the mediation of the rods in the retina that contain visual purple, the cones either being lacking or not functioning' (p. 381). And, Nagel himself argued that: 'the totally colour-blind person sees *regularly* only by means of the elements of the retina that under other circumstances mediate twilight vision' (p. 381; italics ours).

At first, the consistency of the rod only theory with the clinical symptoms of the achromatic disorder (see Chapter 9) seemed to be more or less exact; as did the analogy between total colour-blind vision and twilight vision. As early as 1891, Hering had demonstrated that the photopic luminosity curve of the totally colour-blind was equal to the scotopic luminosity curve of normal observers. Nevertheless, the rod only theory soon began to become seriously compromised by new evidence. The first embarrassment was the inability to demonstrate consistently a central scotoma in the completely colour-blind (see Chapter 10). Later, even more perplexing embarrassments came to light, including frequent reports of inconsistencies (or breaks) in the achromat's dark-adaptation, increment threshold, visual acuity and flicker-fusion curves; dividing the curves into upper and lower branches, where a single, monotonic function was expected. These psychophysical curves suggested that cones, or some other kind of high-intensity receptor, in addition to the rods, were present in the achromat eye and providing a visual signal (for further details see Chapter 10). This second type of photoreceptor was widely speculated about, and was variously described as a *day rod*, a *residual cone*, or a *rhodopsin filled cone*.

7.2.3 Photopic or 'day rods'

In the majority of achromats it has been difficult to demonstrate a central (or photopic) *scotoma* (i.e. an area with reduced or no vision). In fact, a comprehensive survey of 215 cases reported in the literature (François *et al.*, 1955*a*, *b*), lists only 28 cases where a central scotoma was definitely demonstrated, compared with 32 cases where no central scotoma was reported. Faced with the failure of demonstrating in many achromats a central scotoma, which was expected to coincide with the rod-free area of the fovea and to be present if cones were lacking, von Kries (1911/1924) was the first to postulate a modification of the pure rod theory, which became known as the *day rod* or *photopic rod* theory. He argued that in the typical, complete colour-blind there may be two types of rods, one of which is the normal or 'scotopic' rod and the other of which is no more sensitive than a cone, and takes the place of the cones, at least in the fovea.

Subsequent investigators speculated along similar lines, proposing a rod containing either a very dilute concentration of rhodopsin (Hecht *et al.*, 1938, 1948; Sloan, 1954, 1958; Sloan & Feiock, 1972) or having an accelerated rate of photopigment regeneration (Lewis & Mandelbaum, 1943). Having rods with different concentrations of rhodopsin or a faster adaptation rate was thought to offer a valuable advantage, compensating, in part, for the loss of cones. The low concentration receptors would dark-adapt more rapidly and thereby eliminate a prolonged period of relative blindness after exposure to bright light before the usual slow rod dark-adaptation got under way (Lewis & Mandelbaum, 1943). Despite its initial appeal to common sense, the theory based on two types of rods hardly now seems tenable. It is, for instance, not supported by the single-cell recordings from primate rods (Baylor, Nunn & Schnapf, 1984). And, it was largely made irrelevant by the anatomical investigations of the achromat eye, which we will now consider.

7.2.4 The anatomical evidence

As a young woman Mikkeline Nielsen had moved from the island of Fur to Copenhagen. There she died from pneumonia in 1921 (aged 29). Four years before her death (on 5 December 1917), she had been demonstrated by Harald Larsen to *Det oftalmologiske Selskab i Københaun* (The Ophthalmological Society in Copenhagen; Larsen, 1918). (She was not the first achromat, however, to appear before the society: on 26 October 1904, a 21-year-old fisherman, possibly also from Fur, was demonstrated by J. Bjerrum (1904).)

Larsen claimed that Mikkeline Nielsen presented the classical symptoms of typical, complete achromatopsia (see the Taxonomy below). In particular, her corrected acuity was less than 0.1 in both eyes, she was insensitive to long-wavelength light (beyond 640 nm), and her dark-adaptation was monotonic. Surprisingly (to us), her spectral luminosity function peaked at 540 nm, rather than at (the now expected 510 nm (see Larsen, 1918, p. 1131; Holm & Lodberg, 1940, pp. 225–6). This may have been due to measurement errors in the spectroscopic examination performed by Professor Tscherning, since Larsen's own spectral function was found to peak at 570–580 nm. However, when Mikkeline's brother, Anthon Nielsen, was submitted to a spectroscopic examination at the *Rigshospitalet* (January 1937) by P. Møller Ladekarl, his function was also found to peak at a longer (530 nm) wavelength (Holm & Lodberg, 1940, pp. 243–4). The shift to longer wavelengths could be explained by macular pigment absorption, provided Mikkeline and Anthon had central fixation. This, however is inconsistent with the results of the histology, and with the fact that Larsen could not even demonstrate her blind spot because of the strong nystagmus induced when she tried to fixate (Larsen, 1918, p. 1131).

Moreover, ophthalmoscopic examination of both eyes revealed another feature which, in retrospect, is conspicuous. Although her papillae were normal, Larsen reported: '. . . i Centrum paa begge Øjne [ses] en rødlig Plet uden Farvereflex. Tillige ses perifert en Del choroidale Pletter og ejendommelige guirlandeformige choroidale Striber.' ('. . . in the centre of both eyes [can be seen] a reddish spot without a colour [fovea] reflex. Also in the periphery one can see some choroidal spots and strange garland shaped, choroidal stripes.'; Larsen, 1918, p. 1131; see also Holm & Lodberg, 1940, pp. 241–2). These are not normal features of stationary, congenital, total colour-blindness (see the Taxonomy section).

The histological examination of Mikkeline Nielsen's retinae (see Larsen, 1921*a*, *b*) produced results that were contrary to the then-received wisdom of the rod only and day rod theories of total colour-blindness. Although her right eye was improperly fixed and showed unreliable changes, sections of her left eye revealed:

> . . . an der Fovea kurze, plumpe Zapfen, die entweder ein sehr kurzes Außenglied haben oder denen dieses ganz fehlt. Seitwärts der Fovea finden sich fortgesetzt reichlich kurze, dicke Zapfen und dazwischen auch eine Reihe kurzer Stäbchen. Schon wenige Grade vom Zentrum scheint das Retinabild normal zu sein. Es lassen sich lange, schlanke Stäbchen und kurze, kräftige Zapfen, die absolut nicht degeneriert zu sein scheinen, erkennen. In bestimmten Schnitten zeigt sich an den Zapfen sehr gut das kegelförmige Außenglied. Was die Menge der Zapfen anlangt, so ist mit Rücksicht auf den Befund an tangentiellen Schnitten zu sagen, daß sich in diesem monochromatischen Auge nicht weniger Zapfen finden als in einem normalen' (Larsen, 1921*a*, p. 228; 1921*b*, pp. 301–2); '. . . in the fovea, short, plump cones, which have either a very short or totally missing outer segment. To the side of the fovea are found many short, thick cones intermingled with a number of short rods. Within a few degrees of the centre [of the fovea] the retina appears to be normal. It is possible to recognise long, slender rods and short, healthy-appearing cones, which do not at all appear to be degenerated. In several sections, one can easily see the tapered outer segment of the cones. As to the number of cones, in view of the findings from the tangential sections it is possible to say that in this monochromatic eye, no fewer cones are found than in the normal [eye]'.

The three subsequent histological investigations (Harrison, Hoefnagel & Hayward, 1960; Falls, Wolter & Alpern, 1965; Glickstein & Heath, 1975) all fail to confirm Larsen's general findings; for they all document major differences – throughout the entire retina – between the achromat and the normal eye.

The second examination was made of the two eyes of a 19-year-old male achromat, who may have had some residual cone vision, as indicated by his dark-adaptation curves (see Harrison *et al.*, 1960, Figs 2 and 3). The eyes were fixed 40 hours after death, at which time considerable autolysis of the photoreceptor layer had occurred. Nevertheless, the sections were good enough to reveal:

> imperfectly shaped squat cone-like units which lie on the external limiting membrane immediately opposite recognizable cone nuclei. There is considerable thinning of the outer nuclear layer with marked diminution in the numbers of cone nuclei in all parts of the retina. As the macula is approached, the photoreceptor layer almost entirely

> disappears. There is extreme paucity of these abnormal elements in all parts of the retina. (p. 686)

The third histologic study was made on the right eye of a 69-year-old woman, who was known to be totally colour-blind (Falls *et al.*, 1965). The eye was enucleated, before it could be psychophysically tested, because of acute, congestive glaucoma. A subsequent psychophysical investigation of the companion left eye was undertaken. It suggested the presence, in addition to normal rods, of receptors having the dark-adaptation kinetics and spatial summation characteristics of normal, foveal, middle-wave cones, but having the spectral sensitivity of rods 'modified in the blue by a rather marked amount of photostable xanthophile'. As concerns the right eye:

> The retina between the optic disc and 'fovea' contained only very few cones which were well developed . . . There were virtually no cones seen on the temporal side of the fovea. The retina on the nasal side of the disc exhibited only a very occasional cone . . . Many cones between the optic disc and fovea exhibited an outwards displacement of their nuclei from the body into the outer fiber . . . , and true ectopia of cone nuclei was seen in many instances . . . Most of the inner segments containing the ectopic cone nuclei were short and of unusual shapes. (p. 611)

The fourth investigation was of the retinae of an 88-year-old man, whose eyes were removed and fixed within 15 minutes of his death (Glickstein & Heath, 1975). His vision had been extensively tested during his life (Walls & Heath, 1954), and was entirely consistent with a diagnosis of typical, complete achromatopsia (see the Taxonomy section below). The histology revealed:

> . . . no receptors at all in . . . [his] . . . foveas, and . . . between 5 and 10 per cent of the normal number of cones throughout the retina . . . In addition to their abnormally low number, the cones near the fovea . . . [were] . . . abnormal in shape. Those near the fovea . . . [were] . . . characteristically much wider than one would expect in a normal human eye. Also, . . . many central cones . . . [had] . . . their nuclei on the scleral side of the outer limiting membrane. (p. 635)

Obviously the four studies on the histological correlates of total colour-blindness are not uniform in their conclusions. This may be because their subjects were afflicted with different types of total colour-blindness (see the Taxonomy section below), but this is now difficult to establish. Certainly, the clinical and psychophysical findings in the four cases conflict somewhat. In some of the cases, we cannot be certain whether the patient suffered from stationary, congenital colour-blindness or from an early onset, progressive cone degeneration disease, which may also be inheritable. In particular, Mikkeline Nielsen may have been a case of central cone achromatopsia or foveal cone dystrophy (see the Taxonomy section below), because only her fovea had structurally abnormal cones and her fundus showed the macular signs characteristic of these degenerative diseases (see Krill, Deutman & Fishman, 1973).

Setting these objections aside, what is consistent about the four studies is that all confirm the presence of morphologically intact cones, or cone-like structures, in the achromat retina; though three of the studies find that the cone numbers are vastly fewer than those found in the normal retina. The anatomy, therefore, warrants the conclusion that total colour-blindness cannot be caused, *in all cases*, by the absence of cones. However, they do not rule out the possibility that the *cones-that-are-present* are structurally malformed and functionally impaired or that they are too few in number to provide an independent visual signal.

7.2.5 *Residual cone theories*

Even before the anatomical evidence became available, there was speculation about cone sparing in the total colour-blind eye. The earliest theory can be attributed to Hess & Hering (1898). In accord with Hering's theory of *Gegenfarben* (opponent-colours), they believed that the total achromat possessed the cones having the *black-white* visual substance, which supposedly furnished colourless luminosity sensations, but lacked those having the *red–green* and *yellow–blue* substances, which furnished the sensations of colour. Later supporters rejected this view, which if true would make 'numerous peculiarities of the totally colour-blind eye ... completely incomprehensible' (von Kries, 1924, p. 437), such as the poor visual acuity and the absence of a photopic luminosity function. But they held to the belief that at least the periphery of achromat retinae contained functional cones, though they left unspecified the precise photopigment nature of those cones (Lewis & Mandelbaum, 1943; Blackwell & Blackwell, 1961). Nevertheless, it was obvious to presume that the residual cones must be identical in colour-sensitivity and offer no basis for colour-discrimination (Lewis & Mandelbaum, 1943).

Walls & Heath (1954), were the first to hypothesize about the exact nature of the spared cones; suggesting that they were all of the short-wave (or S) type. They supported their hypothesis by a number of 'facts';

which were later shattered by some other facts (see Sloan, 1958). These included the findings that the dark-adaptation, the increment threshold and the flicker-fusion curves of all achromats exhibit the spectral sensitivity of rhodopsin, and that the responses of X-chromosome linked, incomplete achromats (or blue-mono-cone monochromats), who actually do have functioning S cones in addition to rods, are very different from those of typical complete achromats (Blackwell & Blackwell, 1961; Alpern *et al.*, 1971; Green, 1972; Daw & Enoch, 1973; Young & Price, 1985; Hess *et al.*, 1989*a*). That the spared cones are not functioning as S cones does not eliminate the possibility that they are functioning as long-wave (L) or middle-wave (M) cones; as suggested in the case of Falls *et al.*'s (1965) female achromat. But, if so, the spared cones cannot contain cone photopigments in their outer segments because the measured spectral sensitivity in typical, complete achromats, regardless of adaptation level, is always that of the rod photopigment (Alpern, 1974). (If the measured spectral sensitivity at photopic adaptation levels resembles one of the cone photopigments, by definition, the 'totally colour-blind' individual is an incomplete achromat; see Taxonomy below.)

7.2.6 Rhodopsin cones

Given that the measured spectral sensitivity in typical, complete achromats is always that of the rods, but that cones are found in histological sections of the achromat eye, Alpern, Falls & Lee (1960) argued that the 'high-intensity' photoreceptors of the achromatic eye are, in reality, perfectly normal cones, except that instead of the normal cone pigments, their outer segments contain rhodopsin or a 'visual pigment which has an action spectrum indistinguishable from rhodopsin' (Alpern *et al.*, 1960; Falls *et al.*, 1965; Alpern *et al.*, 1971; Alpern, 1974). The second alternative, namely that there is a visual pigment which has an action spectrum indistinguishable from rhodopsin, although plausible, reminds one of Mark Twain's tongue-in-cheek remark that: 'If the Iliad wasn't written by Homer, it was written by another blind poet of the same name'.

The initial and strongest support for this 'rhodopsin-filled cone' theory was Alpern *et al.*'s (1960) own finding that at photopic intensities some achromats displayed a cone-like directional sensitivity function (or Stiles–Crawford effect of the first kind), although their spectral response was that of rhodopsin (for a full discussion see Chapter 10). Later support came from Dodt, van Lith & Schmidt (1967) and from Auerbach (1974). The former found electroretinographic and sensory threshold evidence in an achromat favouring the idea of 'sense cells organized as photopic elements and having rhodopsin as their principal photopigment' (p. 239); though they misleadingly chose to call the cells 'day-rods'. The latter found irregularities in the electro-retinographic (Auerbach & Merin, 1974) and dark-adaptation (Auerbach & Kripke, 1974) data of some achromats which could be explained by assuming residual cone photoreceptors filled with the same 'wrong' pigment, i.e. rhodopsin.

Alpern and other co-workers (Alpern *et al.*, 1971) subsequently reported psychophysical evidence in favour of 'rhodopsin cones' replacing normal cones in the central fovea of X-chromosome-linked, incomplete achromats (see the Taxonomy section below). Their evidence rested once again on directional sensitivity measurements, made at low and high adaptation levels and paired with spectral sensitivity measurements. Pokorny, Smith & Swartley (1970) and Young & Price (1985) cautiously put forward a similar claim, though solely on the basis of spectral sensitivity measurements.

Daw & Enoch (1973) and Hess *et al.* (1989*a*), however, were unable to replicate Alpern *et al.*'s (1971) directional sensitivity finding in other incomplete achromats; and Nordby & Sharpe (1988) were unable to replicate Alpern *et al.*'s (1960) original directional sensitivity findings in a typical, complete achromat (this is discussed at length in Sharpe & Nordby, The photoreceptors in the achromat, Chapter 10). And, it seems likely that Dodt *et al.* (1967) and Auerbach (1974) were not investigating typical, complete achromats; and that Pokorny *et al.* (1970) and Young & Price (1985) had too little evidence to draw their conclusions. Moreover, the theory that rhodopsin cones replace normal cones in the eyes of achromats has always run at least a quarter note off. Like the old Sherlock Holmes enigma of the dog that did not bark, the evidence supporting the rhodopsin cone theory has crucial omissions. It is noteworthy that the rhodopsin in the cones is always assumed to have the bleaching and regeneration dynamics of a cone pigment; and this accords with the idea that such rates are much more dependent on the receptor type than on the pigment itself. But if this is indeed the case, one is led to ask, by analogy; 'Why is the acuity of the typical, complete achromat not better than it is?' and 'Why does the visual system of the achromat saturate at the same levels where the isolated rod visual system saturates in the normal?'. For one would expect the acuity of the achromat to be closer to normal if rhodopsin-filled cones replaced normal cones in the fovea and participated in the process of visual resolution *and maintained the same post-receptoral connexions.* And one would expect the achromat's visual system to be less troubled by hypersensitivity to light and saturation, if cones, regardless of the photopigment in their outer segments, were actually present in large numbers in the peripheral retina, if not in the fovea. This is because the saturation of the rod visual system is largely determined by breakdown of the phototransduction process in the rod outer segment (see Chapter 2). A similar breakdown does not take place in the cone outer segment because it is forestalled by photopigment bleaching.

7.3 A short taxonomy of achromatopsias

Obviously, from the proliferation of theories, there seems to be some confusion about the nature of the photoreceptors in the achromat eye. Part of the confusion has no doubt arisen from the failure in the past to differentiate between the various forms of achromatopsia. Now it is thought that besides *complete achromatopsia with reduced visual acuity*, i.e. the classical or 'typical' type, there are at least three other kinds of congenital achromatopsia: *complete achromatopsia with normal visual acuity*; *autosomal recessive incomplete achromatopsia*; and *X-chromosome-linked incomplete achromatopsia* (Pokorny, Smith & Verriest, 1979; Smith & Pokorny, 1980). Although cerebral achromatopsia and complete achromatopsia with normal visual acuity are extremely rare, the frequency of congenital incomplete or 'atypical' forms may be greater than that of the typical, complete forms (Krastel, Jaeger & Blankenagel, 1983). Thus investigators may have drawn conclusions in the past about typical, complete achromatopsia that pertain only to one of the incomplete, more prevalent forms.

Achromatopsia may also arise adventitiously after brain fever (Boyle, 1688; Mollon *et al.*, 1980), cortical trauma or cerebral infarction (Critchley, 1965; Meadows, 1974; Damasio *et al.*, 1980). Or, it may be associated with progressive macular diseases or retinal disorders that can affect the cones with little or no involvement of the rods (Goodman *et al.*, 1963; Krill *et al.*, 1973; Pokorny *et al.*, 1979).

The classification, inheritance and prevalence of the various congenital forms, insofar as they are known, are shown in Table 7.1 (cf. Pokorny *et al.*, 1979; Smith & Pokorny, 1980; Sharpe, 1985). The prevalence

Table 7.1. *Inheritance, prevalence and classification of congenital achromatopsia*

Type	Classification							Inheritance[a]	Prevalence[b] (%)	
	Colour vision	Discrimination deficit	Absent cone systems	Reduced luminous efficiency	Relative luminous efficiency function (peak) scotopic	photopic	Spectral neutral point		Male	Female
Complete achromatopsia (with reduced visual acuity)	monochromatic	total	S, M and L	long wave-lengths (rod system)	507 nm	—	all wavelengths	autosomal recessive	0.003	0.002
Complete achromatopsia (with normal visual acuity)	monochromatic	total	S and either L or M	long or middle wavelengths	— —	540 nm or 570 nm	all wavelengths	—	0.000001	0.000001
Autosomal recessive incomplete achromatopsia	dichromatic/ monochromatic	various/ total	S and either L or M	long or middle wavelengths	507 nm 507 nm	540 nm or 570 nm	536 nm or none	autosomal recessive	—	—
X-linked incomplete achromatopsia	dichromatic/ monochromatic	red to green/ total	L and M	long wave-lengths	507 nm	445 nm	476 nm	X-linked recessive	—	—

[a] Not known for complete achromatopsia (with normal visual acuity).

[b] For white Europeans. Not known for X-linked incomplete achromatopsia and autosomal recessive incomplete achromatopsia.

given for complete achromatopsia with reduced visual acuity is close to what has been found in a recent survey. Egill Hansen (personal communication) has recorded *c.* 60 cases of complete achromatopsia in Norway, which has a population of a little over four million. Some coastal and rural areas in the North and West are underrepresented in his material, compared to the more densely populated urban and Eastern areas. Conservatively, one could set the number of achromats in Norway at about 80, which yields an incidence of 1 in 50 000 or 0.002%.

7.3.1 Complete achromatopsia with reduced visual acuity

Complete achromats with reduced visual acuity or amblyopia are sometimes referred to as *rod monochromats* or *monochromats*. The former term is used because they are believed to have only functioning rods; the latter because they can match any coloured light to a white light, or to any spectral wavelength, simply by varying the luminance. The term typical, complete achromatopsia is frequently used to describe them, but the use of 'typical' may be ill-advised because instances of atypical complete achromatopsia (better referred to as autosomal, recessive incomplete achromatopsia – see below) may be more frequent. Indeed, strict complete achromatopsia may only be found in every third 'typical', congenital achromat (Krastel *et al.*, 1983).

Besides having poor visual acuity (usually 0.1), which does not change significantly with age, these achromats may lack protective iris pigment (albinism), are usually subject to light aversion (i.e. hypersensitivity to light, also called 'photophobia'), nearly always display pendular nystagmus (i.e. rapid, horizontal oscillations of the eyes), and are unable to maintain foveal fixation. They may have astigmatism, dysplasia of macular yellow, and occasional pallor of the optic discs (Waardenburg, 1963). One must be careful, however, of including eyeground abnormalities and changes as symptoms of stationary, congenital achromatopsia; for such claims seem to be based on 'perpetuation of information from cases originally given this diagnosis which were indeed probably examples of cone degenerations' (Krill *et al.*, 1973, p. 71; see below).

A central scotoma can often be demonstrated with small targets and careful testing, but it may easily be overlooked because nystagmus may make testing difficult. These achromats show no Purkinje shift and no cone–rod transition during dark-adaptation; and they exhibit a shift of the luminosity function to the maximum of the rod visual system and a concomitant shortening of the short- and long-wavelength ends of the spectrum. (The psychophysical evidence is presented in detail in Sharpe & Nordby, The photoreceptors in the achromat, Chapter 10.)

The prevailing view is that typical, total achromatopsia with reduced visual acuity is autosomally, recessively inherited. There is mention in the literature, though, of a possible pseudo-dominant, autosomal inheritance (see Franceschetti *et al.*, 1958; Waardenburg, 1963; Pokorny *et al.*, 1982), and the matter has not been fully resolved. There may, of course, be more than one gene involved in the transmission. Indeed, the occurrence of complete and incomplete achromatopsia in siblings can only be attributed to the influence of a modification-gene, which is located in another chromosone and is acting independently of the achromatopsia-gene (Jaeger & Krastel, 1981). Moreover, an examination of the colour vision of the parents of 'typical', complete achromats has provided evidence that the condition may have a tendency towards a heterozygous manifestation (Pickford, 1957); which would explain some of the strange inheritances reported (see Waardenburg, 1963).

7.3.2 Complete achromatopsia with normal visual acuity

Complete achromatopsia with normal visual acuity is also known as *cone-monochromacy* or *cone-monochromatism* (Pitt, 1944; Weale, 1953) or as *achromatopsia without amblyopia* (Krill, 1977). The incidence is extremely rare, estimated at one case in a million (Weale, 1953). Pitt's (1944) estimate of one in a hundred million, which is frequently cited in the textbooks (e.g. Krill, 1977), is based on assumptions about double dichromatism (i.e. tritanopia combined with either deuteranopia or protanopia). It is theoretically questionable and inconsistent with reported incidences (Weale, 1953; Alpern, 1974). The inheritance of this form of achromatopsia is unknown. Unlike complete, typical achromatopsia with reduced acuity, there is usually no concomitant, reduced visual acuity, nystagmus or light aversion.

Cone monochromats are conventionally assumed to have one type of cone, L or M (long- or medium-wave), but not both. S cones are presumed to be totally absent or nonfunctioning. If the M cones are the only ones functioning, the luminosity maximum is shifted to the short-wavelength end of the spectrum, similar to protanopia (Pitt, 1944; Weale, 1953, 1959; Fincham, 1953; Gibson, 1962; Ikeda & Ripps, 1966), and there is a loss of sensitivity at long- and short-wavelengths. If the L cones are the only ones functioning, the luminosity maximum is shifted to the long-wavelength end of the spectrum, similar to deuteranopia (Vierling, 1928; Crone, 1955; Alpern, 1974), and there is a sensitivity loss at middle- and short-wavelengths.

Residual colour discrimination may occur if the field of view is large enough to involve parafoveal photoreceptors, or if the field is highly saturated or very bright (cf. Sloan & Newhall, 1942; Pitt, 1944; Weale, 1953; Crone, 1956). This has led to the speculation that in some cases there is more than one cone type present and that the defect is post-receptoral in origin (Weale, 1953, 1959; Fincham, 1953; Gibson, 1962; Krill, 1977). Indeed, in some cone-monochromats M and L foveal cone pigments have been demonstrated *in situ* by fundal reflectometry (Weale, 1959); three foveal colour mechanisms have been found by the two-colour increment threshold method (Gibson, 1962), and the accommodation reflex mechanism has been shown to be stimulated by the effects of chromatic aberration in the same way as in the normal (Fincham, 1953). The last of these findings suggest that the effect occurs above the zone at which the paths to the mid-brain concerned with the accommodation reflex leave the visual pathways to the cortex (Fincham, 1953).

However, other evidence, namely the finding of independent protan, deuteran and tritan defects in the relatives of cone-monochromats (Pitt, 1944; Weale, 1953; Crone, 1956; Krill & Schneiderman, 1966), lends support to the hypothesis that cone-monochromacy is a combination (congenital double protan–deuteran) receptor defect.

7.3.3 Autosomal recessive incomplete achromatopsia

Incomplete achromatopsia of autosomal recessive inheritance was first described by Franceschetti (1928, 1939). The condition is sometimes referred to as incomplete achromatopsia with reduced visual acuity, or incomplete, typical, polysymptomatic achromatopsia (Waardenburg, 1963), or atypical, complete achromatopsia. These achromats show all, or most, signs and symptoms of complete achromatopsia – though often to a lesser extent – including poor visual acuity, nystagmus, light aversion, abnormality of the macular yellow pigment and a scotopic luminous efficiency function at low photopic levels. One or more cone type may be partially spared and be functioning with the rods (Jaeger, 1950, 1951, 1953; Jaeger & Krastel, 1983). The sparing of cones permits dichromatic or even trichromatic colour vision at low and moderate photopic luminances and a Purkinje shift at low photopic levels. Hence, these individuals are not, strictly speaking, achromats. Inasmuch as different types of residual colour vision occur in incomplete achromatopsia, the condition appears to comprise multiple genotypes (Jaeger, 1950, 1953; Sloan, 1954; Goodman, Ripps & Siegel, 1963).

Two forms of autosomal, recessive, incomplete achromatopsia are defined and distinguished by whether the M (the protan type) or L (the deuteran type) cones are functioning with the rods (Smith & Pokorny, 1980). When the M cones function with the rods; visual acuity is reduced to 0.1 or less; the fundus appears normal; there is pendular nystagmus and light aversion (Smith, Pokorny & Newell, 1978). The photopic luminosity function is protanopic and Rayleigh matches (on the Nagel anomaloscope) are displaced towards the red primary (Smith *et al.*, 1978). A neutral point may occur in the blue-green region of the spectrum (526 nm). When the L cones function with the rods, visual acuity is less severely reduced (0.33–0.2); the fundus appearance is similar to that of typical, complete achromats; nystagmus may or may not be present and there is a reduced high-intensity scotopic response (Smith, Pokorny & Newell, 1979). The achromat luminosity function is deuteranopic (Sloan, 1954; Fuortes, Gunkel & Rushton, 1961; Siegel *et al.*, 1966; Smith *et al.*, 1979), and Rayleigh matches are shifted towards the red primary, but show normal luminance (Smith *et al.*, 1979). A neutral point may occur in the yellow-green (538 nm) region of the spectrum.

In some cases, two cone types may be spared, L and S, or L and M (Pokorny *et al.*, 1982). These individuals may then be trichromats, with their colour vision being mediated by rods and M and L cones or by rods and S and L cones. In other cases, all three cone types may be spared (van Lith, 1973; Pokorny *et al.*, 1982). The degree of residual cone function found varies considerably between observers and estimates depend on the method of examination. For example, vestigial colour perception and cone function may be more obvious when the observers are tested with large (up to 120° diameter) and/or flickering stimulus fields under selective chromation adaptation conditions (Jaeger, 1950; Baumgardt & Magis, 1954; Pokorny *et al.*, 1979; Krastel *et al.*, 1981, 1983; Jaeger & Krastel, 1983, 1987).

7.3.4 X-chromosome-linked incomplete achromatopsia

Incomplete achromatopsia of X-chromosome-linked inheritance has a different genetic origin than the other form of incomplete achromatopsia (Spivey, Pearlman & Burian, 1964; Spivey, 1965). It is transmitted as a X-linked, recessive trait; and, not surprisingly, all cases reported so far have been male: Blackwell & Blackwell, 1961 (4 cases); Grützner, 1964 (1); Spivey *et al.*, 1964 (1); Spivey, 1965 (5); Alpern, Lee & Spivey, 1965 (1); Pokorny *et al.*, 1970 (1); Verriest, 1971 (1); Alpern *et al.*, 1971 (5); Green, 1972 (1); Daw & Enoch, 1973 (1); Alpern, 1974 (12); Hansen, Seim & Olsen, 1978 (1); Berson *et al.*, 1983 (5); Smith *et al.*, 1983 (5); Young & Price, 1985 (2); Zrenner, Magnussen & Lorenz, 1988 (3); Nathans *et al.*, 1989 (14); Hess *et al.*, 1989*a*, *b* (2). The genes associated with it may also be associated with deuteranomaly (Smith *et al.*, 1983) or with both protanopia and deuteranopia (Alpern, 1974). Minor colour-vision abnormalities have been reported in the female carriers (see Krill, 1977; Table 8-7). Recently, Nathans *et al.* (1989) have reported that the X-chromosomes of 14 individuals with this disorder all had alternations in the gene cluster responsible for the production of the M and L cone visual pigments; either both the M and L visual pigment genes were nonfunctional due to the deletion of DNA or only one of the tandem array remained and was rendered nonfunctional by a point mutation.

The disorder is also known as blue-mono-cone monochromacy (Blackwell & Blackwell, 1957, 1961), blue cone monochromacy (Alpern *et al.*, 1971) or π_1-cone monochromacy (Alpern *et al.*, 1965, 1971). The terms blue and π_1 both refer to the S cones, which are believed to be the only cones functioning with the rods (Blackwell & Blackwell, 1957, 1961; Alpern *et al.*, 1965; Hess *et al.*, 1989*a*, *b*; see also Crone, 1965; Siegel *et al.*, 1966). In confirmation, in some cases, under chromatic adaptation conditions, X-chromosome-linked incomplete achromats fail to exhibit the action spectra of the M and L cones (Zrenner *et al.*, 1988; Hess *et al.*, 1989*a*) and to display transient tritanopia (Hansen *et al.*, 1978; Zrenner *et al.*, 1988), which in normal observers is believed to result from the interaction between the S and the M/L cones. However, in other cases residual L cone function may be revealed if large or even small test fields are used (Smith *et al.*, 1983). It has been suggested that these achromats, in addition to rods and S cones, have rhodopsin cones (see above) in their retinae (Pokorny *et al.*, 1970; Alpern *et al.*, 1971). However, the presence of rhodopsin cones has not been confirmed by Daw & Enoch (1973) and by Hess *et al.* (1989*a*).

As in typical, complete achromatopsia, concomitant signs and symptoms are present, though they may be less pronounced: reduced visual acuity (0.33–0.1; see Green, 1972; Zrenner *et al.*, 1988; Hess *et al.*, 1989*a,b*), pendular nystagmus, aversion to bright light and fundal abnormalities (e.g. macular aplasia). There may be associated myopia (Spivey, 1965; François *et al.*, 1966). A Purkinje shift, however, occurs and there may be residual dichromatic colour perception, as evidenced by reliable colour discriminations (Alpern *et al.*, 1971; Daw & Enoch, 1973; Pokorny *et al.*, 1979; Young & Price, 1985; Reitner, Sharpe & Zrenner, 1990). At scotopic and at low mesopic levels, vision is monochromatic and the luminous efficiency function resembles the spectral response of the rods. At high mesopic and at low photopic levels, vision may be dichromatic and the luminous efficiency function resembles a linear combination of the spectral responses of the S cones and the rods (Blackwell & Blackwell, 1961; Pokorny *et al.*, 1970; Young & Price, 1985; Hess *et al.*, 1989*a*). At high photopic levels, vision is once again monochromatic and the luminous efficiency function resembles the spectral response of the S cones. At all luminance levels, spectral sensitivity is depressed for wavelengths above 550 nm (unless the L cones are also functioning).

To quickly distinguish X-chromosome-linked incomplete achromats from autosomal recessive incomplete achromats, a special four-colour plate test (Berson *et al.*, 1983) and a two-colour filter test (Zrenner *et al.*, 1988) exist. The latter test is based on the observation that the X-chromosome-linked incomplete achromat's spatial acuity is improved by viewing through blue cut-off filters (Blackwell & Blackwell, 1961; Zrenner *et al.*, 1988)

7.3.5 Cerebral achromatopsia

Certain cerebral lesions may cause persisting impairment of colour perception (complete or partial achromatopsia) with preservation of primary visual function. The exact locus of the cortical damage remains unknown, but there is agreement that it is generally localized on the ventral aspect of the occipital and temporal lobes within the lingual and fusi-form (occipitotemporal) gyri. In all cases there is probably damage to part of Brodman's areas 19, 21, 36 and 37 (for reviews, see Critchley, 1965; Meadows, 1974; Damasio *et al.*, 1980; Dubois-Poulsen, 1982).

Cerebral achromatopsia may often be accompanied by *prosopagnosia* (inability to recognize familiar faces), *object agnosia* (inability to recognize familiar objects) and impaired topographical memory, but published reports suggest that the four disorders are usually dissociated from one another, and are probably functionally distinct (Meadows, 1974; Damasio *et al.*, 1980; Heywood, Wilson & Cowey, 1987).

The earliest recorded case is that of the young gentlewoman described above (Boyle, 1688), who is almost certainly the Maid of Banbury seen by Turbervile (1684). She lost all colour vision following a cerebral fever, which was possibly a meningitis or a herpes encephalitis. A small number of modern cases of loss of colour vision in the whole, or in half, of the visual field have been described by Niemetschek (1868), Verrey (1888), MacKay & Dunlop (1899), Critchley (1965), Vola, Riss & Gasset (1973), Meadows (1974), Albert, Reches & Silverberg (1975), Green & Lessell (1977), Pearlman *et al.* (1979), Damasio *et al.* (1980), Mollon *et al.* (1980), Young & Fishman (1980), Dubois-Poulsen (1982), Heywood *et al.* (1987) and Sacks & Wasserman (1987). One of the best investigated is the case of a young policeman who was left with achromatopsia and left homonymous hemianopia, with macular sparing, following a febrile illness (Mollon *et al.*, 1980). The young male could not match, sort or name colours, although his clinical visual acuity was normal and increment threshold measurements indicated that he retained the function of the S, M and L cone-mechanisms.

Individuals with cerebral achromatopsia typically say that they cannot see colours, or in less severe cases they may say that colours have lost their brightness. A common complaint is that everything looks grey, or in varying shades of black and white, or drained of colour. As a consequence, everyday objects, whose identification depends upon discrimination of their exact hue, may prove difficult to distinguish (Meadows, 1974). The loss of colour may be repulsive at first. It is not just that objects are devoid of hues, but that they may have a 'dirty' look, 'the whites glaring, yet discoloured and off-white, the blacks cavernous – everything wrong, unnatural, stained and impure' (Sacks & Wasserman, 1987, p. 26). Although hue discrimination may be entirely lacking, the discrimination of achromatic contrast (i.e. the discrimination of grey levels) may be relatively spared (Heywood *et al.*, 1987; Sacks & Wasserman, 1987).

Cerebral achromats may also claim to have a heightened spatial acuity, as witness by the recent case of a 65-year-old artist, Jonathan I.:

> My vision was such that everything appeared to me as viewing a black and white television screen. Within days [of the concussion producing the colour-blindness], I could distinguish letters and my vision became that of an eagle – I can see a worm wriggling a block away. The sharpness of focus is incredible (Sacks & Wasserman, 1987, p. 25).

Interestingly, these observations parallel, to some degree, those made by Boyle, 300 years earlier, while describing the vision of the young gentlewoman:

> having pointed with my Finger at part of the Margent, near which there was part of a very little Speck, that might almost be covered with the

> point of a Pin; she not only readily enough found it out, but shewed me at some distance off another Speck, that was yet more Minute, and required a Sharp Sight to discern it. And yet, whereas this was done about Noon, she told me, that she could see much better in the Evening, than in any Lighter time of the day.
>
> (pp. 264 and 256; the pagination of Boyle's book is irregular)

Boyle's remarks, however, should be taken with a grain of salt because he himself had quite poor visual acuity and was a patient of the 'great and experienced' Dr Turbervile (John Mollon, personal communication). And so should those of Jonathan I, the artist, since Sacks & Wasserman (1987), who interviewed him, never troubled to assess his astounding claims quantitatively. But, nonetheless, on the basis of his claims, they argue for an 'enhanced, compensatory sensitivity to the nocturnal and scotopic' of the colour-blind; and liken Jonathan I.'s case to that of Kaspar Hauser, the boy who was confined in a lightless cellar for fifteen years (Anselm von Feuerbach, 1832).

Such analogies, however metaphorical, do not seem scrupulous or just. They are not supported by the personal account of one of us, a congenital, typical, complete achromat, who in terms of his visual system is much more like a creature of the night than Jonathan I. or Kaspar Hauser (see Nordby, Vision in a complete achromat: a personal account, Chapter 8). Nor is there evidence for them in the careful studies of other cerebral achromats, whose spatial acuity was merely described as normal (Damasio *et al.*, 1980; Mollon *et al.*, 1980; Young & Fishman, 1980; Heywood *et al.*, 1987).

7.3.6 Progressive cone dysfunction

There are progressive retinal disorders that affect the cones with little or no involvement of the rods (François *et al.*, 1956; Björk, Lindblom & Wadensten, 1956; Steinmetz, Ogle & Rucker, 1956; Sloan & Brown, 1962; Goodman *et al.*, 1963, 1966; Gützner, 1964; Deutman, 1971; Verriest, 1971; Pinckers, 1972; Krill *et al.*, 1973; François *et al.*, 1974; François, De Rouck & Laey, 1976; Neuhann, Krastel & Jaeger, 1978; Pokorny *et al.*, 1979). These cone degenerations, cone dysfunctions or cone dystrophies may involve only the macula, only the periphery, or the entire retina. Sometimes the cone dysfunction is complicated by rod pathology – though the cone impairment usually dominates.

The major symptoms are loss of visual acuity, light aversion and defective colour vision. The severity of the symptoms varies considerably and depends upon the type of the disease – whether the cause of dysfunction is localized macular disease (e.g. Stargardt's disease or juvenile macular degeneration) or optic nerve pathology – and upon the stage of development at the time of examination. The symptoms appear to progress more rapidly in patients with an earlier age of onset. With late onset, the deterioration may progress very slowly and an exact diagnosis may only be possible after many years or even decades of testing.

At disease onset or in localized cases: acuity may be better than 0.2; nystagmus and light aversion may be minimal or absent; the macular changes may be subtle or absent; and the colour vision defect may be only partial. In advanced stages: acuity may deteriorate to between 0.1 and 0.05; nystagmus and light aversion may be present; a non-specific atrophic macular degeneration may be seen (with vascular attenuation); temporal pallor of the optic nerve may be common; and the colour vision defect may be total.

Because of the similarity of symptoms, the cone degeneration disorders in advanced stages are easy to mistake for stationary, congenital complete or incomplete achromatopsia – especially if the disease onset is in early childhood (Goodman *et al.*, 1963). The important distinguishing feature seems to be that congenital, total colour-blindness is stationary and not associated with eyeground (i.e. macula or optic nerve) changes; whereas cone degeneration disorders are progressive and are associated with macular lesions (Krill *et al.*, 1973; Neuhann *et al.*, 1978). The distinction may be missed, however, unless careful ophthalmoscopic examinations are made, and followed-up over an extended period. In fact, it now seems likely that 'cases previously reported in the past as total, congenital colour-blindness with macular and/or optic nerve disease are really examples of cone degenerations' (Krill *et al.*, 1973, p. 75).

7.4 Conclusions

Imagine a rainbow at night: its perfect arc spanning the dark vault of the heavens; its bands, galvanized by moonlight, shimmering from vibrant black to white. Such images allow the colour-normal to enter the world of the colour-blind; a world both share at twilight, when the rainbow's many colours become one. Given the ease of envisaging – nay of experiencing – *total colour-blindness the phenomenon*, it seems surprising that *total colour-blindness the disorder* eluded discovery, or at least public awareness, in Europe until the late eighteenth century. Even then, the evidence for total colour-blindness was entangled with, and not distinguished from, the evidence for deficient colour vision. Only in the late nineteenth century was Western scientific methodology advanced enough to reliably differentiate total colour-blindness from the other colour vision disorders.

In the last hundred years, much more has become known about total colour-blindness and it is now possible to divide those it afflicts into several classes, depending upon whether they have mere rod vision or mere (single) cone vision or joint rod and partial cone vision. These various forms, which were not adequately recognized in the past, may have confused the physiological and anatomical explanations of the disorders, and led to a number of competing and incompatible theories about them. In Chapter 10 and 11 the psychophysical evidence is reviewed concerning the classical or typical type of total colour-blindness and we consider that evidence in terms of the rival theories.

Acknowledgements

The preparation of this manuscript was supported by the Deutsche Forschungsgemeinschaft, Bonn (SFB 325, B4) and the Alexander von Humboldt-Stiftung, Bonn-Bad Godesberg. We thank Dr John Mollon (University of Cambridge), Professor Joel Pokorny (University of Chicago), Dr Andrew Stockman (University of California, San Diego), Professor Robert A. Weale (University of London), Professor W. D. Wright (Radlett, Herts) and Dr Claudia Zrenner (Tübingen) for critically commenting on the manuscript.

8

Vision in a complete achromat: a personal account

Knut Nordby

8.1 Introduction

Being myself a vision scientist who is also a complete achromat, I have, upon demand from friends and collaborators, taken on the task of trying to convey some of my visual experiences and to explain how I cope with my visual handicap. I rely on recollections, both my own and those of my family, and try to separate information that can be documented or is supported by other sources from the mere anecdotal. I also draw on information from interviews with other achromats, but only to supplement or comment on my personal experiences.

My recollections may have become distorted over time, they may not be precise and may also be biased – and they may not, in all cases, apply to other achromats. It is my hope, though, that my account will give both vision scientists and the general reader a glimpse, not only into the manifestations of achromatopsia and rod-vision – topics usually not covered by the learned papers – but also into the practical problems and obstacles encountered by a completely colour-blind person.

8.2 A short biography

8.2.1 Infancy

I was born on 17 November 1942, in Oslo, Norway, as the first child of Kjell Nordby (28.11.1914–30.3.1987) and Mary Camilla Nordby, *née* Bredesen (born 21.12.1914). The pregnancy was normal and the birth went well. My birth-weight was 3845 g and my length 510 mm. There is some early written and photographic documentation showing that, on the whole, I was a healthy baby who seems to have developed normally and, except for a stenosis of the pylorus which was quickly cured, I gave my parents little cause for alarm during the first six months of my life.

Both my parents were born with normal vision and, indeed, excellent colour-vision. I tested both with the *Ishihara* and the *Österberg* pseudo-isochromatic plate tests, and I also tested my father with the *Farnsworth 100 Hue test.* They both performed normally. I have one sister (born 8.10.1943) and one brother (born 5.10.1945) who are both, like myself, typical, complete achromats. This has been confirmed by the *Nagel* anomaloscope.

There is no evidence of consanguinity between my parents, although the possibility cannot entirely be ruled out. My paternal and my maternal grandmother both came from the same small coastal town in southern Norway, but nothing is known with certainty about any relationship between the families. If there is any relationship, it must be at least four generations removed (see Fig. 8.1).

The prevailing view, then and now, is that typical, total achromatopsia with reduced visual acuity is a recessive, autosomal (i.e. not linked to the pair of X–Y or sex-chromosomes) inherited condition. The statistical probability, according to Mendelian laws of inheritance, of all three siblings inheriting and displaying a recessive trait from parents who do not exhibit the phenotype is exceedingly small. On average, and assuming that only one gene is responsible, only one child out of four from heterozygous parents will be homozygous for and display a recessively inherited trait.

No documented case of achromatopsia is known to have existed in either branch of my family. There are, however, rumours of an aunt of my maternal grandmother who, reportedly, had 'very weak eyes' and 'rarely ventured out-of-doors in full daylight'. Despite the suggestive symptoms, such anecdotal evidence cannot be accepted to infer a *bona fide* case of achromatopsia, since no ophthalmological report is known (it is most improbable that any medical assessment of her eyes was ever performed), and her symptoms can be attributed to several other causes (e.g. *retinitis pigmentosa* from diabetes).

According to my parents, I could control my eyes and direct my gaze even at the age of three weeks. Photographs taken of me only a few weeks after birth show me with fully open eyes and not a trace of squinting, or partial closing of the eyes, in bright light (see Fig. 8.2). Nothing unusual was recorded at the time about my visual behaviour (i.e. *light aversion* or 'photophobia') or eye-movements (i.e. *nystagmus*).

Due to enemy actions in Norway, my parents fled with me to Sweden in May 1943, when I was only six months old. One to two months later my

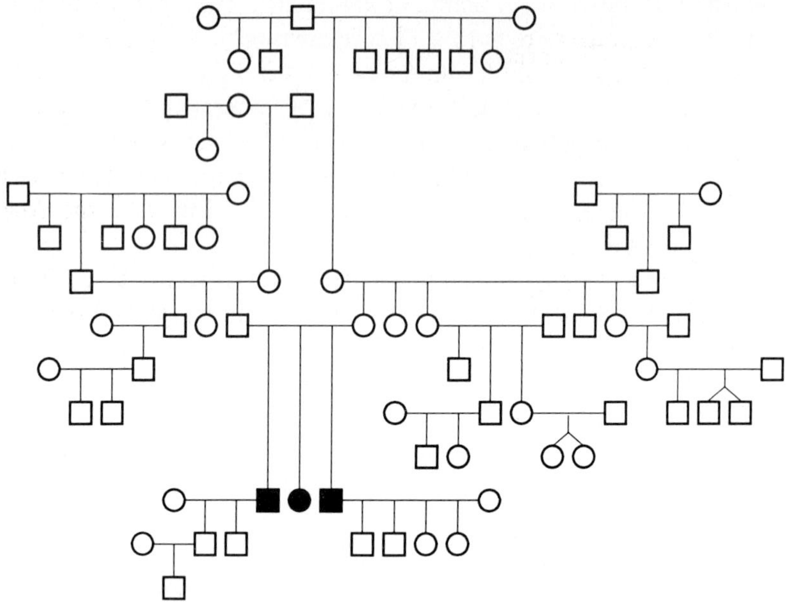

Fig. 8.1 My family pedigree. Solid, black symbols indicate homozygous, typical, total achromats (from left to right; me, my sister and my brother). Open symbols indicate homozygous and heterozygous non-achromats.

parents began noticing that I had developed some strange symptoms. My eyes had started to quiver from side to side (i.e. horizontal, pendular nystagmus) and my eye-movements were irregular. I had begun to blink continuously and partially close my eyes, or squint (looking through the narrow slits between the eye-lids), in bright light, and I habitually avoided bright light, something I had not done before. Earlier, according to my mother, I had sometimes even looked straight into the sun with no signs of distress, and she often had to turn me around, being worried that I would damage my eyes. This special behaviour has also been reported to me spontaneously by the mothers of several other achromats. One mother, in fact, believed that this habit of gazing into the sun had harmed her son's eyes and was the actual case of his achromatopsia and low visual acuity.

After seeing several general practitioners and some ophthalmologists, who could offer no explanation for the symptoms, my parents finally consulted a prestigious professor in ophthalmology (no-one in the family can now recall his name). *Hereditary achromatopsia totalis* [i.e. total colour-blindness] *with concomitant horizontal pendular nystagmus, light aversion, and reduced visual acuity* was diagnosed. He also found that I

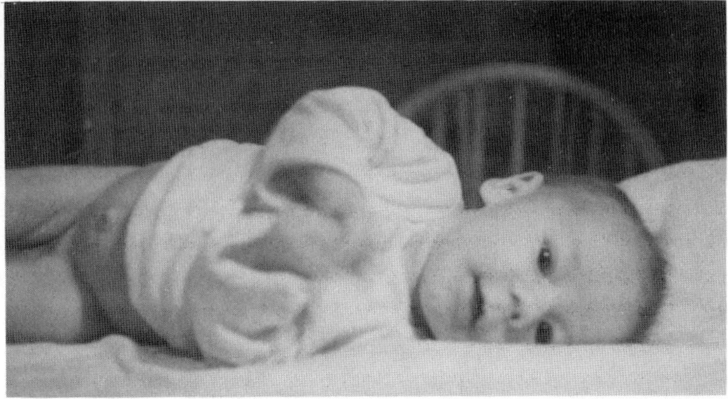

Fig. 8.2. Photograph taken of me 1–2 weeks after birth. I showed no signs of squinting or light aversion at the time, and I fixated normally and kept my eyes fully open, even in bright light.

was hypermetropic with a slight astigmatism. At an age of only nine months I thus received my first pair of spectacles. As far as can now be established these first lenses had a strength of about +3 diopters and had a 1 diopter vertical cylinder.

My parents were told that I was severely visually handicapped, that I was totally colour-blind and that my visual acuity was so low that I would never be able to read and write. They were also told that I would have to attend institutions for the blind and learn to read Braille, and, at best, could be trained for one of the traditional vocations for the blind (e.g. piano tuner, telephone switch-board operator, etc.). As it happens, the authority was disproved in some of his predictions by the course of events, but I am getting ahead of myself.

After hostilities ended my parents decided to stay in Sweden. Because of my father's work we moved many times; living in Stockholm, in Gothenburg, in the small town Töreboda and again in Stockholm; until the summer of 1954, when his work took us to Caracas, Venezuela. There we stayed four years, until the summer of 1958, after which we returned to Norway and settled in Oslo.

8.2.2 Early childhood

My first clear memories seem all to be connected with nights and evenings, or they occur indoors in subdued lighting. As far back as I can remember, I have always avoided bright light and direct sunlight as much as possible. Photographs taken of me, and my siblings, during our

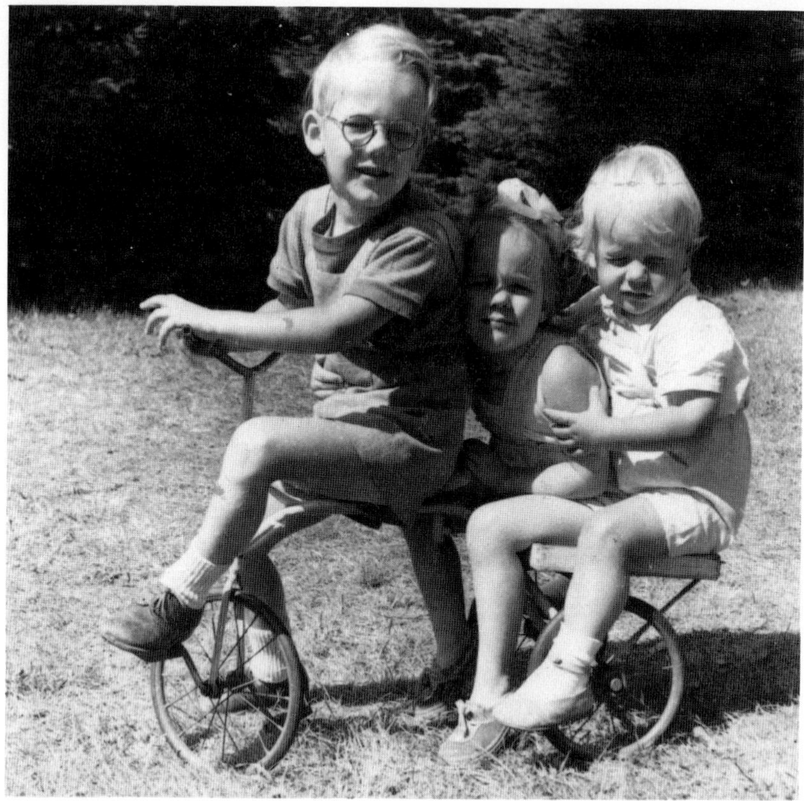

Fig. 8.3. Photograph of me, when I was five, my sister and my brother (from left to right), taken in bright sun-light. We all clearly display the typical squinting and light aversion behaviour shown by all typical, complete achromats.

childhood normally show us with nearly shut eyes, usually looking away from the sun, except when photographers demanded that we look towards the sun for the pictures (see Fig. 8.3). As a child I preferred playing indoors with the curtains drawn, in cellars, attics and barns or outdoors when it was overcast, in the evenings, or at night.

This, of course, was quite the opposite of what well-meaning parents and grown-ups considered to be right for children. My whole childhood was, in fact, a continuous struggle against the prevailing views about what is proper for children; i.e. being out in the sunshine as much as possible, not playing outdoors after dark, not drawing the curtains during the day, not playing in cellars and other dark places, and so on.

It soon became apparent to my parents that the learned ophthalmologist was correct insofar as I was completely colour-blind. My father told me that he had noticed that when sorting my coloured playing blocks in day-light I usually put the red and the black blocks together in one pile, the green and the blue ones in another pile, the yellow were usually, but not always, put in a pile by themselves, and so were the white. Indoors in artificial lighting, on the other hand, I sometimes separated the red and the black in different piles, but frequently confused the green and the blue blocks; the yellow and the white blocks, though, I still put in separate piles.

When using colouring pencils or crayons, I am told, I always confused the colours, breaking all the conventions and 'rules' about what were the 'correct' colours to use: I would happily colour the sky light green, yellow or pink; the grass and leaves orange or dark blue; the sun white or light blue, and so on. I was always corrected in my choice of colours by those who knew better, and, eventually, I gave up painting and colouring my drawings. Unfortunately no coloured drawings from my early childhood seem to have survived.

When I was five we were living in Gothenburg, and from then on my recollections are much clearer. At this time my circle of activity expanded beyond the limits of the house and the garden and into the near parts of the town. I then developed a system for finding my way back, which I still use. The city-block was the basic unit in my system. I always kept myself orientated where I was on the block. When going further away the system consisted of counting the streets I had crossed, keeping count of right and left turns, counting doors or shops along a block, thus forming a mental, topological map of my path. When returning I reversed direction, retracing my path, making turns in the opposite direction, and counting backwards the streets I had crossed.

I also learned to make use of various prominent landmarks, e.g. parks, squares, churches, towers, underpasses, bridges, etc., as important checkpoints along the route. Even today, I find it much easier to orientate myself in cities with rivers, canals, tramways, overground railway lines and other conspicuous and easily identifiable 'boundaries' that divide the city into smaller parts. I cannot remember ever having lost my way returning from a place I had first located myself. On the other hand, it can be more difficult when going with others to keep track of the route, especially when travelling by car.

When five, I nearly fooled my parents into believing that I could read. My parents often read stories and fairy tales to us children, and I was very much intrigued by this activity. I had a children's picture book with a few lines of narrative on each page, all of which I had learned by heart. Sitting with the book at normal reading distance, where, of course, I could not discern the individual letters, I 'read' the text out loud and clear, following the lines with my eyes, turning the pages at the right points. Eventually, I was found out when, by mistake, I turned two pages at a time and continued to read on before realizing my error. This desire to master the art of reading never left me.

8.2.3 School years

When the time came for me to start school we lived in the small village of Töreboda, about halfway between Stockholm and Gothenburg. In Sweden it is compulsory to begin school in the year that children reach the age of seven. The nearest school for the blind and partially sighted was in Stockholm. My parents did not want to send me away to a boarding school at such a young age, and, in defiance of the professor's earlier advice, it was decided that I should try to attend an ordinary school and see if I could manage. Thus, in the autumn of 1949 I started out in the first form of the municipal, primary school in Töreboda.

At this time it became very obvious to me that my vision was different from that of other children. They could see things that I could not see; such as recognizing each other at a distance, spotting ripe berries on bushes and trees, reading cars' licence plates at a distance, etc. They could also take part in activities and sports, especially ball-games, that I could not. Hitting a ball with a bat, or catching a ball thrown towards me, is next to impossible for me, except under the most optimal light-conditions, such as in twilight; when teams were set up, I was always the last one to be taken on.

I must have been a difficult pupil, inquisitive about all that was going on, talkative, always avoiding doing things when my vision would prevent me from performing and thus give me away. I did learn the letters of the alphabet, but I did not really learn to read properly in the first and second form.

The school-books used had ordinary size print, and no-one had thought about getting me books with extra large print, if, indeed, such books existed then. Nor had anyone thought about providing me with a reading-glass. The lenses of my glasses, which by now had been increased in strength to about +6 diopters, did not have enough magnification power for me to read the small print easily.

Since I could actually not discern the individual letters even in ordinary book-print, I again resorted to my old reading hoax; bringing it to new and unprecedented heights. I had developed a very keen memory. It was usually enough if a class-mate or someone in the household read my home-assigment aloud to me once or twice, in order for me to remember and reproduce it, and to perform a rather convincing reading behaviour in class.

An important discovery that I made during my first school-year is worth noting. As an aid for teaching the letters of the alphabet, the teacher placed large cards, each holding a printed letter, in a row over the blackboard as the letters were introduced. To differentiate between the two categories of letters they had different colours; the vowels were red, while the consonants were black. I could not see any difference between them and could not understand what the teacher meant, until early one morning late in the autumn when the room-lights had been turned on, and, unexpectedly, I saw that some of the letters, i.e. the A E I O U Y Å Ä Ö, were now suddenly a darkish grey, while the others were still solid black. This experience taught me that colours may look different under different light-sources, and that the same colour can be matched to different grey-tones in different kinds of illumination. I have since often used this phenomenon of spectral differentiation as an aid to separate colours by their different grey-tones under various light-sources.

A constantly recurring harassment throughout my childhood, and later on too, was having to name colours on scarves, ties, plaid skirts, tartans and all kinds of multi-coloured pieces of clothing, for people who found my inability to do so rather amusing and quite entertaining. As a small child I could not easily escape these situations. As a pure defence measure, I always memorized the colours of my own clothes and of other things around me, and eventually I learned some of the 'rules' for 'correct' use of colours and the most probable colours of various things. As an example, I learned that glass that was very dark to me usually was a dark cobalt-blue, glass that looked a bit lighter was usually bottle-green, and so on. In this way, I could fool some people into believing that I had colour-vision and stop them from pestering me. A friend of the family, though, actually believed that my inability to name colours came from my parents not having taken the trouble to teach me the colour-names. She often tried, but in vain, to train me in naming colours, but had to admit in the end that I could not, in fact, differentiate between the different hues.

When I was eight, my three-year-younger brother was given a small bicycle. This was quite irresistible to me and I soon learned to ride it. At first I only dared to go around the block, keeping to the left-hand side of the road and only making left turns (Sweden had left-hand drive at this time), but as I gained confidence my activity area expanded. Traffic in post-war Sweden was very light, in our village we scarcely saw more than a couple of cars a day, much transport being carried out by horse and cart, and the conditions of the roads in the area did not allow speeding. Riding the bicycle in traffic did not, therefore, constitute too grave a danger to me, despite my visual handicap.

I often 'borrowed' the bicycle, getting up early in the morning, and set out on long journeys visiting out-lying farms, clay-pits, brick-works, factories, railway stations and all kinds of interesting places. When not chased away at once, I would often stay for hours. My curiosity was unbounded, and I learned many wonderful things; how bricks are made, the working of farm machinery, railway operations, etc. When visiting the local railway station the engine driver found it was safest for me (and best for his peace of mind) to take me with him in the cab of the locomotive, rather than have me nosing around the tracks – to which I did not object at all. This inquisitive self-education may have been the origins of my later interest in research.

In the summer of 1951 we moved to Stockholm and I started the third form in a large, municipal school in one of the newly built suburbs south of the city. This did not work out very well. With large classes, the teachers had little time to give me the special tuition and extra training I needed, and after only a month or two it was finally decided that I, and my sister, who had started school the previous year, should attend the state school for the blind and partially sighted at Tomteboda, just north of Stockholm (my brother was not due to start school until the following year). Because the trip each day between the home and the school took too long, my sister and I were forced to live in, seeing our family only on the week-ends and during vacations.

At this school my sister and I were, in all practical matters, treated as blind. Although the staff must have known that I actually could see quite well in some situations, a régime was set up to teach me to write and read Braille. Reading with the tips of my index-fingers I did not find easy and I quickly developed the knack of reading Braille by eye, because the raised dimples of the Braille letters cast shadows on the paper, making them much easier to read by sight than by touch. For this I was punished; it was considered to be cheating, and for a week I was confined to my room after classes, being denied to see the other pupils. And, for the next couple of months I had to wear a heavy, lined, black velvet mask covering my eyes in class when reading – to keep me from peeking. Eventually my Braille reading proficiency increased to such a level that the mask could be dispensed with.

Although I had in many ways become a leader at the school for the blind, having a definite visual advantage over the genuinely blind and the gravely partially sighted pupils, and thus gained much confidence in dealing with other children, I was quite unhappy there and strongly resented being treated as blind. So one day I ran away. Completely on my own I crossed Stockholm, from the north to the far south of the city where we lived. I reached my home by midnight, after more than ten hours of walking, retracing the exact route my father used to take us home by car on the week-ends. This caused a great scandal. Unbeknown to me the bishop was to hold his visitation of the school on that very day, but the staff had to search for me and the police had to be called in to help them, thus ruining the whole event. This in no way improved my popularity with the staff; although, as was later somewhat reluctantly admitted, it was considered to be no mean feat, even for a child with *normal* vision, to find his way across the entire city of Stockholm.

Thus, after only two years at the school for the blind and visually disabled, it was decided that, as an attempt, I should again try to attend an ordinary school for the sighted. I was transferred to a newly opened municipal, primary school very close to where we lived, although it meant being moved down one form to compensate for all I had lost during my two years at the school for the blind.

I have a strong suspicion that at the school for the blind and partially sighted they actually just wanted to get rid of me, since I had always created much turbulence and was considered to be rather detrimental for morale among the more seriously handicapped pupils. My sister and my brother (who had entered the school for the blind the previous year) both continued to attend the school, though, staying for another year until we left Sweden in 1954.

Seen in retrospect, the curriculum at the school for the blind may appear to have been old-fashioned, but it should be borne in mind that at the time this school was considered to be very progressive and one of the world's leading institutions for the blind and partially sighted, and it was run according to the most modern pedagogical principles. Today, 35 years later, we can only be happy that some of these principles now seem to have been abandoned.

During the summer holidays of 1953, before joining my new school, a problem troubled me very much; although I told no-one about it. While at the school for the blind I had forgotten practically all of what little I had learnt before of reading ordinary print, and I did not cherish the prospect of facing my new fourth form class not being able to read and write.

My father, being at that time sales director with a large company, kept a stock of handouts and gifts for customers, which among other things contained lighters, pocket knives, and – *pocket magnifiers*. One day I borrowed a magnifier and used it to look at pictures in a comic-book. I was frustrated at not remembering how to read the text in the speaking bubbles, since I could now clearly discern the individual letters with the help of the magnifier. I then remembered that my parents had been given a sample-sheet with the Braille alphabet embossed on it together with the ordinary printed alphabet. Using the sheet as a 'cipher-key', I managed to 'decipher' and read the text in the speaking bubbles.

This incident was truly a turning-point for me and, more than anything else, opened a whole new world to me, who had always so much wanted to be able to read. In just a few weeks' time I secretly taught myself to read properly and my reading skills very quickly improved. I became a voracious reader who devoured all I could lay my hands on, buying magazines and borrowing books in libraries on practically any imaginable topic.

In my new school I had the unforeseen fortune of having a teacher who had an understanding for my handicap and who really tried to help me overcome my problems in class. He was in many ways a very progressive teacher, ahead of his time. He did not adhere to the strict régime practised in the schools in those days. As an example he let me move my desk up close to the blackboard so that I could actually see what was being written, breaking the regular geometric order of the desks in the classroom, then so much cherished by the other teachers, and he let me move around in the classroom during lessons so that I could inspect at close quarters things that were demonstrated; something completely unthinkable with his colleagues who put their pride in having their pupils sitting attentively at their places. And he made a habit of always telling us what he wrote on the blackboard, which was of great help to me.

Even today, when attending lectures and talks, I always try to sit close to the screen when slides are shown, and I find it easier to follow the presentation when the speaker also tells the audience what is written on the transparencies. When lecturing or giving talks myself, I always do this, showing slides with large print and not crowding too much information into each transparency. In fact, I often treat my audience as visually disabled: if I can see well from a front row seat what I am presenting I know that my audience also will see it.

Because of this outstanding teacher I soon managed to catch up with my peers, regaining much that was lost in the years at the school for the blind. It was also very good for my self-esteem to be able, at least in some fields, to perform like other children of my age, and it also encouraged my parents to try sending my siblings to an ordinary school.

As it happened this was to take place in Caracas, Venezuela. For four years my siblings and I attended a small, private school run by a Scotsman. We had no great problems learning English and otherwise adapting to his somewhat unorthodox style of teaching. During the summer holidays, before starting school, my sister, who had received intensive training in reading and writing ordinary print during the last semester at the school for the blind, taught my younger brother to read and write. He had not received any training at all, and my 10-year-old sister succeeded in bringing him to a level where he could attend the school for the sighted.

After returning to Norway in 1958 we consulted the Department of Opthalmology at the National Hospital in Oslo. Here Dr Egill Hansen confirmed the earlier diagnosis of complete achromatopsia with reduced visual acuity, light aversion and nystagmus in all three of us using the Nagel anomaloscope and the standard battery of tests – and we were entered into the *Registry of Blindness*. In Norway, like in many other countries, people with visual acuities of 6/60 (1/10) or less are *legally* considered as blind. This entitled us to special education and to pensions for the disabled, which we have never made use of.

Instead we started to attend grammar school (*gymnasium* in Norway) where we each, in turn, sat for the General Certificate of Education, Advanced Level (which is required for going to the university). At exams we were given an extra hour for finishing our papers, but little else was done by the school authorities to facilitate us attending a school for sighted pupils. By now, however, we had all become rather expert in coping with the practical problems of attending a school for the sighted. Upon getting our exams we all, in turn, went on to university.

At this time I started my musical education, taking lessons on the clarinet, the cello, and in theory of music at the Oslo Conservatory of Music. I did not have any special plans of becoming a musician, but acquired a professional education along with the gymnasium. Reading printed music proved to be a real obstacle for me, especially *prima vista*, i.e. sight reading. Today I can easily make enlargements of sheet-music on an office copier, but in the early 1960s this was not available to me. For soloists this may not be a great problem, since they often have to learn their parts by heart anyway, but in orchestra play it can be a great handicap.

At university I didn't do too badly. From early on in my studies I was employed by the university as a part-time lecturer, which meant that I could have a study of my own. There I had full control of the light level – drawing the curtains during the day if necessary to shut out sun-light – and I could thus work under conditions that suited me best. When attending lectures and seminars I made a habit of arriving early, not out of courtesy to the lecturer, but to be able to get a good seat, sitting, if possible, with my back to the windows and close to the blackboard or projection screen.

After first having a go at law, which I gave up after one year, I eventually ended up studying psychology at the Institute of Psychology at the University of Oslo. In addition I studied philosophy of science, physiology and music science. My interests soon turned to sensory psychology and perception. As I wanted to work independently, I took up auditory research, partly out of interest for audition, but also because I believed that my visual handicap would not be a big obstacle to me in this field of research.

At this institute also worked Professor Ivar Lie, Svein Magnussen, Bjørn Stabell and Ulf Stabell, all very accomplished vision scientists. They realized that, being trained in psychophysics, I would be a unique subject in research on rod vision, and they tried to persuade me to leave audition for vision. I first wanted to get my Ph.D. (*Mag. art.* in Norway), and after my dissertation (on auditory localization and dichotic time/intensity-trading) I switched to vision research.

I have been in research ever since; first as assistant professor (*stipendiat* in Norway) at the Institute of Psychology, Oslo University, doing vision research and lecturing in perception and neuroscience. I am now a Senior Research Scientist with the Norwegian Telecom Research Department, doing human factors research and development work in telecommunications, and developing telecommunication equipment and services for disabled people.

My vision research activities soon brought me into contact with vision researchers in laboratories outside Norway, some of which I have visited many times and where I have made many good friends. Beside work in Norway with Svein Magnussen and Bjørn and Ulf Stabell, I have also visited and collaborated with Dr Robert F. Hess at the Physiological

Laboratory, University of Cambridge, England, with Dr Lindsay T. Sharpe, in Dr Lothar Spillmann's laboratory at the Klinikum der Albert-Ludwigs Universität, Freiburg, the Federal Republic of Germany, and with Dr L. Henk van der Tweel, at the Laboratorium voor Medische Fysica, Universiteit van Amsterdam, The Netherlands – collaborations that have continued after I joined the Norwegian Telecom. The results of these experiments are dealt with in other chapters of this book (a full list of these works is included in a bibliography with the References for this chapter).

My siblings also entered university; my sister studied Latin, English and music science, and my brother qualified as a psychologist. My sister now works at the library of the Norwegian Association for the Blind in Oslo, being in charge of translation and production of books in Braille; unlike me she has not forgotten her three-year training in Braille at the school for the blind. My brother is employed as a high-ranking civil servant with the Norwegian Directorate for Labour, working mainly in organizational development

In 1965 I met Nina Marie Løberg (born 10.7.1944), who studied psychology, and we were married the following year. There are no known achromats in her family and there are no relations between our families. We have two sons, Cato (born 1.3.1967) and Alexander (born 19.1.1969). Both Nina and the boys have perfectly normal colour-vision as tested with the *Farnsworth 100 Hue Test.* My older son Cato Nordby was married to Anita Ødeby in 1987. Their son, Daniel Nordby (born 27.3.1989) shows normal visual development without the slightest indication of anything unusual at an age of eight months, though, of course, it has not yet been possible to test his colour-vision. My brother is also married and has four children, two sons and two daughters; all with normal colour-vision. My sister is single and has no children.

I have never, nor have my siblings, received any qualified vocational counselling or help in planning my education and my career. What advice I have had has usually been unfounded and ill-conceived. The suggestions have included everything; from simple clerical and assembly-line work to the traditional work for the blind, usually involving simple, manual, low-paying jobs requiring little or no education, and showing complete disregard for what actual tasks the work demanded. Most so-called 'simple' jobs, e.g. filling in forms, sorting mail, filing and retrieving files, assembling components, cleaning, tending machines etc., usually require good visual acuity and colour-vision. No one ever suggested theoretical or academic work requiring higher education.

Luckily, my parents had always wanted their children to have an academic education, and circumstances were highly favourable for this in Norway in the 1960s and 1970s.

In my research work I have had few problems related to my visual handicap. I work in areas where, to a large extent, I can plan my own work and choose my own tasks. In addition to the research activities my work also includes administrative duties, giving interviews, going to meetings and giving talks, both in Norway and abroad, and I also lecture regularly at the University of Oslo. These activities pose few practical problems for an achromat. Typing used to be quite a bother, since I had to lean over the typewriter with my magnifier to be able to read what I had written, but now I use a PC and a word-processing program for all my typing, and this is a very useful tool to me. To overcome my low visual acuity I have to get close (150–200 mm) to the screen, and I have a large (19″) screen installed. With modern printers I can have my documents printed in large type-face, making them easier to read.

8.3 Rod vision

Trying to explain to someone with normal, or nearly normal, colour-vision what it is like to be totally colour-blind, is probably a bit like trying to describe to a normally hearing person what it is like to be completely tone-deaf, i.e. not possessing the ability to perceive tonal pitch and music. My task, though, is probably a bit simpler than the case of the tone-deaf, since practically everyone has had experiences of achromatic (i.e. colourless, or black and white) or monochrome pictures and renderings, and certainly must have witnessed the gradual disappearance of colours when darkness sets in.

A first approximation, then, in explaining what my colour-less world is like, is to compare it to the visual experiences people with normal colour-vision have when viewing a black and white film in a cinema or when looking at good black and white photographic prints (good here meaning sharply focused, high contrast with a long grey-scale, as in crisp, high quality, glossy, technical prints).

This, however, is only part of the story because I have so far only dealt with the achromatic aspect of my perception. To get a fuller understanding of my visual world one must, in addition to my colour-blindness, also take into account my light aversion (i.e hyper-sensitivity to light) and my reduced visual acuity. In the following I will deal in turn with each of these aspects of typical, total achromatopsia.

8.3.1 Total colour-blindness

As mentioned above, I only see the world in shades that colour-normals describe as *black*, *white* and *grey*. My subjective spectral sensitivity is not unlike that of *orthochromatic* black and white film. I experience the colour called red as a very dark grey, nearly black, even in very bright light. On a grey-scale the blue and green colours I see as mid-greys, somewhat darker greys if they are saturated, somewhat lighter greys when unsaturated. Yellow typically appears to me as a rather light grey, but is usually not confused with white. Brown usually appears as a dark grey and so does a very saturated orange. When asking other total achromats to make such matches I get practically the same results from them. In the literature I have found descriptions of colour-determinations made by other typical, total achromats, which all closely match my own judgements (see e.g. Bjerrum, 1904; Larsen, 1918).

Although I have acquired a thorough theoretical knowledge of the physics of colours and the physiology of the colour receptor mechanisms, nothing of this can help me to understand the true nature of colours. From the history of art I have also learned about the meanings often attributed to colours and how colours have been used at different times, but this too does not give me an understanding of the essential character or quality of colours.

Coloured and black and white pictures are usually indistinguishable to me. But sometimes I can, often quite easily, tell coloured and non-coloured pictures apart. Coloured pictures may look less crisp, or slightly less in focus, and often have less contrast than comparable monochrome pictures. Under some conditions I am able to tell a polychrome picture from a monochrome one by noting the different surface textures of the coloured inks used to print the picture. I do this by tilting it so that the light reflects differently in the different inks: coloured inks of various hues show up as duller or glossier patches. I am sometimes able to see the numbers on the Ishihara and Österberg pseudo-isochromatic plate tests by this technique. Given the time I might be able to fool an unwary tester. A few other achromats have also shown me this trick, not because they wanted to deceive me, but because they thought that they had a vestige of colour-vision. However, if I cover the test-plate with a glossy, transparent foil they are unable to do this trick: varnishing or covering pictures with high-gloss films destroys the effect.

I have never experienced 'dirty', 'impure', 'stained' or 'washed out' colours, as reported by the artist Jonathan I. who completely lost his colour-vision after a cerebral concussion (Sacks & Wasserman, 1987). When, occasionally, colour-pictures do look less crisp than black and white pictures, it is usually because of bad printing, lower contrast or faded inks.

Once when Bjørn and Ulf Stabell were measuring my spectral equal-brightness function (using their Wright colorimeter) I felt that I could detect slight differences between colours by distance cues i.e. colour-stereopsis, which could be due to chromatic aberration in the optics. I informed the Stabell brothers about my suspicion and an *ad hoc* experiment was quickly set up to test my conjecture. I was to try any ploy that I could devise to guess the hue of the test field, and they were to counter my ploy, making mock changes or unexpected changes of hue. When the day was over, I had not been able to guess *any* hue beyond pure chance level.

When I know the colour of an object I may often refer to its colour name when describing it or referring to it to other people. Since colour names have meanings for most people, communication is made easier. This, in turn, leads to other people using colour names when addressing me, even those who know of my colour-blindness. Sometimes this can be of help to me, when e.g. they refer to a *red* book among other light-coloured books, but referring to a red book among black and dark-coloured books is of little help to me.

Colours do not help me to distinguish objects from their backgrounds. Since the grey-tone that I can match to a particular colour changes with changing illumination, objects that are partly in bright light and partly in shadow, such as flowers in the mottled sunlight coming through the branches of a tree, can be very hard to see. The same applies to objects under glass, behind windows or under water, since shiny surfaces give off reflections and glare which makes it very difficult to see what is behind them. It is usually impossible for me to recognize people in cars or see if they are waving at me, sometimes even at close quarters, because of the destructive reflections from the windows. Where the colour-normal can make use of the continuity of the hues of an object to perceive the figure through disturbing reflections, I see the reflections *and* the objects behind them translated into different shades of grey, and only when the contrast between the object and its background is very high, or the movements are very distinct, can I see what is behind a strongly reflecting surface as an object. Wearing polarizing clip-on sun-glasses improves things to some extent, and I use them much, although I am often distracted by the mottled *stress*-patterns in some kinds of glass, patterns that are normally invisible.

When I was about 14 I discovered, quite by accident, the use of coloured filters for analyzing and identifying different hues. We had a large salad bowl made of transparent, red-coloured plastic. One day, when holding the bowl before my eyes, I noticed that the pattern of the table-cloth turned nearly white when seen through the bowl. By moving the bowl to and fro, I could make the red-coloured pattern change from light to dark. I was intrigued by my discovery and tried out several other transparent filters of various colours, thinking that I would be able to solve the problem of my colour-blindness by using a few differently coloured pieces of plastic to analyze and thus be able to name any colour. From a purely practical point of view I contemplated the great advantage of being able to determine for myself the name of any hue without having to ask other people. I even envisaged a solution of narrow strips of filters mounted at the upper edge behind the lenses of my glasses, thus dispensing with a set of hand-held filters, and making their use more discreet.

Nothing, however, came out of these ideas of mine as I did not have the resources at my disposal for carrying them through. I have since learned that such filters for analyzing hues are actually made for 'normal' (i.e. anomalous trichromat and dichromat) colour-blind electronic engineers to aid them in reading the colour-coded rings denoting the values of resistors. I have tried, but never succeeded in, obtaining such a set of filters, though the spectral transmission bands of these filters would probably not suit the spectral sensitivity of my rods too well.

Traffic-lights can sometimes pose a problem to me. I have long since learned that *red* is the top light, *amber* is the middle light and *green* is at the bottom. At night, in the evening or in the day, when the traffic-lights are in a shadow, I have no problem in detecting which aspect is shown: by noting its position I can be a law-abiding cyclist or pedestrian. In full sun-light, on the other hand, determining which aspect is shown can be quite impossible; if the traffic-lights are back-lit I am dazzled by the sun and cannot see the weak lights; if the sun is behind me, the reflections in the lenses of the light signals can be so strong that it is impossible to determine which one is showing. In such situations I have to watch the traffic, following the other pedestrians when they cross the street. This can lead to dangerous situations when encountering unexpected cars if I follow someone crossing a street against a red light, believing that the crossing is safe.

I visit art galleries and I am very interested in the visual arts. Looking at paintings I can appreciate form, composition and technique, though of course, I cannot appreciate the colour aspects. Monochrome prints and graphic art I can normally enjoy in the same way as the colour-normal and the same goes for sculpture and architecture. When lecturing on vision and perception I frequently show transparencies with works of art to demonstrate my points.

When painting the house or redecorating I must always make sure that I use the correct colours by carefully reading the labels on the paint tins. My wife normally selects the colours for the house. If the contrast between the new and old colour in terms of grey-tones is not too small, I have no problem painting the house. If I repaint with the same colour, I sometimes have a problem telling the freshly painted areas from the unpainted ones, especially after a break when the fresh paint no longer looks 'wet'. If I repaint with a different colour that is very close to the old one in terms of grey-contrast, I have difficulties in seeing if the new coat covers the old colour properly. Sometimes the only way to resolve this problem is either to paint very systematically, or to look obliquely at the wall for the shiny 'wet' freshly painted parts.

When buying clothes on my own I will only take advice from a sales-person in whom I have high confidence, otherwise I usually ask for 'safe' or neutral colours; white shirts, grey trousers, black socks and shoes: thus, I would never select a tie by myself. For the important colour-choices I have to rely on my wife or on close friends whom I trust and who know my tastes and preferences. To avoid embarrassment I often have to mark my socks in some way so that I will not mix up differently coloured pairs, it can be impossible for me to tell light blue, beige and light grey, or dark blue and black socks apart.

Picking berries has always been a big problem. I often have to grope around among the leaves with my fingers, feeling for the berries by their shape, except in the shade or in the evenings when light levels are low. Then I can usually see the berries; the red ones as small 'black' spheres among the 'grey' leaves. The only berries I can easily see in bright sun-light are the white 'snow-ball' berries of the Guelder-rose bush (*Symphoricarpus rivularis*).

Indoors most flowers are easy for me to discern, out-of-doors, though, I usually only recognize the white and the yellow ones. the oxeye-daisies, not to speak of the dandelions in my lawn, are most conspicuous to me; red roses on bushes I see best in the twilight when I can separate the 'black' flowers from the 'grey' leaves.

Colours are frequently used to code or to highlight information. For me this usually makes matters worse because good colour contrast very often does not transform into good grey-contrast. Sometimes the contrast is so low that the information is next to lost. Black print on red price labels, yellow print on a light blue background, dark green on a bright red background are all extremely difficult for me to read. A teaching aid that has always failed with me is the use of colours, e.g. in arithmetic; adding the red and the green objects, subtracting the blue ones from the yellow ones. Colourful *Venn diagrams* for teaching basic set theory only makes the task more difficult for me. Colour coding of e.g. underground lines maps will often make them more confusing.

8.3.2 Hypersensitivity to light

As far as can be determined, the retinae of my eyes do not contain any cone-receptors at all, only rod-receptors; or cones are present but in such reduced numbers that they do not contribute to the visual process in any measurable amount (see Sharpe and Nordby, The photoreceptors in the achromat, Chapter 10). Since the rods are much more sensitive to light and also saturate at lower light intensities than the cones, my visual system is well adapted for vision only under low light conditions. In fact, my vision will not function at all in very bright light (e.g. out-of-doors in full day-light) if I do not adopt specialized visual behaviour and strategies.

I am easily dazzled and, in effect, blinded if exposed to bright light. If I open my eyes fully for more than one or two seconds under such conditions (about 1000 scotopic trolands and up), the scene I am gazing at is quickly washed out, it turns into a bright haze and all structured vision is lost. It can be very distressing for me, and sometimes even painful, to perform demanding visual tasks in very bright light.

This *hypersensitivity to light*, or *light aversion*, is often referred to as *photophobia*, but has nothing to do with the irrational psychodynamic 'phobias'. In fact, I really enjoy being out in the warm sun, provided I don't have to perform exacting visual tasks. I do not like to read or write in the sun; digging the garden or mowing the lawn, on the other hand, is no problem for me even in bright sun-light.

My main problem, then, is to restrict the intensity of the light entering my eyes. This, as I will show, can be achieved in several ways and I tend to use them all, alone or in combination, according to what the situation demands. In common with nearly all the other achromats I have interviewed, I have developed special visual strategies for restricting the amount of light entering my eyes.

The most obvious strategy is, of course, simply to avoid direct strong light. Staying indoors or in the shade is one way of achieving this if there is no special reason for being in intense sunshine (such as on a bright beach in the summer or in bright sun-lit snow in the winter). Indoors, whenever possible, I try to place myself with my back towards bright windows and strong light sources and avoid having direct sun-light falling on my work-place.

Shading my eyes from direct, intense light with my hand or a visor may be necessary. Ordinarily I wear sun-glasses, *in casu*, the lenses of my glasses are *photo-chromatic* (i.e. tinted lenses which darken in bright light). Out-of-doors I often wear an extra clip-on polarizing filter for cutting down on bright light and for dealing with visually destructive glare and reflections from shiny surfaces. The best sun filters I have tried, though, are the special coloured glasses which are made for the *retinitis pigmentosa* patients. They have a spectral cut-off at 550 nm, passing only the long wavelengths and they give a very pleasant light-attenuation, but they are socially less attractive because of their red appearance.

Actually, it is not only the brightness of what I am looking at that is most bothersome, but the brightness of the total visual field; the larger the part of the field that is illuminated, the more bothered I am. Blinkers or side-shields on the spectacle frame may help in shutting out unwanted light, but they also prevent motion detection in the peripheral visual field, which is important for moving safely about, and I don't use them. If I must see small detail in bright light, e.g. read printed information or look at a map in the bright sun, I turn away from the light, putting the material in my shadow.

The most typical visual strategies, though, that I resort to consists in *squinting*, i.e. partially closing the eyes and looking through the narrow slits formed by the eyelids, and in frequently *blinking* the eyes. This habit has been reported by nearly every author and seems to be universally resorted to by typical, complete achromats (see e.g. Bjerrum, 1904; Larsen, 1918; Krill, 1977). If light levels rise and my retinal illuminance approaches 1000 scotopic trolands, my fully constricted pupils cannot further contract and I have to squint to deal with the higher intensities and to avoid saturating the rods (see Fig. 8.3 above). At higher light intensities even this is not enough, and I also have to start blinking my eyes to shut out excessive light. My blinking is triggered when saturation sets in. The blinking frequency is slow at first, only once every four to five seconds, but the periodicity increases with increasing light intensity, to three to four blinks a second.

At lower light levels, when the blinking rate is slow, the blinks themselves are also rather brief. As light levels go up, the blinking rate also goes up, but the blinks become longer, i.e. the duty-cycle increases. At the very highest light levels where my visual system will function (e.g. new snow in bright sun-light) the blinks are so long that my eyes are, in effect, shut most of the time except for brief opening blinks once every two to three seconds. Whether blinking my eyes briefly at low light levels or extending the length of the blinks at high intensities, I still experience a visually stable world in which I can orientate myself and move about. It should be mentioned, though, that I am able to suppress the blinking on some occasions. In laboratory investigations I have actually sustained retinal luminances of more than 500000 photopic trolands, blinking my eyes only occasionally to keep my corneas moist.

This squinting and blinking behaviour is a strain socially. In bright light people immediately notice that something is wrong with my eyes, and show this by their reactions to me. As a child I was often approached by complete strangers who demanded to know what was wrong with my eyes. Wearing dark glasses or clip-on sun filters can alleviate this social burden to some extent.

At higher light levels the peripheral visual field is much more affected than the central part of the field, which results in a partial tunnel vision. I will still detect movement in the far periphery, but have much more difficulty in identifying what is moving and reacting adequately to it. This makes me move in a rather hesitant and stiff manner, sometimes bumping into people, and to be overcautious when moving about in agitated surroundings or when encountering unmarked steps and stairs. As soon as I am in the shade or in-doors, I again move in a much more relaxed and confident way.

It is very clear to me today that the most debilitating, handicapping and distressing consequence of the achromatopsia is my hypersensitivity to light and the resulting light aversion, which is reported by all other authors. This is also the unanimous verdict of all the achromats I have interviewed so far. The practical problems of being dazzled, the narrowing of the visual fields, resulting in restricted mobility, and the social problems of light aversion and of feeling clumsy in intense light is frequently reported by my informants as being more of a hindrance to them than not being able to experience hues or to discern minute detail.

8.3.3 Reduced visual acuity

In a retina where only rods function, visual acuity will be drastically reduced, since it is the densely packed foveal cones that are responsible for the high acuity of central vision in the normal retina. My visual acuity is 6/60 Snellen (i.e. 0.1 of normal acuity) which means that at a distance of 6 metres I can read those letters on the Snellen chart that people with normal acuity can read at 60 metres. This low acuity is common for all typical, complete achromats reported in the literature and for those I have interviewed. Measured with an interferometer under optimal conditions my acuity may improve to 6/50.

My visual acuity, though, may vary quite a bit depending on the illumination. At higher luminances my acuity very quickly deteriorates, but it may improve slightly at lower light intensities, such as at dusk after the sun has set, but before it gets really dark, or indoors with the curtains drawn during the day, or in the evening with not-too-strong incandescent, tungsten illumination. My best acuity seems to coincide with the illuminance levels at which I do not have to squint or blink my eyes.

I experience a visual world where things appear to me to be well-focused, have sharp and clearly defined boundaries and are not fuzzy or cloudy: I can easily tell the difference between what people with normal vision call a well-focused and a not so well-focused photograph. Once, when giving a talk to the Kenneth Craik Club in Cambridge, one of my slides came up slightly out of focus because of a thinner slide-mount, so I quickly refocused it myself, and Professor Fergus W. Campbell, who attended the talk, commented aloud that to his astonishment I did this as well as any projectionist. Details that are too small for the low resolution of my coarse retinal matrix will disappear, blending into the background, but when they are brought closer and become large enough for me to discern, they are just as sharp and well-defined as other objects.

I am *hypermetropic*, i.e. far-sighted, and the precise refractive power of my ophthalmic correction now is: OS (left eye) +7.74 D. SPH., −0.75 D. CYL. 10°; and, OD (right eye) +8.0 D. SPH., −1.0 D. CYL. 5°. This is rather fortunate since my lenses thus *magnify* the retinal image by a factor of 1.22; it would have been worse if I had been *myopic*, i.e. near-sighted, thus requiring minus-lenses. With my glasses I can read small print by bringing the text close up to my eyes; about 250 mm for 6 mm high letters, 150 mm away for 4.5 mm letters,

80 mm away for 3 mm letters. Letters smaller than 2 mm, as used e.g. in most telephone directories, I cannot read without additional optical magnification.

I use a small, folding, pocket magnifier for reading newspapers, magazines, books, typed documents, etc., even when the print is large enough to read with my glasses alone. My first pocket magnifier (see above) had a +9 diopter, 50 mm ∅ lens set in a transparent perspex frame, rivetted in one corner to a piece of leather. The lens could be folded up into the leather cover to protect it, when unfolded the leather cover served as a handle for holding the glass. Today I use a magnifier with a +16 diopter, 30 mm ∅, biconvex lens, which gives me the necessary magnification for reading large amounts of text without undue visual strain, and makes it possible for me to manage the very small print in telephone directories etc. When reading I usually hold the glass in my right hand, the book in my left, and I always use my dominant left eye. Together with my spectacles, this magnifier is the most important tool I have, and I always carry it with me.

I have, of course, tried many other different loupes, reading glasses and magnifiers of various designs offered by opticians, but they are usually either too large, too obtrusive, not pocketable, too weak or too powerful for my needs. The best design is one that I can easily carry in my shirt breast pocket and is always at hand, one that is small and easy to hold, but with sufficient power for reading small print, as that used in e.g. telephone directories.

I have considered other types of visual aids, such as video-systems etc., but they all seem to fail on one or several points. Usually they are too large and heavy to carry around, they are complicated in use or they are too powerful, giving a very small field of view which makes it rather hard to read continuous text. It is most important to me that I can always take the aid with me and use it wherever I go.

Seeing information at a distance, i.e. street names, destination boards on buses and trains, time-tables in stations, flight-departure indicators in airports, signs and labels in museums, price labels in shop windows etc., is usually impossible or, at best, very difficult. To use my magnifier to make the letters legible to me I have to get close to the material, but this is not possible when signs are placed high up on walls or poles, behind windows, in glass cases or behind barriers. One special problem is reading the destination boards on approaching buses which only stop on signal. Occasionally, as a last resort, I have had to stop every approaching bus until the right one came along, invoking the drivers' wrath and being showered with abuse for my pains.

It can be difficult to find my way in unknown surroundings, a problem when travelling and visiting strange places. I solve this by carrying with me a small, monocular, 8 power, close-focusing telescope, which I can conceal in my hand, and which I use for reading street names, destination signs and other information that I cannot reach. I also make preparations by studying maps and plans, and by inquiring for directions on how to find my way.

Much more serious, though, than the problem of finding my way in strange places, is my disability to identify people only from their facial features at a distance of more than a few metres. I may easily pass people I know well in the street without recognizing them, and those who do not know of my visual handicap may find me aloof or downright rude. Picking out people I know well in a crowd or in a large room, e.g. a restaurant or theatre, is very difficult and socially embarrassing. I usually recognize people from their total appearance, i.e. their clothes, their way of moving, prominent or special features; but first and foremost, from their voices. When expecting people I know well I can manage to identify them at 10–15 metres distance, and if I know what clothes they will be wearing I may even be able to identify them at distances of 20 metres and more. Often, though, I fail to recognize people I know, with embarrassing consequences. Sometimes even people who know about my visual handicap can be offended by my seemingly disinterest and neglect of them. The reason may be that I often, apparently, visually behave rather normally, leading them to believe that my disregard is intentional.

A problem that seemed more serious to me earlier than it does now is that I cannot hold a driver's licence. My brother and I cycle and we have ridden mopeds in Oslo. Driving a car, though, is not possible for us, although my brother actually took some driving lessons. He had to give up, though, after attempting to drive down a flight of steps in a park. Today, I only cycle when I have access to reserved cycle lanes or when traffic is very light.

In other fields, however, low visual acuity has not been an insurmountable obstacle. My sister has since her early teens done all kinds of needlework, producing *tatting*, *bobbin-lace* and *embroideries* to very high standards. To keep her hands free, she uses a clip-on, jeweller's loupe on her working glasses. This provides a high magnification of ×10, but a very small field of view, and is not very suitable for reading. She needs help in selecting the colours of the threads and yarns, but when they have been selected and labelled she manages on her own.

8.4 Closing remarks

From my account it can be seen that I often avoid showing my visual handicap and sometimes simulate normal vision. I often experience negative attitudes if I expose my visual disability before people get to know me. The stigma of being partially sighted can be very unpleasant. If I show my handicap to people who do not know me I will be categorized as a disabled person and will be treated in a patronizing way and often not taken seriously. If, on the other hand, I first expose my visual handicap to people after they get to know me, I get fewer such reactions. With most vision scientists and ophthalmologists I feel at ease, they can even be overcautious in avoiding to offend me, but some ophthalmologists have treated me in a condescending way they often reserve for patients.

In spite of my visual handicap and all the practical and social problems I encounter, I feel that I live a very rich and interesting life. It is my ambition that these very personal and rather private observations I have described here will prove to be of some value to vision researchers and to people dealing with typical, complete achromats.

Acknowledgements

I wish to thank my close friend Dr Lindsay 'Ted' Sharpe for his critical comments on the manuscript. Further I want to thank my friends and collaborators Bjørn Stabell and Ulf Stabell for many helpful suggestions, and last, but not least, my sister Britt Nordby for reviewing the manuscript and for setting me right where my memory had failed me.

9

Clinical aspects of achromatopsia

Egill Hansen

Achromatopsia is a unique and infrequent colour vision deficiency which has special clinical significance. In recent years it has been realized that cone pathology is often present in patients with low vision of obscure etiology. Cone dysfunction syndromes, is a term introduced by Goodman, Ripps & Siegel (1963) that comprises several forms. The typical total achromatopsia is the best known. This is a congenital, stationary condition which is specific to one retinal receptor system. Therefore it is of great physiological interest.

Despite the total lack of colour discrimination, this being the most extreme of the colour vision deficiencies, the condition is, however, often missed by clinicians. The explanation for this is that it is frequently combined with more serious symptoms. Furthermore, the patient himself may often be ignorant of his colour vision defect. The diagnosis is important for correct evaluation of the patient, and also for socio-medical counselling. Among 55 achromats registered in the Norwegian Registry of Blindness, 45% were partially sighted (visual acuity less than 0.3) and 55% were socially blind (visual acuity not better than 0.1). The incidence of achromatopsia in the population has variously been estimated to vary between 1:30000 and 1:100000. From the Norwegian material the calculated incidence is 1:80000.

9.1 Classification

Congenital achromatopsias may occur with and without amblyopia. The latter condition is extremely rare (Pitt (1944) estimated the incidence at 1:100000000). This form is termed cone monochromacy. A satisfactory explanation of cone monochromacy has not been advanced. It is probably a defect of post-receptoral nature (Weale, 1953). Visual acuity is normal and no nystagmus (i.e. rapid oscillations of the eyes) or photo-

Table 9.1. *The congenital colour vision defects*

Monochromacy	Cone monochromacy
	Rod monochromacy
	  Complete (typical) achromatopsia
	  Incomplete (atypical) achromatopsia
	    with protan luminosity
	    with deutan luminosity
	    blue cone monochromacy

Dichromacy	Protanopia (P) Deuteranopia (D) Tritanopia (T)

Anomalous trichromacy	Protanomaly (PA)
	  Extreme protanomaly (EPA)
	Deuteranomaly (DA)
	  Extreme deuteranomaly (EDA)
	Tritanomaly (TA)

phobia (i.e. aversion to intense light) is noticed. In three known cases ERG (electroretinography) was normal (Krill, 1968), supporting the notion of a more central defect in cone monochromacy. In support of this is also the presence of three cone mechanisms which could be shown in a patient with total achromatopsia following encephalitis (Mollon *et al.*, 1980).

Total achromatopsia in its usual form is combined with amblyopia. This is the typical achromatopsia, or rod monochromacy, with the classical findings: low visual acuity, photophobia and nystagmus. In most reports, the achromatopsia is complete with a total loss of colour discrimination. Exceptionally, unilateral cases have been described. An extensive survey of the congenital forms of achromatopsia is given by François, Verriest & De Rouck (1955) and detailed laboratory investigations are outlined in Chapters 10 and 11.

Many reports of incomplete forms of achromatopsia have appeared in the literature, especially during recent years. Blue cone monochromacy is an example of an incomplete form (the term was introduced by Blackwell & Blackwell (1957) to describe the condition with functioning blue cones in addition to the rod receptors). The incomplete forms have been called atypical achromatopsia, in contrast to the complete form, the typical achromatopsia or the typical total colour blindness. Different types of incomplete achromatopsia have been described by Jaeger (1953), François *et al.* (1955) and Crone (1956). Smith & Pokorny (1980) demonstrated an autosomal recessive form with protan luminosity function (see Fig. 9.1) as well as a form with deutan luminosity function.

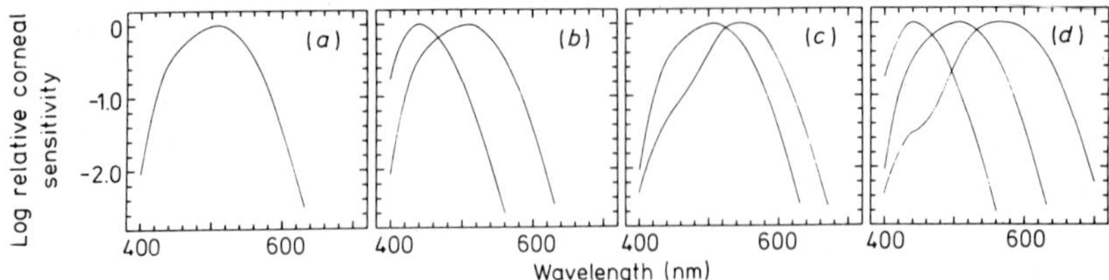

Fig. 9.1. Postulated spectral sensitivities of the visual photopigments for different classes of achromatopsia. (*a*) Complete achromatopsia; (*b*) X-chromosomal linked recessive incomplete achromatopsia (blue cone monochromacy); (*c*) autosomal recessive incomplete achromatopsia with protan luminosity; (*d*) autosomal recessive achromatopsia with deutan luminosity. (From: Smith, V. C. & Pokorny, J. (1980), with permission from Adam Hilger.)

Fig. 9.1 shows the luminosity functions postulated for typical and atypical forms of achromatopsia. The classification of congenital colour vision deficiencies is shown in Table 9.1.

Loss of discrimination and shortening of the red end of the spectrum (i.e. scotopization of vision) which commonly occurs in type I of acquired colour vision defects may result in a total achromatopsia. However, this form of achromatopsia is not included in this chapter, nor are the different types of progressive cone dystrophies.

9.2 Heredity

The reports of cone monochromacy suggest an autosomal, recessive inheritance. Also rod monochromacy is inherited as an autosomal, recessive trait. There may be an accumulation of cases in certain areas (Holm & Lodberg, 1940; Nordstrøm & Polland, 1980). Quite commonly, other cases are known to occur in the same family and, not infrequently, there is consanguinity between the parents. Among the registered 55 cases in the Norwegian material, 56% occurred in families with other known cases; and in 24% of the cases the parents were related.

Different forms of inheritance were reported in the incomplete forms. These defects can be inherited either as an X-linked recessive trait, as in the blue cone monochromacy, or as an autosomal recessive trait. The blue cone monochromacy is generally regarded as a stable, nonprogressive, developmental anomaly, affecting the red and green cone functions. A black child with this disorder was reported by Fleischman & O'Donnell (1981) as a slowly, progressive abiotrophy. Also, in reports by Blackwell & Blackwell (1961) and Feiock, Maumenee & Sloan (1977), it is suggested that X-linked achromatopsia is a slowly, progressive abiotrophy, which, possibly, can evolve into complete achromatopsia. Two clinically distinct types of incomplete achromatopsia, one with protan and one with deutan luminosity function, are inherited as an autosomal recessive trait.

Franceschetti *et al.* (1958) suggested that both typical, complete and incomplete achromatopsia may be different expressions of the same gene. Or they may be multiple allelism with regard to genes causing achromatopsia, with dominance of the complete form over the incomplete form. The results of Nordstrøm & Polland (1980) support the theory that complete and incomplete achromatopsia are different expressions of the same autosomal, recessive gene.

9.3 Associated somatic defects

Achromatopsia typically occurs as a solitary defect. In the literature some few concomitant defects have been reported, however, without proved connections (François *et al.*, 1955). Some patients have hearing defects (Jan *et al.*, 1976: Ferguson & MacGregor, 1949). Hearing defects may also be combined with arterial hypertension.

Among our patients, one patient had a slight cerebral palsy, while unilateral hearing defects were found in another patient. Congenital dysplasia of the hip joint occurred in one patient, and also in two of her normally sighted siblings. One blue cone monochromat had erythroblastosis at birth. His maternal grandfather and granduncle were both protanopic.

9.4 Natural history

Achromatopsia may be recognized at an early age. It becomes apparent by light aversion (photophobia), unsteady fixation and nystagmus. In families or in areas where people are familiar with this condition, it may be recognized in the infant. However, it is only at a later stage, when colour vision tests can be performed, that the condition is usually identified and can be properly diagnosed.

Due to rod saturation and lack of inhibition from cones, as a fundamental defect, the patient exhibits light aversion, or photophobia, under moderate and bright light intensities. This is a main symptom and is present in most cases. It is noticed by the patient's tendency to avoid bright light, especially sunlight (see Chapter 11 for detailed analysis of photopic function). The patient compensates by blinking or partially shutting the eyes. The complaint is chiefly one of dazzling, though usually not associated with pain. The patient prefers twilight, where he may function as well as normals (see Chapters 10 and 11 for detailed evaluation of scotopic function). This preference for faint light to good illumination is hard for other people to understand, and is often difficult for the patient to explain satisfactorily to others. Therefore some patients prefer to ignore or explain away this peculiarity. This symptom, therefore, may sometimes be concealed.

Likewise, the other fundamental defect, the lack of colour discrimination, may be even less evident. Many colour-blind persons learn to associate colours with objects and, apparently, they may function satisfactorily in many situations, even when colour choices are necessary. Therefore it might not be obvious to connect their visual problems with a total colour-blindness. In many cases uncertainty and misunderstandings may arise due to colour confusions. In some instances children will function inadequately in school, and a mental retardation is sometimes suspected. Typically, red is confused with black, and the brightest colours are chosen in the green range of the paint-box. Sometimes this may appear as a characteristic feature in the childrens' paintings. However, the patients' difficulties may be disguised, as they try to get their school-fellows to pick out the right colours for them.

Paradoxically, in some instances the achromats may actually do better than colour-normals in seeing faint smudges or stains in clothes, or in seeing slight differences between colours of the same hue, while in other instances, obvious confusions are made, such as knitting with an incorrectly coloured yarn.

Nystagmus is present in nearly all achromats (see appendix to Chapter 10 for more details), and can be observed from an early age. It is typically of the pendular or ocular type, as in albinism, and is commonly of the conjugate form and in the horizontal direction. The nystagmus is often rapid. It is also generally more pronounced in bright light, while it is reduced, and may even disappear, in the darkness. Nystagmus is also dependent on fixation. As a rule, it is less marked and has a higher frequency when the eye is fixating (François *et al.*, 1955), but the contrary may also be seen. Nystagmus may differ very much in severity. It is generally observed that the nystagmus tends to diminish with age, and will often disappear.

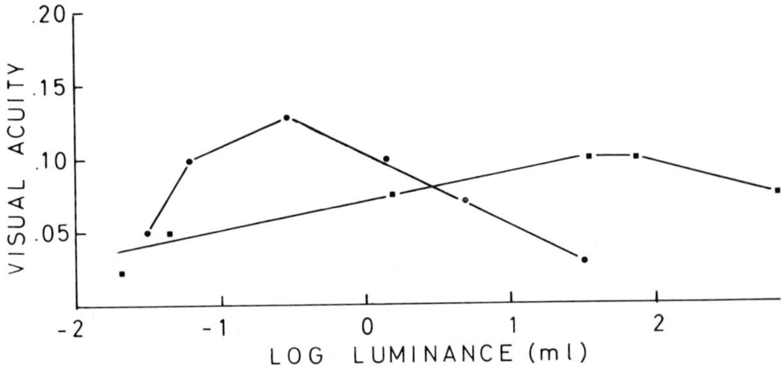

Fig. 9.2. The variation of visual acuity with the room illumination in two complete achromats, redrawn from Sloan & Feiock (1972). Notice that the visual acuity in both observers is reduced in high illumination. In one observer, the optimal illumination acuity is very low. (After: Sloan, L. L. & Feiock, K., 1972.)

9.5 Clinical findings

Visual acuity is reduced in the typical, total achromat as well as in the incomplete forms. Values about 0.1 (6/60 or 20/200) are typical. A somewhat better visual acuity is usually found in the incomplete forms than in the total achromats. Their performance, in general, is markedly worse with illuminated screen tests of the transparency type than with printed test charts. Improvement of visual acuity can be demonstrated both in the complete, as well as in the incomplete, forms when illumination levels are reduced (Sloan & Feiock, 1972; see Fig. 9.2). Fig. 9.2 shows the variation in visual acuity with room illumination for two achromats. Optimal values are defined individually. The refraction does not differ significantly from other groups. However, myopia is often reported to be combined with the X-linked recessive form. A regular astigmatism is a common finding in achromats (François *et al.*, 1955).

Visual fields may be normal or slightly constricted. Sometimes a central scotoma can be demonstrated, but this may be masked by the nystagmus. Tube vision in bright light was reported by Crone (1965) in an incomplete achromat, who also could see colours under the same conditions. In reduced illumination, however, enlargement of the visual fields was recorded; at the same time reduction of visual acuity and disappearance of the colour vision occurred in this patient (see Fig. 9.3). The variation in visual field size with illumination is shown in Fig. 9.3 for an incomplete and a typical achromat, compared with a normal trichromat.

The same feature was seen in one of our achromats who exhibited

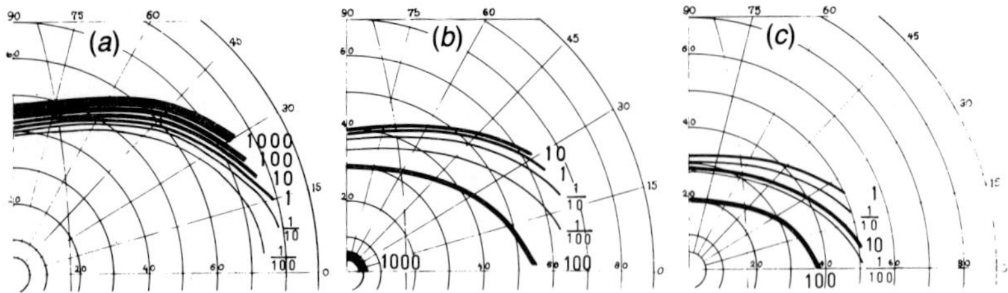

Fig. 9.3. Change in visual field size with illumination: (*a*) in a normal trichromat; (*b*) in an incomplete achromat, and (*c*) in a typical achromat. Characteristically, the largest visual field is registered in the highest illumination in the normal observer, while the opposite is true for the two achromats. The largest field for the typical achromat was registered in a 1 lux background illumination. The figure is reconstructed from Crone (1965), and is based on data from the upper temporal meridian (right eye), using the same object size (16 mm^2) under constant contrast (150%). The numbers indicate the lux values of the background. (After: Crone, R. A., 1965.)

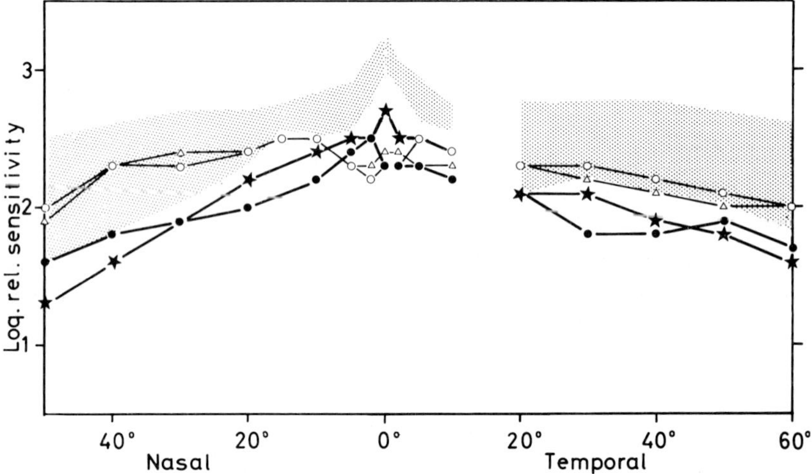

Fig. 9.4. The sensitivity to light increment thresholds measured across the visual field by static perimetry. Perimetric profiles of two typical achromats (open symbols) and two blue cone monochromats (filled symbols) were obtained with the Goldman perimeter in white background light (10 cd/m^2) along the horizontal meridian. Angular diameter of target was 54′. Shaded area indicates the normal variation (mean ± 2 SD). (From: Hansen, E. (1979), with permission from *Acta Ophthalmologica*.)

extreme tube vision in bright light, though, without any improvement in colour vision. While perimetry in reduced illumination reveals visual field defects more easily in a number of eye diseases, the reverse pattern is seen in achromats of the typical and total form, who actually perform better in reduced illumination (Crone, 1965; Krastel *et al.*, 1981*b*). In automatic perimeters of the Octopus type, a normal threshold sensitivity

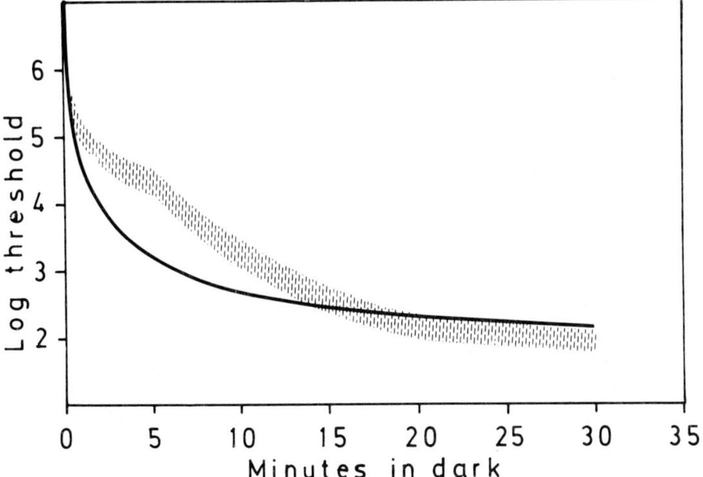

Fig. 9.5. Dark-adaptation curve of a typical, total achromat, showing a monophasic course, obtained in the Goldman-Weekers adaptometer. A great increase in sensitivity is seen during the first 5 minutes. The shaded area indicates the mean normal level.

is registered in typical and atypical achromats in the peripheral field. A relative central scotoma can be demonstrated in some cases. By static perimetry the curves are characteristically deflected and irregular in the central part (see Fig. 9.4). Fig. 9.4 shows the perimetric profiles of two typical achromats and two blue cone monochromats under standard conditions.

Dark-adaptation is generally good (see Chapter 10 for detailed evaluation of bleaching adaptation). Typically there is a monophasic curve with a rapid drop during the first minutes, as shown in Fig. 9.5. Biphasic and polyphasic curves have also been described. There may be an elevated first part of the curve as well as other variants (François *et al.*, 1955; Goodman *et al.*, 1963). Immediately after extinction of a bright light, the typical achromat may show fast recovery of light sensitivity, which may be even better than in normals (Hansen, Seim & Olsen, 1978). This could be because of either the lack of inhibitory impulses from the cone system, or incomplete light adaptation due to photophobia. It is in accordance with the practical experience of some achromats, who have noticed a greater ability to regain their visual capacity compared to other people when entering dark rooms from bright light.

The *fundus picture* is usually normal, but may show a variety of lesions, none of which can be considered pathonomonic of the condition (Goodman *et al.*, 1963). A weak foveal reflex, accompanied by slight

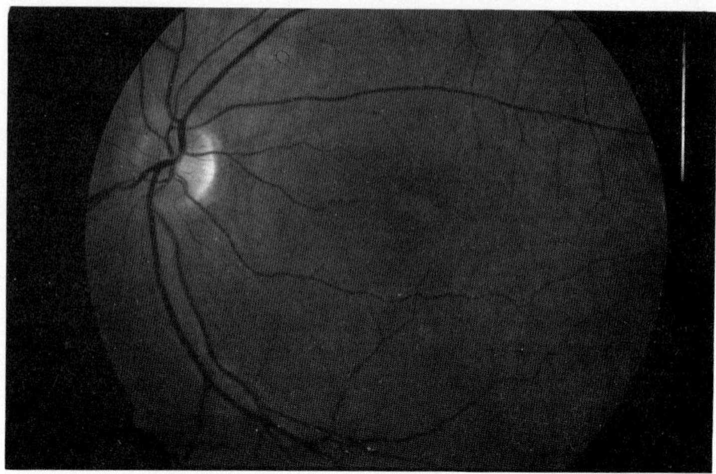

Fig. 9.6. Fundus photograph of a typical achromat showing slight irregular pigmentation in the macula. The optic disc and the vessels have a normal appearance.

pigmentary irregularities, is not infrequently observed (Sloan, 1954; François *et al.*, 1955). Slight temporal pallor of the optic disc is described in some patients, while the typical finding is normal disc colour. As opposed to the common finding of attenuated retinal vessels in progressive cone dystrophy, normal retinal vessels are found in congenital achromatopsia, which is seen in the fundus photograph of a typical achromat shown in Fig. 9.6.

The *choroidal circulation*, as recorded by the corneal identation pulse amplitudes (dynamic tonometry), has been found to be normal in a series of typical achromats (which is contrary to the typical finding of low amplitudes in the pigmentary rod dystrophies) as well as in some cases of progressive cone dystrophy (Hansen, Frøyshov Larsen & Berg, 1976).

9.6 Electrophysiological examinations

Electrooculography (EOG) and visual evoked response (VER) has been reported to be normal (see also Chapter 10). Electroretinography (ERG) shows significant changes. The photopic ERG is extinguished, while a normal scotopic ERG can be recorded. The photopic ERG response is shown as a minimal (or absent) single flash response, or may be demonstrated as a very low flicker fusion frequency, usually below

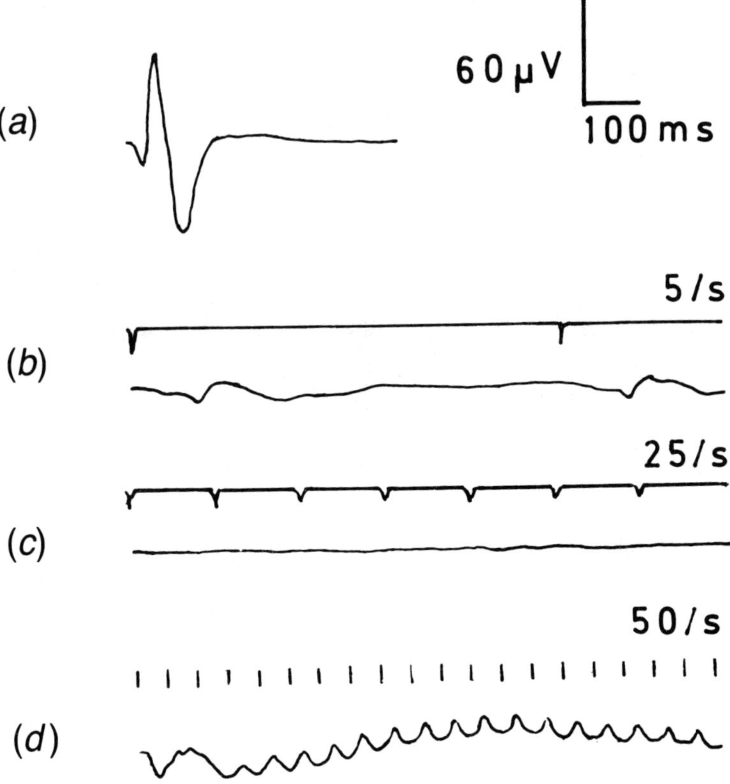

Fig. 9.7. ERG registered in a typical achromat under different conditions. (*a*) An ERG of normal appearance is obtained under scotopic conditions. (*b*) Likewise, an ERG is obtained at slow flicker stimulation of 5 cycles per second. (*c*) No ERG response, however, is obtained at a flicker frequency of 25 cycles per second in the achromat, while (*d*) a flicker response at 50 cycles per second is easily registered in the normal observer.

25 Hz (see Fig. 9.7). Fig. 9.7 demonstrates the ERG response of a typical achromat under different conditions. The fusion frequency becomes lower as the stimulus intensity increases (Krill, 1968). ERG is similar in the complete and the incomplete types of rod monochromacy. In cone monochromacy the photopic ERG-response pattern has been found to be normal or subnormal.

9.7 Colour vision tests

The pseudo-isochromatic type test charts clearly demonstrate the lack of colour discrimination in the typical and atypical achromats to most charts. Apparently, as a paradox, some of the test charts may also be

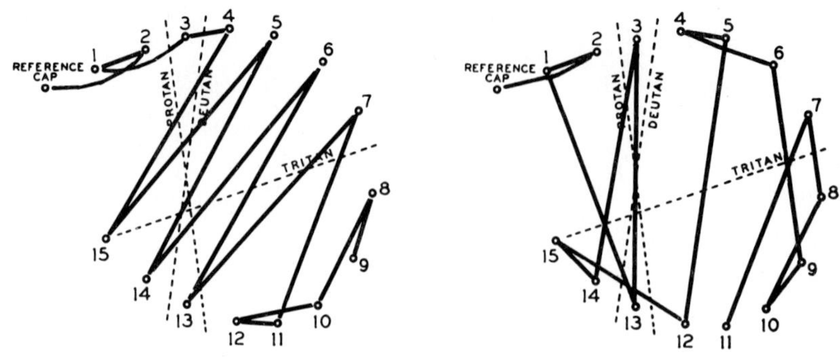

Fig. 9.8. The performance with the Farnsworth D-15 test of a typical achromat (left) and of a blue cone monochromat (right). The coloured caps were arranged along a scotopic axis by the typical achromat, while the blue cone monochromat mode irregular arrangements along a red – green axis. The normal sequence of the caps is in accordance with the numbers indicated.

seen by the achromats, which is due to the tests being designed to diagnose the colour vision defects of persons with a photopic luminosity function and not a scotopic one.

The arrangement tests, especially the Farnsworth Panel D-15 test, show grave confusions of colours and are also easy to use. Characteristically, the FD-15 test shows confusions along a scotopic axis. Very high error scores are obtained with the Farnsworth–Munsell 100 Hue test, usually showing an irregular pattern. The incomplete achromats may show a more distinct pattern and other confusion axes on the FD-15 test. Fig. 9.8 shows a typical scotopic pattern on the FD-15 test for a total achromat (left) and confusions along a red–green axis for a blue cone monochromat (right). With confrontation tests, such as the Holmgren wool skein test and the colour lantern tests, being administered in a way to eliminate the brightness contrast, a complete loss of colour discrimination can be demonstrated. Also the Sloan achromatopsia test (Sloan, 1954) demonstrates the total lack of hue discrimination in typical achromats. Here a set of greatly saturated pigment colours are matched by the achromat to a series of grey values. In incomplete achromats a perfect match with the grey scale may or may not be obtained. In addition this test demonstrates in an easy way the characteristic spectral sensitivity of scotopic vision (see Fig. 9.9). Fig. 9.9 shows the perfect matches of different colours with a grey scale as performed by a typical achromat (see Hess *et al.*, 1989*b*, for atypical achromatopsia).

Tissue paper contrast tests are generally not well suited for demonstrating colour defects in achromats because of a false clue introduced

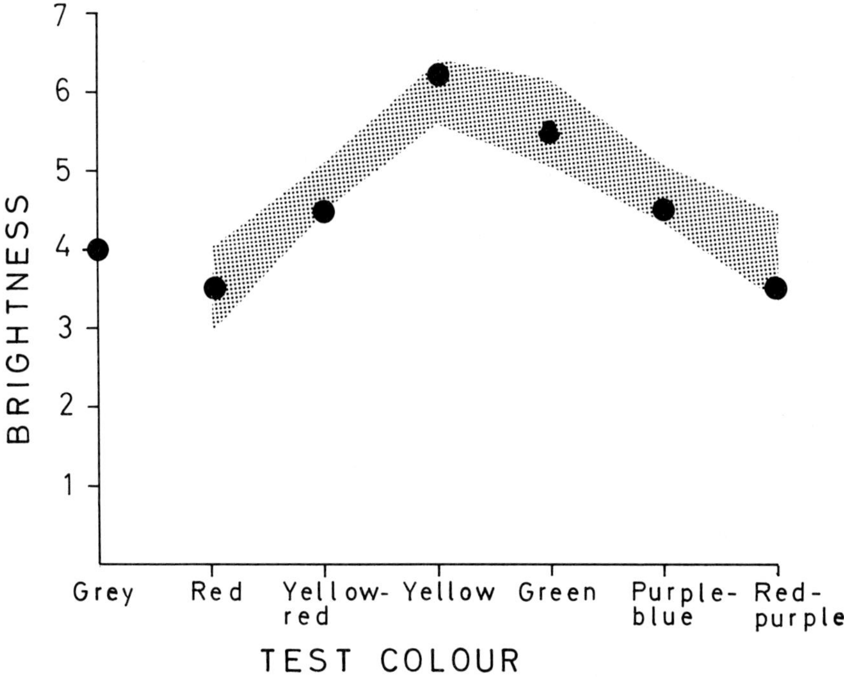

Fig. 9.9. Performance with the Sloan achromatopsia test of a typical achromat. A selection of pigment colours can be perfectly matched with shades of greys by the typical achromat, reflecting the scotopic luminosity function. The shaded area indicates the range (mean ± 1 SD) of 9 achromats according to Sloan (1954). The performance of one achromatic patient is indicated by filled circles. In persons with preserved colour discrimination no matches can be obtained.

with their special luminosity function. Therefore charts with green, blue and yellow backgrounds may be seen by the achromats and hence can not be used for diagnosis. However, the achromats typically miss the red background chart (Hansen, 1976).

Colour matching performed in anomaloscope examination shows a peculiar set of matches. The yellow field is matched with a mixture of red and green in all combinations all over the long wavelength spectral range as can be demonstrated by the Rayleigh equation ($\lambda_{546\,\text{nm}} + \lambda_{670\,\text{nm}} = \lambda_{589\,\text{nm}}$) in the same way as for protanopes and deuteranopes (see Fig. 9.10). Characteristic matching patterns made in the Nagel anomaloscope are shown in Fig. 9.10 (left panel) for protanopes, deuteranopes and normal trichromats, where also the matches made by typical and atypical achromats are shown, the latter displaying a totally different pattern. However, to the achromat, the green light appears to be very

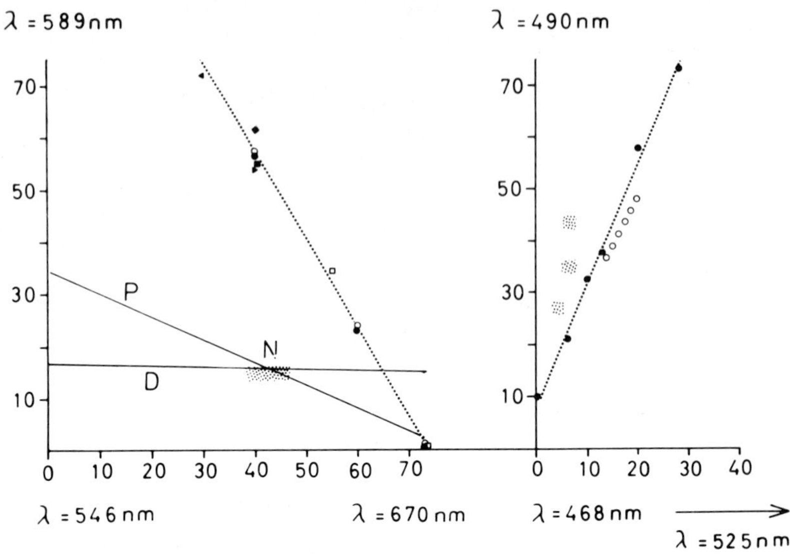

Fig. 9.10. Colour matches made with the Nagel type II anomaloscope by typical achromats (filled symbols) and blue cone monochromats (open symbols). The *left panel* shows the standard Rayleigh equation: Here a mixture of red ($\lambda_{670\,\mathrm{nm}}$) and green ($\lambda_{546\,\mathrm{nm}}$) is matched to monochromatic yellow ($\lambda_{589\,\mathrm{nm}}$). The mixture values are indicated on the abscissa and the brightness values are indicated along the ordinate. Both types of colour vision deficiencies show the same kind of response, i.e. a true monochromacy in this spectral region. The shaded areas indicate the limited range of accepted typical matches by normal observers, and the lines P and D indicate the average match values from protanopes and deuteranopes, respectively. Also shown (*right panel*) is the cyan blue equation ($\lambda_{468\,\mathrm{nm}} + \lambda_{525\,\mathrm{nm}} = \lambda_{490\,\mathrm{nm}}$) demonstrating a true monochromacy in the typical achromats, as matches (filled circles) are accepted all along the dotted line, while matches are accepted only within a limited region by a blue cone monochromat (indicated by open circles), demonstrating a dichromatic response type in this spectral region. Shaded areas indicate normal matches.

bright and, as a rule, can not be matched with any yellow value, which appears too dark. Furthermore, the red light is seen to be very dark and is matched with a nearly extinguished yellow light. The spectrum is shortened in the long-wavelength end, as for the protanopes, but to an even greater extent. In Fig. 9.10 (right panel) only matches within a limited range are shown for a blue cone monochromat (open circles), demonstrating a dichromatic pattern in this spectral region.

9.8 Tests for incomplete achromatopsia

1. The Nagel type II anomaloscope may be used over a wider spectral range than the type I anomaloscope, including also the short wavelength part. In some blue cone monochromats a dichromacy can be shown (see Fig. 9.10). Colour vision in those patients is supposed to be mediated by normal short-wavelength sensitive cones and cone photoreceptors filled with rhodopsin (Alpern *et al.*, 1971). Another possibility is that some residual colour sensation can be achieved by a comparison of rod and blue cone signals (see Hess *et al.*, 1989*a*, *b*).

2. Spectral sensitivity measurements under high and low photopic levels may show a change in the luminosity function in incomplete achromats. While the rod sensitivity function dominates under moderate light adaptation, a *reversed* Purkinje phenomenon can be seen in blue cone monochromats in bright illumination, i.e. there is a displacement of the peak sensitivity towards shorter wavelengths. In some atypical achromats maximum sensitivity is displaced to the normal photopic maximum in bright illumination – i.e. a *Purkinje shift* (Smith & Pokorny, 1980). Under certain conditions, such as selective chromatic adaptation, the response of colour receptors may be recorded – even in cases where colour vision is rudimentary. Fig. 9.11 shows the blue cone response in an incomplete achromat during adaptation to a green background, which brings forward the blue cone response. With a white background this patient only had a rod response luminosity function.

3. In some patients with rudimentary cone function the cone impulses may be so weak that their colour perception can be shown only with very large stimulus fields. By presenting large stimuli during chromatic adaptation cone response patterns can be demonstrated in some patients who originally may have been classified as total achromats (Krastel, Jaeger & Blankenagel, 1981*a*; see Fig. 9.12). Fig. 9.12 shows the effect of selective chromatic adaptations, using very large, coloured stimuli. The patient, originally diagnosed as a typical achromat, now also demonstrates a red cone response. These cases present a 'crypto-incomplete' variation of achromatopsia. Like the manifest, incomplete achromatopsia, the 'crypto-incomplete' achromatopsia may occur among siblings with complete achromatopsia (Jaeger & Krastel, 1983).

(Also, in some forms (see also Hess *et al.*, 1989*a*) of so-called blue cone monochromacy, there is evidence for residual red cone function which can only be revealed under conditions of chromatic adaptation.)

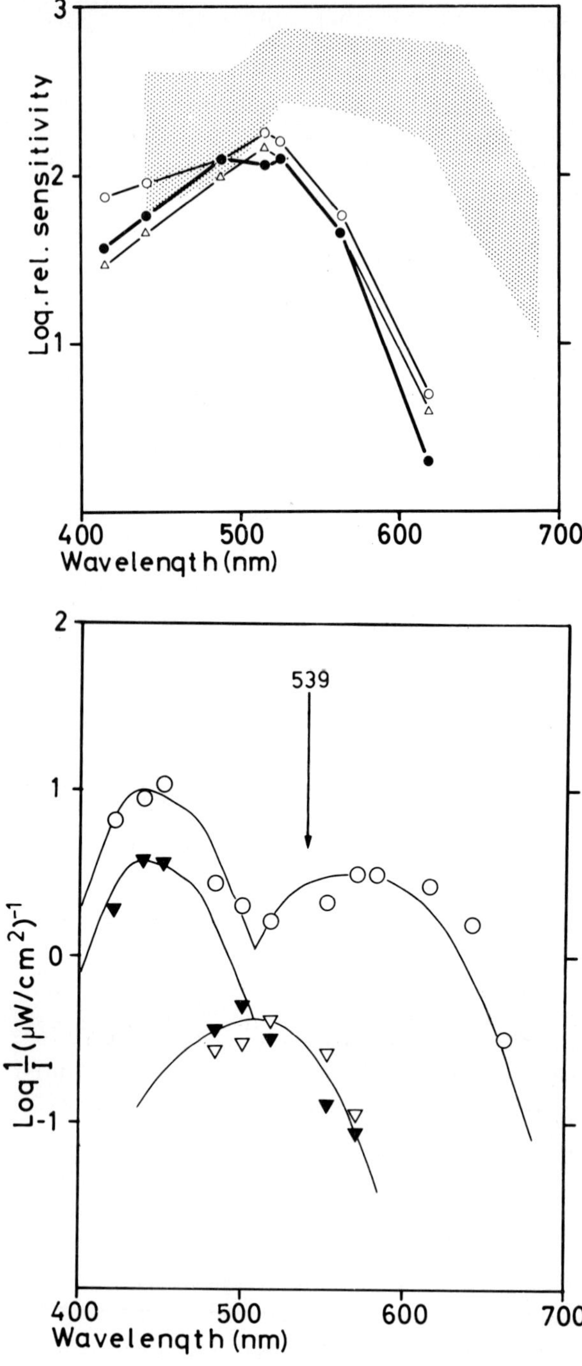
3
2
1
Log. rel. sensitivity
400
500
600
700
Wavelength (nm)
2
1
0
-1
539
Log $\frac{1}{I}$ ($\mu W/cm^2$)$^{-1}$
400
500
600
700
Wavelength (nm)

9.9 Diagnosis

Lack of awareness of the clinical manifestations of achromatopsia has resulted in frequent misdiagnoses. Some cases have been diagnosed as optic atrophy, macular degeneration, cerebral pathology or albinism. Especially the incomplete, uniform form of albinism or ocular albinism may easily be confused with achromatopsia (Krill, 1965). In some instances suspicion of cerebral pathology has led to cumbersome and extensive examinations for the patient. Hysteria has been suspected in some cases.

Congenital nystagmus, or unexplained amblyopia, may easily be misdiagnosed in cases of achromatopsia (Goodman *et al.*, 1963). This was experienced in our material. Here a large percentage of the patients were originally registered under the diagnosis of congenital nystagmus or congenital amblyopia. Photophobia in small children may justify the suspicion of congenital glaucoma. The diagnosis of achromatopsia is based on the colour vision tests, where the typical feature is the perception of red as a very dark quality, and where a characteristic scotopic luminosity pattern is revealed (see Figs 9.8 and 9.9). Such findings in a patient with normal dark-adaptation and normal visual fields, low vision and photophobia (with otherwise normal findings) is highly suspicious of total achromatopsia. Verification with ERG should be done in suspected cases in children.

A difficult differential diagnosis of the progressive cone dystrophies can arise in cases with a very slow progression of the dystrophic process (Neuhann, Krasbel & Jaeger, 1978). The functional disturbances, diminution of visual acuity, deterioration of colour sense and the appearance of central scotoma, may precede any visible fundus changes by years.

Smith & Pokorny (1980) evaluated the differences between the cone

Fig. 9.11. *Upper panel.* Spectral sensitivity of a blue cone monochromat (filled symbols) and of typical achromats (open symbols) obtained under neutral adaptation conditions. For both types of deficiency the response curves are close to the scotopic luminosity curve ($V'\lambda$) when registered against a neutral white background of low luminance (10 cd/m^2). *Lower panel.* When registered against a bright monochromatic green surface (λ_{max} = 539 nm, 73 cd/m^2), the typical achromat still demonstrates a pure rod luminosity function (open triangles), while the blue cone monochromat responds according to a combined function of the rod and the blue cone mechanisms (filled triangles). The normal response is indicated by the shaded area in the upper panel and by open circles in the lower panel. (From: Hansen, E. (1979), with permission from *Acta Ophthalmologica*.)

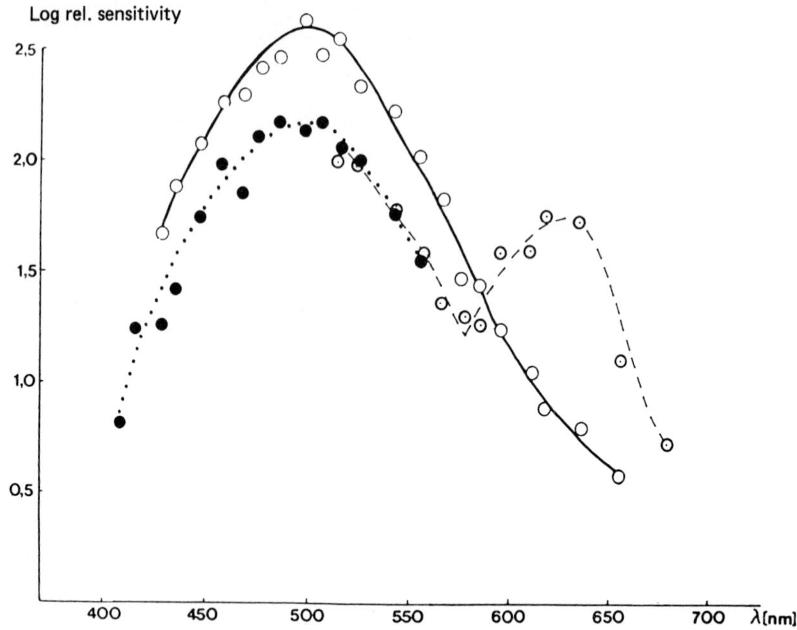

Fig. 9.12. Spectral sensitivity obtained by use of large stimuli lights (120°) under different chromatic adaptation in a patient originally diagnosed as a typical achromat. Filled circles, dotted line: yellow background (Schott OG 515). Open circles, full line: purple background (Schott KV-Magenta). Dotted circles, stippled line: blue-green background (Schott BG 18). Equal energy spectrum. Adaptation: yellow 71 fL, purple 53,5 fL, blue-green 70 fL. The curves are fitted by eye. (From: Krastel, H. *et al.* (1981*b*), with permission of J. F. Bergmann Verlag.)

degeneration and the cone–rod dystrophy versus the congenital forms of achromatopsia. The question as to whether low vision in a child reflects an achromatopsia or a progressive cone or cone–rod dystrophy may be a difficult one. Here specialised psychophysical testing of colour vision may be useful.

Scotopization of vision, which commonly develops in the severe forms of acquired colour vision defects type I, is seen in a number of cases with severe ocular pathology. This type of acquired colour vision defect may be difficult to distinguish from the congenital form.

The subdiagnosis of complete and incomplete forms of congenital achromatopsia may be difficult. Spectral sensitivity curves, obtained during different adaptation conditions, and the use of large-field stimuli could be necessary for a correct classification.

9.10 Visual habilitation

In addition to low vision, photophobia constitutes a definite handicap (see also Chapter 8 for a personal account of disability). However, if bright light can be avoided, the patient functions very well. Occupations requiring a good visual acuity, especially for distance, are naturally to be avoided. It is more often difficult to find occupations where illumination is or can be adjusted to optimal levels for the achromat. Work in brightly illuminated factories, sports-halls etc., should be avoided. Concerning sporting activities, ball games are generally difficult because of the poor fixation of moving objects. Skiing is likewise often difficult because of the high level of reflected light and the low contrast of objects in the snow. In particular, the difficulties can be considerable when skiing in sunny conditions. In the same way, some patients have experienced great difficulties with white stairs at low contrasts, which can be dangerous.

A reduction of the light level can be obtained with tinted glasses, if the light level cannot otherwise be adjusted. A hat with a brim or spectacles with side shields may give sufficient shadow to reduce the high light intensity. Tinted glasses can be used for an overall reduction in light intensity. Sunglasses, transmitting chiefly in the mid-wavelength range, are inappropriate and should not be recommended; transmission in the long-wavelength range is to be preferred. Such red, tinted glasses have been tried and are recommended, as are purple glasses (Weder, 1975; Young, Krefman & Fishman, 1982). These are cosmetically better than the usual glasses with high overall absorption. Improvement is solely a function of the reduced illumination level obtained with the glasses and not the wavelengths transmitted. Tinted contact lenses are used by some patients to great advantage. Here, also, cosmetic considerations should be taken into account, and brown coloured lenses have been well accepted.

Use of colour coding should obviously be avoided in work and education, and, also, coloured writing should be restricted as much as possible. With one patient, for instance, writing was completely illegible when green ink was used on white paper. In achromats the near vision is generally better than the distance vision. Classification based on visual acuity may therefore not be appropriate for evaluating a patient's ability to perform some specific work. Magnifying optical aids can be used for reading. In many situations just a hand magnifying glass is the most practical device. For distance, some kind of telescope or telescopic glasses may be preferred for special purposes.

9.11 Prognosis

The medical prognosis is generally good. Typical, total achromatopsia, is a stationary condition, and need not worry the patient nor the doctor regarding further development. It is, however, important that the condition is correctly diagnosed. For appropriate genetic counselling, correct diagnosis is essential. However, in patients with X-linked incomplete achromatopsia a deterioration of the residual colour vision may take place.

The occupational and educational prognosis has proved to be good (Norn, 1968), despite the classification of many patients as socially blind. In education, limiting factors due to achromatopsia can often be compensated for, and this is especially true for the lack of colour discrimination. The reader is referred to Chapter 8 where a personal account is given by one typical and complete achromat.

10

The photoreceptors in the achromat

Lindsay T. Sharpe and Knut Nordby

10.1 Introduction

In 1868, Galezowski proposed a physiological theory of the origins of total colour-blindness based on M. Schultze's (1866, 1867) functional distinction between rods and cones two years earlier:

> 'Selon notre hypothèse, ces éléments [les cones de la rétine] devraient être ou incomplétement développés, ou peut-être même ils seraient complétement absent, et les fonctions visuelles se passeraient toutes dans les bâtonnets' (Galezowski, 1868, pp. 146–7).
> ('According to our hypothesis, the elements [the cones of the retina] are deviant or incompletely developed, or perhaps even completely absent, and the visual functions take place wholly in the rods.')

This *pure rod theory* is generally consistent with the clinical symptoms of typical, complete achromatopsia (see Chapters 7 and 9); and it has been enthusiastically taken up or independently put forward by other researchers for more than 100 years (see, for example, König, 1894; von Kries 1897*a*, *b*; Nagel, 1911). In spite of its popular appeal, however, the pure rod theory has not gone unchallenged. In fact, several sorts of evidence have seriously compromised the theory by suggesting that cones or some other type of high-intensity receptor, in addition to the rods, are present in the achromat retina and are providing a visual signal. This second type of receptor has been variously described as a 'day rod' (i.e. a rod-like cone), a residual cone or a 'rhodopsin cone' (i.e. a cone whose outer segment is filled with rhodopsin) (for references and further details, see Chapters 7 and 11).

In this chapter, we consider the evidence gathered from many achromat observers that has been used to support these rival interpretations. And we attempt to reconcile it with extensive new evidence gathered from a single achromat observer (co-author K.N.). Our aim is to show that Galezowski's 120-year-old hypothesis is still viable today and that it is more persuasive in explaining the behaviour of the achromat visual system than are its more recent rivals.

We consider it a good research strategy to investigate in depth the response functions of a single achromat observer, rather than to collect a small number of observations from a large sample of achromats, who may be only superficially similar in terms of clinical tests and behavioural deficits. Our opinion is that a single case study of a well-trained, motivated observer provides a more compelling, less ambiguous, database for inferring about the underlying visual process of complete achromats; and further, that this view is warranted given that cases of incomplete achromatopsia may largely outnumber cases of complete achromatopsia (Krastel, Jaeger & Blankenagel, 1983) and may be mistaken, on the basis of conventional clinical tests, for complete cases. Nevertheless, we concede the danger of drawing general conclusions from a single achromat observer; for there may be more than one variety of the typical, complete achromat. Although typical, complete achromatopsia is usually deemed to be a case of recessive autosomal inheritance, it may well be the end product of several different genetic entities, or it may be a case of polyallelic inheritance (Pokorny *et al.*, 1982). In some families, such as K.N.'s, all affected members (i.e. he and his brother and sister) are typical, complete achromats; in others, however, the affected members may include both complete and incomplete forms of achromatopsia (Franceschetti *et al.*, 1958; Waardenburg, 1963; Jaeger & Krastel, 1981).

Be that as it may, we can still consider whether or not Galezowski's hypothesis is valid for achromat K.N. Accordingly, if K.N.'s vision is mediated solely by normal rods, one would expect the following to be true (cf. Alpern, 1974): (1) rods should be the only morphologically intact photoreceptors found in the retina; (2) the central fovea, which is rod-free in the normal eye, should be blind (i.e. have a central scotoma); (3) rhodopsin should be the only photo-pigment found in the eye; (4) the visual system should saturate at mesopic levels; (5) only a small directional sensitivity to light or Stiles–Crawford effect should be elicited; (6) psychophysically measured functions, such as increment threshold, dark-adaptation, flicker fusion and spatial acuity, should follow the course of rods alone; and (7) the electroretinogram should only be composed of scotopic (i.e. rod) components. We will consider, in turn, how well each of these propositions are fulfilled by the achromat observer K.N. and by the achromat observers investigated by others.

10.2 The histology

Although we lack direct anatomical information about K.N.'s eyes, we can still make inferences about the morphological nature of his photoreceptors on the basis of histological sections obtained from other achromat eyes. The first histological investigation of the achromat retina was made by Larsen (1921*a*, *b*). Contrary to Galezowski's hypothesis and the then-received wisdom, he found that the cones were neither completely absent, nor completely deviant, nor incompletely developed. Although the cones were scarce and malformed in the fovea, they were normally distributed and normally shaped in the periphery.

Three subsequent studies (Harrison, Hoefnagel & Hayward, 1960; Falls, Wolter, & Alpern, 1965; Glickstein & Heath, 1975) confirmed Larsen's findings, insofar as establishing that cone-like structures are indigenous to sections of the complete achromat retina. However, the later studies differed considerably from Larsen's and from each other in their descriptions of the morphological conditions and spatial distributions of the cone structures. The discrepancies may, in part, be due to differences in the cone dysfunctions of their subjects (see Sharpe & Nordby, Total colour-blindness: an introduction, Chapter 7). In one study (Harrison *et al.*, 1960) cones were found to be imperfectly shaped and markedly reduced in numbers throughout the entire retina; in another (Falls *et al.*, 1965) cones were found to be normally-distributed, though abnormally shaped, in the foveal region, and scarce, though less often malformed, in the periphery; and in the third (Glickstein & Heath, 1975) cones were found to be completely absent in the fovea, abnormally shaped near the fovea and severely reduced in number throughout the entire retina.

The histological studies, their differences notwithstanding, oblige us to reject the first premise about K.N.'s eyes – namely, that they have no morphologically intact cones – and to abandon any version of Galezowski's theory of achromatopsia that would have us believe otherwise. Even though the best evidence (Glickstein & Heath, 1975) indicates that there are no cones whatsoever in the foveola of the achromat, and only reduced numbers in the rest of the retina (5–10% of the normal complement), we cannot reasonably attribute total achromatopsia to the complete anatomical absence of cones (the strictest version of Galezowski's theory). Moreover, since most of the spared cones in the histologically investigated achromat eyes appear to be morphologically intact, we are obliged to question the version of Galezowski's theory which presupposes that the cones are completely nonfunctioning and to consider the evidence for residual cone function. For, as Walls & Heath (1954) argue:

> The simple truth is that in the face of Larsen's actual findings [the only histological study published at the time], the pure-rod theory can be retained only by one who is willing to believe that a structurally perfectly normal cone population can be perfectly functionless, and yet not proceed to degenerate and disappear in a very few years at most.
>
> (Walls & Heath, 1954, p. 264)

Fair enough, but the presence of morphologically intact cone-like structures is only a necessary and not a sufficient condition for supporting the proposition of residual cone function. The visual functions of the achromat could still take place wholly in the rods, despite the presence of physiologically unimpaired cones, if the spared cones are too diminished in number and too anomalous in distribution to provide an independent post-receptoral signal. Since it is our aim to verify this version of Galezowski's theory, we must demonstrate not only that *the cone-like structures* (which we are assuming to be present in all achromat eyes) *are not mediating vision nor moderating rod-mediated vision as normal cones*, but also that *they are not doing so in an altered form* as 'rhodopsin cones'.

10.3 The scotoma

Before the histological sections became available, the debate about the anatomical nature of the achromat eye centred on the issue of whether or not achromats exhibited an absolute, central scotoma. (Like normals, achromats were expected to display a relative, central scotoma or Arago's phenomenon, i.e. the disappearance of foveally fixated, very low luminance, targets.) Cases in which an absolute central scotoma could be demonstrated were taken as support for the pure rod theory (König, 1894; von Kries, 1897*a*, *b*). The scotoma was assumed to coincide with the normal rod-free area, which should be empty if cones were lacking and were not replaced by other receptors. Cases in which a scotoma could not be demonstrated were taken as proof either that cones must be present, though incapable of signalling colour (Hess & Hering, 1898; Hess, 1902), or that day-rods had replaced the cones in the centre of the fovea (von Kries, 1897*a*).

Although each side collected its successes, the issue was never convincingly settled. Of the 215 cases reported in the literature, surveyed by François, Verriest & De Rouck (1955), 28 reported an absolute central scotoma, while 32 did not. The fact that in the remaining 155 cases, the matter was not fully investigated or left unresolved is not surprising: small central scotomas often evade detection; especially when measurements are confounded by the achromat's nystagmus and eccentric fixation. A case in point is the achromat whose retinae were histologically studied by Glickstein & Heath (1975). During the achromat's lifetime, no central scotoma could be demonstrated, at any illumination level, even though it was later revealed that he had no receptors at all in his foveae.

What about achromat K.N.? Both static (Goldmann) perimetry (E. Mehdorn, 1979, private communication) and campimetry (Sharpe, Collewijn & Nordby, 1986) indicate that he has a small, central scotoma. In his left eye, which is his preferred experimental eye, the scotoma is approximately 0.3 deg in diameter and is located about 14.1 deg nasal to the centre of the blind spot, and 0.9 deg above it in the external field of view (Sharpe *et al.*, 1986). The scotoma corresponds closely in size and position to the rod-free island within the foveola (Polyak, 1941; Wyszecki & Stiles, 1982), whose position could be inferred from the fundal photographs used to estimate K.N.'s preferred area of fixation (Sharpe *et al.*, 1986; see Fig. A/10.1). Therefore the presence of the scotoma is consistent with the hypothesis that K.N. entirely lacks functioning cones within his foveola; and it is consistent with the histological findings of Glickstein & Heath (1975) described above. However, it tells us nothing about whether K.N. has functioning cones elsewhere in his retina. To find out about that, we must look at other measures of sensitivity.

10.4 The photopigment: fundal reflectometry and spectral sensitivity

One way to reveal more about the nature of the photoreceptors in the achromat eye is to investigate the nature of their photopigments. This can be done, either with densitometry, to determine if normal cone photopigments are actually present, or with psychophysics, to determine if the photoreceptors containing them are providing a visual signal. Both types of measurements have been made in K.N.'s eyes.

10.4.1 Fundal reflectometry

Consider first the densitometric measurements made in K.N.'s left eye with the Utrecht continuous recording, densitometer (Sharpe, van Norren & Nordby, 1988*b*). Fig. 10.1 (panel (*a*)) shows the results

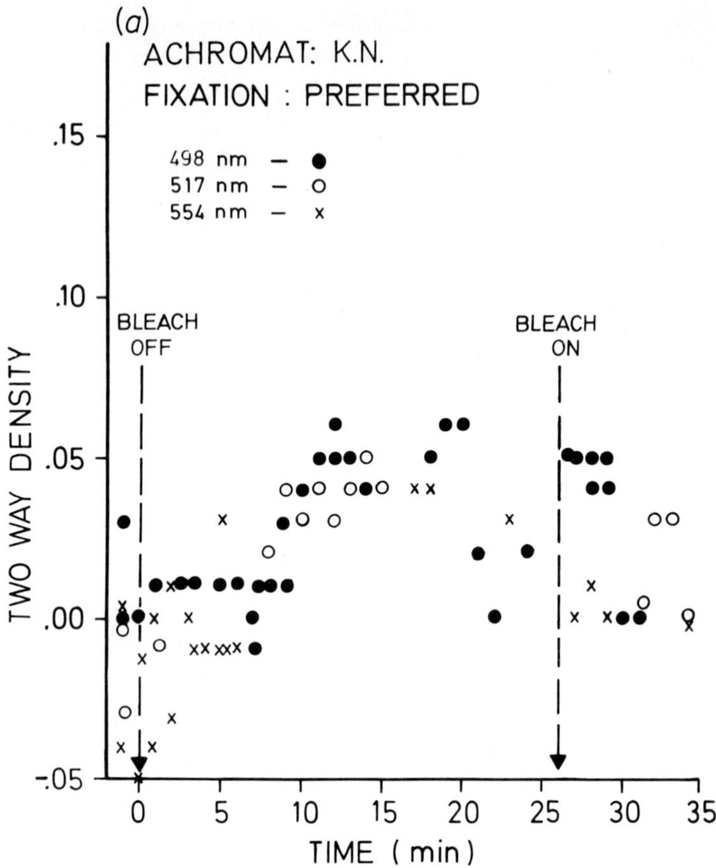

Fig. 10.1. Two-way, optical (photopigment) densities from the area of the fundus where the achromat K.N. prefers to fixate (*a*) and from his peripheral retina, 12 deg temporal to the fovea (*b*). Pigment regeneration is plotted as a

obtained from K.N.'s preferred area of fixation which is located 0.99 deg temporal to and 3.45 deg below the optic axis in his external field of view (Sharpe *et al.*, 1986; see Fig. A10.1). Pigment regeneration is plotted as a function of time following the extinction and onset of a bleaching light which was sufficiently intense to photolyse more than 99% of all photopigments in normal subjects (see Chapter 12).

Very low total two-way densities (i.e. the maximum change in measured density of pigment concentration between the fully bleached and fully dark-adapted retina) were obtained for measuring beam wavelengths of 498 nm (0.03), 517 nm (0.02) and 554 nm (0.03). The presence of cone photopigments would lead one to expect larger

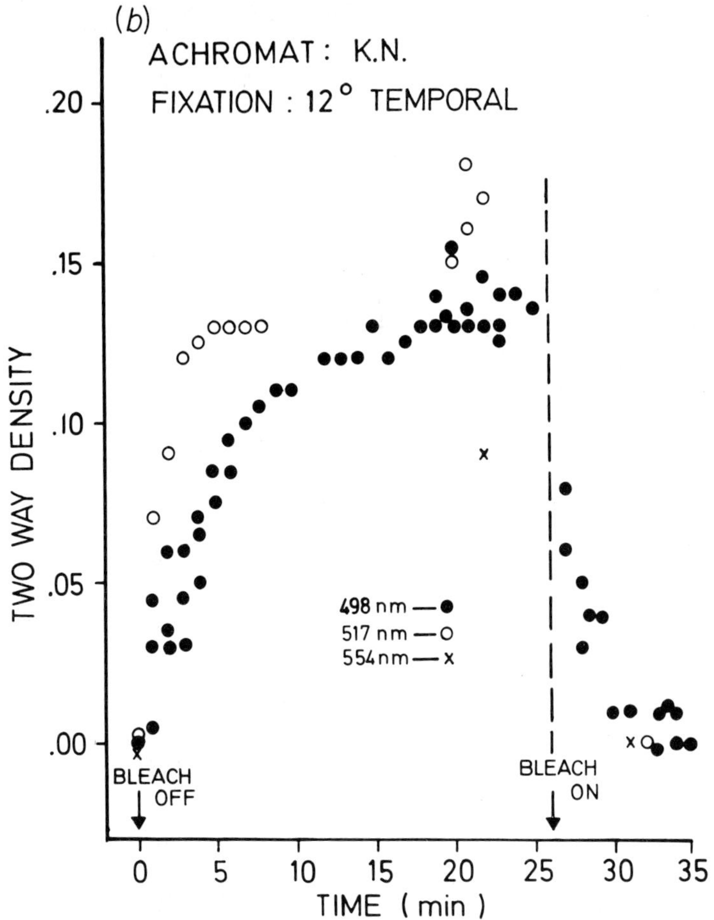

function of time in the dark, following a full bleach of 6.0 $\log_{10}$ td, for measuring beam wavelengths of 498 (●), 517 (○) and 554 (×) nm. (From Sharpe *et al.*, 1988*b*.)

two-way density values; especially for the 554 nm measuring beam, which is close to the peak of the CIE photopic luminosity function. However, the finding of such small two-way density values is not conclusive evidence for the absence of cone photopigments because at the same retinal locus in trichromatic control observers near-marginal two-way density values are also found: 0.05 ± 0.01 for 498 nm, 0.07 ± 0.03 for 517 nm, and 0.06 ± 0.01 for 554 nm.

Because it is difficult, even in the normal observer to measure cone pigments in this retinal region, we cannot conclude that there are no cone photopigments present in the vicinity of K.N.'s retinal area of fixation. Nevertheless, our results do suggest that if cone photopigments are present in the achromat eye, their amounts are extremely low. This conclusion is confirmed by the results of Alpern (1974), who made densitometric measurements in a centrally fixating, female achromat. He found the difference spectrum between her fully bleached and fully dark-adapted retina reasonably well described by the Dartnall photopigment nomogram (see Wyszecki & Stiles, 1982, p. 592) with a peak wavelength of 510 nm (the peak of the CIE scotopic luminosity function; see Alpern, 1974, Fig. 3); and her time constant of regeneration (i.e. the time required for the measured density of pigment concentration to return to 1/e of the total two-way density) to be that of rhodopsin (380 s) and not that of a cone photopigment.

Figure 10.1 (panel (*b*)) shows the total two-way densities obtained from an area centred 12 deg in the periphery of K.N.'s temporal retina. The values are much larger than those obtained for his area of preferred fixation: 0.13 $\log_{10}$ unit for 498 nm; 0.16 $\log_{10}$ unit for 517 nm; and 0.09 $\log_{10}$ unit for 554 nm. The time constant of regeneration is about 290 s for the 498 nm measuring beam and 240 s for the 517 nm measuring beam (not enough data points were available to make an estimate for the 554 nm measuring beam). Both time constants are considerably longer than the standard values for the cones (about 100 s). Normal subjects, tested with the Utrecht densitometer, at the same retinal locus, have a mean density of 0.15 ± 0.02 (SD) and a mean time constant of 226 ± 33 s for a 517 nm measuring beam (Keunen, van Meel & von Norren, 1988). (Time constants measured with the Utrecht densitometer are typically shorter than those measured with Alpern's densitometer in Ann Arbor; see van Norren & van der Kraats, 1981.)

For the peripheral location, the difference spectrum between the fully bleached and the fully dark-adapted retina could be determined. This is shown in Fig. 10.2, in which the optical density is plotted as a function of wavenumber (the reciprocal of wavelength). The optical density values have been standardized to a peak value of 507 nm. The continuous line represents the Dartnall nomogram set to a value of 507 nm. No correction has been made for light that did not pass the photoreceptors twice; nor for self-screening effects (cf. Ripps, Mehaffy & Siegel, 1981; Smith, Pokorny & van Norren, 1983); nor for bleach products at short wavelengths, where the two-way densities fall below the curve. Despite these limitations (the corrections would improve the fit), the density values at middle and long wavelengths reasonably approximate the Dartnall

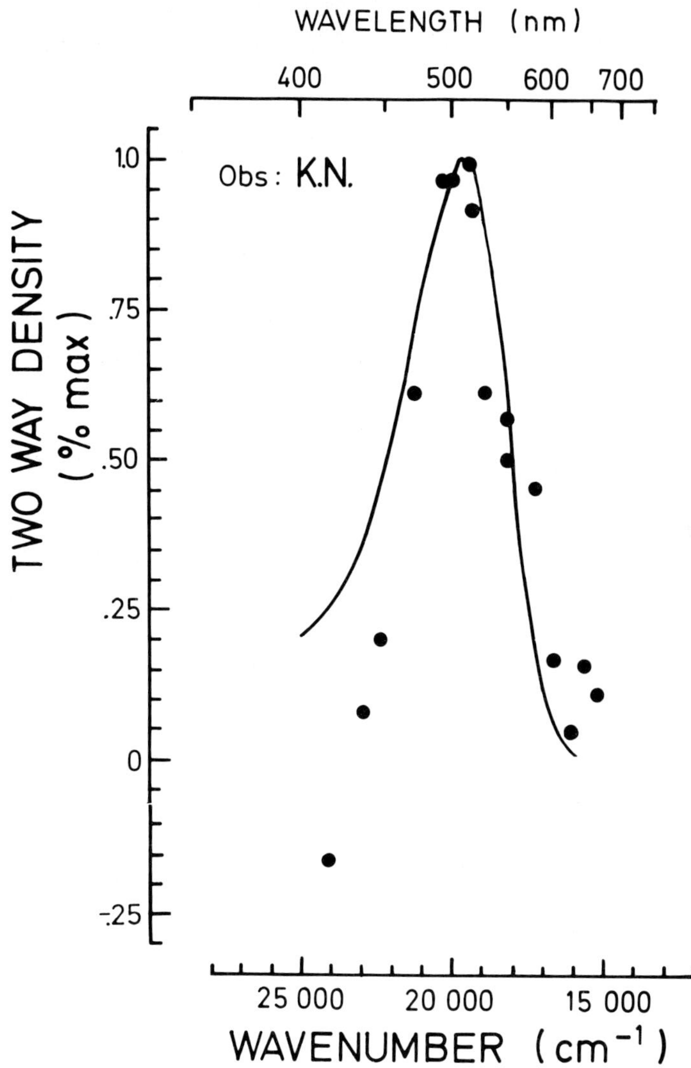

Fig. 10.2. The difference spectrum of achromat K.N. measured in the peripheral retina, 12 deg temporal to the fovea, following a full bleach of 6.0 $\log_{10}$ td. Total two-way density, standardized to a peak vaue of 507 nm, is plotted as a function of wavelength. The continuous curve is the Dartnall nomogram with its peak set equal to 507 nm. (From Sharpe *et al.*, 1988*b*.)

nomogram calculated for the rod photopigment. The density values at short wavelengths are too small to be reliable.

Thus the only two densitometric results so far made in achromats (Alpern, 1974; Sharpe *et al.*, 1988*b*) support the interpretation that their

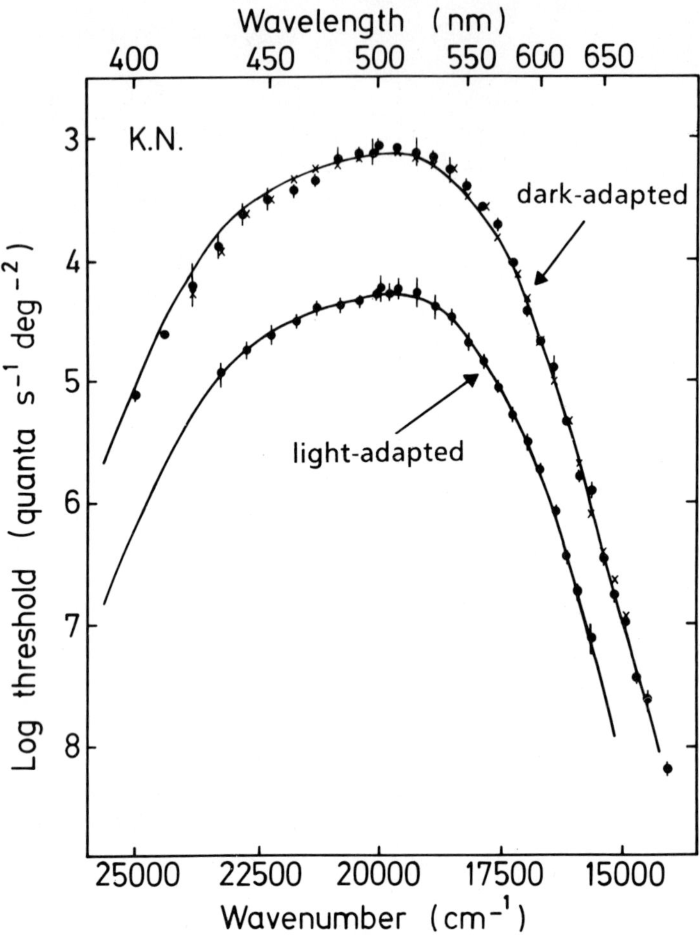

Fig. 10.3 The achromat K.N.'s dark-adapted (upper curve) and light-adapted (lower curve) spectral sensitivities. The target and adapting field (499 nm; 3.79 $\log_{10}$ scotopic td) were centred at a point 12 deg temporal to his fovea. The error bars indicate two standard errors of the mean. The continuous curve fit to the upper and lower thresholds is the (quantized) CIE luminous efficiency function for scotopic vision. The crosses (upper curve) represent the achromat K.N.'s dark-adapted (absolute) sensitivities as measured by Nordby *et al.* (1984). (From Sharpe *et al.*, 1988*b*.)

retinae contain normal amounts of the rod photopigment (rhodopsin) but no amounts of the cone photopigments or, at least, amounts so small that it is impossible to measure them with present-day densitometers. This is consistent with the best histological findings, indicating that the number of cones (and hence the amount of cone pigment) in the achromat eye is at most 5% to 10% of the normal complement.

10.4.2 Spectral sensitivity

The densitometric results are supported by the spectral sensitivity measurements made in K.N. at 6 deg (Nordby, Stabell & Stabell, 1984) and at 12 deg (Sharpe *et al.*, 1988*b*) in the temporal retina. At both retinal eccentricities, measurements were made against a zero background (i.e. dark-adapted) and against a high mesopic background. For the light-adaptation measurements, Nordby *et al.* used a white 3.46 $\log_{10}$ scotopic td background; Sharpe *et al.* a 499 nm, 2.79 $\log_{10}$ scotopic td background. Fig. 10.3 shows the dark- and light-adapted detection sensitivities obtained by Sharpe *et al.* (1988*b*; ●) and the dark-adapted sensitivities obtained by Nordby *et al.* (1984; upper curve, ×). The Nordby *et al.* measurements have been converted to quantal units and shifted downwards by 0.26 $\log_{10}$ unit to provide the best fit with the Sharpe *et al.* measurements. The agreement between the two sets of dark-adapted measurements is excellent; in both cases, the peak sensitivity is found between 500 and 510 nm. The continuous line, fitted through the data points, represents the (quantized) CIE luminous efficiency function (V'_λ) for scotopic vision, adjusted vertically by eye to provide the best fit.

The lower curve in Fig. 10.3 (●) shows the spectral sensitivities obtained for K.N. against a 499 nm, 2.79 $\log_{10}$ scotopic td adapting field (the curve has been shifted upwards by four $\log_{10}$ units). As for the dark-adapted measurements, the peak sensitivity is between 500 and 510 nm. Thus, at absolute threshold and at high mesopic luminances, K.N.'s spectral sensitivity is that of the rods.

These results, indicating that K.N. only displays the spectral sensitivity of rhodopsin and displays no Purkinje shift, confirm results made in other achromats (Hecht *et al.*, 1948; Sloan, 1958; Alpern, Falls & Lee, 1960; Falls, Wolter & Alpern, 1965; Blakemore & Rushton, 1965; Alexandridris, 1970; Alpern, 1974; Auerbach & Kripke, 1974). Alpern (1974), in fact, asserts that in typical, complete achromatopsia;

> . . . all action spectra, independent of criterion, fit the CIE scotopic spectral sensitivity curve reasonably well, allowing only for measurement error and differences in pre-receptor absorbances. This observation is so well established as to make additional spectra documenting it redundant . . . (p. 650)

We agree and would only add that the densitometric and spectral sensitivity measurements all accord with the version of Galezowski's theory (that we favour) in which the rods function alone because the normal cone signals are utterly compromised by low cone densities. The spectral sensitivity measurements, taken by themselves, however, do not rule out the possibility that the residual cones are functioning as 'rhodopsin cones' and providing a signal that is spectrally indistinguishable from that of the rods (Alpern *et al.*, 1960; Falls *et al.*, 1965; Alpern, 1974).

10.5 Saturation

A good way to test the 'rhodopsin cone' hypothesis and to determine at the same time whether or not K.N.'s vision is mediated solely by normal rods is to measure the extent of his operating range. If only rods are mediating his vision then his psychophysical response curves, as a function of background intensity, should saturate at the same adaption levels as the psychophysically isolated rod mechanism in normal observers; and that level should approximately correspond to the level at which the electrophysiologically measured saturation of isolated rod photoreceptors occur in the primate. On the other hand, if physiologically normal cones, regardless of the photopigment contained in their outer segment, are mediating his vision under photopic conditions, then there is no reason why his dynamic range should be constrained by the saturation limits of the rods.

The saturation of the rod visual system can be defined psychophysically in terms of the increment threshold function or contrast sensitivity. According to Aguilar & Stiles (1954), the rod system is effectively saturated in normal observers (in the sense that it is incapable of responding to an increment stimulus, however intense) when the Weber–Fechner fraction is 100 times the nearly constant value it has in the 0.01–100 scotopic td range of a threshold versus intensity (t.v.i) curve (see Chapter 2). For the four subjects of Aguilar & Stiles, saturation occurred between 3.59 and 3.77 $\log_{10}$ scotopic td. For K.N., by the same criterion, saturation occurs at 3.68 and 3.65 $\log_{10}$ scotopic td, respectively, for central (i.e. preferred fixation) and 12 deg temporal stimulation (Sharpe *et al.*, 1988; Sharpe (1989*a*). His values agree well, not only with those of Aguilar & Stiles (1954), but also with the estimates made from the t.v.i. data of an incomplete achromat (about 3.3 $\log_{10}$ scotopic td, Fuortes, Gunkel & Rushton, 1961), and five other achromats (3.0 $\log_{10}$ scotopic td, Blakemore & Rushton, 1965; 2.5–3.0 $\log_{10}$ scotopic td, Hayhoe, MacLeod & Bruch,

1976; 3.0 $\log_{10}$ scotopic td, Sakitt, 1976*a*; 3.0 $\log_{10}$ scotopic td, Klingaman, 1979; 3.2 $\log_{10}$ scotopic td, Baker & Donovan, 1982). These other estimates, it should be noted, are slightly lower than K.N.'s because they are based on qualitative assessments of where changes in the slope of the t.v.i. functions occur and not on the hundredfold criterion change (for a discussion of rod saturation, see Chapter 2).

That K.N.'s visual system exhibits no cone-driven, post-receptoral function is further confirmed by the unitary way in which his sensitivity to all spatial and temporal frequency stimuli declines as illuminance is increased (see Chapter 11). In contrast to what would be expected for residual cone function, there is neither a lateral displacement of his spatial and temporal contrast sensitivity functions during saturation nor a discontinuity in the saturating limb of his spatial acuity (see Fig. 10.13) and temporal resolution (see Fig. 10.14) functions. Instead all his functions saturate at about 3.3 $\log_{10}$ scotopic td.

This abrupt fall-off in K.N.'s psychophysical sensitivity is consistent with electrophysiological estimates of rod saturation, which take as their measure the steady intensity needed to reduce the flash response of the rod-photocurrent to half its dark-adapted value (Baylor, Nunn & Schnapf, 1984). In the cynomolgus monkey (Macaca fascicularis), the intensity required is in the region of 100 photoisomerizations s^{-1} rod $^{-1}$ (Baylor *et al.*, 1984). We can make a comparable estimate for K.N. by determining the background intensity at which his threshold rises by a factor of 2 above the line of constant slope in the t.v.i. function (Hayhoe *et al.*, 1976). The change, which corresponds to the onset of saturation rather than to saturation itself, occurs at backgrounds of about 2.6 $\log_{10}$ scotopic td for both central and peripheral viewing (see Fig. 10.12) or an effective isomerization rate of *c*.2900 quanta [507 nm] s^{-1} rod^{-1} (for the conversion factors, see Chapter 2). Such estimates are highly prone to the assumptions made about rod density, lens absorption, etc., and can only be considered as rough approximations. Nevertheless the value for K.N. is close enough to the electrophysiological measurements to strengthen the case that K.N.'s spatial and temporal vision is driven solely by rods (see Chapter 11 for proof); and, correspondingly, to weaken the case that cones are providing a signal with the spectral sensitivity of rhodopsin. For if cones afford any functional advantage to the visual system of the complete achromat, why should their signals stop at the same light levels as the rods'? After all, the cone systems, as opposed to the rod system, do not saturate under steady-state conditions in the normal. Photopigment bleaching that conveniently stops further photon absorptions at light levels above 4.0 $\log_{10}$ scotopic td (or 5.0 $\log_{10}$ scotopic td, when the conversion is made at 507 nm) enables the cones, but not the rods, to operate up to the light-damage limit. The inescapable conclusion, therefore, seems to be that, even if cones are present, their numbers and post-receptoral connexions do not suffice to stave off the consequences of rod saturation.

10.6 Directional sensitivity

A further way to test the validity of the 'rod only' theory and to rule out the 'residual cone function' and 'rhodopsin cone' theories, at least for K.N., is to investigate the directional sensitivity of K.N.'s photoreceptors. This involves measuring the visual effectiveness of light stimuli as a function of their angle of incidence on the retina, the so-called Stiles–Crawford Effect of the first kind, the SCE_1 (Stiles & Crawford, 1933). The magnitude of the SCE_1 (i.e. the visual effectiveness of obliquely incident light rays relative to normally incident rays) is associated with the shape of the photoreceptors. It is most pronounced for the squat, parafoveal cones (Westheimer, 1967), slightly smaller for the elongated (i.e. rod-like), central, foveal cones (Westheimer, 1967), and considerably smaller for the rods (Crawford, 1937; Stiles, 1939; Flamant & Stiles, 1948; van Loo & Enoch, 1975; Alpern, Ching & Kitahara, 1983). In fact, the differences between the directional sensitivities of rods and cones are so pronounced that the SCE_1 effectively can be used to differentiate between the photopic and scotopic systems (Donner & Rushton, 1959; Fuortes *et al.*, 1961; Alpern *et al.*, 1983). Thus, the SCE_1 can be used to determine if the cone-like structures, found histologically in the achromat eye (and presumed to be present in K.N.'s eye), are functioning and providing an independent post-receptoral signal.

Measurements of K.N.'s directional sensitivities (filled symbols) are shown in Fig. 10.4 for comparison with the directional sensitivities of a normal trichromat (open symbols) obtained under identical conditions (Nordby & Sharpe, 1988). Both the test and adapting fields were 621 nm to favour photopic vision and were centred on the temporal parafoveal retina. The sensitivities are plotted (ordinate) as a function of the test field's point of entry along the horizontal meridian of the pupil (abscissa).

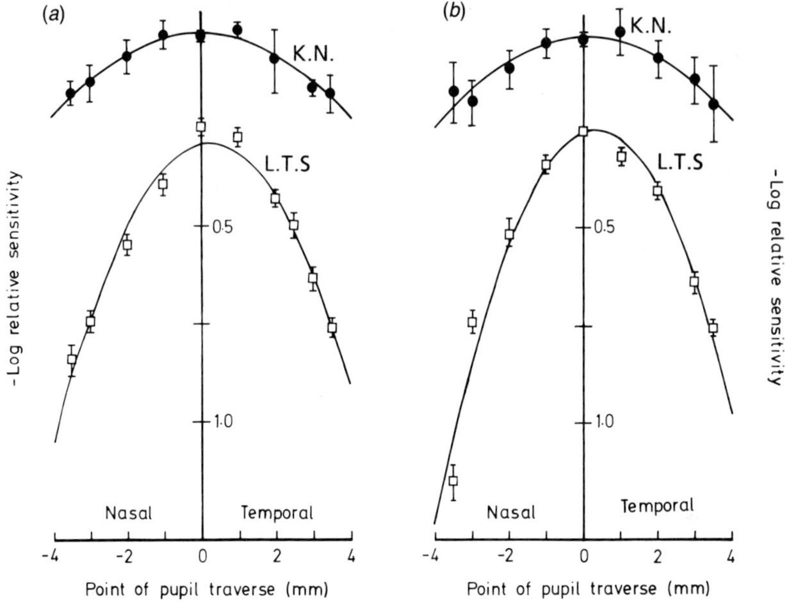

Fig. 10.4. Directional sensitivities obtained with a zero background (panel (*a*)) and with a high mesopic background (panel (*b*)) for achromat K.N. (●) and for a normal trichromat observer L.T.S. (□). The data have been corrected for losses by absorption in the lens of the eye. Each data set has been standardized separately to the abscissa reference zero (the first Purkinje image of the test). The data sets for the normal observer have been arbitrarily displaced 0.25 $\log_{10}$ unit below those of the achromat. The parabolic curves fit through the data sets are defined by the empirical formula introduced by Stiles & Crawford (1933). The error bars indicate ±1 standard error of the mean. (From Nordby & Sharpe, 1988.)

The curves in the left panel correspond to SCE_1 functions measured against a zero background when both K.N. and the normal observer were fully dark-adapted. The data points have been corrected for losses in the eye, resulting from absorption in the lens (for details, see Nordby & Sharpe, 1988). The effect is qualitatively similar for both observers; i.e. test flashes through the pupil centre are more effective than those reaching the retina from the margins of the exit pupil. However, the effect is quantitatively much larger for the normal observer. The total range of the effect for the horizontal traverse, from the centre of the pupil to ± 3.5 nm in the periphery, is about 0.16 $\log_{10}$ unit for K.N. (p = 0.014; where p is a measure of the curvature determined from a parabolic least-squares fit to the data), and 0.60 $\log_{10}$ for the normal observer (p = 0.043).

The curves in the right panel of Fig. 10.4 correspond to SCE_1

measured when both observers were light-adapted with a mesopic background field of 1.75 $\log_{10}$ scotopic td. The total range of the effect is about 0.20 $\log_{10}$ unit for K.N. ($p = 0.013$) and 0.90 $\log_{10}$ unit for the normal control ($p = 0.054$). For the normal observer the SCE_1 increases slightly in magnitude with the brighter (mesopic) adapting field. This is probably because in the parafovea, where the measurements were made, there is a larger contribution from the cones when the eye is light-adapted (see Stiles, 1939; Nordby & Sharpe, 1988). For K.N., on the other hand, the effect has the same magnitude both for dark- and light-adapted measurements.

The p-coefficients, 0.014 and 0.013, for K.N.'s dark- and light-adapted functions, respectively, are much smaller than those Stiles found for the parafoveal cones, and compare very favourably with the p-coefficients he found for the parafoveal rods of normal observers (whose values, uncorrected for light losses due to the lens, range from 0.010 to 0.015). Thus, although the SCE_1 effect (at 621 nm) for the normal observer is being determined exclusively by the cone photoreceptors at the high adapting level and by possibly both the rod and cone photoreceptors in absolute darkness, it seems clear that the SCE_1 effect for K.N. is being solely determined by the rod photoreceptors at both adapting levels.

This is confirmed in Fig. 10.5 (left panel), which shows directional sensitivity functions obtained with a series of adapting field luminances. The backgrounds ranged from absolute darkness to a level near K.N.'s saturation limit (2.12 $\log_{10}$ scotopic td). On the right of each curve are shown the $\log_{10}$ scotopic td values of the adapting field, which like the test field was always fixed at a wavelength of 621 nm. Each data set has been corrected for losses by absorption in the lens of the eye, standardized to the abscissa reference zero and arbitrarily displaced from the adjacent sets by 0.25 $\log_{10}$ unit along the ordinate. Over a range covering more than seven $\log_{10}$ units, there is very little change in the position of the peak and in the magnitude of the directional sensitivity functions. The p-coefficients of the best fitting parabolas vary from 0.013 to 0.019, indicating that the rod receptor system is mediating the directional sensitivity functions at all adapting luminances. For if the cone-like structures, found histologically in the achromat eye, were functioning normally (and in densities large enough to mediate detection), then a large difference in magnitude should be obtained between the SCE_1 measured with low- and high-adapting field luminances; the former rod-like in magnitude and the latter cone-like.

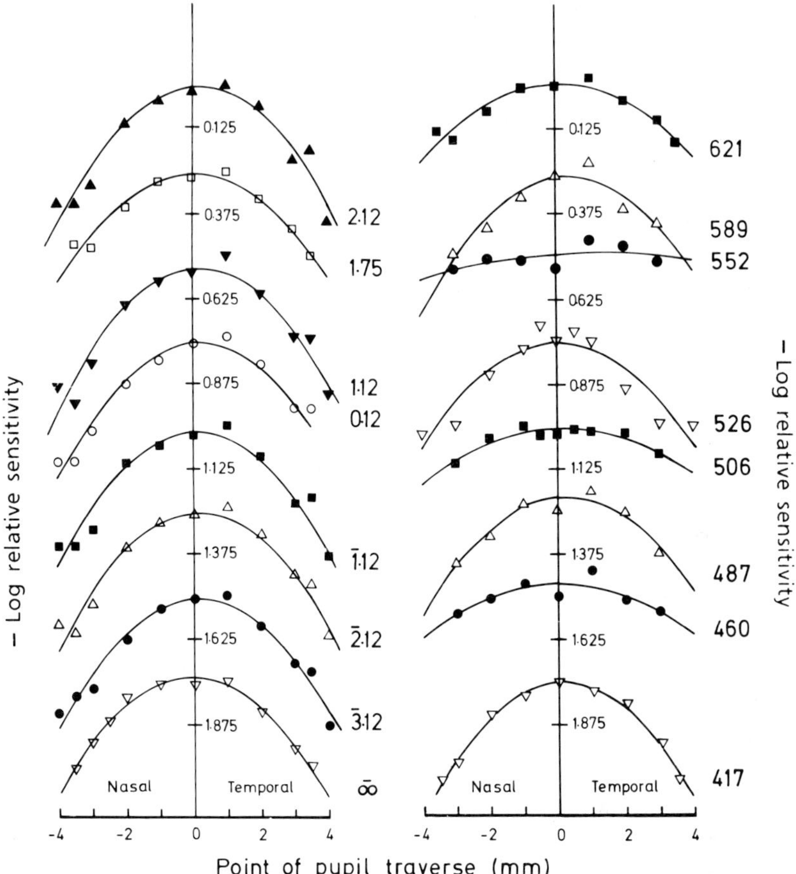

Fig. 10.5 Directional sensitivities obtained for achromat K.N. as a function of retinal illuminance (left panel) or wavelength of the adapting field (right panel). The $\log_{10}$ scotopic td values (left panel) or the wavelengths (right panel) of the adapting fields are shown on the right of each curve. The individual data sets have been corrected for losses by absorption in the lens of the eye and have been separately standardised to the abscissa reference zero. Each set has been arbitrarily displaced from the adjacent sets by 0.25 $\log_{10}$ unit along the ordinate. The parabolic curves fit to the corrected data sets are defined by the empirical formula of Stiles & Crawford (1933). (From Nordby & Sharpe, 1988.)

Fig. 10.5 (right panel) presents results for K.N. at eight monochromatic test and adapting-field wavelengths. The wavelengths are noted on the right of each curve. In each case, the background luminance was high enough to elicit a cone SCE_1 in the normal eye. The largest directional sensitivity is found for 417 nm light (due to the large correction factor for lens absorption; see Nordby & Sharpe, 1988). At this wavelength, the

Table 10.1. *Directional sensitivity of the rods (p-coefficients[a]), as a function of wavelength*

Wavelength (nm)	Achromat K.N. (Nordby & Sharpe, 1988)	Normal observer (Stiles, 1939)
417	0.023	0.067
460	0.010	0.064
487	0.019	0.061
506	0.009	0.058
526	0.019	0.052
552	0.003	0.047
589	0.021	0.047
621	0.013	0.052

[a] The *p*-coefficient is a measure of the directional effect found by solving the equation $\log_{10}\eta = -p(r-r_m)^2$, where η is the directional sensitivity, r is the point of entry (in nm) for maximal η (Stiles, 1937)

p-coefficients has a value of 0.023, but this is still only a third of the value that Stiles (1937) obtained for dark-adapted parafoveal cones (> 0.067). Directional sensitivity values obtained for K.N. at other wavelengths (and the estimates of Stiles, 1939, for the dark-adapted fovea, interpolated from his Fig. 8) are given in Table 10.1.

Since K.N.'s values are all much less than half of Stiles's, they suggest that only very reduced (i.e. rod-like) directional sensitivity functions are being measured. (The difference in shape with wavelength are probably in part due to noise in the measurements caused by K.N.'s nystagmus and to inaccuracies in the factors used to correct for lens absorption.) Furthermore, the average *p*-coefficient (across the 8 wavelengths) for K.N., 0.015, is very close to the average value, 0.011, that Alpern *et al.* (1983, see their Fig. 5) obtained for the rod directional sensitivity in three normal observers. Again, this strongly indicates that cones are not influencing K.N.'s functions. Thus, K.N.'s directional sensitivity data support the 'rod only' interpretation of the complete achromat's visual system, and lend no support to the 'residual cone function' and 'rhodopsin cone' theories.

These results are at odds with those of Alpern *et al.* (1960), who inferred that four achromats – though data were only given for one (F.B.) – had a photoreceptor type with the directional sensitivity of the cones and the spectral sensitivity of the rods (i.e. a rhodopsin cone). However, Alpern *et al.*'s results and/or interpretation are called into question for several reasons. First of all, Blackwell & Blackwell (1961), on the basis of spectral sensitivity functions, independently diagnosed Alpern *et al.*'s subject F.B. as possessing blue (or short-wave sensitive) cones as well as rods (see Alpern *et al.*, 1960, footnote p. 996). Their diagnosis of blue-mono-cone monochromacy (or X-chromosome-linked incomplete achromatopsia; see Chapter 7) would straightforwardly explain why F.B. shows the directional sensitivity of the cones at higher illuminances; for this is indeed what is found for the blue-mono-cone monochromat (cf., Alpern *et al.*, 1971; Daw & Enoch, 1973; Hess *et al.*, 1989).

Even if achromat F.B. is not a blue-mono-cone monochromat – the spectral sensitivity evidence of Blackwell & Blackwell may not support their interpretation (M. Alpern, private communication) – he still may not have been a typical, complete achromat, but rather an example of cone degeneration (Krill, Deutman & Fishman, 1973). This possibility arises because the (corrected) acuity measured in his left eye (the test eye) was rather high (0.25); whereas that in his right eye was closer to typical values (0.1). Moreover he showed 'slight pigment degeneration and clumping situs inversus O.U.' in his left eye (Alpern *et al.*, 1960, p. 1009); which is not characteristic of typical, complete achromatopsia (cf. Krill *et al.*, 1973; see the Taxonomy of Chapter 7).

Secondly, the directional sensitivity measurements of F.B. were made without monitoring his pendular, conjugate nystagmus, even though it was very pronounced at the light levels used to make the measurements (excursions of *c.* 4 deg). The effects of such eye movements can markedly alter directional sensitivity functions. For instance, the fall-off in the slopes of the achromat's SCE_1 function may be exaggerated due to the test beam being vignetted by the pupil during his nystagmoid excursions.

Thirdly, directional sensitivity measurements have not confirmed the presence of rhodopsin cones in X-chromosome-linked incomplete achromats/blue-mono-cone monochromats (Daw & Enoch, 1973; Hess *et al.*, 1989), despite Alpern *et al.*'s (1971) claim that these achromats also possess them.

10.7 The psychophysics

The evidence, reviewed above (see also Chapter 11), suggests that typical, complete achromats, such as K.N., have only normal rod receptors providing a post-receptoral signal to the visual system. It

Table 10.2. *Psychophysical studies of the complete, typical achromat*

Study	Total no. of cases	No. of cases for which bipartite functions were measured			
		Dark adaptation	tvi	spatial acuity	flicker
1. Best (1917)	1	0	—	—	—
2. Wøfflin (1924)	1	1	—	—	—
3. Snyder (1929)	1	0	—	—	—
4. Waardenburg (1930)	1	0	—	—	—
5. Bunge (1936)	2	0	—	—	—
6. Hecht *et al.* (1938, 1948)	1	—	1	0	1
7. Barbel (1938)	3	0	—	—	—
8. Kolycev (1940)	1	0	—	—	—
9. Sloan & Newhall (1942)	1	1	—	—	—
10. Lewis & Mandelbaum (1943)	4	3	—	—	—
11. Ferguson & MacGregor (1949)	4	1	—	—	—
12. Walls & Heath (1954)	2	2	—	—	—
13. Sloan (1954)	14	11	—	—	—
14. Peskin (1954)	3	1	—	—	—
15. Francois *et al.* (1955)	3	3	—	—	—
16. Goodman & Bornschein (1957)	1	0	—	—	—
17. Sloan (1958)	5	5	—	—	—
18. Alpern *et al.* (1960)	5	5	5	5	5
19. Blackwell & Blackwell (1961)	3	3	—	—	—
20. Goodman *et al.* (1963)	17	7	—	—	—
21. Falls *et al.* (1965)	1	0	—	—	—
22. Blakemore & Rushton (1965)	1	1	1	—	1
23. Dodt *et al.* (1967)	1	—	1	—	—
24. Alpern (1971)	1	0	—	—	—
25. Sloan & Feiock (1972)	4	2	—	—	—

26. van der Tweel & Spekreijse (1973)	1	0	—	—	—
27. Auerback & Kripke (1974)	5	3	—	—	—
28. Alpern (1974)	1	0	0	—	—
29. Hayhoe *et al.* (1976)	1	—	0	—	—
30. Sakitt (1976*a*)	1	0	0	—	—
31. Klingaman (1977, 1979)	1	—	0	—	—
32. Skottun *et al.* (1980)[a]	1	0	—	—	—
33. Nordby *et al.* (1984)[a]	1	0	—	—	—
34. Hess & Nordby (1986*a*)[a]	1	—	—	0	1
35. Stabell *et al.* (1986)[a]	1	0	—	—	—
36. Stabell *et al.* (1987)[a]	1	—	0	—	—
37. Sharpe *et al.* (1989*b*)[a,b]	1	—	0	—	—

[a] In these studies the co-author K.N. was the observer.
[b] These data have been reanalyzed. See discussion in text.

thus supports the modified version of Galezowski's pure-rod theory, which presupposes that all the visual functions of the achromat take place wholly in the rods. However, evidence gathered from other achromats suggests that there is more than one post-receptoral signal in the achromat visual system. The seemingly discordant evidence consists of discontinuities in dark-adaptation, spatial acuity, critical flicker fusion (CFF) and increment threshold (t.v.i.) functions. According to our current assumptions about the behaviour of the scotopic visual system, we would expect such functions to be monophasic, exhibiting only a single rod branch. Yet, the functions often appear as if they are biphasic; divided into low-intensity (scotopic) and high-intensity (photopic-like) sections, although their dynamic range is usually that of the scotopic system.

Table 10.2 provides a summary of 37 psychophysical investigations, which have measured dark-adaptation, spatial acuity, flicker sensitivity and increment threshold in the achromat. Many more studies of the achromat's vision have been published (for a survey of studies up to 1955, see François *et al.*, 1955). The table, however, lists only those in which the subjects were clearly identified as typical, complete achromats and in which the measurements were quantitative enough to decide whether the functions were biphasic or not. The majority of the achromats whose dark-adaptation (49 of 90 cases), spatial acuity (5 of 7), critical flicker frequency (8 of 8), or increment threshold sensitivity (8 of 14 cases) was measured, had duplex curves as a function of the independent variable, adapting level or time in the dark.

What is to be made of this? To start with, it is unlikely that the discontinuities or breaks are due to independent receptor systems. This is because, at both low- and high-intensity adaptation levels, almost all typical, complete achromats show only the spectral sensitivity of the rods (Alpern, 1974). Moreover, their dynamic range of function is almost invariably limited by rod saturation. Still, it is possible that variation may exist among achromats. Some may have rod-like cones, whereas others, like K.N., have not.

10.7.1 Dark-adaptation

If cone or cone-like activity in the complete achromat is normally suppressed or masked by rod activity, the best chance to find it or its remnants would seem to be during the first seconds or minutes in the dark after an adapting or bleaching light has been extinguished. If some cones are functioning, their activity might be revealed by a fast recovery branch or high-intensity plateau of the dark-adaptation curve. As indicated in Table 10.2, this is what is frequently found in many achromats. Is there evidence for a fast cone recovery branch in the dark-adaptation curves of K.N. as well?

Figs. 10.6–10.8 summarize dark-adaptation thresholds measured in K.N. (filled symbols) and in a normal trichromat (open symbols), under the same conditions (Nordby *et al.*, 1984). The target was a 1 × 2 deg, 500 ms flash presented 7 deg nasally to the fixation point in the visual field (for K.N., this would be about 6 deg nasally). The following parameters were varied: (1) retinal illumination during pre-adaptation (Fig. 10.6; target wavelength 490 nm); (2) duration of pre-adaptation at a retinal illumination of 143 200 scotopic td (Fig. 10.7; target wavelength 550 nm); and (3) target wavelength (Fig. 10.8; pre-adaptation 143 200 scotopic td for 3 min). Depending on the intensity and duration of the bleach and the wavelength of the target, the normal curves are either biphasic, containing both cone (upper) and rod (lower) branches, or monophasic, containing only a rod branch. But K.N.'s curves are all monophasic, containing a single rod branch, regardless of the bleach and target conditions. The sets of curves nicely illustrate how rod adaptation proceeds undelayed by cone adaptation. The alpha (or Kohlrausch) break in the normal observer occurs as a passive consequence at a time and threshold where the cone curve of the normal is intersected by the descending rod curve of the achromat.

The similarly shaped curves, shown in Fig. 10.6–10.8, were all measured at about 6 deg in K.N.'s nasal field of view. It seems reasonable to ask whether or not differently shaped curves (i.e. curves with two branches) might be measured at other retinal eccentricities, since the distribution of a second type of high-intensity receptor might change with retinal location. Sloan, for instance, maintained that she almost invariably found kinks in the dark-adaptation curves of complete achromats when the rate of dark-adaptation was measured at 15 deg from fixation in the nasal field (Sloan, 1954, 1958; Sloan & Feiock, 1972). For K.N., however, retinal eccentricity does not seem to make any difference. Similarly shaped curves were measured with a 1 × 2 deg, 125 ms target at K.N.'s area of preferred fixation and at about 6 deg and 45 deg in his nasal field of view (Stabell, Stabell & Nordby, 1986). Thus, there is no evidence from K.N. that the dark-adaptation process in the achromat is bipartite, differentiating into high- and low-intensity sections similar to those found in the normal trichromat.

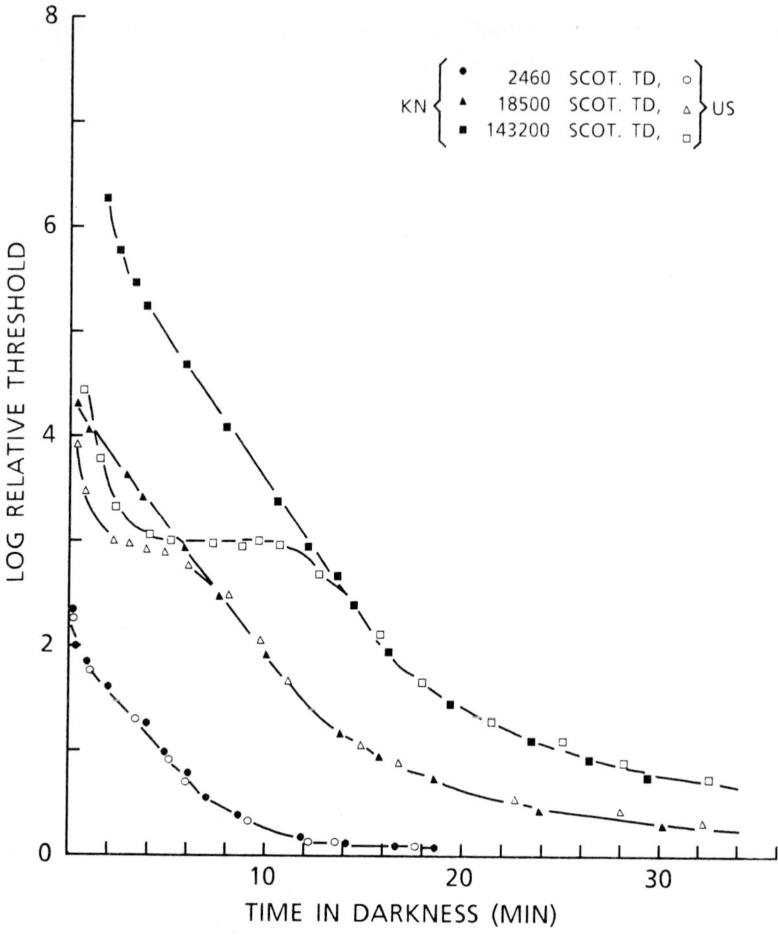

Fig. 10.6. Dark-adaptation thresholds for the achromat K.N. (filled symbols) and a normal trichromat observer U.S. (open symbols) measured following various retinal illuminations during pre-adaptation. The target wavelength was 490 nm. The zero ordinate represents the absolute threshold measured in the completely dark-adapted state. (From Nordby *et al.*, 1984.)

This is markedly different from the results often reported in other achromats; and there are a few points to be made about why this may be so. In some cases, but by no means all, it is possible to discount the finding of double-branched dark-adaptation functions as spurious or as over-interpreted. For instance, the evidence for breaks at high intensity levels in the curves presented by Sloan & Newall (1942) and Blackwell & Blackwell (1961) is very slight. In other cases, the evidence for breaks is not wholly presented, but only referred to (Blakemore &

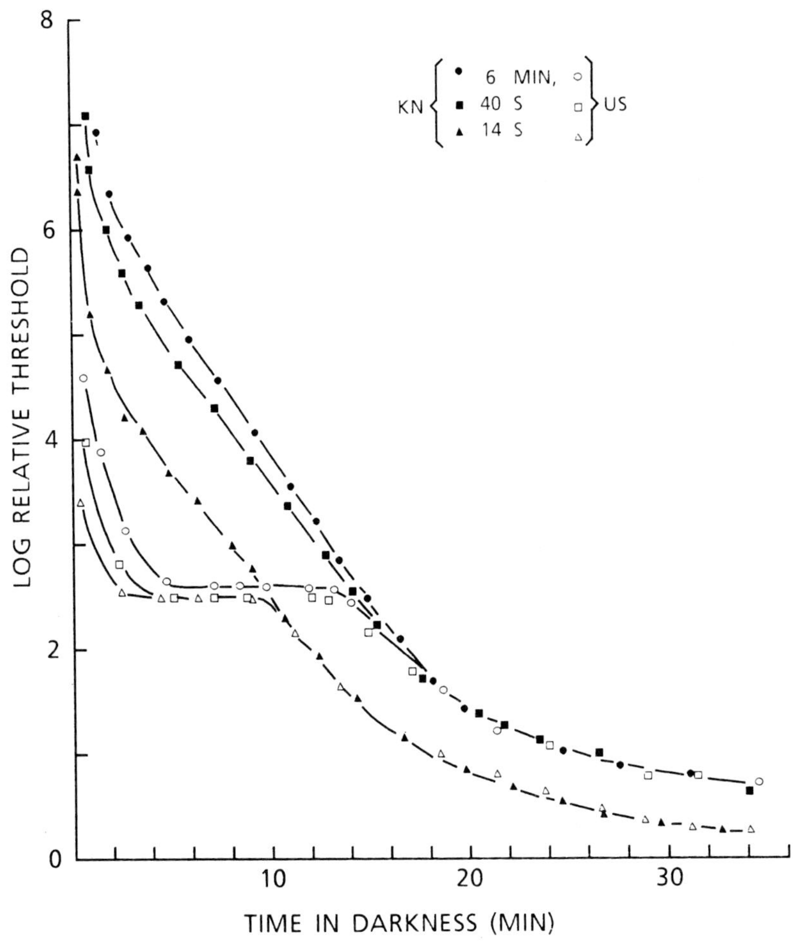

Fig. 10.7. Dark-adaptation thresholds for the achromat K.N. (filled symbols) and a normal trichromat observer U.S. (open symbols) measured following various durations of pre-adaptation at a retinal illumination of 143 200 scotopic td. The target wavelength was 550 nm. The zero ordinate represents the absolute threshold measured in the complete dark-adaptation state. (From Nordby *et al.*, 1984.)

Rushton, 1965, p. 616) or given in part (Alpern *et al.*, 1960, p. 1002). Sometimes the evidence for breaks is only found in the fovea (e.g. Walls & Heath, 1954), where the histology of achromats suggests there are no receptors; sometimes the evidence is found in both the fovea and periphery. In some cases, the upper part of the curve (i.e. the part of the curve above the kink) lies more than a $\log_{10}$ unit higher than the upper part of the curve of the average colour-normal subject (Sloan, 1954;

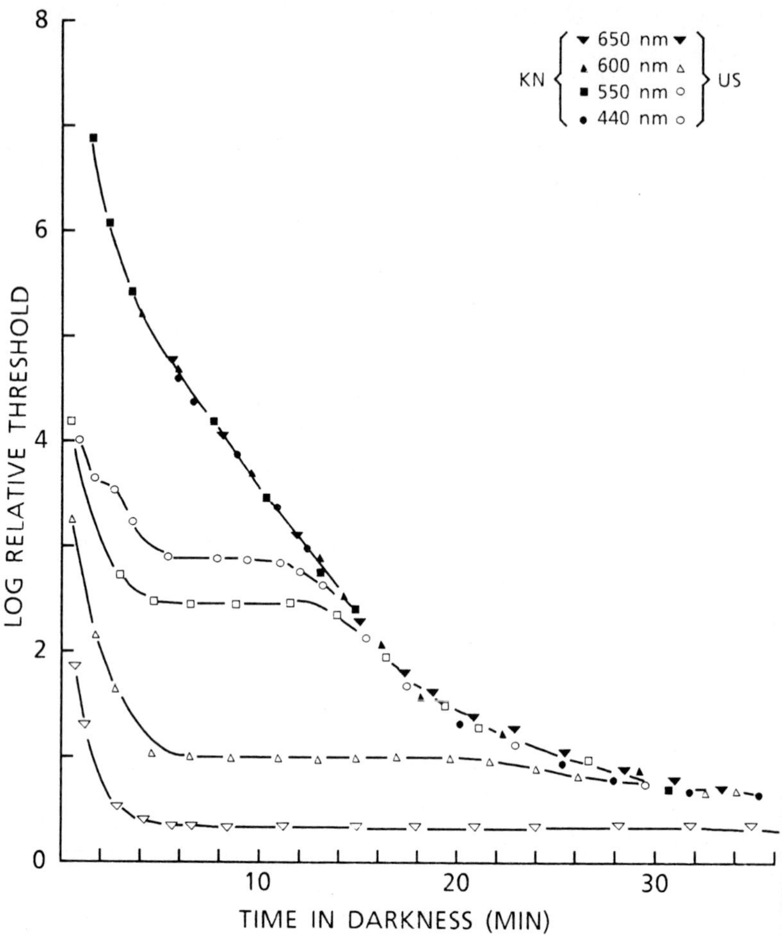

Fig. 10.8 Dark-adaptation thresholds for the achromat K.N. (filled symbols) and a normal trichromat observer U.S. (open symbols) measured with several target wavelengths. The intensity of the white pre-adapting field was 143200 scotopic td and its duration was 3 min. The zero ordinate represents the absolute threshold measured for each wavelength in the completely dark-adapted state. (From Nordby *et al.*, 1984.)

1958). This last discrepancy may be explained by the finding that many subjects assumed to be typical, complete achromats, may actually be incomplete types with sparing of cone function in the peripheral retina (Pokorny *et al.*, 1982; Krastel *et al.*, 1983) or they may be examples of cone degeneration (this may especially be true of some of the patients described by Sloan, 1954; see Krill *et al.*, 1973, pp. 71–2). Residual cone function may be revealed in such cases if large test stimuli are used

(Krastel *et al.*, 1983; see Sharpe & Nordby, Total colour-blindness: an introduction, Chapter 7).

Even if definite breaks are measured, they might be caused by other factors. It is possible that the early or upper branch of the achromat's dark-adaptation curve is an artefact, resulting from the achromat's unstable fixation or from his use of scattered light to define threshold. For instance, if the retinal area exposed to the bleaching light is limited, the rods outside this area will not be bleached, and hence will remain fairly dark-adapted and capable of being excited by stray light if sufficiently intense (Rushton, 1961). Or, it is possible that the early branch is an artefact arising from too frequently sampling threshold during dark-adaptation, which can elevate threshold and give the appearance of false plateaux and false bumps. A long training period may be necessary to obtain valid results.

The importance of training is highlighted by what seems to us to be misleading reports that the final rod threshold in typical, complete achromats is reached much sooner than in normals (Rushton, 1961; Alpern, 1971; Sakitt 1976*a*; Krill, 1977). Faster recovery also appeared to be the case for K.N. In the earliest measurements made with him as an observer, his half-recovery times (i.e. the time required for the threshold to reach half the fully dark-adapted value) were about half as long as those of normal observers. But in the latest measurements his half-recovery times are similar to those of normals (Nordby *et al.*, 1984). The difference may be due to less effective pigment bleaching in the untrained subject. Nystagmus and light-avoidance behaviour (such as squinting and blinking) will tend to reduce the amount of light that enters the eye and must be taken into account when determining retinal illumination and thresholds. K.N. is now aware of this problem and takes measures to reduce his squinting and blinking during pre-adaptation (see Chapter 8). Infra-red monitoring of his eye with feedback during threshold experiments helps prevent him from decreasing retinal illumination by partially closing his eyelids, particularly at high adaptation levels. During threshold measurements, he also guards against using information from the target after-images which are enhanced by blinking. Sakitt (1976*b*) has shown that such after-images provide information that differs from that obtained from real images.

10.7.2 Increment threshold

Save for the dark-adaptation curves, the most frequently cited evidence for double-branching in the achromat comes from increment threshold functions. Although Table 10.2 lists three studies giving evidence in support of double-branching, two of these studies (Alpern *et al.*, 1960; Blakemore & Rushton, 1965) actually present no curves. The third study (Hecht *et al.*, 1948) presents functions measured for a completely colour-blind observer, with blue (450 nm) and red (670 nm) light. The two functions are double-branched, with the transition occurring at a level near 0.5 $\log_{10}$ scotopic td. Both branches have the spectral sensitivity distribution of the rods. On the basis of this and similarly double-branched critical fusion frequency data (see below), Hecht and his co-workers concluded that two kinds of rods are present in the achromat eye: one kind containing the usual concentration of rhodopsin and functioning at low intensities; the other containing rhodopsin in much lower concentration and functioning at higher intensities. Their results have been used to support the 'day rod' theory of the achromat visual system (see Chapter 7). But there are problems with the interpretation that Hecht *et al.*'s observer is a typical, complete achromat. For one thing, his visual acuity is rather high: it reaches a value of 0.18 measured with square-wave gratings (see below). For another thing, Hecht *et al.* were able to measure his acuity at a log retinal illuminance of 4.54 $\log_{10}$ photopic td or 5.59 $\log_{10}$ scotopic td (see Hecht *et al.*, 1948, Table II; the conversion was made at a dominant wavelength of 490 nm according to the factors given in Wyszecki & Stiles, 1982, p. 104). This intensity is more than 2.0 $\log_{10}$ units above the saturation limit reported in all other typical, complete achromats (see above). It may be, therefore, that the colour-blind observer of Hecht *et al.* (1948) was not a typical, complete achromat, but rather a blue-cone monochromat (see Sharpe & Nordby, Total colour-blindness: an introduction, Chapter 7); and that their tests were not sensitive enough to reveal the participation of the short-wavelength sensitive cones in his visual functions.

The results for K.N., our subject and model, on the other hand, are consistent with no residual cone function and with the 'rod-only' theory. Stabell, Nordby & Stabell (1987) measured many t.v.i. functions for K.N. and compared them with curves measured under the same conditions for two normal trichromats. Fig. 10.9 shows the results obtained with a 520 nm, 125 ms duration target superimposed on a 525 nm, 7.5

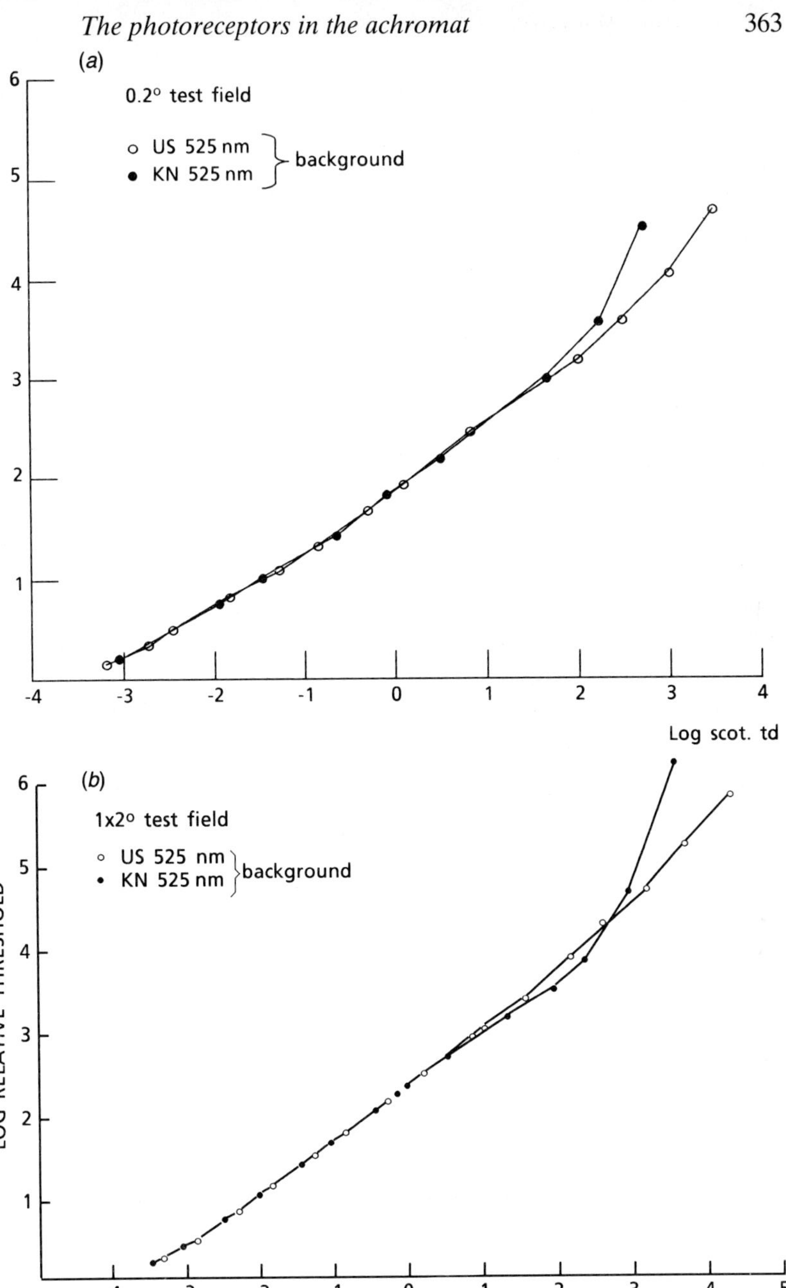

Fig. 10.9 Increment threshold is plotted against background intensity for the achromat K.N. (●) and a normal observer U.S. (○). A 520 nm, 125 ms target was presented at 7 deg in the nasal visual field. It was centred on a 525 nm, 7.5 deg diameter background. In panel (*a*), the target subtended 0.2 deg in diameter; in panel (*b*), it subtended 1×2 deg. The increment thresholds are given in log threshold units relative to the absolute threshold. (Modified from Stabell *et al.*, 1987.)

deg diameter background; the target was either small (0.2 deg in diameter; Fig. 10.9*a*) or large (1 × 2 deg; Fig. 10.9*b*). For the smaller target (*a*), the curves for K.N. and the normal (U.S.) are essentially identical over almost the entire range of adapting luminances; even the absolute dark-adapted thresholds are in close agreement (note, only $\log_{10}$ relative threshold values are given in the figure). Only when the retinal illuminance of the background rises above 2.0 $\log_{10}$ scotopic td do the two curves diverge. The achromat's curve rises steeply, presaging the onset of saturation in the rod visual system (see Aguilar & Stiles, 1954; Baylor *et al.*, 1984). The normal observer's curve, on the other hand, shows no sign of saturating because the cones supersede the rods in detecting the target.

For the larger target (*b*), a similar course of desensitization is found for the two observers. At the lower adapting backgrounds, the slope of both curves is steeper (*c.* 0.65) than that found with the smaller target (*c.* 0.5). This is to be expected for a change in target parameters (see, for example, Barlow, 1958). What is not expected is that the trichromat's curve proceeds above K.N.'s shortly before K.N.'s onset of saturation. This deviation can be readily explained, however, by assuming that cones activated by the background are reducing the sensitivity of the rods in the normal to the target (Sharpe *et al.*, 1989*a*).

Similar t.v.i. functions were measured against backgrounds of 425 nm and 640 nm (not shown). For K.N., the t.v.i. curves coincided over the whole adapting range, when equated for rod quantal absorptions, suggesting that the rod system completely determines his sensitivity (Stabell *et al.*, 1987). In contrast, for the trichromats, the curves measured against the 640 nm background had a much steeper slope than the curves measured against the 425 nm and 525 nm backgrounds. The source of this deviation, as with the 525 nm background, must be signals from the cones in the normal. The effect may be larger for the 640 nm than for the 525 nm background because the absolute sensitivities of the rods and cones lie closer together at long wavelengths (for a fuller explanation, see Chapter 2).

That K.N. displays no double-branching in his curves is further confirmed by increment thresholds measured for various durations (8–1000 ms, Fig. 10.10) and retinal eccentricities (7–40 deg, Fig. 10.11). In each case, below the background intensities at which the rods saturate in the achromat and at which rod–cone interactions occur in the normal

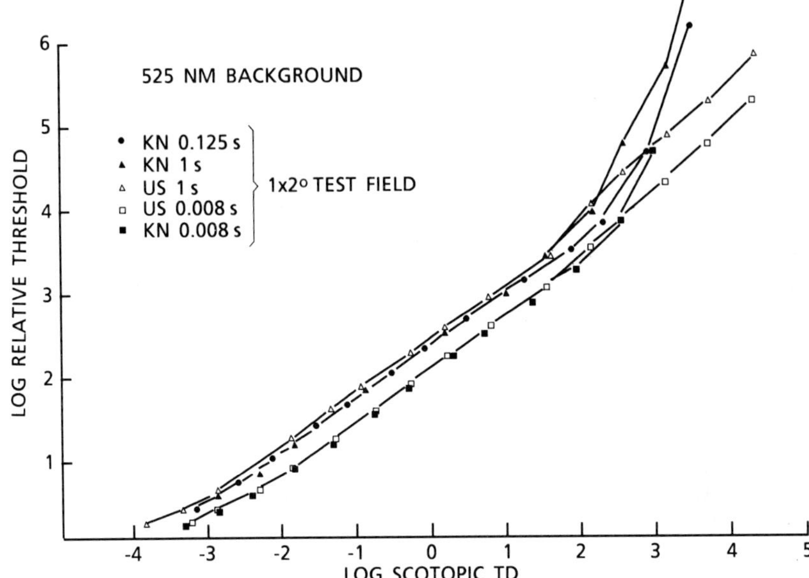

Fig. 10.10. Increment threshold curves measured with different target durations for the achromat K.N. (filled symbols) and a normal observer U.S. (open symbols). The 520 nm target, subtending 1 × 2 deg, was presented at 7 deg in the nasal field of view. It was centred on a 525 nm background subtending 7.5 deg in diameter. (From Stabell *et al.*, 1987.)

(*c.* 1.5 $\log_{10}$ scotopic td), the t.v.i. curves of K.N. and the normal are essentially identical in shape. (For the target and background conditions chosen, the normal also shows single-branched curves.)

Stabell *et al.* (1987) interpret all the t.v.i. curves of K.N. as consisting of two major ascending sections below the region where his rod visual system saturates. The first section, they argue, has a slope that may change with test parameters. At 7 deg eccentricity, for small test field sizes (0.12–0.4 deg), it is close to 0.5. This finding is in accord with fluctuation theory, which predicts that the threshold should rise as the square root of background illuminance (see Chapters 1 and 2). For larger test field sizes and even for small test field sizes at greater retinal eccentricities, Stabell *et al.* (1987) find that the slope increases, attaining a value as large as 0.65. The second section, they argue, has a slope of about 0.65, which is approximately independent of size (0.2–2 deg), exposure time (0.008–1 s) and eccentricity (7–40 deg nasally) of the test field.

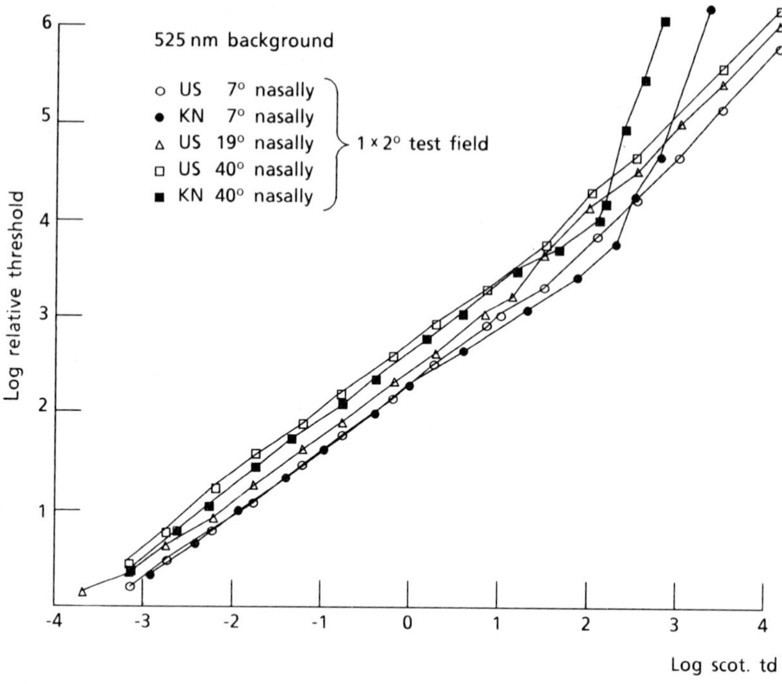

Fig. 10.11. Increment threshold curves measured at different retinal eccentricities for the achromat K.N. (filled symbols) and a normal observer U.S. (open symbols). The 520 nm, 125 ms target subtended 1 × 2 deg. It was centred on a 525 nm background subtending 7.5 deg in diameter. (Modified from Stabell *et al.* 1987.)

The difference in slope between the two sections is consistent with the notion that the rod visual system switches from being quantum-limited to being gain-control limited, depending upon the target parameters and the background illuminance (see Chapter 2). However, one would not expect the slope of the second section to remain invariant for larger target sizes and longer target durations. In fact, one would expect the second section – and the first section as well – to have a slope closer to 1.0, the value predicted by Weber's Law (i.e. threshold is directly proportional to background intensity). This is what is found in the normal observer when the increment threshold function is measured under the classic rod-isolation conditions of Aguilar & Stiles (1954); i.e. a large area (9 deg in diameter) and long duration (200 ms) target.

What about curves measured in K.N. for the conditions of Aguilar &

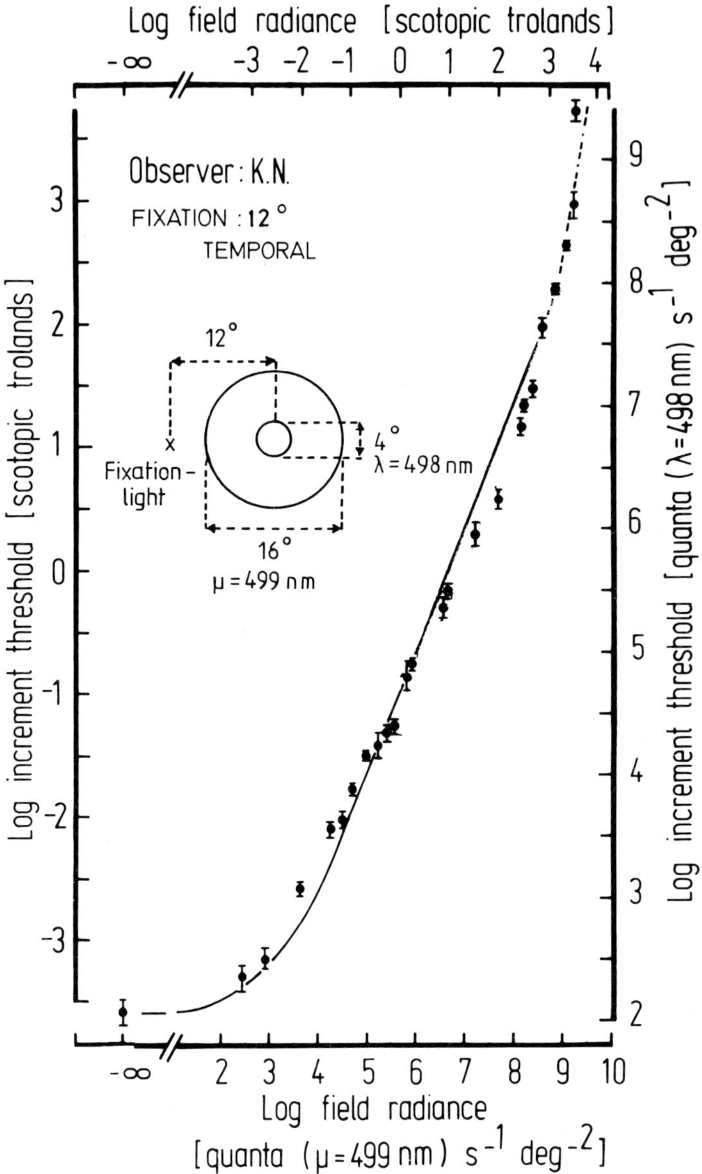

Fig. 10.12. Increment thresholds for achromat K.N. plotted as a function of background intensity. The 498 nm, 197 ms, 4.0 deg in diameter, target and the 499 nm, 16 deg diameter, background were imaged at a point 12 deg temporal from his fovea. The error bars indicate two standard errors of the mean. The continuous curve fit through the threshold data is a rod mechanism template derived from Aguilar & Stiles (1954). The inset shows K.N.'s field of view. (Modified from Sharpe *et al.*, 1988*b*.)

Stiles (1954)? Sharpe *et al.* (1988*b*) investigated t.v.i. curves in K.N. under conditions closely approximating those of Aguilar & Stiles (1954). They presented a 4 deg diameter, 197 ms, 498 nm target, centred 12 deg nasally in the external visual field against a 16 deg diameter background. The only important departures from the classic Aguilar & Stiles conditions were that the target entry in the pupil was central and the background was blue-green (499 nm), not red (see Chapter 2). The results for achromat background are shown in Fig. 10.12, where they are compared with the average curve Aguilar & Stiles obtained from four normal observers (see Wyszecki & Stiles, 1982, p. 547). Clearly the thresholds rise steeper for the Aguilar & Stiles (1954) mean observer than for K.N. The long linear desensitization region (i.e. from −2.0 to 2.0 $\log_{10}$ scotopic td) of the Aguilar & Stiles function has a slope of 0.95 on logarithmic coordinates, whereas that for K.N. has a slope of 0.84 (repeated measurements of K.N.'s function now indicate that it has a fixed slope of 0.77 ± 0.3; see also Chapter 2).

The Aguilar & Stiles function, however, provides an excellent fit to the function of a normal trichromat measured under the same conditions (see Sharpe *et al.*, 1989*a*). Confronted with this problem, Sharpe *et al.* (1988*b*; see their Fig. 4) originally took the deviations to mean that a second rod process was intruding in K.N.'s curve; an interpretation consistent with the flicker sensitivity functions measured in the achromat and the normal (see below) and with the results of Hecht *et al.* (1948). They divided K.N.'s data into two branches, without allowing for the possibility of cone intrusion affecting the normal curve. The extensive comparisons made by Stabell *et al.* (1987) between K.N.'s and the normal's results, however, patently require that allowances for cone interactions be taken into account. For if the Aguilar & Stiles function is contaminated by cone signals, arising from the long-wavelength background, bending the curve upward at high adapting intensities, then there is no reason why it should provide a good fit to K.N.'s t.v.i. functions (see Chapter 2).

That cone intrusion is elevating the rod increment threshold in the normal has since been confirmed by t.v.i. functions measured under the full rod isolation conditions of Aguilar & Stiles (Fach & Sharpe, 1988; Sharpe *et al.*, 1989*a*). As expected, against a 640 nm background, which strongly adapts the long-wavelength cones in the normal, the slope is shallower for K.N. (0.77 ± 0.03) than for a normal trichromat (0.96 ± 0.03); whereas, against a short-wavelength (450 nm) background, which does not strongly adapt the cones, the slope is identical for K.N. (0.75 ± 0.04) and the trichromat (0.75 ± 0.04). Similarly low gradients are found for K.N.'s curves measured against backgrounds of 520 nm (0.78) and 560 nm (0.79); and for the normal (520 nm: 0.76 ± 0.05; 560 nm: 0.77 ± 0.06). In none of these curves is there evidence for double-branching. Thus, all the t.v.i. results measured for K.N. confirm the hypothesis (after Galezowski) that all his visual functions take place wholly in the rods.

10.7.3 Spatial sensitivity

Alpern *et al.* (1960) assert, but present no data, that in the achromat measurements of acuity as a function of intensity for various coloured lights differentiate into low- and high-intensity sections, both having the spectral sensitivity of the rods. This dichotomy was not found by König (1894), nor by Hecht *et al.* (1948). In fact, Hecht *et al.* (1948) reported only a monotonic relation between visual acuity (measured with square-wave gratings) and retinal illuminance in the achromat eye. The function, which levelled off at a visual acuity of about 0.16 for intensities above 0.5 $\log_{10}$ scotopic td, corresponded to the rod acuity function of the normal eye.

Spatial contrast sensitivity measurements made in K.N., who has a visual acuity of about 0.1 with the Snellen and Ostberg charts and 0.12 with the laser interferometry test, corroborate Hecht *et al.* (Hess & Nordby, 1986*a*, *b*). The data are summarized in Fig. 10.13, in which the spatial acuity of K.N. and a normal trichromat are compared at various levels of retinal illuminance (see also Chapter 11 for complete spatial contrast sensitivity functions). The spatial acuity was defined as the highest spatial frequency of a 100% contrast sine-wave grating that could be resolved at each level. The gratings subtended 10 × 15 deg and were centred at 2 deg in the nasal field of view. The results for the normal eye show the well established double-branched function representing rod- and cone-mediated function (Hecht & Mintz, 1939). The lower scotopic branch of the acuity function is identical for the normal and K.N. However, just above the point of intersection of the photopic and scotopic acuity branches for normal vision, the acuity of K.N. ceases to increase with increasing illuminance. A plateau (approximately 6 cycles deg^{-1}) is reached between 13 and 130 scotopic td, after which acuity falls abruptly, asymptoting at 1800 (3.26 $\log_{10}$) scotopic td. Hess, Nordby & Pointer (1987) confirmed these results at other retinal

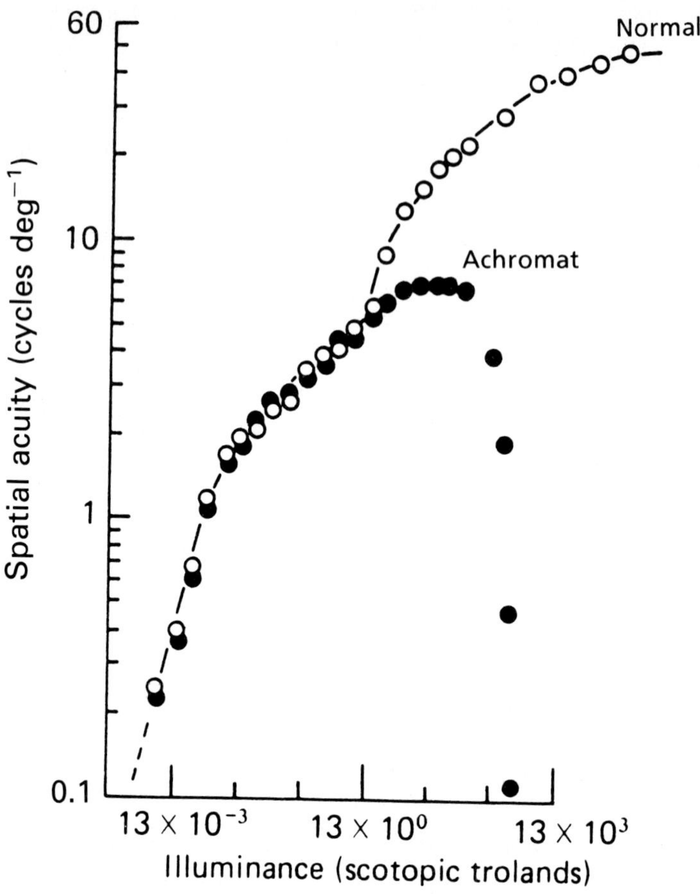

Fig. 10.13. Spatial acuity for a sine-wave grating of 100% contrast is plotted against mean retinal illuminance for the achromat K.N. (●) and a normal observer (○). (From Hess & Nordby, 1986*a*.)

eccentricities, always finding that under scotopic conditions the regional fall-off in spatial sensitivity was similar for K.N. and the normal trichromat. The abrupt drop in K.N.'s sensitivity at 1800 scotopic td is consistent with saturation of the rod visual system (for more details, see Chapter 11). Thus, the spatial properties of the scotopic mechanism are similar for the normal and achromat; whereas the photopic mechanism possessed by the normal is absent in the achromat.

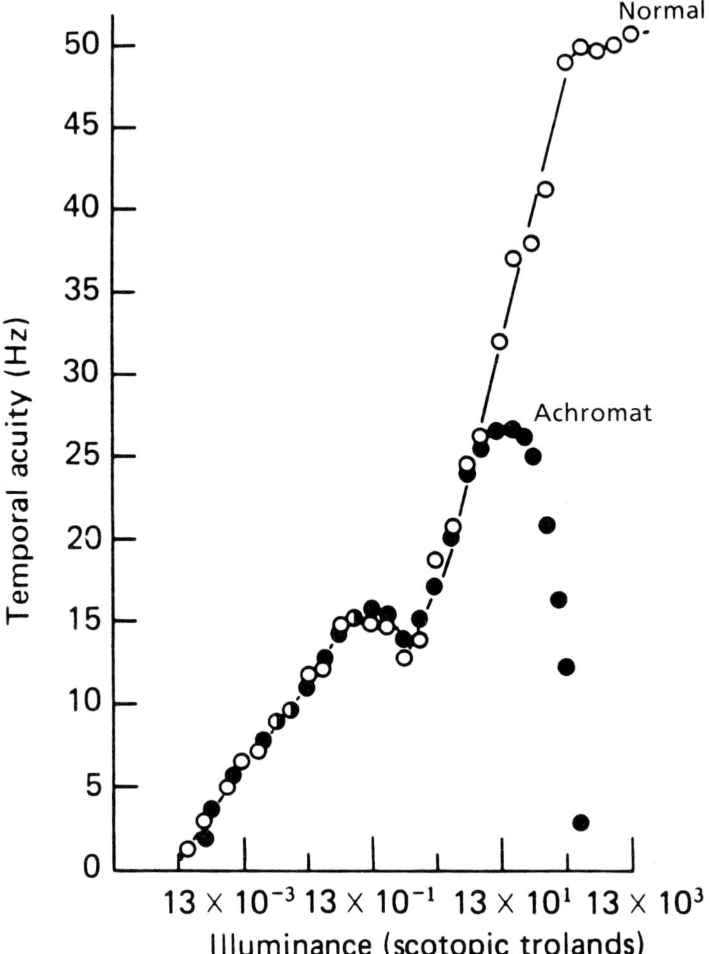

Fig. 10.14. Temporal resolution (here labelled acuity) for an unpatterned 10 deg circular test field sinusoidally modulated in time is plotted against illuminance for the achromat K.N. (●) and a normal observer (○). The test field was presented with a 40 × 60 deg surrounding field matched in mean illuminance. (From Hess & Nordby, 1986*a*.)

10.7.4 Flicker sensitivity

Discontinuities in the flicker sensitivity curve have also been taken to indicate that the achromat's vision is not mediated purely by the rods. And, indeed, every achromat so far tested has shown double-branching (Hecht *et al.*, 1948; Alpern *et al.*, 1960; Blakemore & Rushton, 1965). This is also true for K.N. His temporal resolution (i.e. critical flicker fusion or CFF) as a function of illuminance, as well as that of a normal observer, is shown in Fig. 10.14. The stimulus was a centrally fixated, sinusoidally flickering (modulation depth of 0.95), 10 deg diameter, unpatterned field presented within a mean luminance-matched surround (Hess & Nordby, 1986*a*).

Two things are worth noting about the curves. The first is that the results for K.N. are identical to those for the normal from the absolute threshold up to a mean illuminance of around 80 scotopic td (yielding a temporal resolution of 28 Hz); whereafter K.N.'s resolution, unlike the normal's, levels off and then rapidly falls to zero at around 2000 scotopic td. Thus K.N.'s temporal resolution attains only half that of the normal (*c.* 55 Hz) and its precipitous fall-off at higher intensities, like that of his spatial acuity, accords with the saturation of the rod visual system (for more details see Chapter 11). This result, confirmed at other retinal eccentricities (Hess *et al.*, 1987), is consistent with comparisons that have been made between K.N.'s and the normal's ability to temporally summate light energy for detection (Sharpe, Fach & Nordby, 1988*a*). At low background luminances where the rods mediate detection, the critical duration (i.e. the longest value at which target duration and luminance are reciprocal in their effects upon threshold) is the same for K.N. and the normal (see Fig. 10.15); decreasing from approximately 200 ms in darkness to approximately 130 ms against a background of 0.6 scotopic td. At a moderately high background of 813 scotopic td, however, where the cones mediate detection in the normal, the critical duration of K.N. does not further decrease, whereas that of the normal does by a factor of 3 (to about 40 ms).

The second thing to note in Fig. 10.14 is that, for both subjects, the function is double-branched, with the kink in the curve occurring around 5 scotopic td. (There is no comparable kink in the spatial acuity curve.) This kink must be characteristic of both the achromat and normal visual systems since it is found in both for stimuli of different modulation depth (0.6, 0.8 and 0.95), angular subtense (0.2, 0.8, 2 and 2.4 cycles deg^{-1}) and retinal position (0, 5, 10, 15, 20 and 25 deg temporal and nasal) (Hess & Norby, 1986*a*,; Hess *et al.*, 1987). Originally, the kink was thought to be due to a transition from rod- to cone-mediated vision (Hecht & Shlaer, 1936) or, in the case of the achromat, to a transition from rod to a high-intensity receptor-mediated (i.e. day rod or rhodospin cone) vision (Hecht et al., 1948). However, since the double-branched function is observed for both the rod response of K.N. and the rod-

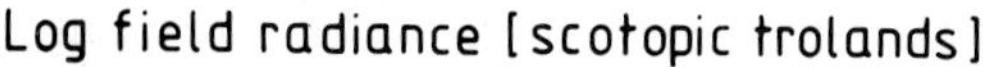

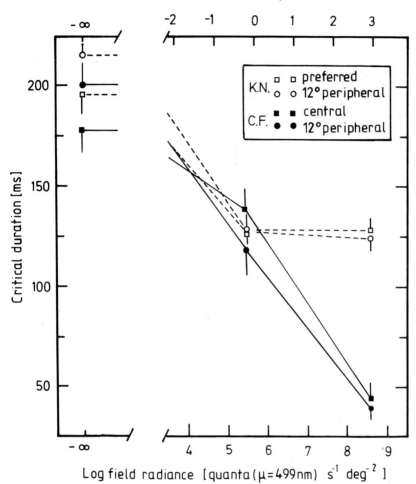

Fig. 10.15. The critical duration values (± 2 SEM) for K.N. (open symbols) and for a normal observer (C.F.; filled symbols) plotted as a function of adapting field radiance. The squares indicate central viewing (or preferred fixation for K.N.); the circles, 12 deg peripheral viewing. (From Sharpe *et al.*, 1988*a*.)

isolated response of the trichromat, it must be due solely to the normally functioning rods. Similar breaks can be seen near 8 scotopic td in the CFF thresholds of Hecht *et al.*'s colour-blind observer (their Fig. 6), measured with both large (19 deg diameter) and small (3 deg diameter) fields of 450 nm and 670 nm.

The breaks may signify an internal duplexity of organisation in the rod

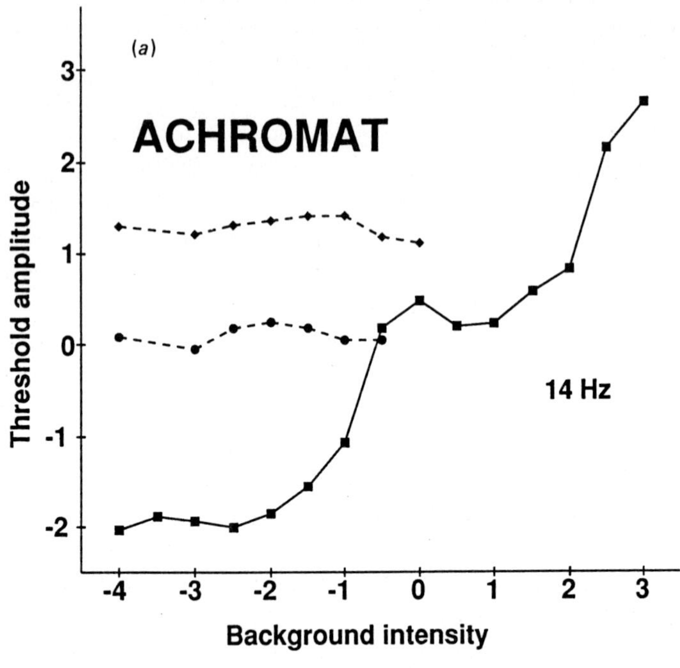
(a)
ACHROMAT
14 Hz
Threshold amplitude
Background intensity
3
2
1
0
-1
-2
-4
-3
-2
-1
0
1
2
3

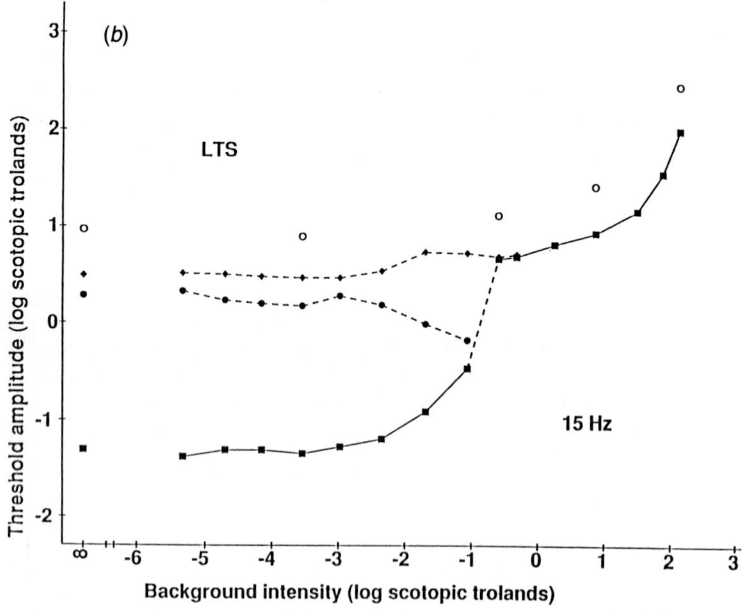
(b)
LTS
15 Hz
Threshold amplitude (log scotopic trolands)
Background intensity (log scotopic trolands)
3
2
1
0
-1
-2
∞
-6
-5
-4
-3
-2
-1
0
1
2
3

visual system (Conner & MacLeod, 1977; Conner, 1982; Sharpe, Stockman & MacLeod, 1989*b*). Supporting evidence for this hypothesis comes from the flicker detectability data of K.N., which like that of the normal, exhibit at certain frequencies a region well above the conventional flicker threshold within which no flicker is seen (Stockman *et al.*, 1990; Sharpe *et al.*, 1989*b*). This region can be attributed to destructive interference between rod signals transmitted along two pathways; one of which is sluggish and sensitive, functioning in dim light, and the other of which is quick and less sensitive, functioning in mesopic light (Conner & MacLeod, 1977; Conner, 1982; Sharpe *et al.*, 1989*b*). (A null region due to destructive interference between rod and cone signals can also be demonstrated in the normal observer with a mesopic yellow target flickering around 7.5 Hz; see MacLeod, 1972, 1974.)

Fig. 10.16 shows the average flicker thresholds (scale of the ordinates) measured with a 500 nm, 6 deg in diameter, target flickering at 14 Hz for K.N. (panel (*a*)) and at 15 Hz for a normal observer (L.T.S.; panel (*b*)). The scale of the abscissae indicates the intensity of a red background field, upon which the target was superimposed. For both observers, the conventional flicker function (squares) contains two distinct branches. The transition from one branch to the other occurs at about 0.25 $\log_{10}$ scotopic td (total time-average intensity). Both branches are due to the rods and fall below the cone flicker thresholds measured in the normal for the same target conditions (panel (*b*); open circles). The cone thresholds, which are being mediated by the middle-wavelength sensitive cones, were measured during the plateau that terminates the cone phase of recovery from a white bleaching light of about 7.7 $\log_{10}$ scotopic td-s.

Fig. 10.16. The 14–15 Hz flicker detectability data for K.N. (panel (*a*)) and for a normal observer (L.T.S.; panel (*b*)). The 500 nm, square-wave flickering target subtended 6 deg of visual angle in diameter and was centred 13 deg temporally from the observer's fovea. It was superimposed upon a steady background, which subtended 18 deg (K.N.) or 11.5 deg (L.T.S.) of visual angle and which had a wavelength of 640 nm (K.N.) or 684 nm (L.T.S.). The squares represent the lowest amplitude at which flicker can just be seen, measured as a function of intensity. The filled circles and diamonds designate the lower and upper limits, respectively, of a nulled region, within which flicker cannot be seen. Strong flicker is seen both above and below this region. The open circles (only for L.T.S.) are cone thresholds measured during the cone phase of recovery following a 7.7 $\log_{10}$ scotopic td-s bleach. (Modified from Stockman *et al.*, 1990), and from Sharpe *et al.*, 1989*b*.)

For both the normal and K.N., who does not have any cone thresholds, the upper and lower branches are separated by a range of luminance within which the flicker is completely invisible. The lower and upper limits of this nulled region are denoted by the filled circles and diamonds, respectively. Above and below these limits, strong flicker can be seen. We assume that within the null region both the sluggish and fast rod processes are active, but that their signals, which are similar in magnitude, are 180 deg out of phase and interfere destructively to cancel the perception of flicker (Stockman *et al.*, 1990; Sharpe *et al.*, 1989*b*). This interpretation has been confirmed by electroretinographic recordings (Stockman *et al.*, 1990).

10.8 The electroretinogram

The psychophysical results reviewed above are based on tests that probe the sensitivity of localized areas of the retina. The tests were made at several retinal eccentricities to determine if cone or cone-like responses are confined to one small central or paracentral region. However, the areas of the retina tested may have been too small to yield a measurable cone signal; especially since the cones shown by histological studies seem to be widely separated from one another and confined to peripheral regions. The possibility remains, therefore, that the function of the remaining cones may only be detectable when large areas of the retina are simultaneously tested.

The Ganzfield electroretinogram (ERG) offers a means of testing this possibility. It is a mass response of the whole retina (see Chapter 12). When elicited by flickering light, the ERG normally consists of an initial (cornea-) negative response or a-wave, believed to originate in the receptor layer, followed by a (cornea-) positive response or b-wave, believed to originate in the inner nuclear layer. Both the a-wave and b-wave are composed of a rapid photopic component (referred to as a_p and b_p, respectively) and a slower scotopic component (referred to as a_s and b_s, respectively). The conspicuousness of these components depends, in part, upon the wavelength, frequency and intensity of the flickering light and the state of adaptation of the eye. The components are best distinguished when elicited by long-wavelength light stimuli of high intensity.

In achromat observers, the most frequent observation is that the faster photopic components of the ERG are extinguished, while the scotopic components are normal (Waardenburg, 1963; Krill, 1977*a*). In particular, the a_p component is reported as missing or severely reduced and the b_p component (or photopic x-wave) as completely absent (Vukovich, 1952; Dodt & Wadensten, 1954; Wadensten, 1954; Goodman & Bornschein, 1957; François, Verriest & Renard, 1959; François, Verriest & de Rouck, 1956; Schappert-Kimmijser, 1958; von Assen, 1960; Pabst & Echte, 1962; Jayle, Boyer & Aubert, 1962; François, de Rouck & Verriest, 1963; Goodman, Ripps & Siegel, 1963; Krill, 1966; Berson, Gouras & Hoff 1969). Photopic components in the ERG, however, have been reported in some congenital achromats (see, for example, Goodman *et al.*, 1963; Dodt, van Lith & Schmidt, 1967; Auerbach & Merin, 1974); though it might be argued that when the ERG indicates photopic system responses – even if the case is clinically diagnosed as complete achromatopsia – the diagnosis should be changed to incomplete achromatopsia.

Abnormalities of the scotopic components of the ERG have been found in only a few complete achromats. One reported abnormality is a much more rapid increase in amplitude of the b_s component during the course of dark-adaptation (Elenius & Heck, 1957; Elenius & Zewi, 1958; Yonemura & Aoki, 1960; Frey, Heilig & Thaler, 1973; Auerbach & Merin, 1974). But this most likely is a measurement artefact. The reported advantage is small when compared as a percent of maximum amplitude (cf. Auerbach & Merin, 1974) and seems to be reasonably explained either by a slight reduction in the overall amplitude of the achromat b-wave (due to the absence of the cones) or by the achromat not receiving the full effectiveness of the preliminary light adaptation, by reason of a strongly contracted pupil and frequent blinking. Another reported abnormality is a change in the culmination time between the peak of the negative a-wave and the peak of the positive b-wave; and a corresponding change in the implicit time between the stimulus onset and the peak of the b-wave. Both the culmination and the implicit times of the achromat have been reported as being intermediate between those of the normal b_p and b_s components (François *et al.*, 1956). But this shift in latency may be due to a reduction in the b_s component in (mistakenly identified) incomplete achromat subjects, rather than to a speeding up of the a_s and b_s components in the typical complete achromat. A third reported abnormality is a supernormal amplitude of the achromat's b-wave (Krill, 1968). However, the larger amplitudes that have been shown are well within the range of inter-observer variability.

Neither photopic components nor abnormal scotopic ones are to be found in achromat K.N.'s ERG at any adapting level. As an example, Fig. 10.17 shows K.N.'s electroretinographic (b-wave) responses for three scotopic intensities of a 0.5 Hz flickering target: 0.97, 2.39 and 2.77 log scotopic td. The culmination times between the trough and peak of the b-wave at the three levels for K.N. (and the range for normal observers ± 2 SDs measured under the same conditions) are 68.0 (65–88 ms), 45.6 (47–71 ms) and 50.4 ms (32–47 ms). The amplitudes measured between the trough and peak of the b-wave for K.N. (and the range for normal observers ± 2 SDs) are 185.5 (125–225), 253.9 (185–290) and 249.0 (250–530) μV. Thus, K.N.'s scotopic components display neither a larger b-wave amplitude, nor a faster culmination time than those of normal observers.

Fig. 10.18 shows the ERG recordings from K.N. (right panel) and a normal observer (left panel), under photopic conditions. The stimulus conditions were chosen to suppress the activity of the rods and to favour the response of the long-wavelength sensitive (L) cones. Accordingly, a red (Wratten filter 29; Illuminant C, dominant wavelength 639 nm), test was presented against a blue background (Wratten filter 44; 6000 K, dominant wavelength 489 nm). The background had a luminance of 11.5 cd m^{-1} (3.60 log scotopic td). The test flickered at a rate of 1.5 Hz and was presented at four luminance levels: 0.23, 0.61, 0.91 and 1.18 log scotopic td. At all four intensities of the test stimulus, the normal observer shows a clear-cut, L-cone response. The latency and amplitude of the response for the four test intensities are: (1) 27.2 ms, 33.20 μV; (2) 28.0 ms, 42.96 μV; (3) 26.80 ms, 35.15 μV; and (4) 30.40 ms, 87.89 μV. K.N., on the other hand, shows no L-cone response at any of the four levels. This is emphasized by the fact that the voltage scale in the right panel is expanded eight times relative to that in the left panel. The small peak at the start of the response, within the first 10 ms, is a flash artefact. The large change in shape at the highest flash intensity is due to a pupillary response or large eye movement. If K.N. had residual cone function one would expect to find a consistent photopic ERG response with a similar latency to that found in the normal, but with a much reduced amplitude.

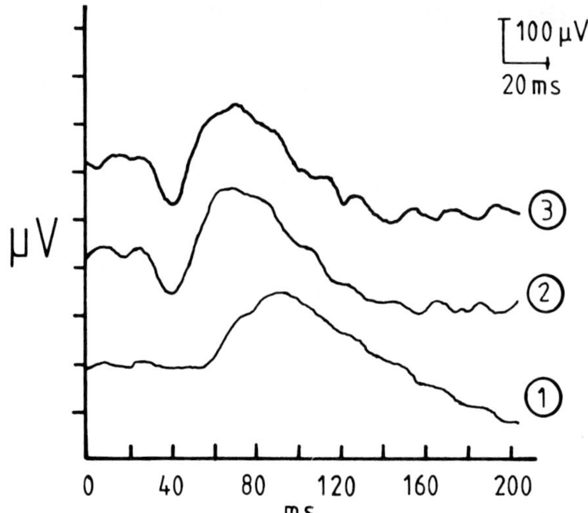

Fig. 10.17. Electroretinographic recordings made in achromat K.N., under scotopic conditions favouring the responses of the rods. A 0.5 Hz flickering test stimulus (6000 K) was presented at three intensity levels: (1) 1.03, (2) 2.45 and (3) 2.83 log scotopic td. K.N.'s pupil was fully dilated with a mydriatic.

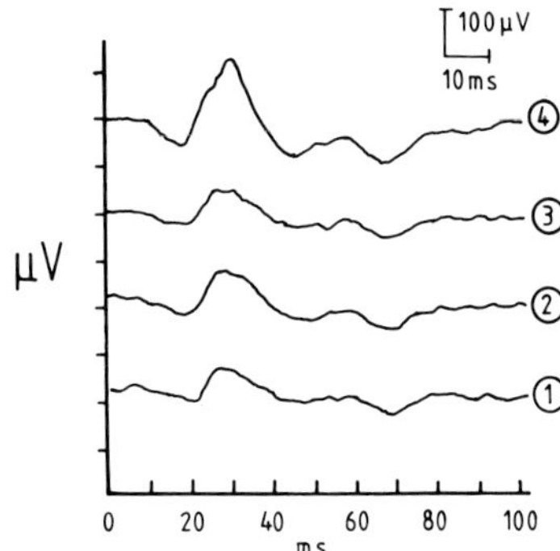

Fig. 10.18. Electroretinographic recordings obtained from a normal trichromat (above) and achromat K.N. (overleaf), under photopic conditions favouring the responses of the L-cones. The background, a xenon source filtered by Wratten filter 44 (6000 K, dominant wavelength 489 nm), had a luminance of 3.69 log

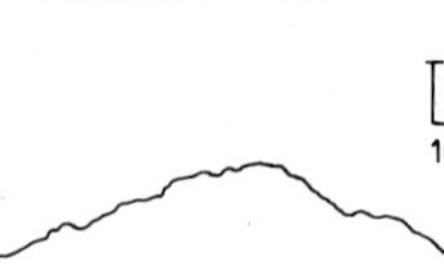

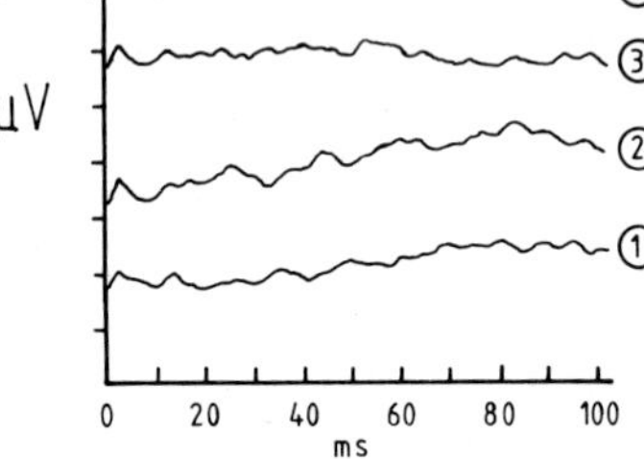

Fig. 10.18 (*cont.*)

scotopic td. The 1.5 Hz flickering test stimulus was filtered by Wratten filter 29 (6000 K, dominant wavelength 632nm). For each observer, four intensity levels of the test were presented: (1) 0.23, (2) 0.61, (3) 0.91 and (4) 1.18 log scotopic td. The observer's pupil was fully dilated with a mydriatic.

10.9 Concluding remarks

Nagel, in his appendix to the second volume of Helmholtz's monumental treatise on Physiological Optics (1911, 3rd edition), concluded, on the basis of the then available evidence, that:

> there is a perfect analogy between the vision of the achromatope [viz. the typical, complete achromat] and twilight vision and . . . support for the assumption, that the totally colour-blind person sees regularly only by means of the elements of the retina that under other circumstances mediate twilight vision. (1962, p. 381)

This analogy may not be perfect for all typical, complete achromat observers (Pokorny *et al.*, 1982), but it certainly seems to hold for the thoroughly investigated achromat observer K.N.

True, the histological evidence forces us to abandon the strictest version of the pure rod theory (Galezowski, 1868). For we must presume that some cone receptors are present, perhaps 5–10% of normal numbers, and most likely functioning in all achromat eyes. Nor can we dismiss out of hand, though we find them unconvincing, the case Alpern (1974) makes for the achromat observers he investigated – namely, that the few cones present are functioning with a rhodopsin action spectrum – and the case Hecht *et al.* (1948) make for their complete colour-blind observer – namely, that 'day rods' replace cones and complement the normal rods. It seems to us more likely that the subjects in these experiments were not typical, complete achromats.

Despite these caveats, which restrict the generality of our findings, the observer K.N. appears to be, as far as all available psychophysical data are concerned, not only a typical complete achromat, but also a rod monochromat in the functional sense of the term. That is, in his eye only the threshold responses of normal rod receptors containing the normal rod pigment can be measured. Thus, it seems fair to presume that any cone receptors present in his retina are too few in number and too anomalous in distribution (e.g. they are missing from the foveola) to contribute a measurable signal to post-receptoral sites.

The very strong possibility that at least some typical, complete achromats, such as K.N., have no functional cone-driven, post-receptoral system holds out to vision scientists the opportunity to study the nature of rod vision, uncomplicated by simultaneous cone activity. It illustrates Occam's razor at work; giving them the chance to explore to the fullest the operation of single visual mechanisms. Their confidence in doing so should be upheld by the investigations reviewed in the next chapter (see Chapter 11), which demonstrate that the post-receptoral function of K.N. is similar, in sensitivity and underlying organisation, to that of normal vision under scotopic conditions.

Acknowledgements

The preparation of this manuscript and the execution of many of the experiments described in it were supported by the Deutsche Forchungs-gemeinschaft, Bonn (SFB 70, A6; SFB 325, B4) and the Alexander von Humboldt-Stiftung, Bonn–Bad Godesberg. We thank Professor Joel Pokorny (University of Chicago), Professor Lothar A. Spillmann (University of Freiburg im Breisgau), Dr Andrew Stockman (University of California, San Diego) and Professor Henk van der Tweel (University of Amsterdam) for critically commenting on the manuscript.

10.10 Appendix

The purpose of this appendix is to present briefly some material about achromat K.N.'s fixation, eye-movements and pupillary light reflex; some of which was referred to in the main text.

10.10.1 Preferred area of fixation

K.N.'s central foveola contains a scotoma and his preferred area of fixation is, resultingly, displaced (Sharpe *et al.*, 1986). This is shown in Fig. A10.1, which is a montage of 21 fundal photographs of K.N.'s left eye. The small crosses are estimates of where he fixates (for the method, see von Noorden, Allen & Burian, 1959). The large scatter is partly due to K.N.'s spontaneous nystagmus, which increases in frequency during fixation and which is markedly accentuated in amplitude by the high luminances required to focus and photograph the fundus (see below). The large cross marks the approximate location of K.N.'s preferred area of fixation: 0.29 ± 0.21 mm (± 2 SEM) nasal to the foveola (i.e. 0.99 ± 0.70 deg to the left or temporal in the external field of view) and 1.01 ± 0.19 mm superior to the horizontal meridian (i.e. 3.45 ± 0.64 deg below in the external field). (For more details, see Sharpe *et al.*, 1986.)

10.10.2 Fixation and pursuit eye movements

K.N.'s fixation is generally unsteady and his pursuit is very imprecise, especially in the horizontal direction. This is shown in Fig. A10.2. The upper part displays *X–Y* plots of K.N.'s eye position while he binocularly fixated a stationary red laser target, while in total darkness and while he fixated the target monocularly with his left and right eyes. In all cases, the distribution of eye movements is much wider than in normal observers. The lower part of Fig. A10.2 displays *X–Y* plots of K.N.'s pursuit of circular and diamond trajectories. His vertical and horizontal pursuit eye movements are highly irregular; especially when the tracking is discontinuous as in the case of the diamond with its inversion points. When the circular trajectory is slowed down (bottom row, middle), K.N.'s vertical tracking improves considerably, but his horizontal tracking does not: large, irregular horizontal eye movements still remain. (For more details, see Sharpe *et al.*, 1986.)

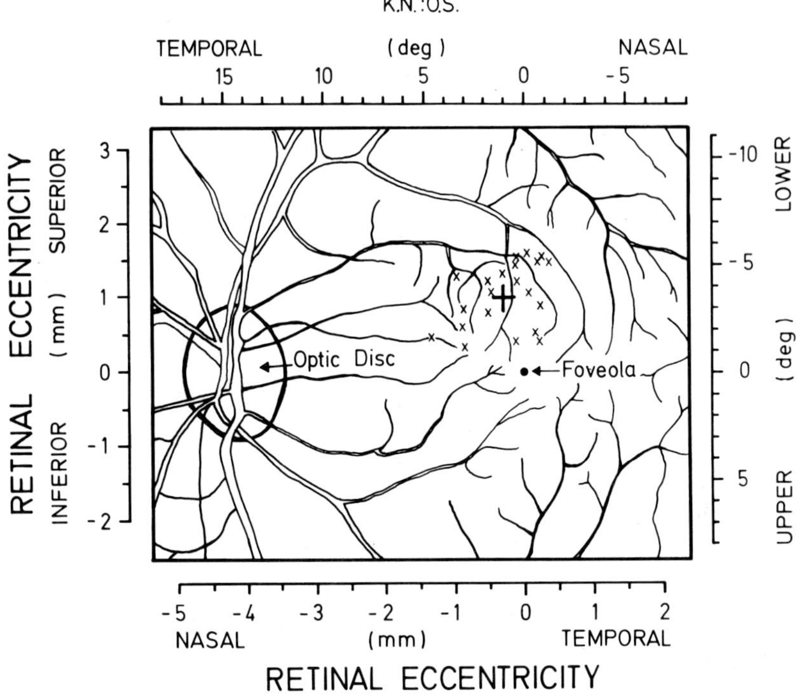

Fig. A10.1. Schematic reproduction of a montage of 21 superimposed fundal photographs of observer K.N.'s left eye. Distances are expressed in both mm of retinal eccentricity and deg of external visual angle. The positions of the foveola and the optic disc and the distribution of the larger retinal blood vessels are indicated. The small crosses indicate the separate photographic estimates of K.N.'s preferred area of fixation; the large cross indicates their approximate centre. (From Sharpe *et al.*, 1986.)

10.10.3 Spontaneous nystagmus

Fig. A10.3 displays representative recordings of K.N.'s monocular and binocular fixation of a stationary, red laser, target and his spontaneous eye-movements in darkness (same conditions as in Fig. A10.2, upper row). The basic nystagmus type is dual-jerk, according to the classification of Dell'Osso & Daroff (1975). It is a mixture of a jerk nystagmus which has fast phases, mostly to the left, and pendular nystagmus which varies in amplitude and has a period of about 5–7 Hz. K.N. displays this nystagmus type, not only when deliberately making an effort to fixate, but also when making no special fixation effort or when pursuing a moving target. In general, the vertical nystagmus is much smaller than

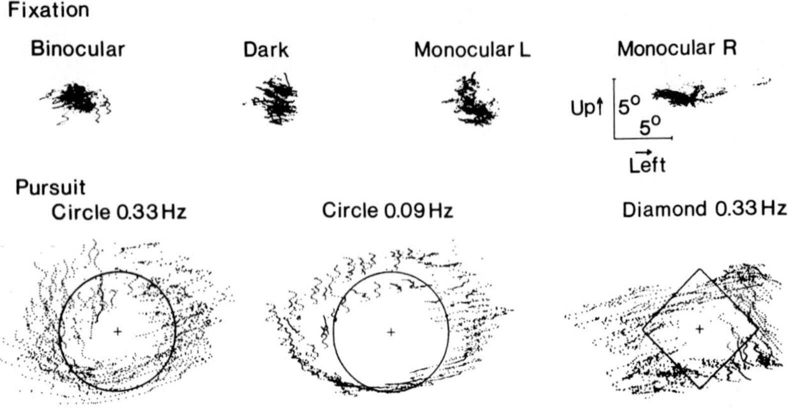

Fig. A10.2. The upper part shows *X–Y* plots of K.N.'s eye position (from left to right) while he binocularly fixated a stationary red laser target, while in darkness, and while he fixated the target monocularly with the left and the right eyes. Each trial lasted 32 s. The lower part shows *X–Y* plots of K.N.'s pursuit of three trajectories: (left to right) a fast circle (0.33 Hz), a slow circle (0.09 Hz) and a fast diamond (0.33 Hz). The excursions of all three trajectories had a radius of 5 deg. (From Sharpe *et al.*, 1986.)

the horizontal nystagmus. It is mainly of the jerk type with a very small superimposed pendular component.

During binocular fixation (upper left), the jerk component almost completely disappears and a more or less pure pendular component remains. In contrast, in darkness (upper right) the pendular component totally disappears (even in the velocity traces) and only a pure jerk nystagmus is evident. Only during monocular fixation (lower left and right) can both components be clearly seen. It should be noted that the direction of the jerks does not invert when the viewing eye is alternated: the fast beats are always to the left and the slow drifts are always to the right. It should also be noted that the changes in type of nystagmus are not related to change in the average position of the eye in the orbit. (For more details, see Sharpe *et al.*, 1986.)

10.10.4 Optokinetic nystagmus

Fig. A10.4 shows recordings of K.N.'s optokinetic nystagmus (OKN) elicited by downward, upward, rightward and leftward movement of a square-wave grating. The grating, which had a spatial frequency of 0.1 c deg^{-1}, was presented binocularly at a velocity of 47.6 deg s^{-1} on

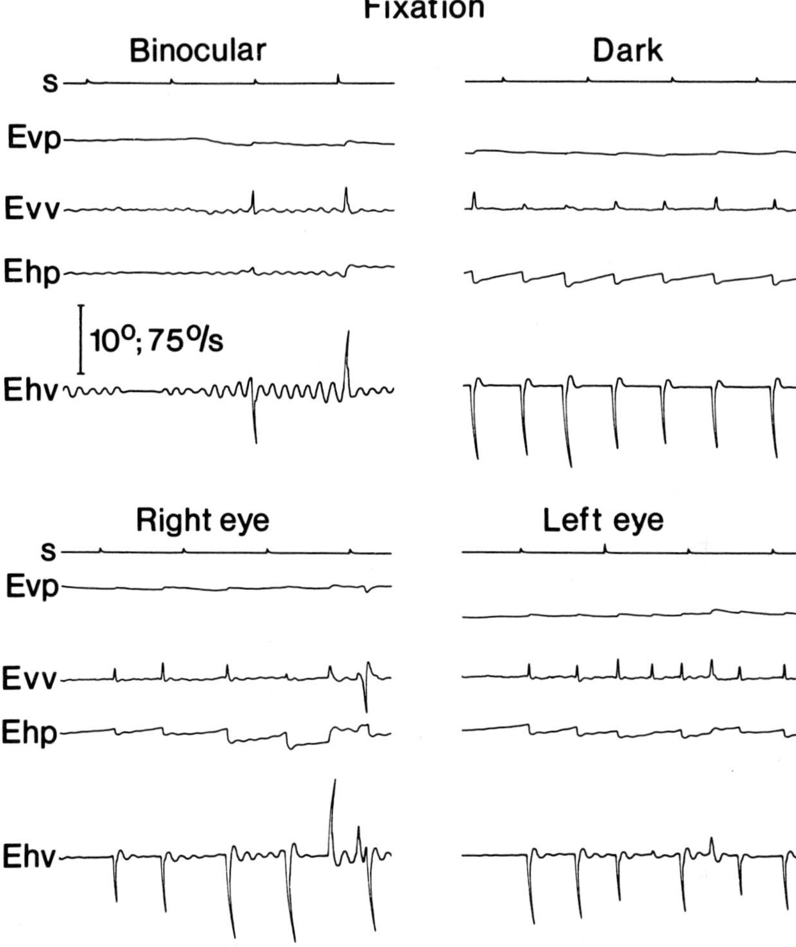

Fig. A10.3. Representative recordings of K.N.'s fixation while he monocularly and binocularly fixated a stationary red laser target and while in darkness (same four conditions as shown in Fig. A10.2, upper row). Time is marked in seconds (s). Evp indicates eye vertical position; Ehp, eye horizontal position; Evv, eye vertical velocity; and Ehv, eye horizontal velocity. Pen displacement upward corresponds to rightward or upward eye motion; pen displacement downward corresponds to leftward or downward eye motion. (From Sharpe *et al.*, 1986.)

the tangent screen. K.N.'s vertical OKN, elicited by the downward and upward movement, is essentially normal in structure. The slow phase velocities fluctuate considerably with maxima of slightly more than 40 deg s^{-1} for downward movement and 45 deg s^{-1} for upward movement. K.N.'s horizontal OKN, elicited by the rightward and leftward

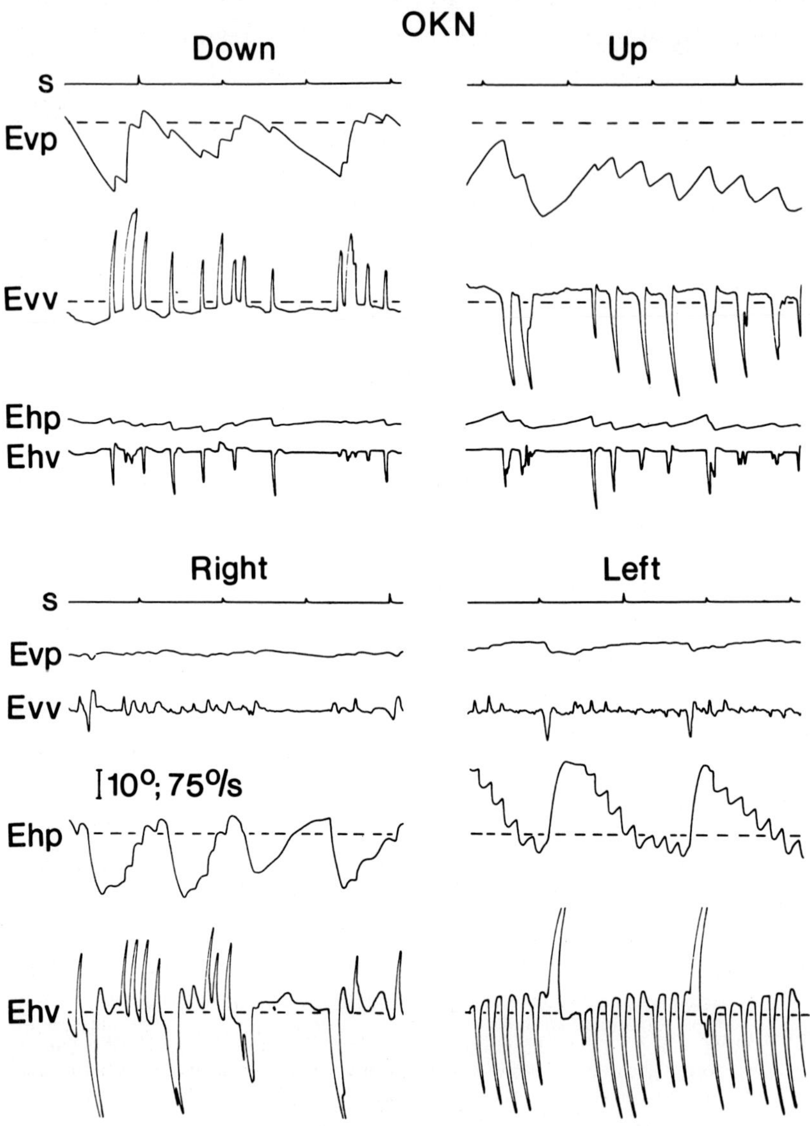

Fig. A10.4. Recordings of K.N.'s optokinetic nystagmus (left eye) elicited by downward, upward, rightward and leftward movement of a square-wave grating. The grating, which had a spatial frequency of 0.1 c deg^{-1}, was presented binocularly at a velocity of 47.6 deg s^{-1}. The abbreviations are the same as in the caption to Fig. A10.3. (From Sharpe *et al.*, 1986.)

movement, however, is abnormal. His best performance is for stimulation to the right. This is the same direction as the slow phase of his spontaneous nystagmus. Occasionally, the tracking is smooth; but more typically, it is very jerky and saccadic. The smooth components, interspersed between the saccades, tend to beat in the wrong direction, running to the left, in the direction opposite to the spontaneous nystagmus. Leftward stimulation elicits only apparent OKN, in which the tracking is totally saccadic, and the interspersed smooth components are inverted at high velocities (i.e. they run to the right in the direction opposite to the stimulus motion). The fast phases of his horizontal OKN often appear to be abnormally slow.

Yee and his co-workers have reported that the OKN in complete achromats has two characteristic features not found in individuals with other varieties of spontaneous congenital nystagmus: a temporal to nasal directional preference and a gradual build-up in slow phase velocity with time (Baloh, Yee & Honrubia, 1980; Yee, Baloh & Honrubia, 1981; Yee *et al.*, 1982; Yee *et al.*, 1985). This is at odds with our findings; the OKN recordings of K.N. displays neither a preference for temporal-to-nasal motion, nor a gradual acceleration in pursuit velocity. Rather, both his binocular and monocular recordings display a general preference for rightward over leftward motion and a constant pursuit velocity. (For more details, see Sharpe *et al.*, 1986.)

10.10.5 Pupillary light reflex

It is frequently asserted that the pupillary light reflex in the typical, complete achromat is 'sluggish' or abnormally 'extensive' (Engelking, 1921, 1922; Walls & Heath, 1954; Waardenburg, 1963; Lowenstein & Lowenfeld, 1969; Krill, 1972, 1977). Although the precise interpretation of the term 'sluggish' is not clear, it would seem to imply a disorder in the time constants of the activating mechanisms, the pupillary sphincter and dilator muscles, because they primarily limit the speed of the light reflex, both in the normal and in the complete achromat eye.

In Fig. A.10.5, K.N.'s pupillary reflexes (solid line) are directly compared with those of a normal trichromat (stippled line), chosen for similar values of the resting pupil (Sharpe *et al.*, 1988). (The adapting field level was 18 scotopic td for K.N. and 56 scotopic td for the trichromat.) The upper panel (*a*) shows mean traces for a 700% increment pulse superimposed upon a steady-state adapting field; the lower panel (*b*) mean traces for a 100% increment pulse. The differences

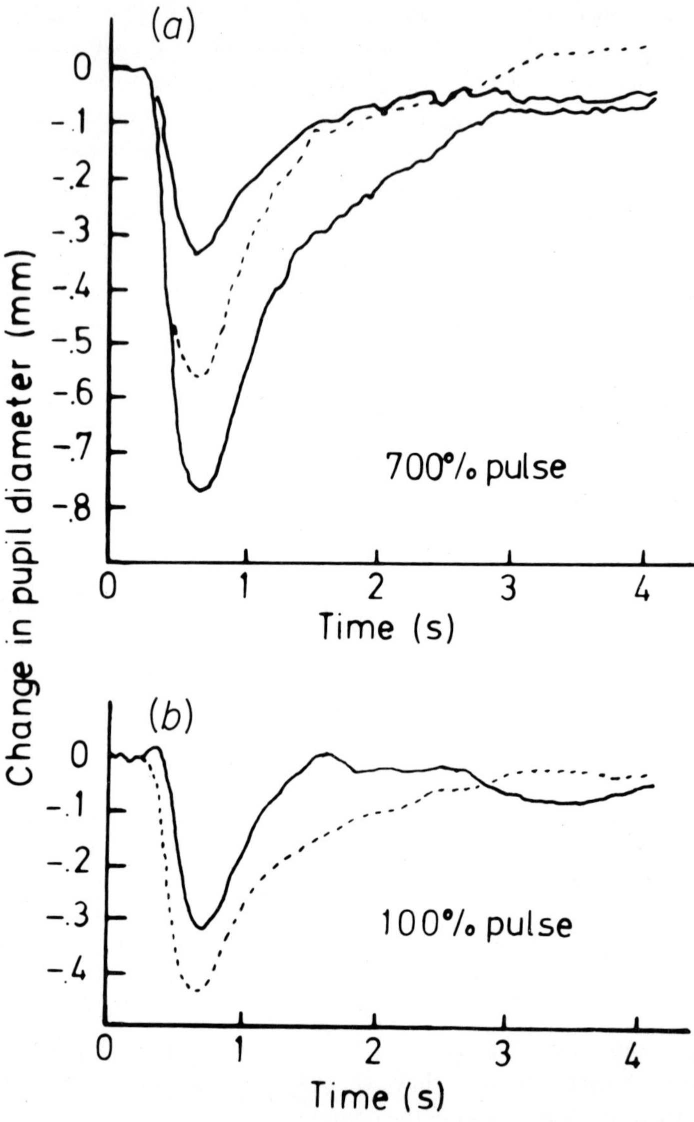

Fig. A10.5. The average pupillary light reflexes of K.N. (solid line) and a normal trichromat observer (stippled line). Change in pupil diameter is shown as a function of time following exposure to (*a*) 700% (two traces for K.N.) and (*b*) 100% incremental light pulses. The abscissa zero indicates the time of pulse presentation. The rectangular pulses were 100 ms in duration and were repeated once every 4 s. They were 18 deg in diameter and were superimposed on an 18 deg diameter adapting field, which had a retinal illuminance of 18 scotopic td for K.N. and 56 scotopic td for the trichromat. The retinal illuminances were chosen to yield similar value of the resting state pupil. The pulses and the adapting fields had a colour temperature of 3000 K. (Modified from Sharpe *et al.*, 1988.)

between the traces of K.N. and the normal observer fall within the experimental accuracy of pupillary measurements. Thus pupillary light reflexes with typically normal response parameters can be elicited in K.N., implying that he has normal pupillary sphincter and dilator dynamics. It seems likely that the impairments of the pupillary light reflex reported in other achromats (Engelking, 1921, 1922) resulted from the saturation of the rods during intense light adaptation. (For more details, see Sharpe *et al.*, 1988.)

This explanation accords with the findings of Alexandridis & Dodt (1967) in a totally colour-blind female. They found that her pupillary responses to a white light flash (0.1 s in duration, 5 deg in diameter) were quite normal in the dark-adapted state and at adaptive illuminations up to about 10 photopic td. At higher levels of adaptation, however, her pupillary response was absent, regardless of the luminance of the test light. Moreover, following light adaptation, the re-dilation of her pupil was rather slow: 90% of the full diameter being reached only after 3–4 min in darkness as compared to less than 1 min in the normal eye. In another totally colour-blind observer, Alexandridris (1970) found that the spectral sensitivity of the pupillary light reflex, as well as that of the psychophysical threshold, at all adaptation levels, agreed with the CIE (1951) scotopic luminosity function.

11

Post-receptoral sensitivity of the achromat

Robert F. Hess

11.1 Introduction

Achromatopsia has been the subject of continual research over the past three decades, yet we know very little about the associated post-receptoral sensitivity of achromats. This is even more surprising when one considers that during this same period there has been substantial progress in delineating the post-receptoral sensitivity of the photopic visual system. Over this same period there has been a preoccupation with the more receptoral aspects of the achromat's visual function such as bleaching adaptation (see Chapters 9 and 10), spectral sensitivity and directional sensitivity. These were the obvious implements with which to assess whether achromatopsia of the total and complete form was equivalent to rod monochromacy. However, it is worth remembering that while these are the implements of first choice they are not the only implements and in fact, when used in isolation can even be misleading. As we will see shortly this question can also be resolved if we assess *post-receptoral* measures of visual performance.

If the vision of the achromat of the typical, complete kind can be shown to be functionally equivalent to rod monochromacy then the study of this condition can tell us how the rod mechanism of normal vision is organized without the need of using elaborate isolation procedures. Furthermore within the post-receptoral arena, the rod monochromat can supply unique information about two particular aspects of sensitivity which are not amenable from a study of the normal Duplex retina. These concern mesopic function and suprathreshold function. The first is important because it represents the illuminance where rod sensitivity is at its best, while the latter is intimately concerned with everyday visual perception. This chapter will concentrate on these two aspects. Photopic and scotopic function will be mentioned only briefly because they tell us about the limits of rod vision and address the issue of whether the achromat is a rod monochromat. Since our present view of rod vision is limited to detection thresholds and scotopic illuminances the emphasis placed on mesopic function and suprathreshold information should help redress this imbalance.

11.2 Are there high intensity receptors in the achromat's retina?

11.2.1 Saturation

One of the main obstacles to equating achromatopsia and rod monochromacy has been the psychophysical hypothesis that high intensity receptors containing rhodopsin are present in the achromat's retina (Alpern, Falls & Lee, 1960). This proposal was advanced in an attempt to reconcile the cone-like Stiles–Crawford effect seen in some achromats (for counter case see Chapter 10 and Nordby & Sharpe, 1988) with rhodopsin-like spectral sensitivity and bleaching adaptation. This can only be adequately tested by investigating psychophysical sensitivity under photopic conditions where all vision should cease due to saturation if only rods are functioning (Aguilar & Stiles, 1954; Fuortes, Gunkel & Rushton, 1961; Adelson, 1982; Baylor, Nunn & Schnapf, 1984). If there are high intensity receptors present, some cone-mediated residual vision should remain at this light level. The results are very clearly in favour of there being only rods because sensitivity 'saturates' completely no matter what the spatio-temporal properties of the stimuli used to assess it. This is shown in Fig. 11.1*a*, *b* for contrast sensitivity for a variety of spatial and temporal stimuli. The normalized fall-off in sensitivity above 180 Ts for these spatial (*a*) and temporal (*b*) stimuli is seen in Fig. 11.2*a*, *b*. It is described by a unitary function of exponential form (solid curve) which begins at around 100–400 Ts and is complete by 2000 Ts. Similar results were found by Blakemore & Rushton (1965). Above 2000 Ts, achromats of this type see nothing with their eyes open, the world appears an even grey. They can, however, 'derive' some rudimentary vision by attending to the after image when their eyes are closed. This suggests that there is some storage in the outer segment which can be retrieved when the receptor comes out of saturation (Sakitt, 1976). It is this that enables achromats to get about during the day and it is this that might have misled earlier workers who thought that they had found evidence for cone function in the eyes of achromats.

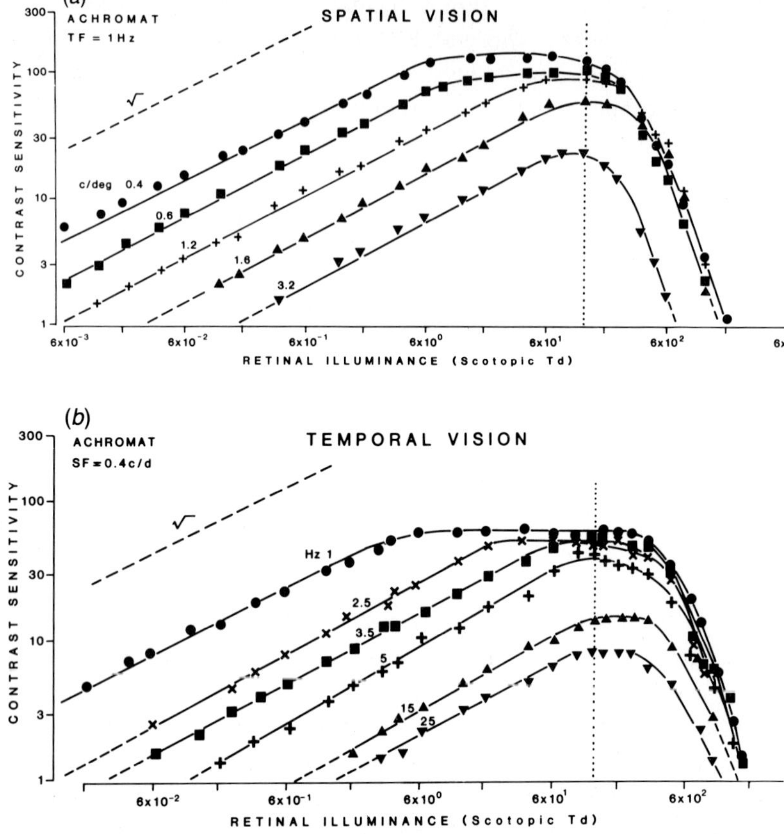

Fig. 11.1. Contrast sensitivity of the achromat is plotted against mean retinal illuminance for grating stimuli of different spatial (*a*) and temporal (*b*) frequency. Notice that the form of the rod response is not critically dependent on the spatial or temporal properties of the sinusoidal gratings used. Sensitivity rises to a plateau in the mesopic and then falls rapidly as the mean retinal illuminance is futher increased. Contrast vision cannot be measured above 2000 Ts. (From Hess & Nordby, 1986*a*.)

The results displayed in Fig. 11.3 show that this photopic decline in sensitivity also occurs in a unitary manner across the retina. Here the results for a number of retinal eccentricities (nasal as well as temporal) have been combined and compared with the solid curve in Fig. 11.2. The stimulus is a 0.8 c/deg grating temporally modulated at 1 Hz (*a*) or 5 Hz (*b*). There are two reasons why this precipitous drop in sensitivity above 400 Ts in the achromat is likely to be due to saturation of the rod photoreceptors. First, the illuminance range over which it occurs corresponds reasonably well to where Aguilar & Stiles (1954) found rod

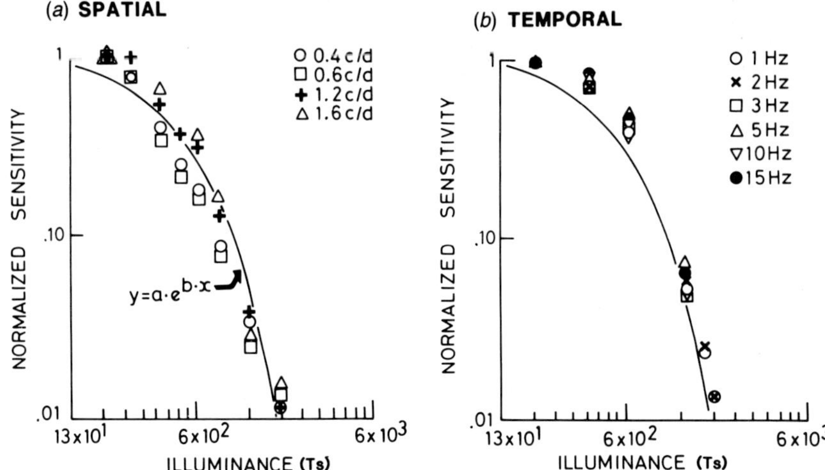

Fig. 11.2. Contrast sensitivity of the achromat for different spatial (*a*) and temporal (*b*) frequencies from the high luminance regions of Fig. 11.1 has been normalized and replotted. The sensitivity fall off is similar for all stimuli and well fitted by an exponential with a decay constant of 0.0024. (From Hess & Nordby, 1986*a*.)

saturation in the normal Duplex retina (marked by horizontal bar in Fig. 11.3). Second, it has an exponential (solid curve in Figs 11.2 and 11.3) form ($y = ae^{-bx}$, where a is the normalization constant and b is the decay constant). The form of this response is what Baylor *et al.* (1984) find for the saturation response of isolated primate rod photoreceptors. However, the histology (Larsen, 1921*a*, *b*; Harrison, Hoffnagel & Hayward, 1960; Falls, Wolter & Alpern, 1965; Glickstein & Heath, 1975; see also Section 10.2 of Chapter 10) suggests that at least some cones do exist in the achromat's retina. Thus we can interpret the psychophysics to mean that there are no cone post-receptoral signals contributing to perception.

11.3 Do the rods in the achromat's retina make normal post-receptoral connections?

11.3.1 Detection sensitivity

Studying the post-receptoral sensitivity of the achromat under scotopic conditions is unlikely to contribute much to our understanding of normal rod vision. It is here that the rod mechanism of normal vision can be

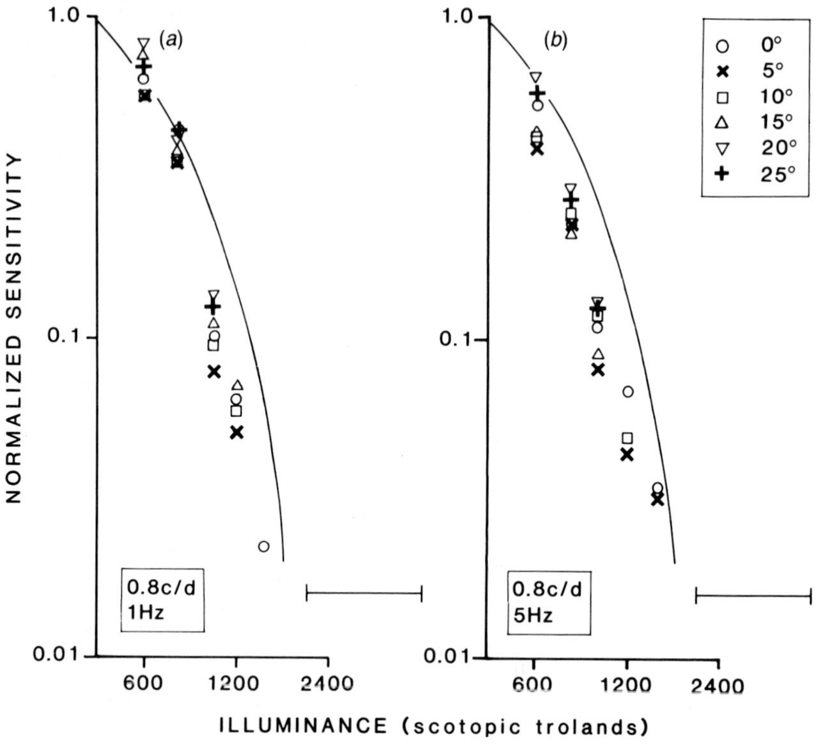

Fig. 11.3. Contrast sensitivity of the achromat for different retinal regions has been normalized and plotted against mean retinal illuminance. Two sinewave stimuli were used, each had a spatial frequency of 0.8 c/deg and a temporal frequency of either 1 or 5 Hz. At high illuminance the rate of fall off in sensitivity is similar in different retinal regions. The solid curve is that which best describes the data of Fig. 11.2 and the horizontal bar represents the upper limit of saturation for rods in the duplex retina, from the work of Aguilar & Stiles (1954). (From Hess, Nordby & Pointer, 1987.)

easily isolated because of the difference in the operating range of rod and cone mechanisms. It is for this reason that almost all we know about the rod mechanism of the Duplex retina comes from studying it under scotopic conditions. However, studying the post-receptoral sensitivity of the achromat under scotopic conditions will tell us a great deal about how the achromat's rods are connected to post-receptoral neurons. In particular it will tell us whether the achromat's rods make the same types of post-receptoral connections as do the rods in the normal Duplex retina. If they do, then scotopic sensitivity should always be the same in trichromat and achromat independent of the type of stimulation. The only excusable exception would be for those relatively uncommon

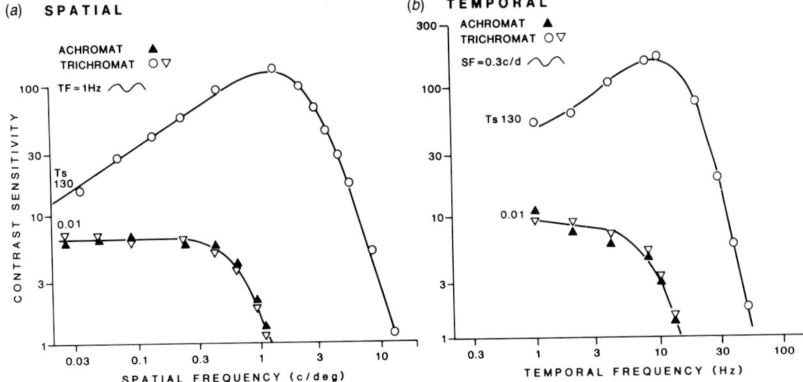

Fig. 11.4. Contrast sensitivity for a large field sinewave gratings is plotted against spatial frequency (*a*) or temporal frequency (*b*) of the stimulus. The open circles are for the photopic mechanism of normal vision. The open and filled triangles represent the scotopic results of trichromat and achromat respectively. Notice that the scotopic transfer functions are more low pass in form and sensitivity is matched for trichromat and achromat. (Replotted from Hess & Nordby, 1986*a*.)

situations where destructive or facilitative rod–cone or cone–rod interactions modify normal sensitivity. In one such case, it has been shown that the achromat does have slightly better than normal sensitivity (Hess & Nordby, 1981).

The spatial (*a*) and temporal (*b*) scotopic sensitivity functions for *large*, centrally located stimulus fields are displayed in Fig. 11.4. In each of these and subsequent figures the scotopic results of trichromat and achromat are compared. The data depicted with unfilled circles represent the normal photopic contrast sensitivity curve. For these large stimulus fields, the spatial and temporal scotopic sensitivity functions have a low-pass shape and shift down and to the left as illuminance is reduced to scotopic levels. More importantly, notice that the results for trichromat and achromat are matched in terms of spatial and temporal sensitivity within the scotopic range. The results displayed in Fig. 11.5 show another comparison of scotopic spatial and temporal sensitivity for achromat and trichromat but this time for small *localized* stimulus fields imaged on central retina. Again in terms of spatial and temporal sensitivity functions, the achromat and trichromat are matched in sensitivity. There is one important difference between the results of Figs 11.4 and 11.5 which relates to the stimulus area. For localized stimuli (<3 deg) the spatial and temporal functions have a more bandpass shape. In all cases, the results for trichromat and achromat are similar

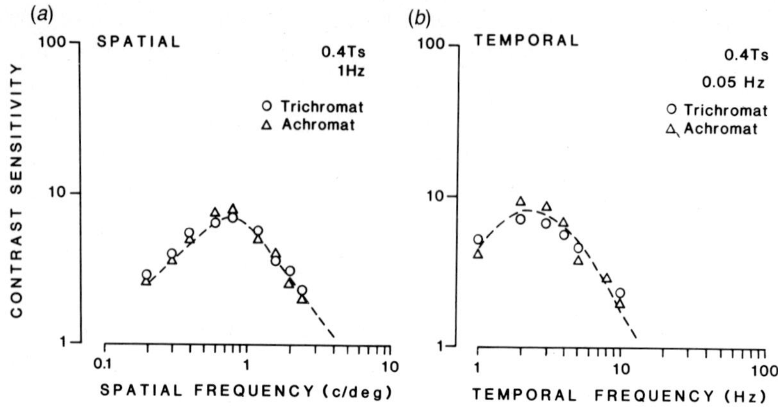

Fig. 11.5. Scotopic spatial (*a*) and temporal (*b*) contrast sensitivity functions for achromat and trichromat are compared for localized patches of sinewave gratings imaged on the fovea. Notice that for localized stimuli the scotopic transfer functions are more bandpass and that sensitivity for achromat and trichromat are in register. (Replotted from Hess *et al.*, 1987.)

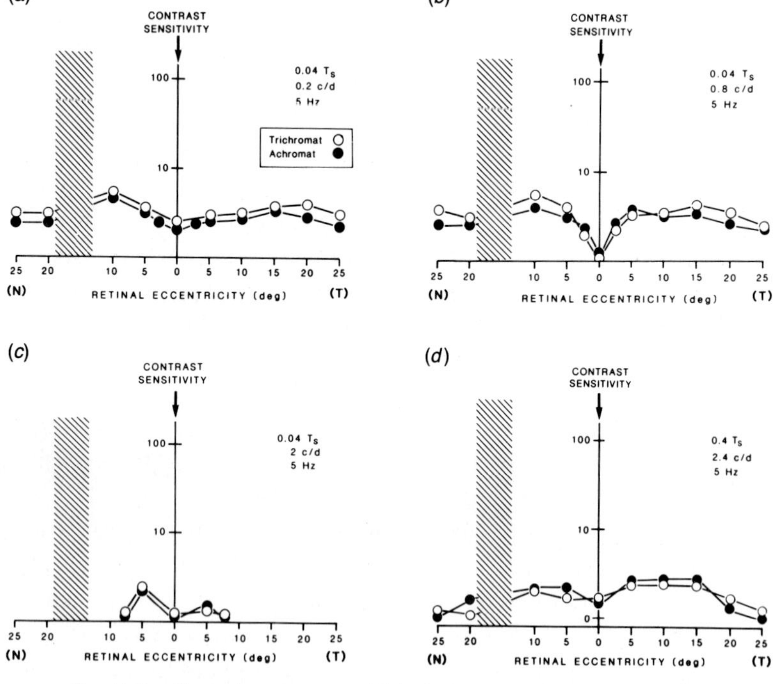

Fig. 11.6. Scotopic contrast sensitivity is plotted against retinal eccentricity for four different spatial frequency stimuli, namely 0.2 c/deg (*a*), 0.8 c/deg (*b*), 2 c/deg (*c*) and 2.4 c/deg (*d*). The results of the achromat (●) and trichromat (○) are compared. Notice that sensitivity is better at mid peripheral locations and that it is comparable for achromat and trichromat. (From Hess *et al.*, 1987.)

under scotopic conditions. Another important feature of scotopic vision is that sensitivity is maximal not in the central foveal region of the retina, but in a mid-peripheral region. Results that show this for a variety of spatial and temporal stimuli are seen in Fig. 11.6. Here contrast sensitivity is plotted against eccentricity for four spatial frequencies, namely 0.2 c/deg, 0.8 c/deg, 2 c/deg and 2.4 c/deg. Although the form of results does depend on the spatial frequency of the stimulus, notice that sensitivity is reduced in the fovea and that the scotopic sensitivities for trichromat and achromat are in register across the retina.

When these results are taken together (see also supporting evidence in Chapter 10) they suggest that the rods in the retina of the achromat and trichromat make similar post-receptoral connections. The spatial sensitivity *function* tells us about how rod signals are pooled in the same region of the retina and spatial sensitivity *profiles* tell us how rod signals are pooled in different retinal regions. Temporal sensitivity also contains a large post-receptoral component because isolated primate rod photoreceptors show neither a low frequency decline in sensitivity nor greatly reduced dynamics as illuminance is reduced to scotopic levels (Baylor *et al.*, 1984, and B. J. Nunn, personal communications).

One is forced to conclude on the basis of this information on the post-receptoral photopic and scotopic sensitivity of the achromat that firstly, only rods determine vision and secondly, they make normal neural connections as per the Duplex retina. Thus the achromat in these studies is a functional rod monochromat and offers an ideal opportunity for exploring aspects of rod function that are not able to be easily or adequately studied using psychophysical isolation procedures in the normal trichromat. This first such aspect involves mesopic function.

11.4 Mesopic vision

11.4.1 Detection sensitivity

The spatial and temporal contrast sensitivity functions for achromat and trichromat are displayed in Fig. 11.7, each at their respective optimal illuminance. For the achromat the mesopic illuminance corresponds to the contrast sensitivity plateaux seen in Fig. 11.1*a*, *b*. The field size is large (20 deg × 30 deg) and the stimuli are imaged on the central retina. For spatial vision (Fig. 11.7*a*) achromat and trichromat have similar sensitivity for low spatial frequencies where it can be assumed that their signals are conveyed along common pathways in a Duplex retina. As the

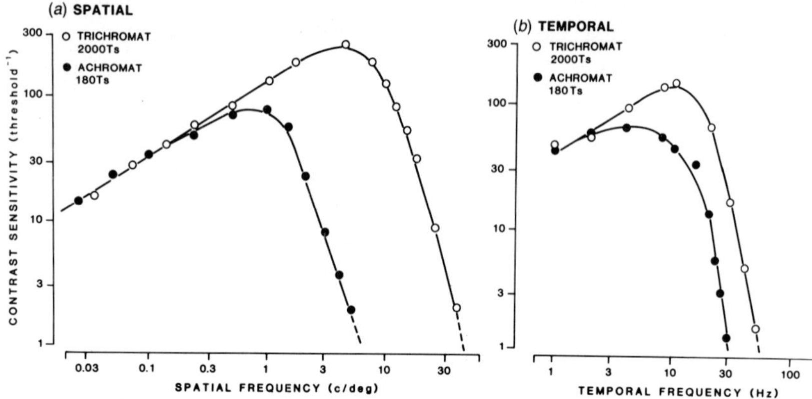

Fig. 11.7. Spatial (*a*) and temporal (*b*) contrast sensitivity functions for large field grating stimuli are compared for achromat and trichromat at their respective optimal illuminances. For cone vision this is 2000 Ts, whereas for rod vision it is 180 Ts. Notice that contrast sensitivity is similar for stimuli of low spatial and temporal frequency. Cone acuity is around 50·60 c/deg whereas rod acuity is around 6–7 c/deg. (From Hess & Nordby, 1986*a*.)

spatial frequency of the target increases, sensitivity for the achromat rapidly falls below that of the photopically adapted trichromat. Presumably this is because neurons with smaller receptive fields in the trichromat receive sole input from cones. Spatial acuity in the achromat is around 6–7 c/deg and sensitivity for intermediate stimuli reaches 80. This acuity estimate has been verified for other achromats (Daw & Enoch, 1973; Green, 1972); however, the sensitivity estimate depends on the stimulus conditions and especially its field size. For example, Aguilar & Stiles (1954) used an increment threshold task for a large (9 deg), eccentrically located spot (9 deg) and reported incremental threshold sensitivity of 0.2 (i.e. an equivalent Weber contrast of 20) for the rod mechanism of normal vision. A similar study of normal rod vision by D'Zmura & Lennie (1986) using grating stimuli found contrast sensitivities of 30. In the achromat, Green (1972) reported a peak sensitivity of 50 and Daw & Enoch (1973) reported a peak sensitivity of 60. The field sizes used in all of these studies are much smaller than that used for the results of Fig. 11.7. The spatial position of peak sensitivity under mesopic conditions occurs at 0.8–1 c/deg in all studies of the achromat and normal rod vision. The temporal sensitivity function of the achromat (Fig. 11.7*b*) exhibits similar sensitivity to that of the trichromat at low temporal frequencies. The temporal position of peak sensitivity is around 5 Hz and temporal acuity is around 30 Hz. The achromat's

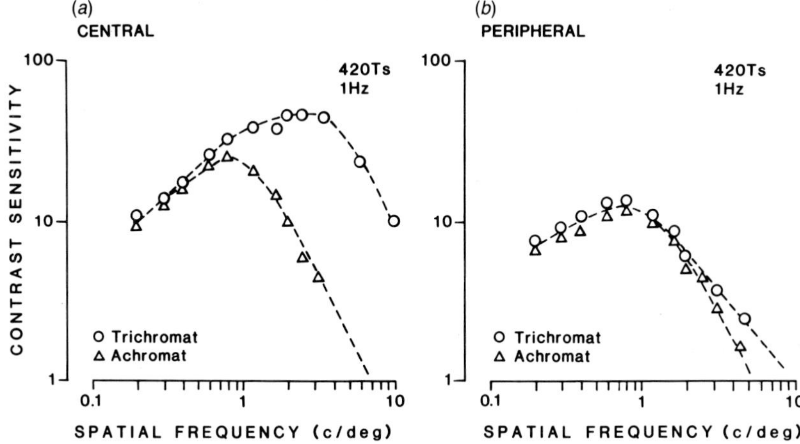

Fig. 11.8. Mesopic spatial contrast sensitivity functions for central (*a*) and peripheral (*b*) retinal regions are compared for achromat and trichromat. In the central retina sensitivity is similar for achromat and trichromat only at low spatial frequencies whereas at peripheral sites it is comparable over most of the spatial range. The stimuli were localized patches of sinewave gratings. (From Hess *et al.*, 1987.)

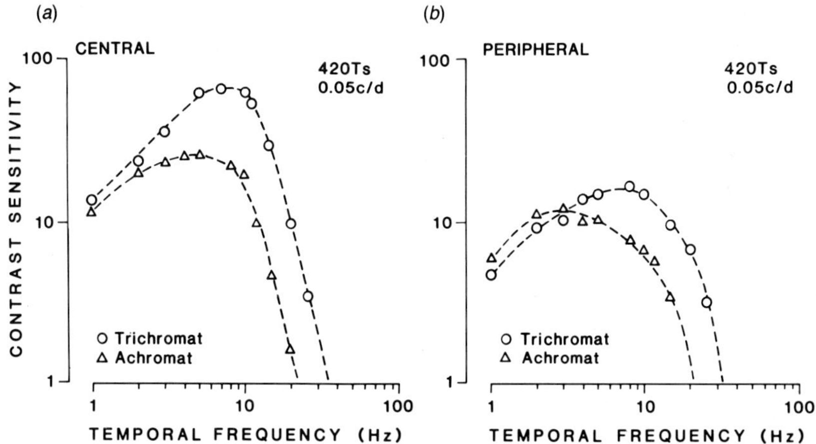

Fig. 11.9. Mesopic temporal contrast sensitivity functions for central (*a*) and peripheral (*b*) retinal regions are compared for achromat and trichromat. Notice that for both central and peripheral retinal sites temporal contrast sensitivity of achromat and trichromat are only similar in the low temporal frequency range. The stimuli were localized patched of sinewave grating. (Replotting from Hess *et al.*, 1987.)

sensitivity under mesopic conditions is a low-pass version of the trichromat's sensitivity under photopic conditions. Originally it was thought that the rod mechanism of normal vision had a temporal acuity of around 10–15 Hz (Hecht & Shlaer, 1936) but the more recent results of Conner & MacLeod (1977) and Conner (1982) have firmly established that under mesopic conditions it can reach 30 Hz. These results concerning temporal acuity of the achromat are consistent with this recent claim.

All of the results discussed so far have involved the use of large stimulus fields, central retinal regions and comparisons between the achromat and trichromat each operating at their respective optimal illuminance. The results displayed in Figs 11.8 and 11.9 are for small patches of stimuli (<3 deg) which are imaged on peripheral as well as central retinal regions and for which the sensitivities of the achromat and trichromat are compared at the *same* mesopic illuminance. The main difference between these results for central vision (Figs 11.8*a*, 11.9*a*) and those previously described (Fig. 11.7) is that peak contrast sensitivity has now fallen to around 30. The spatial acuity is still 6–7 c/deg, the correspondence of sensitivity at low spatial frequencies and the spatial position of the peak remains unchanged. The spatial sensitivity of the achromat's peripheral retina is identical to that of the central retina except that it is shifted in its overall sensitivity. Interestingly the peripheral spatial contrast sensitivities of achromat and trichromat are now in register except at the highest frequencies. It would seem that the acuity of the cone mechanism is superior to that of the rod mechanism under these conditions, a result also found for the Duplex retina (D'Zmura & Lennie, 1986). The results of Fig. 11.9 are for a similar comparison of temporal contrast sensitivity in central and peripheral regions of the achromatic and trichromatic retina. Again, these findings are essentially similar to the previous findings for central vision (Fig. 11.7*b*). The temporal acuity of the achromat for smaller stimulus areas is around 25 Hz, peak sensitivity occurs at around 5 Hz and the sensitivity of trichromat and achromat are similar at low temporal rates when measured at the same mesopic illuminance. The overall sensitivity is, however, reduced from that displayed in Fig. 11.7*b*. The achromat's temporal sensitivity function in the peripheral retina is a high-pass version of that found for central vision. That is, temporal acuity remains unaltered but there is a reduction of sensitivity at lower temporal frequences. Actually, the same is true for the trichromat so that as a consequence the relative temporal sensitivities of achromat and trichromat remain the same across the retina.

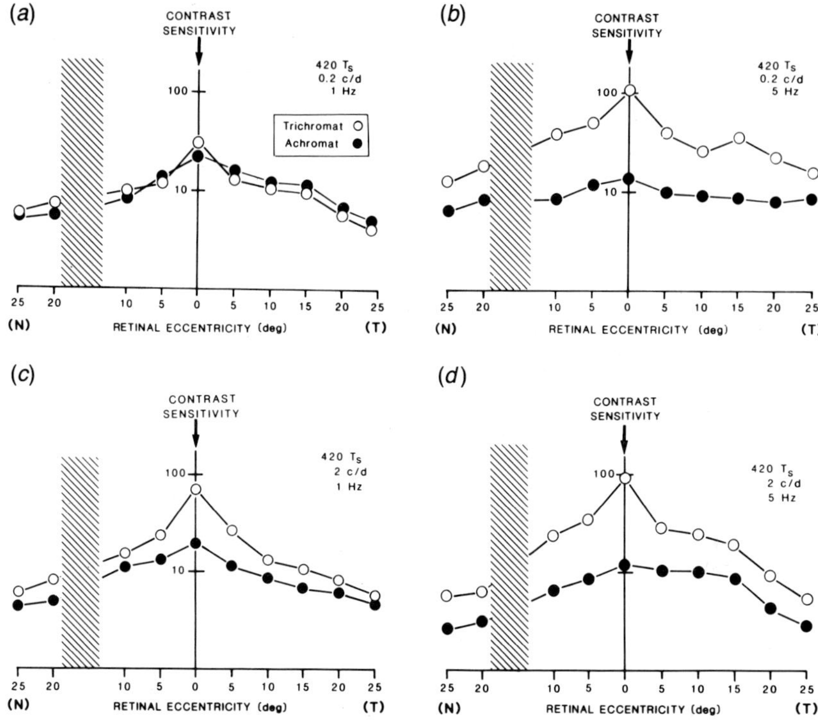

Fig. 11.10. Mesopic contrast sensitivity is plotted against retinal eccentricity for localized patches of sinewave gratings. Results are compared for achromat and trichromat. In all cases sensitivity is maximum in the central region. It is only for targets of low spatial and temporal frequency that mesopic sensitivity of achromat and trichromat are matched. (From Hess *et al.*, 1987.)

These results suggest that under mesopic conditions no matter what the stimulus (except for one corresponding to the temporal limit), the sensitivity of the rod mechanism is greater in the central retina. This is better seen in the results displayed in Fig. 11.10 where mesopic sensitivity for different spatial and temporal stimuli (field size <3 deg) has been measured as a function of retinal eccentricity. In all cases, the mesopic sensitivity of the achromat is greatest for the central retina and falls off as a function of retinal eccentricity. Furthermore, the fall-off of sensitivity is, to a first approximation, independent of the spatial parameters of the stimulus when the fall-off is compared on a scale of absolute eccentricity (i.e. in degrees). The fall-off is approximately 6 dB per 10 deg of eccentricity. The regional distribution of sensitivity is quite different for the cone mechanism under photopic conditions where the fall-off in sensitivity is only independent of the stimulus spatial parameters when

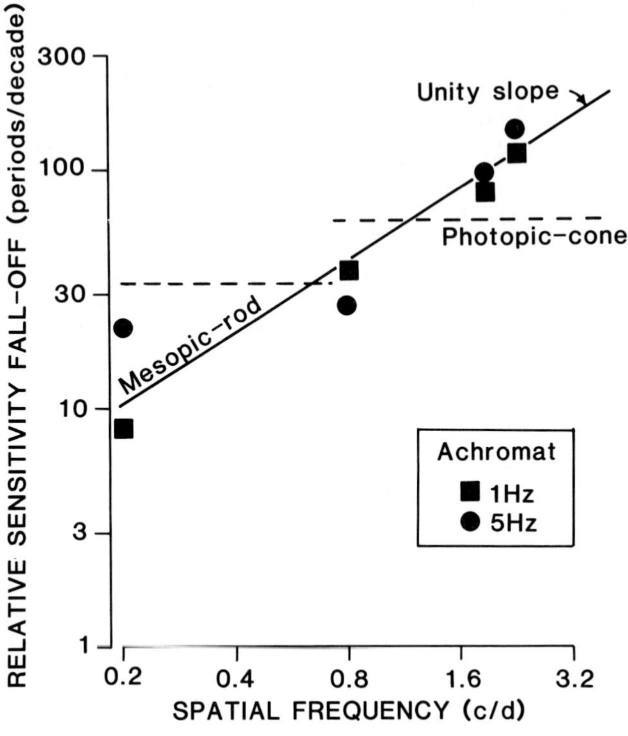

Fig. 11.11. The relative fall-off in sensitivity with eccentricity in periods per decade of sensitivity for the mesopic results displayed in Fig. 11.10 is plotted against the spatial frequency of the stimulus for the achromat. The results are well fitted by a line of unity slope indicating that rod sensitivity for different spatial targets falls off at a constant rate when considered in terms of absolute eccentricity (in degrees). The dashed lines represent the results of Robson & Graham (1981) and Pointer & Hess (1989) for the photopic system. Photopic sensitivity for different spatial targets falls off at a constant rate only when considered in terms of relative eccentricity (i.e. periods of eccentricity). The rate depends on the spatial frequency range (see text).

compared on a scale of relative eccentricity (in periods of eccentricity for a particular spatial frequency). The fall-off for the photopic system for spatial frequencies above 1 c/deg is approximately 20 dB per 60 periods of eccentricity (Robson & Graham, 1981) and 20 dB per 35 periods for spatial frequencies in the range 0.8–0.2 c/deg (Pointer & Hess 1989). This difference in the regional distribution of sensitivity for rod and cone mechanism each operating at their optimal illuminance is illustrated in Fig. 11.11. The data for the achromat have been derived from

Fig. 11.10 while the photopic results (dashed line) are from Robson & Graham (1981). These results concerning the regional distribution of sensitivity in the achromat under mesopic conditions raise two questions. First, why do we not see a loss of foveal sensitivity corresponding to the 1 deg rod-free area? This is because eccentricity is not sampled finely enough owing to the field size and eye movement instability. To do this adequately one would need to use image stabilization in the achromat. The second question is more fundamental. What underlies the dramatic change in the regional distribution of sensitivity in the achromat (and hence for the rod mechanism of normal vision) as the light level is reduced from mesopic to scotopic? (Compare the results in Figs 11.6 and 11.10). One possibility is that it follows the average convergence of rod receptors to ganglion cells. This can be assessed by dividing Osterbergs' (1935) data on human rod photoreceptor distribution by Perry & Cowey's (1984) data on primate ganglion cell distribution. The result is that averaged convergence increases monotonically from fovea to far periphery. This fits neither the mesopic nor the scotopic sensitivity profiles for the achromat or trichromat (Figs 11.6 and 11.10). Could it be that these losses in central sensitivity under scotopic conditions are compensated for by gains in acuity? In other words, do the rules concerning receptor convergence change as a function of light level? Again, the answer is no, spatial acuity is independent of retinal eccentricity under scotopic conditions as is also temporal acuity (see Fig. 11.5). Could it be a consequence of the finding that light flux and not retinal illuminance determines neural adaptation of retinal ganglion cells (Enroth-Cugell & Shapley, 1973)? An argument could be advanced by taking the results of Enroth-Cugell & Shapley's experiments at face value and postulating that central rod-driven neurones have smaller receptive fields and hence always determine threshold under more light adapted conditions. However, this is unlikely to be the case for the stimuli used in these psychophysical experiments. Enroth-Cugell & Shapley (1973) used very small stimuli compared with the receptive field centre of the neurones which they studied, and plotted their results in terms of impulses per quantum. In terms of the psychophysics the relevant measure is impulses per receptive field centre and unless the sensitivity of neurones with larger receptive fields is limited by additional factors which are located more central to the adaptation pool, the adaptation gain curves of different sized receptive fields will never cross and can therefore not offer an explanation for the present results. In lieu of a better explanation one is forced to conclude that the operating range of centrally located rod-driven neurones is 'adapted' to more mesopic conditions than those in the mid-periphery. This suggests a duplicity of function within the rod mechanism of the achromat and hence the rod mechanism of normal vision (see also Chapter 10 and Sharpe, Stockman & MacLeod, 1989).

There is evidence from spatial adaptation studies that the rod spatial sensitivity curve is the envelope of a number of more spatially selective mechanisms or channels (Kranda & Kulikowski, 1976; Graham, 1972). The bandwidth of these mechanisms remains unchanged as illuminance is reduced (Kranda & Kulikowski, 1976; Graham, 1972) and it is likely that their neural counterpart are cortical cells whose spatial properties are also invariant with illuminance (Bisti *et al.*, 1977; also see Fig 3.6 in Chapter 3) unlike those seen in the retina which become more low-pass as illuminance is reduced (Barlow, Fitzhugh & Kuffler, 1957; Enroth-Cugell & Robson, 1966). The lowest channel or largest rod summation area has been estimated to be around 0.1 c/deg (Kranda & Kulikowski, 1976; see also Fig. 1.3*b* in Chapter 1) whereas the highest frequency channel or smallest summation area is around 1.5 c/deg (Hess & Nordby, 1986*b*). This would suggest that the size of rod pools extend from 40 minutes to 5 deg in any one region of the visual field.

11.4.2 Discrimination at threshold

So far we have discussed only the post-receptoral sensitivity of the achromat in terms of detection thresholds. While these are experimentally convenient, they do not tell us about what limits the later processing of detectable information. To do this we need to assess discrimination sensitivity. Discriminations at threshold are not just the limiting case but since there is evidence for more selective spatial and temporal mechanisms or channels in vision they take on a special significance. If we assume that a channel has a threshold and gives a 'labelled signal' to later visual centres then if two stimuli can be perfectly discriminated apart when each is at its respective threshold then two channels must be active. Thus, given the above assumptions, by looking at the number of discriminable steps across the spatial and temporal ranges an estimate can be derived of the number of channels which underlie spatial and temporal vision (Watson & Robson, 1981).

Let us first consider spatial vision. As will be seen later it is necessary to consider spatial discrimination at low and high temporal frequencies separately. The results in Fig. 11.12 and 11.13 compare discriminations at threshold for a trichromat (results of Watson & Robson, 1981) and

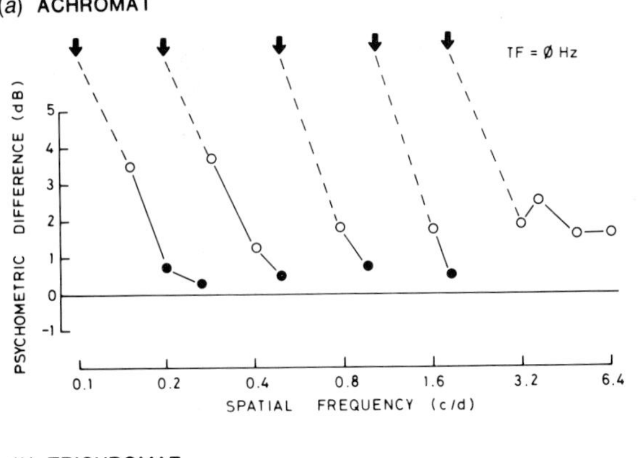

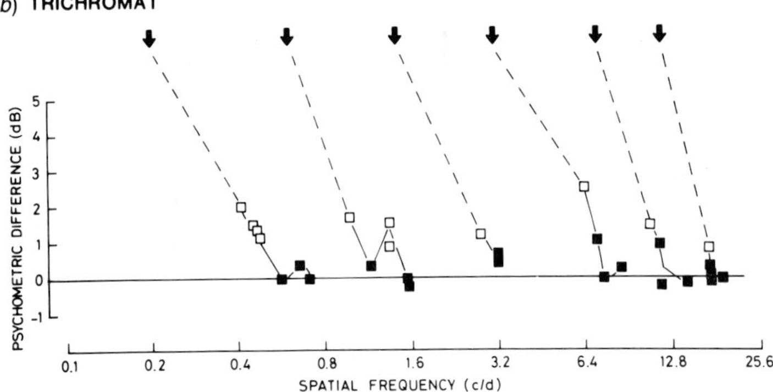

Fig. 11.12. Difference between the psychometric functions for detection and for discrimination are plotted as a function of the spatial frequency of one of the stimuli. Results are compared for the achromat operating at 180 Ts (*a*) and for the trichromat operating at photopic levels (*b*). The comparison stimulus is indicated by the filled arrow. Differences below 1 dB (●, ■) satisfy the criterion of perfect discrimination at detection threshold. Notice that between 0.1 and 2 c/deg four discriminable steps of comparable size can be made by achromat and trichromat. The photopic results are taken from Watson & Robson, 1981. The stimuli have a temporal frequency of 0 Hz. (From Hess & Nordby, 1986*b*.)

achromat (Hess & Nordby, 1986*b*). For each individual the difference between the psychometric functions for detection and discrimination is plotted against spatial frequency of the test stimulus. The fixed, comparison stimulus (sinewave grating) is indicated by the arrow, while each datum represents a different comparison grating. Filled symbols represent comparison stimuli whose detection and discrimination functions relative to the test stimulus are within 1 dB and thereby fulfil the criterion for perfect discrimination. In other words their psychometric functions are statistically indistinguishable. At low temporal frequencies (Fig. 11.12), Watson & Robson (1981) found that 6 discriminable steps

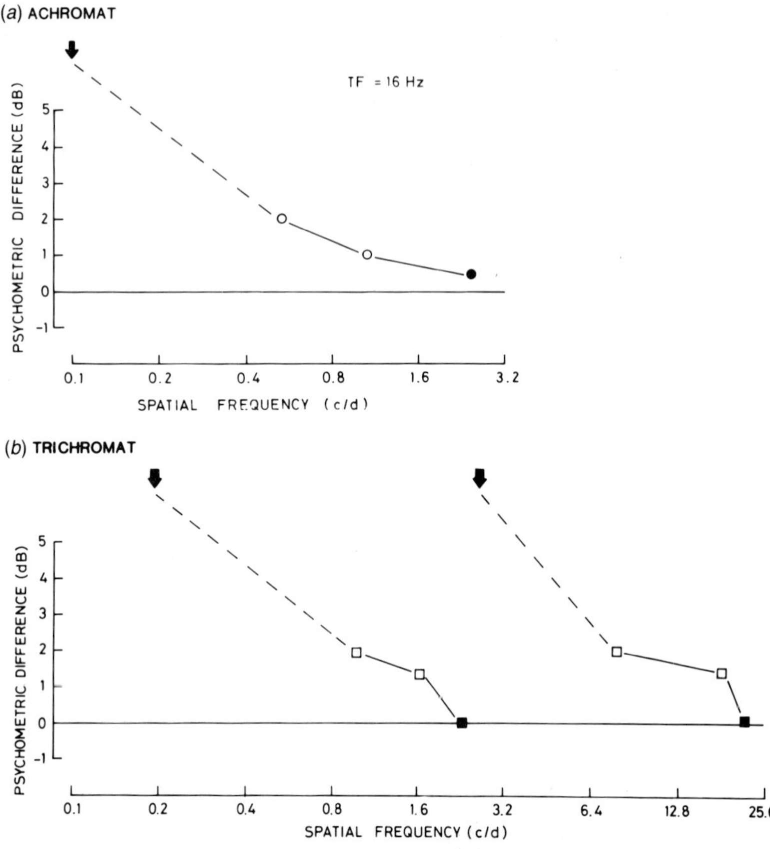

Fig. 11.13. A spatial discrimination experiment similar to that described for Fig. 11.12 is carried out for stimuli of high temporal frequency (16 Hz). The trichromat (data from Watson & Robson, 1981) can make only two discriminable spatial steps at threshold whereas the achromat, because of his restricted spatial range can only make one. (From Hess & Nordby, 1986*b*.)

could be made across the entire spatial range under photopic conditions (Fig. 11.12*b*). Under mesopic conditions the achromat can make 4 discriminable steps at threshold across the spatial range (Fig. 11.12*a*). These steps for both trichromat and achromat are about 1 octave wide. Since it is likely that the photopic system can also make the discriminable step from 0.1 to 0.25 c/deg (not tested by Watson & Robson, 1981), one can conclude that the same labelled lines or channels subserve rod and cone vision over their shared range. A similar conclusion has been arrived at by D'Zmura & Lennie (1986) for rod vision isolated in the normal trichromat. The highest channel for the achromat is located at

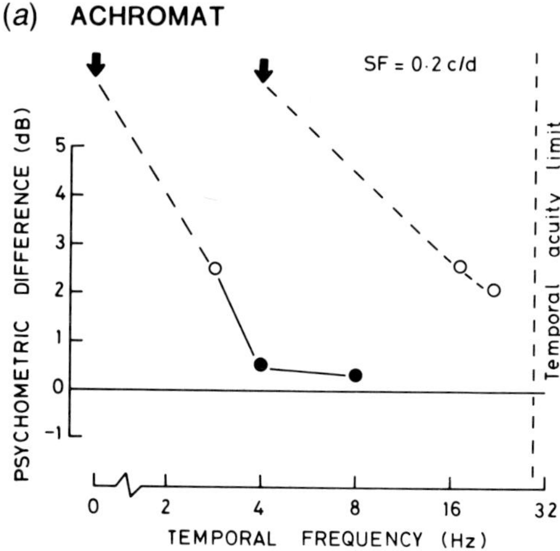

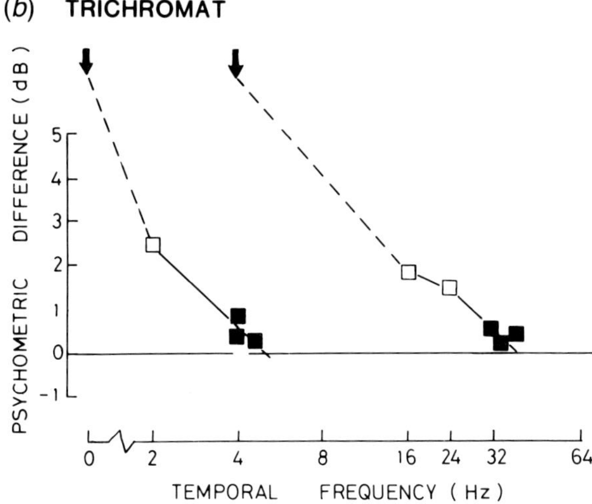

Fig. 11.14. Differences between the psychometric functions for detection and for discrimination are plotted as a function of the temporal frequency of one of the stimuli. All stimuli have a spatial frequency of 0.2 c/deg and the results for the achromat were obtained at 180 Ts and the trichromat at 2000 Ts (replotted from Hess & Plant, 1985). The temporal frequency of the comparison stimulus is represented by the filled arrow. Differences of less than 1 dB (●, ■) represent perfect discrimination at detection threshold. Over the same spatial range (0–30 Hz), the achromat and trichromat can make the same number of discriminable steps at threshold. Above 30 Hz a second discriminable step can be made by the trichromat. (From Hess & Nordby, 1986*b*.)

around 1.6 c/deg whereas it is around 20 c/deg for the trichromat. A similar picture is seen for spatial discriminations at high temporal frequencies, although many fewer discriminable steps can be made (Fig. 11.13). The photopic system (Fig. 11.13*b*) is capable of just two discriminable steps each of about a decade in size whereas the achromat (Fig. 11.13*a*) is capable of only the first of these, the second being outside his spatial range. So within their shared spatial range the same number and size of discriminable steps can be made by achromat and trichromat at threshold. Hence, the underlying neural mechanism subserving spatial vision are similar over this range.

When considering temporal discriminations it is also worthwhile separating them into those at low and high spatial frequencies. At low spatial frequencies the photopic system can make just two discriminable steps (Fig. 11.14*b*), 0 Hz can be discriminated from 4 Hz, and 4 Hz can be discriminated from 32 Hz (Hess & Plant, 1985). Under mesopic conditions, the achromat (Fig. 11.14*a*) can make only the first of these, the second being outside the temporal range. At high spatial frequencies (Fig. 11.15*a*, *b*) the trichromat and achromat can make only one discriminable step at threshold, namely 0 Hz from 4 Hz (Watson & Robson, 1981).

These results suggest that the number and size of the discriminable steps that can be made *at threshold* is similar for trichromat and achromat across their shared spatial and temporal ranges. Thus the underlying neural properties are likely to be the same and possibly shared between rod and cone receptors. The threshold discriminations that only the trichromat can perform most probably represent the information carried by the cone-only projection in the Duplex retina. Finally, although these results have been considered against the context of spatial and temporal channels in vision, this is not the only interpretation. For example, consider that the visual system contains an infinite number of extensively overlapping spatial and temporal filters. These quantal steps in discrimination would then reflect the statistical criteria adopted by a more central processing device needed to separate the different distributions of neural activity produced by the two stimuli to be discriminated. However, one still must conclude that these and more central neural properties are shared by the rod and cone receptors of the Duplex retina.

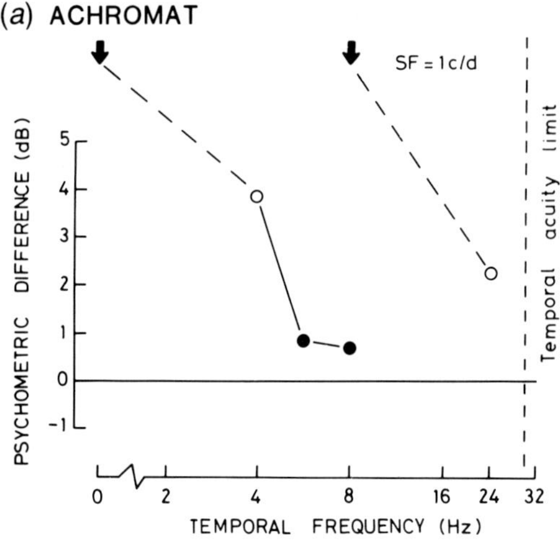

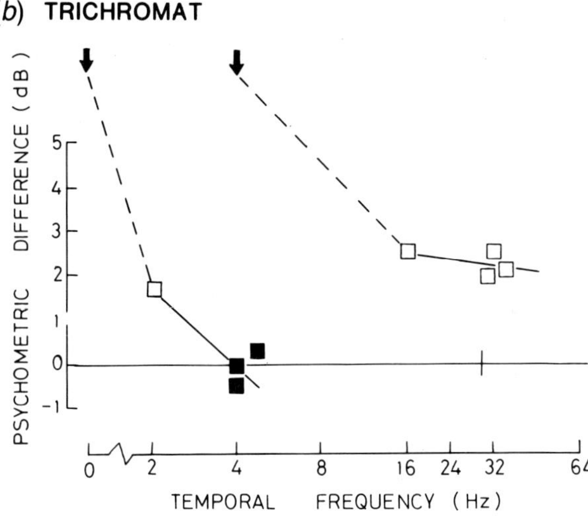

Fig. 11.15. A temporal discrimination experiment similar to that already described in Fig. 11.14 except that now the spatial frequency is 1 c/deg. Achromat and trichromat are capable of only one discriminable step across the entire temporal range. (From Hess & Nordby, 1986*b*.)

11.4.3 Discriminations above threshold

One of the most obvious ways of comparing visual performance of the trichromat and achromat is to examine spatial and temporal discrimination above detection threshold. Such a comparison bears upon whether rod and cone signals share a common pathway and hence are

(*a*)

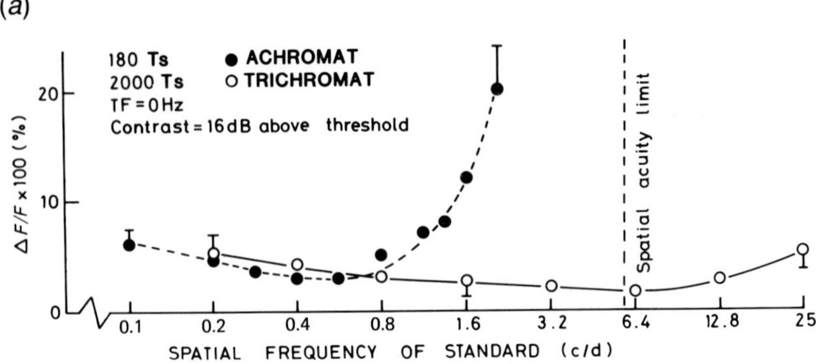

(*b*)

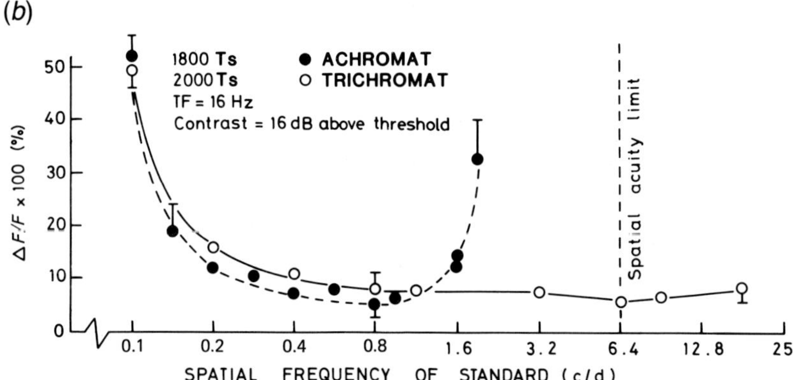

Fig. 11.16. Spatial discriminations for suprathreshold sinewave gratings of low (*a*) and high (*b*) temporal frequency are compared for the achromat and trichromat, each operating at his optimal illuminance. Discriminable sensitivity is comparable for achromat and trichromat up to a factor of 3 from the acuity limit of the achromat. (From Hess & Nordby, 1986*b*.)

limited by the same, central neural processes. While discrimination *at* detection threshold might be limited by more peripheral factors discrimination *above* detection threshold is likely to be limited by more central computations.

Spatial discriminations for achromat and trichromat are compared in Fig. 11.6 where the discriminable ratio $\Delta F/F$ expressed as a percentage is plotted against the spatial frequency of the comparison stimulus. This is done for two temporal conditions (11.16*a* – 0 Hz; and 11.16*b* – 16 Hz), each subject is working under his/her best conditions of illumination. The contrast is set to a factor of 6 times the contrast threshold. The contrast is

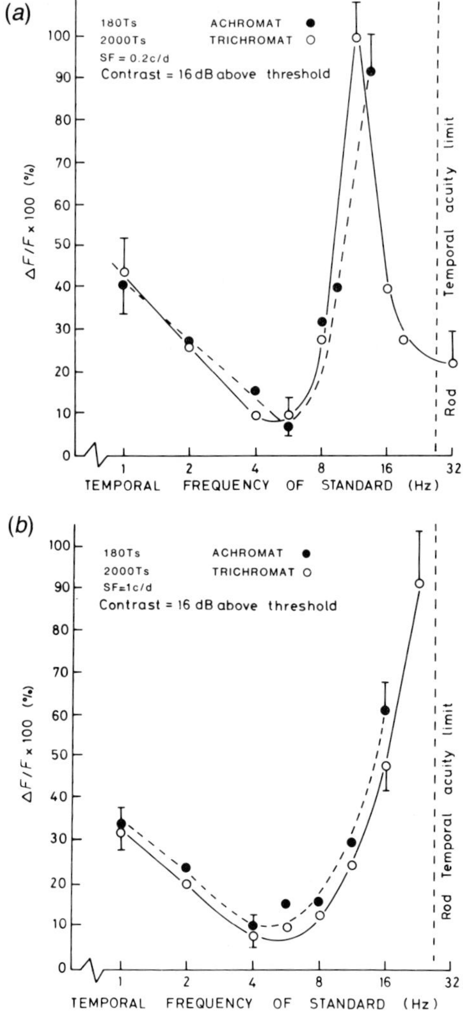

Fig. 11.17 Temporal discriminations for suprathreshold sinewave gratings of low (*a*) and high (*b*) spatial frequency are compared for achromat and trichromat, each operating at his optimal illuminance. Discriminable sensitivity is comparable for the achromat and trichromat up to a factor of 2 from the acuity of the achromat. (From Hess & Nordby, 1986*b*.)

jittered within narrow limits to ensure that subjective contrast cues are not being used to aid discrimination. It can be seen that under both types of temporal stimulation, spatial discriminations of the achromat and trichromat are very similar over a decade of their shared range (0.1–7 c/deg). Beyond 1 c/deg, spatial discriminations in the achromat fall-off rapidly.

Similar temporal frequency discriminations for the achromat and trichromat are displayed in Fig. 11.17 for two spatial conditions, namely 0.2 c/deg (11.17*a*) and 1 c/deg (11.17*b*). A similar supra-threshold contrast level is used together with a control (randomly varying the contrast level) to guard against subjective contrast cues. The results again show that the discrimination performance is comparable for achromat and trichromat when each is operating under his/her best illumination. These results are comparable over 1.5 decades of their shared range. It is only within a factor of 2 of the temporal resolution of rod mesopic vision that achromat and trichromat exhibit different sensitivities.

The reason why cone spatial and temporal vision extends to higher limits than those of rod vision is because some ganglions receive only cone input and presumably their spatial and temporal properties are biased to the higher part of the range (Gouras & Link, 1966). If this underlies the difference in rod- and cone-mediated acuity (spatial and temporal) it probably also underlies the difference in spatial and temporal discriminative sensitivity. The present results lead one to suspect that the cone-only projection has a dominant influence in conveying visual information in the spatio-temporal range above 1 c/deg and above 16 Hz.

11.5 Concluding remarks

Recent psychophysical investigations of the typical, complete achromat suggest that vision is mediated only by rod receptors. Furthermore, the rods of the achromat make similar post-receptoral connections to those of their counterparts in the normal Duplex retina. Thus the achromat is a functional rod monochromat and provides an excellent model of normal rod function where it is most difficult to isolate in the Duplex retina, namely under mesopic and suprathreshold conditions.

The data from the achromat suggest that the detection sensitivity of rod and cone mechanisms is similar in the low spatial and temporal range. Furthermore, rod- and cone-mediated vision is capable of comparable levels of discrimination for spatial and temporal stimuli at and above threshold across most of their shared ranges. These results suggest that the neural mechanisms subserving rod vision are a subset of those subserving cone vision.

Acknowledgements

This work was supported by the Wellcome Trust, the Medical Research Council and the European Science Foundation. I am especially grateful to all of my colleagues here and abroad for enlightening discussion. R.H. is a Wellcome Senior Lecturer.

Part III

Clinical and applied

12

The loss of night vision: clinical manifestations in man and animals

Harris Ripps and Gerald A. Fishman

12.1 Introduction

It is appropriate for a volume devoted to the subject of night *vision* to include a section on night *blindness*. There are numerous instances in which studies on the pathophysiology of disease processes have furthered our understanding of the factors contributing to normal function, and some notable examples can be found in the literature on night blindness. Indeed, the night-blinding disorders selected for discussion serve to illustrate the rather diverse ways in which various types of abnormalities result in defective night vision. In this connection, we should mention that because of its subjective connotation, a generally acceptable definition of the term 'night blindness' is difficult to formulate. From a clinical standpoint, however, it is convenient to regard any defect in the rod-mediated segment of the dark-adaptation curve as a form of night blindness. This includes conditions in which thresholds remain elevated irrespective of the time in darkness, as well as those in which rod threshold eventually returns to normal but the time course of the adaptation process is prolonged.

It is important to recognize that the many well-documented cases of night blindness are attributable invariably to disorders that affect (directly or indirectly) photoreceptors and second order elements of the neural retina; by contrast, defects at or central to the ganglion cell layer have not been implicated thus far in the selective loss of rod-mediated vision. However, even the issue of selectivity requires some qualification. Few, if any, of the night-blinding retinal disorders encountered in clinical practice entirely spare the cone mechanism, and it is often a question of the degree of impairment that separates the so-called night-blinding diseases from the progressive cone–rod dysfunctions (cf. Goodman, Ripps & Siegel, 1963*a*; Krill & Martin, 1971). There are of course non-retinal factors which can lead to the complaint of night blindness, e.g. lenticular sclerosis, night myopia etc. (Owens & Leibowitz, 1976), but these conditions will not be considered further.

12.2 Non-invasive tests of visual function

Perhaps the greatest obstacle to the investigation of retinal disorders in man is the requirement for non-invasive test procedures. Unlike the array of powerful biochemical and cell biological methods that are suitable for research on post-mortem (donor) tissue and animal 'models', the methods available for *in vivo* study are subject to the limitations of ophthalmoscopic examination, the complexities of remote recording techniques, and the variability of subjective responses in psychophysical tests. Nevertheless, a cooperative patient and the judicious application of such methods can provide some insight as to the sites of abnormal function, the cellular origins of the defects, and the nature of the underlying disorder. Before discussing the findings obtained in the various forms of night-blinding disease, it is appropriate to consider briefly the fundamentals of several of the procedures that have been used clinically to examine the functional status of the rod and cone mechanisms.

12.2.1 Electroretinography

The electroretinogram (ERG) is regarded generally as a reliable, objective method for detecting widespread dysfunction of the rod and cone mechanisms, and for charting the deleterious changes that accompany progressive degenerative retinal conditions (cf. Goodman, Ripps & Siegel 1963*b*; Berson, Gouras & Hoff, 1969; Fishman, 1980). Although first recorded in humans more than a century ago (Dewar, 1877), it was not until the development of the contact lens electrode (Riggs, 1941; Karpe, 1945) that the electroretinographic technique became practicable for clinical use. There are now a number of methods in use for special purposes, e.g. computer-average responses to focal and/or alternating pattern stimuli, but retinal function is usually evaluated in patients by means of the light-evoked, full-field (ganzfeld) ERG. This simple stimulus configuration provides relatively uniform illumination of the entire retina, and elicits a mass electrical response that represents the summation of several component potentials generated by cells throughout the retina (cf. Ripps & Witkovsky, 1985). Although in these

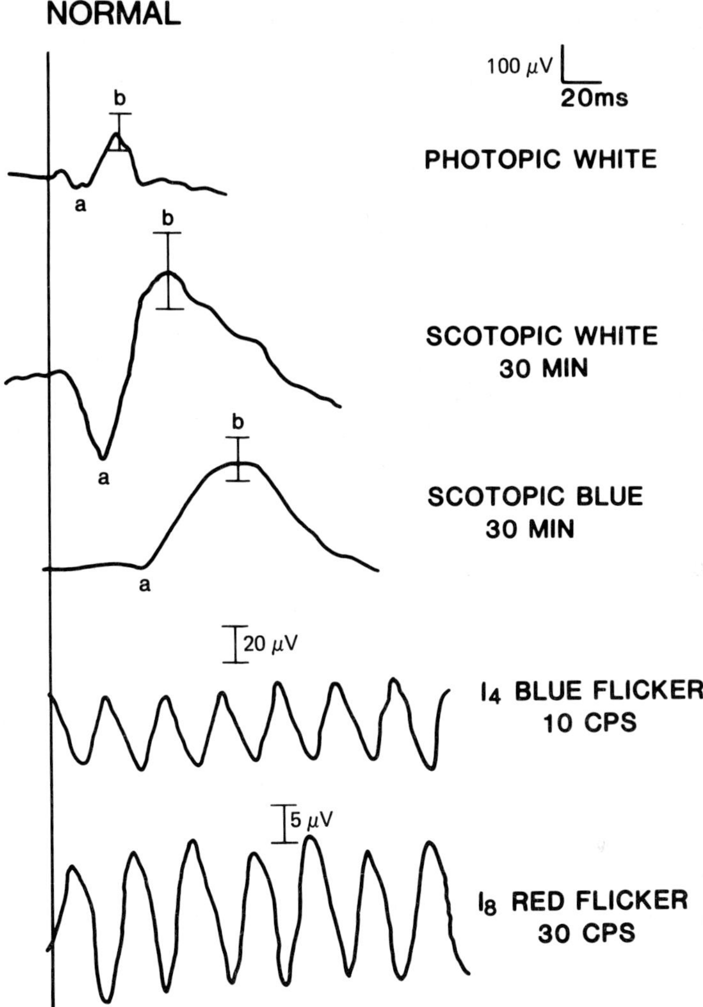

Fig. 12.1. ERG recordings from a normal eye under various stimulus conditions. Cone-mediated responses were elicited by a white test flash delivered under light-adapted (photopic) conditions, and by a flickering (30 Hz) red stimuli. On the other hand, rod-mediated potentials were evoked under dark-adaptated (scotopic) conditions by a dim blue test flash or by a 10 Hz flickering blue stimulus. The bright white stimulus to the dark-adapted retina generates a combined rod and cone response that is rod dominant.

circumstances it is apparent that isolated focal lesions will not affect the recorded response, two of the main objectives of clinical electroretinography can be satisfied reasonably well. The first is to distinguish receptoral from post-receptoral activity and thereby provide information on the depth within the retina that abnormal function is encountered; the second is to assess separately responses generated by the rod and cone mechanisms.

As shown in Fig. 12.1, the ERG waveform consists of two main components, the a- and b-waves, when obtained under the recording conditions used generally for patient studies, namely, capacitance-coupled, limited band-pass electronics. There is good evidence that the leading edge of the cornea-negative a-wave reflects the light-evoked response of the photoreceptors, i.e. a conductance decrease across the outer segment membrane that mediates the cell's hyperpolarizing potential (Penn & Hagins, 1969; Sillman, Ito & Tomita, 1969). On the other hand, the cellular basis of the b-wave remains somewhat of an enigma, although its post-receptoral origins are not in question (Furakawa & Hanawa, 1955; Dowling & Ripps, 1971). The light-induced hyperpolarization of the photoreceptor diminishes the release of neurotransmitter at the cell's synaptic terminal (Dowling & Ripps, 1973; Ripps, Shakib & MacDonald, 1976) which produces, in turn, activation of post-synaptic neural elements (Kaneko & Shimazaki, 1975). As a result, there is a transient increase in the extracellular concentration of K^+ (Kline, Ripps & Dowling, 1978, 1985; Karwoski & Proenza, 1980) that alters the ionic balance across the membrane of the radially-oriented glia (Muller cells), and produces a current flow along the length of the cell. Based on the results of a broad range of studies (Farber, 1969; Newman, 1980) it appears that the large cornea-positive b-wave derives primarily from the K^+-mediated trans-retinal currents that circulate through the Muller cells (cf. Newman & Odette, 1984; Ripps & Witkovsky, 1985). The electrical activity of ganglion cells or their optic nerve fibers do not contribute to the a- or b-waves of the ganzfeld ERG.

Since the ERG b-wave is dependent upon electrochemical events that generate the ERG a-wave, it follows that any retinal disorder that interferes with the response properties of the photoreceptors will also affect the b-wave potential. The converse, however, does not apply. Disorders that result in diffuse dysfunction of cells within the inner nuclear layer, e.g. bipolar and Muller cells, can selectively depress the b-wave without diminishing the ERG a-wave. It should be noted also that with d.c. electronics and a cooperative patient it is sometimes possible to record a late-onset positive potential (the c-wave) that is generated in part by ionic currents across the apical membrane of the retinal pigment epithelium (RPE) (Steinberg, Linsenmeier & Griff, 1983). Although c-wave recordings may eventually prove useful in assessing abnormalities of the RPE, there are difficulties, apart from recording stability that may preclude a valid interpretation of the data (cf. Taumer *et al.*, 1976; Hock & Marmor, 1983).

The second objective of clinical electroretinography, namely, to distinguish rod- from cone-mediated responses, is realized by appropriate variation in the spectral and temporal characteristics of the photic stimuli, and by varying the levels of light- and dark-adaptation under which the recordings are made. For example, cone function can be evaluated by using either a red or white flickering stimulus at 30 cps, a frequency at which rods are unable to respond. Cone-mediated responses can be elicited also with a bright flash of white light superimposed on a steady background luminance that desensitizes the rod mechanism (usually 7–10 foot lamberts). On the other hand, this same stimulus delivered to the dark-adapted retina will evoke mixed (rod–cone) response that, in normal subjects, is rod dominated. It is possible, however, to isolate rod activity by using a relatively dim, short-wavelength (blue) stimulus, and allowing at least 30 min of dark adaptation before testing. Alternatively, a low-intensity blue, intermittent (10 per second) stimulus can be used to obtain the flicker response of the rod mechanism. Representative ERG recordings, obtained under the conditions described above, are illustrated in Fig. 12.1.

In addition to amplitude information, temporal factors may also be of importance in ERG analysis. In this regard, the implicit time, i.e. the time from stimulus onset to the peak of the a- or b-wave, is the most often used index of response kinetics. More detailed discussion of waveforms, stimulus conditions, and the effects of age, sex, refractive error, etc., on the ERG can be found in other publications (Peterson, 1968; Pallin, 1969; Fishman, 1975; Weleber, 1981).

12.2.2 Electro-oculography

The electro-oculogram (EOG) records changes in the 'standing' potential that exists between the cornea and the back of the eye. Electro-oculography was seen as a potentially valuable clinical procedure when it became apparent that abnormal results could be detected in various retinal diseases (Riggs, 1954; François, Verriest & de Rouck, 1956), and that a reliable index of the EOG was readily obtained by determining the light peak to dark trough ratio (LP/DT), i.e. the ratio of the amplitudes recorded under light- and dark-adapted conditions (Arden & Fojas, 1962). Recording procedures have been described in a number of previous reports (François *et al.*, 1956; Arden & Fojos, 1962; Fishman, 1975). Retinal elements that contribute to the potential changes include the retinal pigment epithelium, photoreceptors, and cells of the inner nuclear layer (Gouras & Carr, 1965; Steinberg *et al.*, 1983).

Because the RPE figures prominently in the generation of the light peak of the ERG (Steinberg *et al.*, 1983), the technique has been of diagnostic value in patients with hereditary disorders that induce widespread abnormalities in the RPE while sparing most of the sensory retina, e.g. Best's (vitelliform) macular dystrophy. But there is less than complete agreement as regards the importance of EOG recordings in the screening of patients with night-blinding disorders. The LP/DT ratio is predictably abnormal in patients with progressive retinal diseases that induce widespread destruction of photoreceptors, e.g. retinitis pigmentosa (RP) and choroideremia. However, abnormal EOG results are not usually seen before significant changes have occurred in the ERG, particularly in the amplitudes of rod-mediated responses (Gouras & Carr, 1964). Thus, although the EOG is abnormal once there is appreciable damage to the photoreceptors and/or RPE, it is not an especially sensitive method for detecting early stages in the disease process. In sum, the EOG probably does not offer any advantage over the ERG, and does not provide much by way of additional information in assessing functional loss in patients with progressive night-blinding disorders.

The technique is even less revealing in stationary night-blinding disorders. For example in recessively-inherited stationary nyctalopia with normal fundus, and in Oguchi's disease, normal LP/DT values are recorded, whereas gross abnormalities in the scotopic b-wave of the ERG reveal the presence of widespread defects in the neural retina. In fundus albipunctatus, normal results will be obtained if a prolonged period of dark adaptation is given prior to determining the dark trough, but a normal ERG is also recorded after adequate dark adaptation. Thus, although the EOG has been applied widely to the study of night-blinding disorders, the other test procedures discussed here appear to provide more definitive information.

12.2.3 Psychophysical testing

Visual function can be evaluated clinically with a variety of subjective methods, but there are several which are particularly appropriate for the night-blinding disorders. Determining the detection threshold for a stimulus after 30 min of dark adaptation, or charting the rod- and cone-branches of the dark-adaptation curve after bleaching are among the most frequently used techniques. However, important additional information is obtained by making measurements at more than one retinal locus (a 'retinal profile'), and using chromatic stimuli to separate contributions from the rod and cone mechanisms (Sondheimer *et al.*, 1979). Fig. 12.2 presents an example of threshold data at several retinal loci in the vertical meridian of a patient with retinitis pigmentosa; thresholds were measured with alternating blue and orange stimuli. Note the marked difference in the thresholds obtained at different locations, and the fact that had only one locus (e.g. at 15° in the superior retina) been measured, the patient's dark-adapted threshold would have erroneously been considered normal. Fig. 12.3 shows the retinal profile of a patient with congenital stationary night blindness; measurements were made with blue and red test lights in the horizontal meridian after 45 min of dark adaptation. In this case, absolute thresholds are elevated, except in the central fovea, and it is apparent by comparing the chromatic thresholds that rods are mediating the threshold responses, i.e. thresholds for blue test stimuli lie appreciably below those for the red stimuli. Had white test stimuli been used exclusively at 10° from the fovea, the examiner might have mistakenly concluded that cones were mediating the threshold response. These examples illustrate how psychophysical testing with a white test field at only one locus gives limited, and sometimes misleading, information regarding the functional status of the retina.

Psychophysical tests of scotopic threshold are plagued by the lack of sensitivity for detecting altered rod function and inherent variability in the results obtained even on normal subjects. For example, a 50% reduction in rod outer segment length would be expected to induce a threshold increase of approximately 0.3 log unit based solely on the corresponding reduction in quantal absorption. However, the short term variability in test–retest results on the same observer may vary by 0.2–0.3 log units, and the range of normal values for absolute rod threshold spans nearly 1 log unit (Sloan, 1947). Therefore, appreciable damage to rod outer segments could theoretically occur without a significant elevation of rod thresholds as determined psychophysically. Fundus reflectometry offers a potentially more sensitive means of monitoring this type of visual cell abnormality.

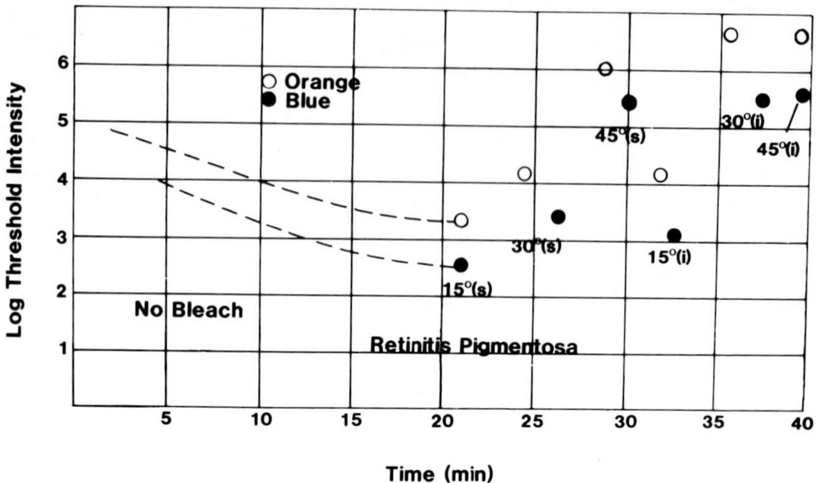

Fig. 12.2. Thresholds for blue (●) and orange (○) stimuli recorded on a modified Goldmann–Weekers adaptometer in a patient with retinitis pigmentosa. Measurements were made in the vertical meridian above (s) and below (i) fixation. The data obtained during the first 20 min period (dashed lines) represent thresholds measured at 15° above the fovea as the patient dark-adapted following exposure to the ambient (waiting room) illumination. At this locus, final thresholds for both chromatic stimuli were normal. However, note the very significant threshold elevations at other loci in the vertical meridian.

12.2.4 Fundus reflectometry

If we are to attempt functionally to 'dissect' the retina, i.e. examine the integrity of successive stages in the visual process, it is clearly desirable to have some means of testing the initial stage of that process: namely, the light-induced photochemical changes in the rod pigment, rhodopsin. Fortunately it is a relatively straightforward matter to record some of the principal reactions in the complex sequence of events that accompany the bleaching and regeneration of rhodopsin. Although a number of rather sophisticated instruments have been devised for this purpose (cf. Kemp & Faulkner, 1981; Kilbride *et al.*, 1983), all are based on the fact that rhodopsin undergoes dramatic spectral changes following exposure to light, and all utilize the well-known principle of the ophthalmoscope to detect and measure light reflected from the fundus oculi – hence 'fundus reflectometry'.

The principle of the method and a sample of the results obtained with a rapid-scan fundus reflectometer are illustrated in Fig. 12.4; earlier papers (Ripps & Weale, 1965, 1969; Ripps & Snapper, 1974) provide

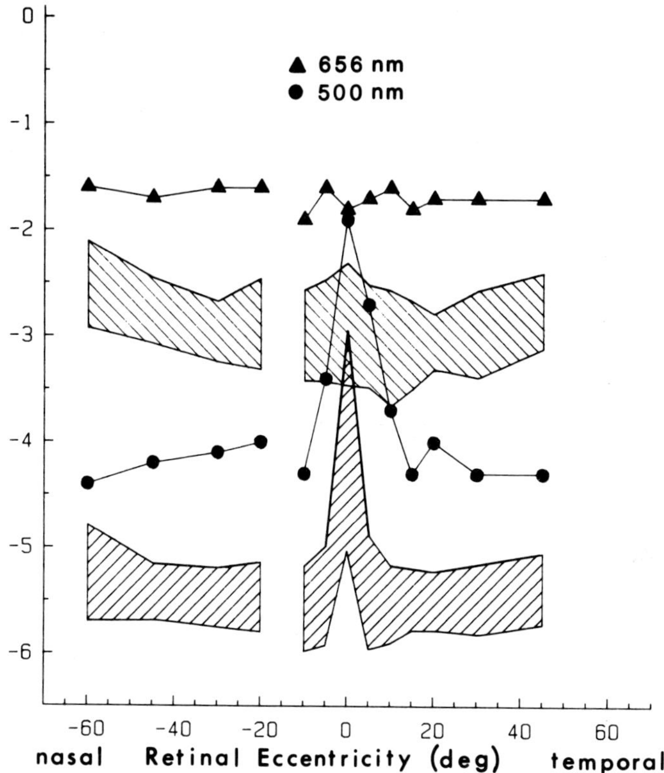

Fig. 12.3. Dark-adapted retinal profiles measured on a Tübinger perimeter with blue (= 500 nm) and red (= 656 nm) test stimuli for a patient with congenital stationary night blindness. Note that except for the fovea, where threshold is cone-mediated, the much lower thresholds (by >2 log units) for the 500 nm stimulus indicate that the rod mechanism subserves visual threshold throughout the other regions of the retina.

more detailed descriptions of the technique. As shown in Fig. 12.4*a*, a beam of monochromatic light enters the dark-adapted eye, returns through the pupil after twice traversing the retina, and strikes a sensitive photocell that records its intensity. In so doing, the beam has passed through the pigment-bearing outer segments of the photoreceptors, and is attenuated to a degree that depends upon the amount of photopigment present and the absorption properties of the pigment for the particular test wavelength. After exposing the same retinal area to a very intense light that bleaches the pigment to a relatively transparent photoproduct, a second measurement with the test beam gives a higher reading on the photodetector. The logarithm of the ratio of these two measurements

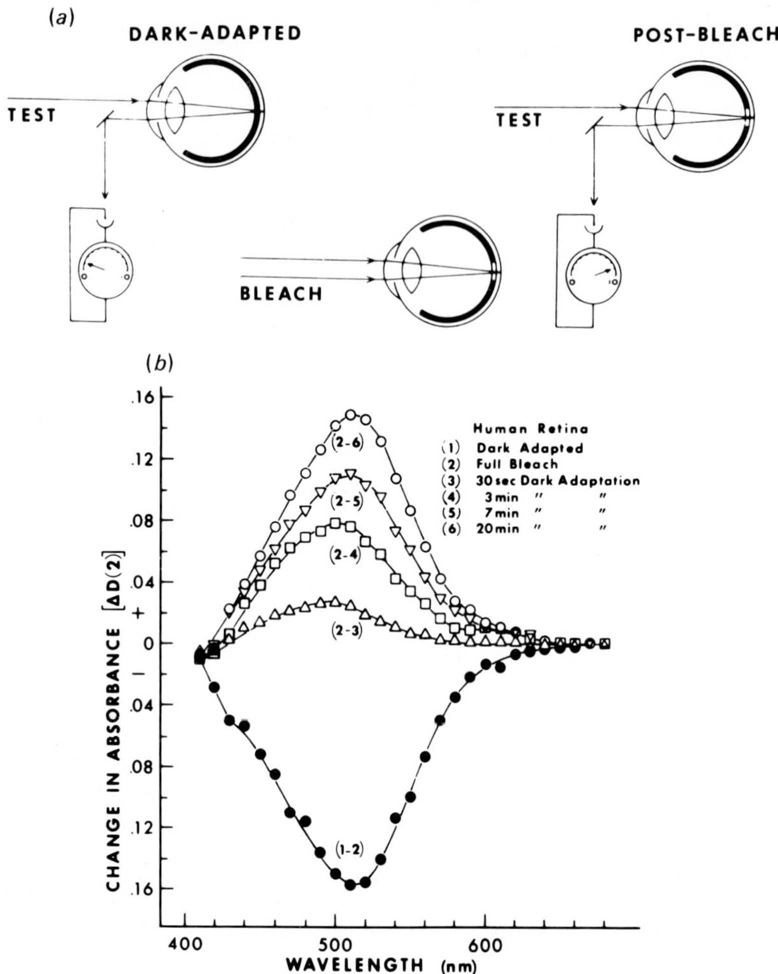

Fig. 12.4. (*a*) The principle of fundus reflectometry. Measurements are made before and after exposure to an intense beam that bleaches a large fraction of the visual pigment. (*b*) Absorbance changes (*D*) due to the bleaching and regeneration of rhodopsin in the mid-peripheral human retina. Density losses due to bleaching (filled circles) are plotted as negative values; open symbols show the progressive gain in density as the pigment regenerates during dark adaptation.

yields the density difference for the wavelength (*D*).

In practice, a range of test wavelengths is used to obtain the bleaching difference spectrum (Fig. 12.4*b*). Repeating the spectral measurements at various times during the course of dark adaptation provides data on the kinetics of the process by which pigment is regenerated (Fig. 12.4*b*); i.e. the values for the half-time of regeneration ($t_{1/2}$), and the time constant (τ) of the ostensibly exponential function.

12.3 Vitamin A in night vision

The role of vitamin A (retinol) in vision, and the consequences of prolonged vitamin A deficiency are too well known to be belabored here. Nevertheless, it may be useful at this juncture to summarize the main features of the rhodopsin cycle, the link between these events and electrogenesis, and the possible involvement of these processes in night-blinding disorders.

12.3.1 The rhodopsin cycle and visual transduction

Quantal absorption – the initial event in vision and in the photolysis of rhodopsin – induces an instantaneous change in the isomeric form of the visual pigment chromophore, converting 11-*cis* to all-*trans* retinaldehyde (Hubbard & Kropf, 1958). The molecule then degrades thermally through a series of spectrally identifiable intermediates (see also Chapter 5) that lead ultimately to the formation of a colorless ('bleached') photoproduct. In the final stages of this process the chromophore is hydrolyzed from the protein moiety (opsin) and rapidly reduced to retinol (cf. Ostroy, 1977, for a more complete description of the bleaching sequence).

During the course of these changes, probably in the transition to metarhodopsin II (Bennett, Michel-Villaz & Kuhn, 1982), the conformational state of the photoactivated rhodopsin (R*) catalyzes the exchange of GTP for GDP on the GTP-binding protein, transducin, which activates in turn a cGMP-specific phosphodiesterase that induces hydrolysis of the nucleotide (cf. Liebman & Pugh, 1981; Kuhn & Chabre, 1983; Stryer, 1986). This enzymatic cascade provides the amplification required of the transduction mechanism, and there is convincing evidence from recent studies that cGMP serves as the internal transmitter that controls the light-sensitive membrane conductance of the rod outer segment (Fesenko, Kolesnikov & Lyubarky, 1985; Nakatani & Yau, 1985).

However, if vision is to be maintained, a further requirement is the renewal of the rhodopsin content of the rod outer segment; i.e. the restoration of 11-*cis* retinal to the disc membranes where it reacts with opsin to regenerate rhodopsin. In this, the retinal pigment epithelium (RPE) plays a vital role (Kuhne, 1878). The all-*trans* retinol formed in the visual cell is transported, presumably by means of an interstitial retinoid-binding protein (IRBP) (Lai *et al.*, 1982; Liou *et al.*, 1982), to the apical surface of the RPE, and transferred to a cellular retinoid-binding protein (CRBP) for esterification and delivery to storage depots within the cell (Krinsky, 1958; Futterman, 1974; Berman *et al.*, 1980). The all-*trans* retinyl ester (mainly palmitate and stearate) must then by hydrolyzed to the corresponding alcohol, oxidized to the aldehyde, isomerized to the 11-*cis* form, and returned to the rod outer segment for regeneration to take place. Where and in what order these events occur, the forms of vitamin A involved at each stage in the sequence, and the precise mechanism by which retinoids are translocated from intra- to extracellular compartments (and vice versa) are still unknown. Nevertheless, it is clear that a defect at any stage in this complex cyclical process will affect the normal behavior of the visual cells.

12.3.2 Vitamin A deficiency, rhodopsin and visual threshold

In addition to the retinol acquired from the photoreceptors, the ocular stores of vitamin A are replenished from the choroidal vasculature and delivered by a serum retinol binding protein (RBP) to receptor sites on the basal surface of the RPE (Bok & Heller, 1976). The source of this supply derives from the ingestion of carotenoids and vitamin A esters which penetrate the mucosa of the small intestine, are stored in the liver, and released into the circulation where it combines with RBP and transthyretin to form a complex molecule that is transported to target organs.

Although vitamin A deficiency as part of a general malnutrition syndrome is still prevalent in some parts of the world, its occurrence in modern societies results most often from chronic diseases of the liver and gastrointestinal tract (Petersen, Peterson & Robb, 1968; Ong, Page & Chytil, 1975; Main *et al.*, 1983), tissues involved in the absorption, storage and mobilization of vitamin A and in the production of its serum transport proteins (Smith & Goodman, 1971). In such cases, as well as in vitamin deficiencies resulting from malabsorption due to intestinal by-pass surgery (Partamian, Sidrys & Tripathi, 1979; Brown, Felton & Benson, 1980; Perlman *et al.*, 1983), night blindness is a frequent concomitant, and the marked elevation of threshold is readily demonstrated by dark adaptometry and electroretinography.

To our knowledge, however, only one vitamin A-deficient patient has been reported in whom the rhodopsin density was estimated by fundus reflectometry (Ripps, Brin & Weale, 1978). Although rod threshold in an area of the mid-peripheral retina was indeterminate (lying above the cone plateau and 3 log units above the normal rod threshold), the rhodopsin content of that same retinal region was reduced by only 20%. Had the loss of visual pigment represented simply a reduction in the efficacy of quantal absorption, threshold should have been raised a mere 0.1 log unit. Clearly, the results indicate a severe upset in the functional integrity of the rod mechanism quite apart from its light-absorbing capacity. In fact, the profound effects of vitamin A deprivation on rod structure and function were shown first in the experiments of Dowling & Wald (1958) and Dowling & Gibbons (1961) on the rat, and it seems likely that a similar situation obtains in the human condition.

Interestingly, bleaching a fraction of the available rhodopsin also induces a disproportionate rise in rod threshold that persists through dark adaptation (Rushton, 1961; see also Chapter 5). While the physiological basis of this phenomenon is probably quite different from that seen in vitamin A deficiency, it illustrates again the requirement of the visual cell for its normal complement of visual pigment.

12.4 Inherited night blindness in man and animals

Inherited night-blinding disorders can be either stationary or progressive. Progressive diseases are often associated with deterioration of the RPE and choroid in addition to photoreceptor cell dystrophy. Stationary disorders, on the other hand, do not show signs of degeneration or evidence of the loss of neural cells.

Within both categories, there appears to be a wide range of functional abnormalities affecting the rod system and leading to the subjective complaint of poor night vision. In the following sections we will cite the findings (and interpretations) in a few examples from each category.

12.4.1 Stationary disorders

Fundus albipunctatus

Hereditary night-blinding disorders are not usually associated with abnormal visual pigment kinetics (cf. Ripps, 1982). Fundus albipunctatus provides a notable exception (Carr, Ripps & Siegel, 1974). In this unusual autosomal recessive disorder characterized by large numbers of yellowish-white spots scattered throughout the fundus (Fig. 12.5), both the cone- and rod-mediated segments of the dark-adaptation curve are grossly abnormal. As shown in Fig. 12.6, final thresholds for both systems eventually reach normal levels, but the time course of adaptation

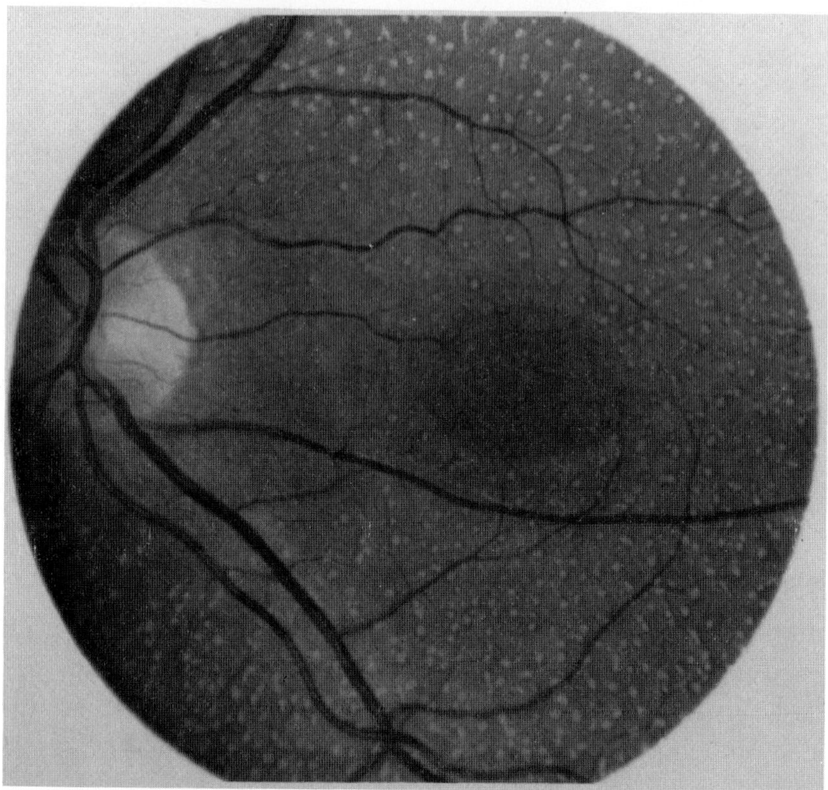

Fig. 12.5. Fundus albipunctatus. The fundus photograph shows the distribution of punctate spots with some sparing of the macular region.

is extremely slow. Similar kinetics are seen in the regeneration of rhodopsin and the cone pigments measured by fundus reflectometry (cf. Carr *et al.*, 1974).

In view of these findings, and the fact that other indices of retinal function, e.g. the electroretinographic a- and b-waves, EOG, also await the slow regeneration of visual pigments before returning to normal sensitivity, it seems likely that the condition results from a defect at some stage in the visual pigment cycle. However, serum levels of vitamin A and RBP are normal in patients with fundus albipunctatus (Carr, Margolis & Siegel, 1976), as they are in most inherited night-blinding diseases (Futterman, Swanson & Kalina, 1974; Maraini, Fadda & Gozzoli, 1975; Massoud, Bird & Perkins, 1975; but cf. Carr, 1969). Nevertheless, it is possible that the disturbance involves proteins responsible for the exchange of retinoids between the photoreceptors and RPE,

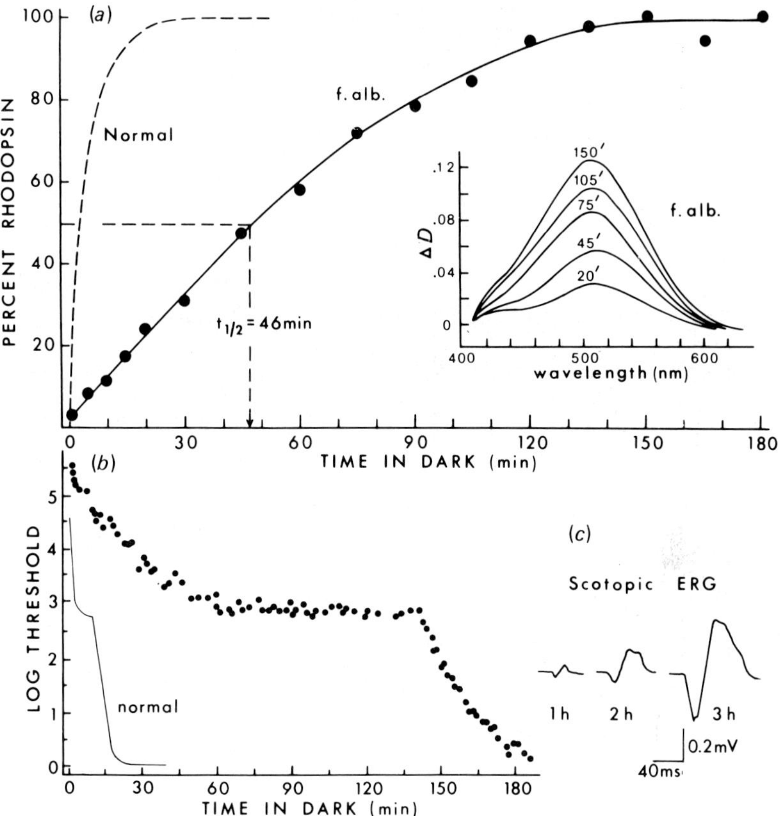

Fig. 12.6. Experimental results in fundus albipunctatus. (*a*) Kinetics of rhodopsin regeneration for 540 nm obtained from difference spectra (inset) recorded at various times in the course of dark adaptation. (*b*) Visual thresholds during dark adaptation for the same region of the mid-peripheral retina. (*c*) ERG recordings to a bright test flash (white) recorded after 1, 2, and 3 h of dark adaptation.

i.e. IRBP or its receptor sites. But there are clearly a number of equally plausible alternative explanations that could account for the findings in this condition, e.g. deficiencies in cellular retinoid binding protein, esterification enzymes, etc.

Oguchi's disease

Another uniquely aberrant form of stationary night blindness occurs in Oguchi's disease, a relatively rare autosomal recessive condition in which the fundus exhibits a metallic, phosphorescent-like sheen that disappears

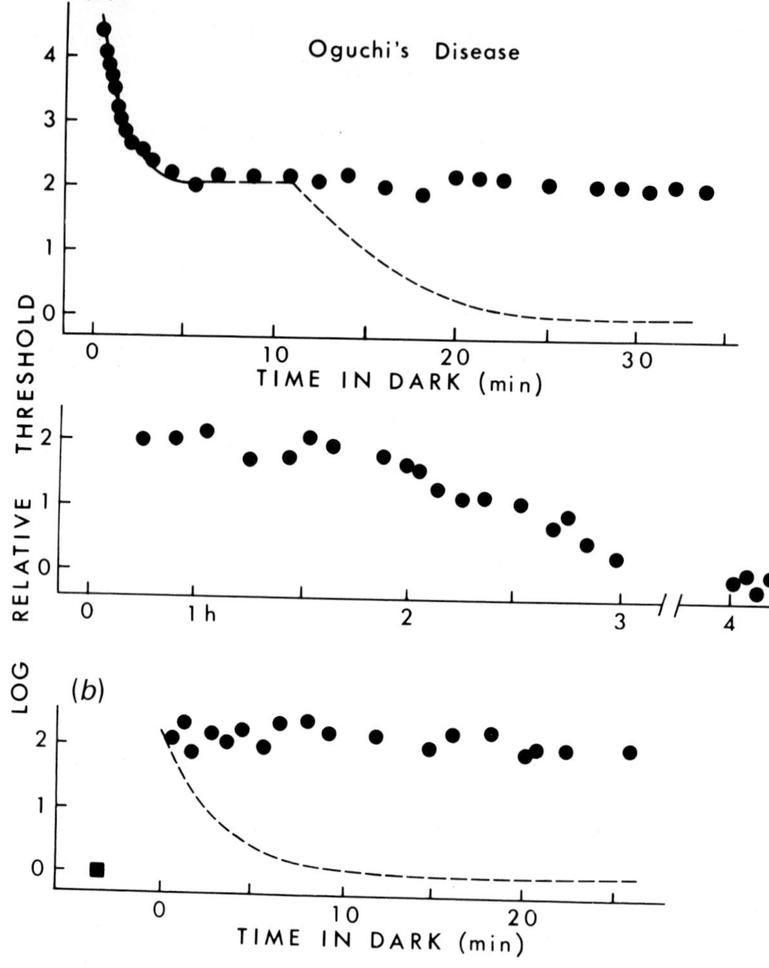

Fig. 12.7. (*a*) The course of dark adaptation in the mid-peripheral retina of a normal eye (dashed curve), and in a patient with Oguchi's disease (data points). Note the change of time base between the upper and lower panels of the graph; the data were obtained following a 7 min exposure to 8900 cd/m^2. (*b*) Dark adaptation following a 1 min exposure to a retinal illuminance (1250 td) that bleached less than 1 percent of the rhodopsin within the test region. Threshold measurements in Oguchi's disease (circles) are compared with results obtained for a normal subject (dashed curve). The black square indicates the visual threshold for both observers just prior to the period of light adaptation.

or becomes less apparent after prolonged dark adaptation (Mizuo–Nakamura phenomenon). Several histopathological studies have been reported (Yamanaka, 1924, 1969; Oguchi, 1925; Kuwabara, Ishihara & Akiya, 1963), but the findings are quite disparate, and the cause of the strange color change is still not known. As regards the night-blinding disorder, the cone-mediated branch of the dark-adaptation curve appears to be normal, but the rod branch resembles that seen in fundus albipunctatus; its onset is delayed by nearly 2 h, and the time course it follows to final threshold is greatly prolonged (Fig. 12.7*a*). However, unlike fundus albipunctatus, rhodopsin kinetics, the EOG, and the growth of the ERG a-wave after bleaching are normal (Carr & Gouras, 1965; Carr & Ripps, 1967); i.e. rhodopsin is fully regenerated and the a-wave grows to its maximum amplitude in less than 30 min of dark adaptation. On the other hand, the ERG b-wave fails to develop normally (Ripps, 1976), and in some cases may be markedly suppressed even after the eye is allowed to dark adapt for 4 h (Gouras & Carr, 1965).

With both the rhodopsin cycle and the electrical activity of the visual cells performing well, it appears reasonable to suggest that the normal adaptation process in Oguchi's disease is being compromised by some post-receptoral abnormality that affects the cellular elements responsible for generating the ERG b-wave (Carr & Ripps, 1967). There is, in fact, good evidence from animal experimentation that a post-receptoral neuronal 'network' controls an important phase of the dark-adaptation process (Green *et al.*, 1975; Tranchina, Gordon & Shapley, 1984; Chapter 1 and 3 contain specific details of network adaptation). For example, when the all-rod retina of the skate is exposed to a very dim adapting light, one that has practically no effect on the sensitivity of the a-wave (receptor) potential, it produces a sharp rise in b-wave and ganglion-cell thresholds. And after the exposure, the receptors dark-adapt almost instantaneously, whereas the b-wave and responses of ganglion cells (the fibers of which form the optic nerve) require about 10 min to reach maximum sensitivity. Clearly *visual* adaptation in these circumstances will reflect the slowly adapting network mechanism and not the status of the rod photoreceptors.

Applying the same protocol to the subjective study of human dark adaptation, with both a normal observer and one with Oguchi's disease, gives strikingly different results (Fig. 12.7*b*). After exposure to the weak adapting light, the normal eye, like that of the skate, recovers maximum sensitivity in about 10 min. But in Oguchi's disease, the dim pre-adapting field causes thresholds to remain elevated for at least 30 min. The profound long-lasting depression of visual sensitivity following illumination that exerts no effects on the rod photoreceptors, supports the notion that this condition results from a defect in the processes that control network adaptation.

12.4.2 Congenital stationary night blindness

In the more common types of non-progressive inheritable night-blinding disorders, referred to generally as congenital stationary night blindness (CSNB), the fundus appearance is normal, the rod-mediated branch of the dark-adaptation curve is absent or greatly elevated, and the scotopic ERG is distinctly abnormal. However, the results obtained in the different genetic forms of the disorder can be quite variable, particularly with respect to the ERG responses (Schubert & Bornschein, 1952; Carrol & Haig, 1952) which may exhibit remarkably different waveforms, even among patients with the same mode of inheritance (cf. Armington & Schwab, 1954; Auerbach, Godel & Rowe, 1969). Indeed, the most consistent finding thus far is in the results obtained by fundus reflectometry. Only a few patients have been studied with this technique, but in each instance the *in situ* density of rhodopsin as well as its photosensitivity and regeneration kinetics were entirely normal (Carr *et al.*, 1966*a*; Alpern, Holland & Ohba, 1972). In this section we have chosen two examples from Carr *et al.* (1966*a*, *b*) to illustrate not only the extremes in the range of ERG responses encountered in CSNB, but also the differences in retinal loci at which functional impairment is thought to occur.

CSNB (dominant inheritance)

The first patient represents a case of dominant inheritance in which eight members from three generations of a family were night blind. Dark adaptometry showed the typical monophasic curve, with the cone-mediated branch lying about 0.4 log unit above the normal plateau (Fig. 12.8*a*). And as already noted, the results of fundus reflectometry were entirely normal (Fig. 12.8*b*). However, a most unexpected finding was obtained by electroretinography. Despite the fact that rhodopsin was present in normal amounts, light flashes, no matter how intense, failed to elicit even a trace of a rod-mediated potential from the dark-adapted retina (Fig. 12.9). At best, only a small cone-like potential was recorded in response to the brightest stimulus. It appears likely, therefore, that there is a breakdown in the mechanism whereby quantal absorption is linked to the generation of a receptor potential. Quite possibly the defect involves one of the light-activated enzymatic stages in the transduction process (see above), or perhaps one of the mechanisms responsible for the synthesis and transport of related proteins to the

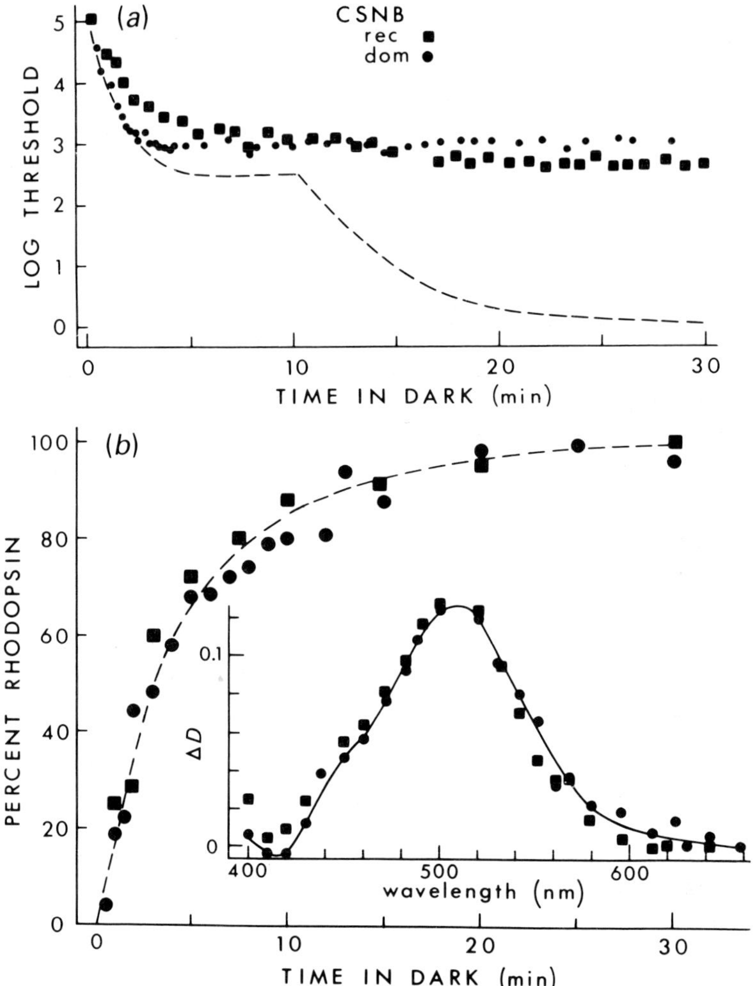

Fig. 12.8. Dark adaptometry (*a*) and fundus reflectometry (*b*) in two patients with CSNB; results were obtained at 12° in the temporal retina. In both the recessive (rec) and dominant (dom) forms of the disorder, the dark-adaptation curves are monophasic, and both the rhodopsin content and the kinetics of photopigment regeneration are normal.

receptor outer segment. On the available evidence, it is not possible to decide between these and a score of other alternatives. In any event, a disturbance at the initial stage of the visual process will exert its effect upon the entire train of events leading to visual perception.

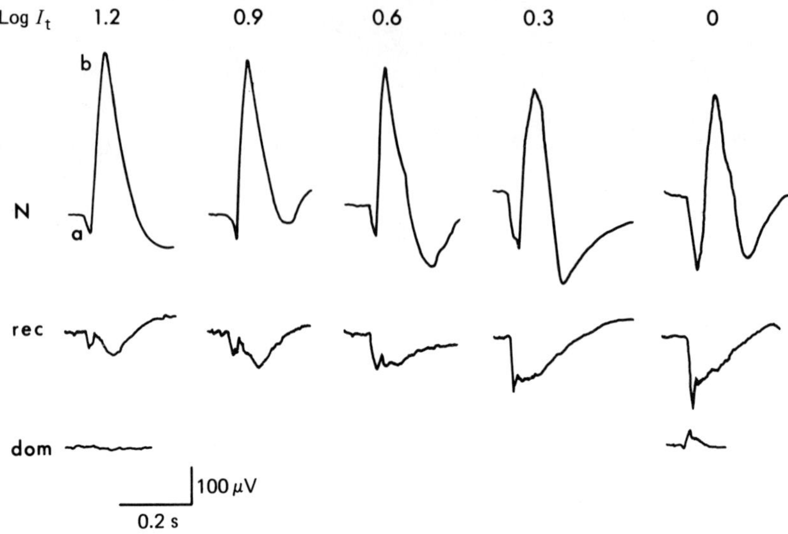

Fig. 12.9. ERG recordings in response to test flashes of increasing intensity in a normal subject (N) and in two forms of CSNB. In the normal, the b-wave amplitude over this range of intensities is relatively constant, but the a-wave grows with each increment in flash intensity. In the recessively-inherited night blind (rec), the scotopic b-wave was not recordable, but a-waves of increasing amplitude were elicited with successively brighter flashes. In dominantly-inherited CSNB (dom), the brightest test flash evoked a small response, which had the characteristics of a rapid, cone mediated potential.

CSNB (recessive inheritance)

The other case of CSNB we wish to consider inherited the night-blinding disorder as a recessive trait. The dark-adaptation curve, like that of the previous subject, was monophasic with no evidence of the rod-mediated segment of the normal function (Fig. 12.8*a*). And here too, fundus reflectometry was used to demonstrate the presence of a normal supply of rhodopsin that bleached and regenerated with normal kinetics (Fig. 12.8*b*). There was, however, an important difference in the type of abnormality seen electroretinographically. The a-wave of the ERG, i.e. the cornea-negative component derived from the light-evoked voltage change across the photoreceptor membrane, was readily elicited by photic stimuli, and its amplitude increased with increasing flash intensity (Fig. 12.9). Thus, all testable aspects of receptor function were normal.

On the other hand, evidence of the scotopic b-wave, a useful index of

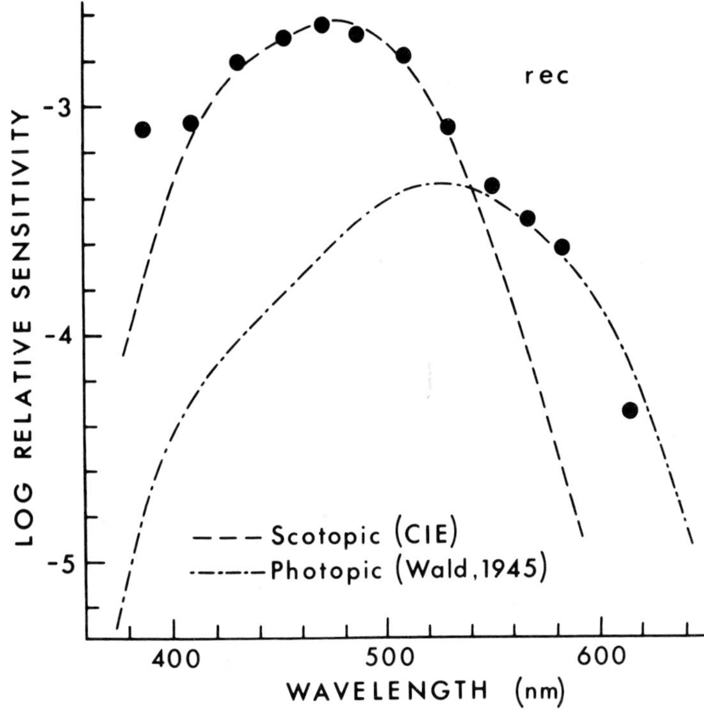

Fig. 12.10. Spectral sensitivity in recessively-inherited night blindness. At long wavelengths (>540 nm) the data follow the photopic sensitivity function of the peripheral retina. At shorter wavelengths, threshold is mediated by the rod mechanism.

rod-mediated, post-receptoral activity, was completely lacking, a finding strongly suggestive of a defect involving the mechanism by which the receptor potential is coupled to the generation of the b-wave, i.e. at a distal stage in the visual pathway. But the break in signal transfer was apparently not complete. A psychophysical determination of the eye's dark-adapted spectral sensitivity function showed that the rod mechanism was not totally inactive (Fig. 12.10). In the short-wavelength region of the spectrum, where the data departed from the photopic curve, it was fit well by the CIE (Commission International de L'Eclairage) scotopic function, indicating that rod signals were being transmitted to higher visual centers, although the sensitivity of the system was reduced by nearly 1000-fold compared with the normal.

The Appaloosa horse

Because the visual cell is often implicated in night-blinding disorders (cf. Ripps, Siegel & Mehaffey, 1985) it was assumed at first that the 'decoupling' between receptors and their second-order cells results from a failure in the modulation of transmitter release at the receptor terminal. While this remains a possibility in the human condition, it appears not to be the case in an animal model of recessive CSNB, the night-blind Appaloosa horse (Witzel *et al.*, 1978). Using HRP as a tracer for detecting the exocytotic release of synaptic vesicles (cf. Ripps *et al.*, 1976), it was possible to show that light and dark adaptation affected vesicle recycling in the normal way, i.e. a dark-release of transmitter and its suppression by light (Ripps, 1982).

Vincristine-induced night blindness

There is still reason to suspect that the visual cell is the defective element in the recessive form of CSNB, although the rationale is based on studies performed on a patient who had developed night blindness after treatment with vincristine, a widely used anti-tumor agent. The drug exerts its oncolytic effect by interfering with the assembly of microtubles, a class of cytoskeletal proteins involved in cell division as well as in an axonal transport of synaptic vesicles, neurotransmitters and their precursors. The surprising observation in this case was the fact that the test results (Fig. 12.11) were nearly identical in every detail to those obtained in the patient with the recessively inherited condition described previously. The dark-adaptation curve was monophasic, with final thresholds elevated more than 3 log units above the normal rod plateau; rhodopsin bleached and regenerated with normal kinetics; the ERG gave precisely the same response pattern, i.e. normal a-wave potentials and the absence of a rod-mediated b-wave; and finally, the short wavelength shoulder in the spectral sensitivity data showed the remnants of rod-mediated vision (Ripps *et al.*, 1984).

The remarkable parallel with inherited stationary night blindness suggests the possibility that both the iatrogenic and genetically-acquired visual anomalies stem from the same functional defect, namely, an abnormality in the axoplasmic transport machinery that serves to deliver to the receptor terminal the molecular and vesicular constituents required for neurotransmission. The consequences are obvious: failure of the cell to maintain normal function at its synaptic terminal, and the

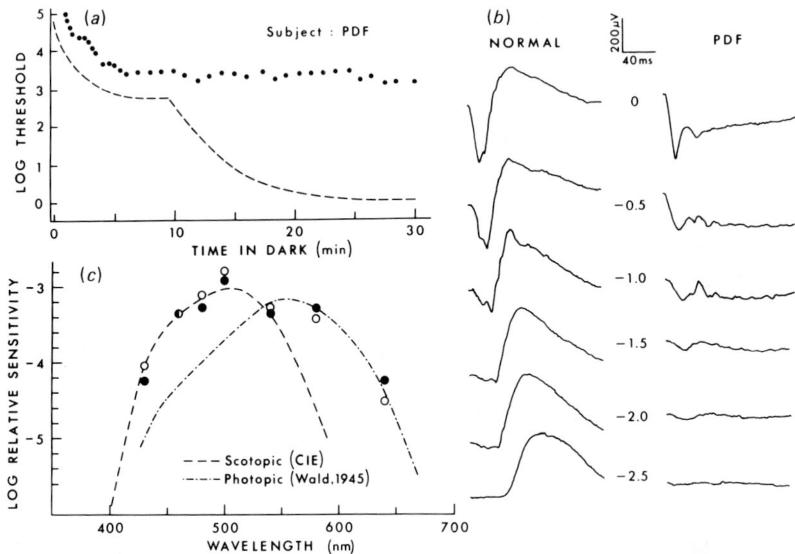

Fig.12.11. Test results from a patient with vincristine-induced night blindness. (*a*) Thresholds during dark adaptation (filled circles) are compared with the results obtained in the normal (dashed curve). (*b*) As in the case of recessively-inherited CSNB, the a-wave of the ERG grows with increasing flash intensity, and (*c*) the dark-adapted spectral sensitivity data show a hump at short wavelengths indicating the presence of rod-mediated function.

development of electrophysiological and visual abnormalities like those seen in our patients. It is noteworthy that studies on the arterially-perfused cat eye have demonstrated similar ERG abnormalities after short-term perfusion with vincristine, and EM (electron microscopic) examination of the retina indicated that the principal site of drug damage was the microtubular elements of the visual cells (Ripps *et al.*, 1985).

12.4.3 Inherited progressive night-blinding diseases

Humans and animals with progressive night-blinding diseases typically show signs of photoreceptor degeneration, most probably due to the greater susceptibility of these neurons to genetically-mediated abnormalities (Ripps *et al.*, 1985). Although as a rule rod receptors are affected earlier, cone cells are also appreciably impaired in the majority of these diseases. In the animal models it is obviously not always possible to establish unequivocally whether the animal experiences night blindness. However, the evidence from electrophysiological and histological

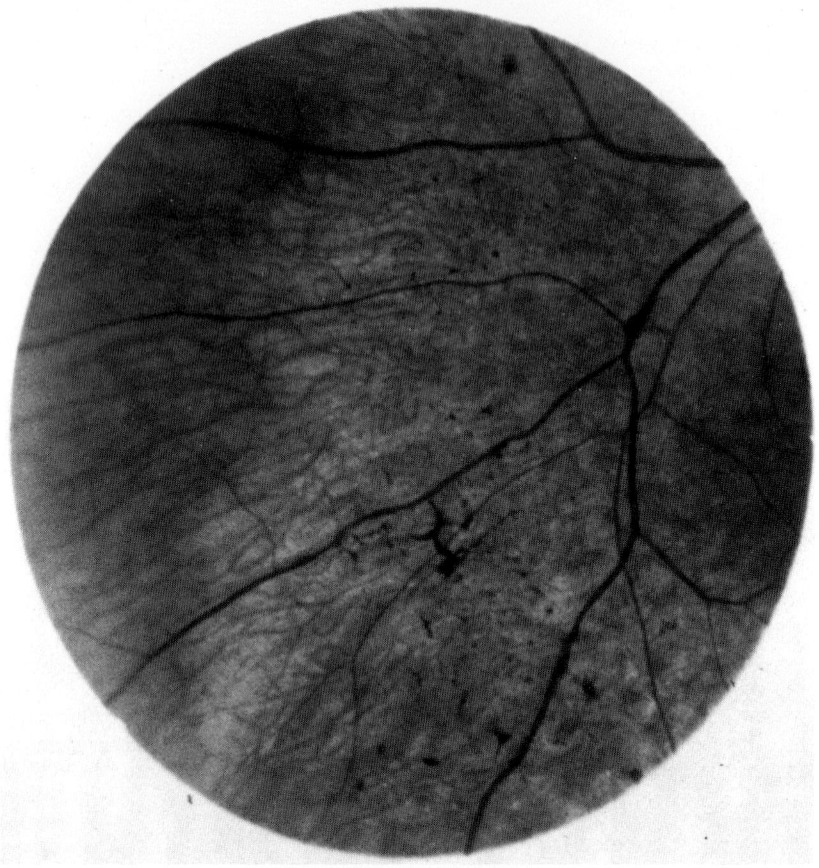

Fig. 12.12. Fundus photograph of the mid-peripheral retina in a patient with retinitis pigmentosa. Note regions of hypopigmentation and 'bone-spicule'-like pigmentation.

studies, as well as observations of the animal's nocturnal behavior, indicates early, widespread involvement of the rod mechanism.

12.4.4. Retinitis pigmentosa

The term retinitis pigmentosa (RP) refers to a genetically and clinically heterogeneous group of degenerative diseases; there is probably appreciable heterogeneity also in the pathogenetic mechanisms that underlie the various forms of RP. Patients complain of night blindness and peripheral field loss usually within the first two decades of life, and fundus examination typically reveals attenuated retinal vessels, a variable degree of 'bone-spicule' pigmentation most extensive in the mid-peripheral retina (Fig. 12.12), and eventually a pale, atrophic-looking optic disc.

The disease was first described by Donders in 1857 soon after the invention of the ophthalmoscope, but despite its long history and frequent occurrence, differential diagnosis remains an important consideration. An RP-like fundus picture has been described in a variety of syndromes, e.g. Usher's, Bardet–Biedl, Refsum's and Bassen–Kornzweig (cf. Stiggelbout, 1972; Fishman, 1980; Campo & Aaberg, 1982; Berson, 1982; Fishman *et al.*, 1983), and signs and symptoms resembling RP may occur secondarily to inflammation, drug toxicity, trauma, malabsorption, etc.

RP and vitamin A

Vitamin A therapy has been tried in patients with RP but without success (cf. Chatzinoff *et al.*, 1968). This is hardly surprising in view of experimental results indicating that retinol transport in the general circulation of RP patients is unimpaired; i.e. there are normal levels of serum retinol and its binding protein (Wagreich, Lasky & Elkan, 1961; Krachmer, Smith & Tocci, 1966; Futterman *et al.*, 1974; Maraini *et al.*, 1975; Massoud *et al.*, 1975). However, this does not preclude the possibility of a defect in some local (ocular) phase of the rhodopsin cycle, e.g. the isomerization process, or the intercellular transport of retinoids. In fact, there are reports of extremely low levels of 11-*cis* retinyl ester in the RPE (Bridges & Alvarez, 1982), and depletion of IRBP (Bridges *et al.*, 1985; Rodrigues *et al.*, 1986) in donor eyes with retinitis pigmentosa. It is not clear yet whether these changes are primary events, or occur secondarily to the photoreceptor cell degeneration. In either event, abnormalities of this kind could result in the accumulation of toxic levels of free retinol, and accelerate the destructive process. Histological evidence tends to support the view that at least some types of RP are diseases of the visual cell, with secondary changes occurring within the RPE (Kolb & Gouras, 1974; Szamier *et al.*, 1979; Bunt-Milam, Kalina & Pagon, 1983).

Functional classification of RP

There is a need for more precise means of classifying RP patients so that biochemical and morphological findings from donor eyes can be correlated with functional data obtained with non-invasive methods. Massof & Finkelstein (1979, 1981) have noted that most RP patients fall into one of two categories, based on the relative losses in rod- and cone-mediated function. In the Type I category, there is a diffuse and fairly uniform loss of rod function; the cone mechanism, which is not as severely affected, therefore mediates threshold in both the light- and dark-adapted retina. In Type II patients, both cone and rod mechanisms are affected early in the course of disease, and rods tend to mediate threshold despite the marked loss in sensitivity. These subtypes also show differences in the age of onset of night blindness (earlier in Type I), in the degree of rod function seen in the ERG (absent in Type I, but recordable in Type II patients) (Lyness *et al.*, 1985), and in the distribution of pigment deposits seen ophthalmoscopically (diffuse in Type I as compared to a more regional localization in Type II patients (cf. Fishman, Alexander & Anderson, 1985).

Although the pathogenesis of the various forms of RP is still obscure, some progress has been made, in part due to results obtained with non-invasive *in vivo* methods, from histological studies of donor eyes, and from investigations on animal models (see below). In RP patients in whom the disease is not too advanced, measurements of rhodopsin density and visual threshold in mildly affected areas of the visual field showed that although visual sensitivity was only moderately depressed in these regions, the rhodopsin content of the rods was severely depleted (Highman & Weale, 1973; Ripps *et al.*, 1978; Perlman & Auerbach, 1981). When graphed (Fig. 12.13), the data indicated that threshold elevation was attributable to the reduced quantal absorption by rods containing less than their normal complement of rhodopsin. This led to the suggestion that the disease process, at least in some RP subtypes, probably results in a progressive shortening of rod outer segments, due most likely to an upset in the normal balance between disc shedding and new disc formation, i.e. the rate of degradation exceeds the rate at which new discs are synthesized (Ripps *et al.*, 1978). By whatever means this upset is brought about, the outcome for the photoreceptor is entirely predictable: a progressive loss of function and cell death.

It is noteworthy that in their ultrastructural study of the retina of a patient with advanced, dominantly-inherited RP, Szamier & Berson (1977) were unable to find any rod photoreceptors, but the outer segments of the remaining cones were absent or significantly shorter than normal, and autophagic vacuoles were seen frequently in the myoid region of these elements. Somewhat similar findings were reported for both rods and cones in a later study of sex-linked RP (Szamier *et al.*, 1979). It is entirely possible that the synthetic machinery for disc formation located in the myoid region of the receptor inner segment, or the cytoskeletal system by which membrane is delivered to the outer segments is affected early in the disease process. However, this is unlikely to represent a general pattern

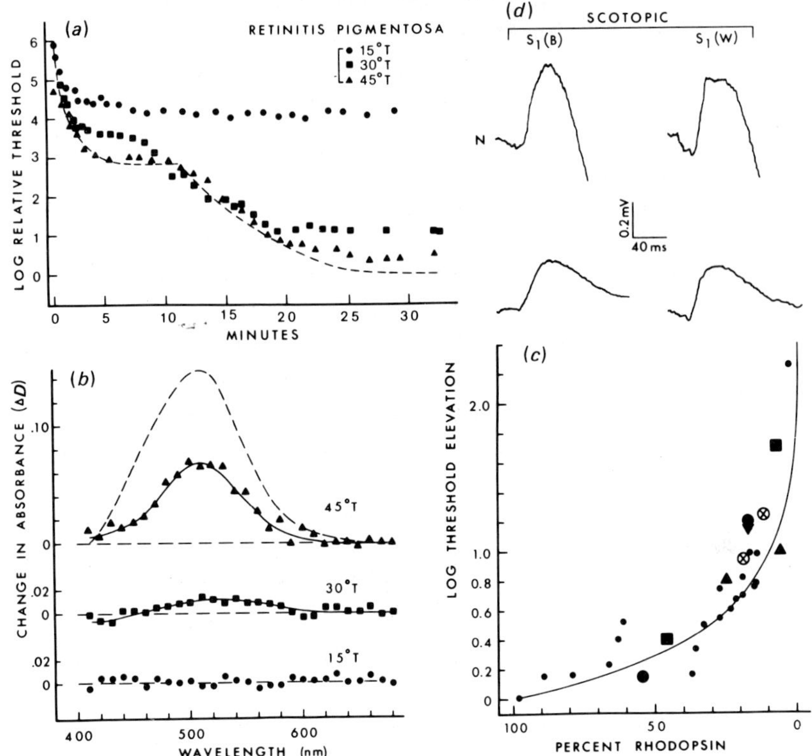

Fig. 12.13. Experimental findings in a patient with dominant RP. Dark adaptation (*a*) and rhodopsin difference spectra (*b*) were measured in the same regions of the mid-peripheral retina. At 30° and 45°, where final thresholds are elevated above the normal (dashed line) by only 1.0 and 0.3 log unit, respectively, the corresponding rhodopsin levels are markedly reduced to 10 and 50 percent of normal. (*c*) Log of the absolute (dark-adapted) threshold plotted as a function of the percent rhodopsin measured at various retinal loci. The data fall along a curve that describes the visual sensitivity solely in terms of the probability of quantal absorption. (*d*) Electroretinographic responses to brief flashes of blue and white light in the patient are only moderately reduced compared with those obtained from a normal subject.

for all RP-like diseases, and evidence that very different findings may be otained in some forms of RP has been reported (Perlman & Auerbach, 1981).

Advancements in molecular genetics will likely extend our understanding of this group of disorders. X-chromosome-specific probes have already been used to localize the X-linked retinitis pigmentosa gene to a subregion of the short arm of the X-chromosome (Bhattacharya *et al.*, 1985; Musarella *et al.*, 1988; Chen *et al.* 1989).

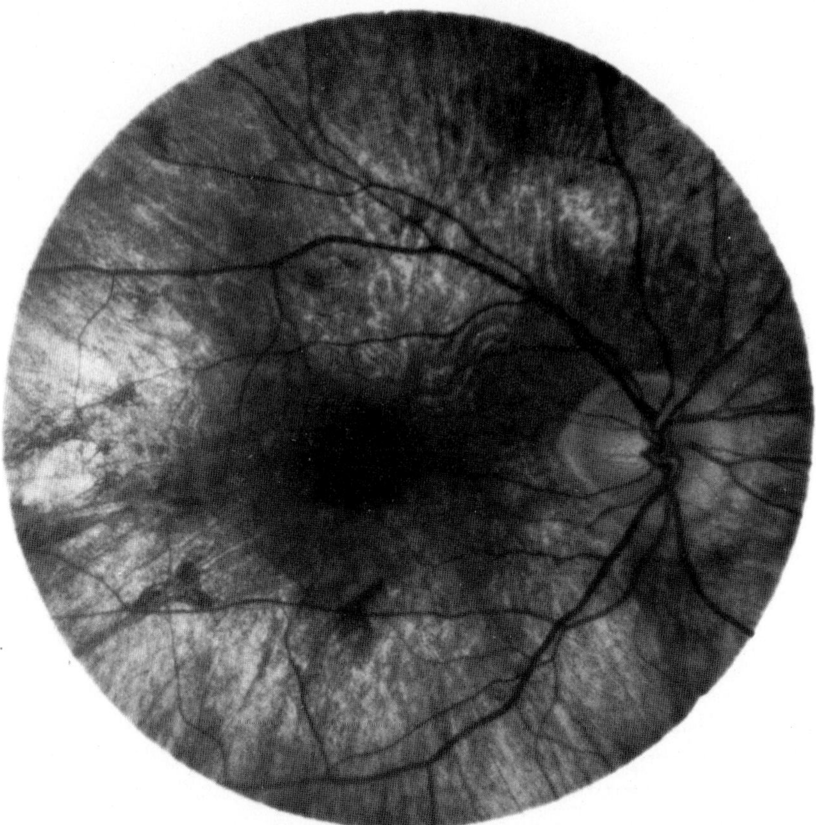

Fig. 12.14. Moderately severe fundus changes in a patient with choroideremia. Note atrophy of the retinal pigment epithelium and choroidal vasculature (choriocapillaris).

12.4.5 Choroideremia

Choroideremia is a diffuse X-linked recessive chorieretinal dystrophy first described by Mauthner (1871). Affected males show bilateral progressive degeneration of the choroid and retina and complain of poor night vision within the first 10–20 years of life. At first, central acuity is normal or nearly so, but it eventually undergoes progressive deterioration. Peripheral fields are usually moderately contracted even at an early age, with severe peripheral field restriction occurring in the fifth and sixth decades. In early stages of the disease, the ERG and EOG are markedly abnormal. In more advanced stages, atrophic changes are seen within the choroid and retinal pigment epithelium, but unlike RP, there is little or no migration of spicule-like pigment into the anterior layers of the retina (Fig. 12.14).

There is some clinical evidence to suggest that the disease originates in the retinal pigment epithelium. For example, the initial pigmentary changes occur in regions where the choroid is normal both by ophthalmoscopic examination and fluorescein angiography. Moreover, the fundi of carrier females may reveal a 'moth-eaten' appearance of the retinal pigment epithelium where no clinically-detectable choroidal changes are evident, and in the presence of normal photoreceptor cell function as determined by the ERG (Sieving, Niffenegger & Berson, 1986). Although the evidence is not conclusive, these observations tend to support the notion that the photoreceptor and choroidal degenerations are secondary to a disease of the RPE.

Linkage studies have demonstrated that a DNA fragment polymorphism (DXYSl) located on the long arm of the X-chromosome shows reasonably close linkage with the X-linked gene for choroideremia (Nussbaum *et al.*, 1985; Lewis, Nussbaum & Ferrell, 1985). Eventual isolation of the actual gene could lead to further identification of the specific cellular defect responsible for this night-blinding disorder.

12.4.6 Gyrate atrophy

Gyrate atrophy, an autosomal recessive chorioretinal dystrophy, is one of the few progressive night-blinding disorders in which a metabolic defect has been implicated, and for which therapeutic measures are currently under investigation. Except in cases where the family history is positive, patients with the disease are first seen when they present with the complaint of poor night vision, usually between 20 and 30 years of age. Although considered at first to be an atypical form of RP (Cutler, 1895; Fuchs, 1896), the atrophic fundus changes involve initially the RPE and choriocapillaris of the mid-periphery, and usually appear as sharply defined areas with scalloped margins (Fig. 12.15); the latter may be bordered by clumps of pigment. With time, the larger choroidal vessels become atrophic, the lesions tend toward confluence as the disease extends both centrally and peripherally, and eventually the fundus assumes the whitish color of the bared sclera. ERG, EOG, and visual field changes parallel the course of the disease as it progressively destroys the neural retinal. Other clinical features of the disease have been reviewed *in extenso* by Kurstjens (1965).

Although rare – approximately 90 cases have been reported in the world literature – interest in gyrate atrophy escalated when it was shown that the disease is associated with hyperornithemia resulting from a

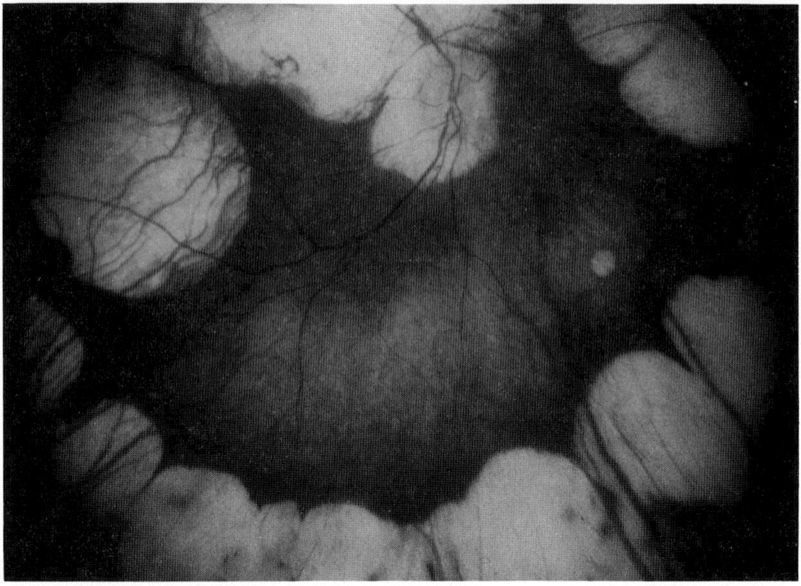

Fig. 12.15. Gyrate atrophy of the choroid and retina. The several areas of sharply defined atrophy with rounded or scalloped margins are characteristic of the fundus lesions seen in this disease.

deficiency in ornithine alpha-aminotransferase (OAT) (Simell & Takki, 1973). This mitochondrial matrix enzyme utilizes pyridoxal phosphate (vitamin B_6) as a co-factor. Vitamin B_6 and/or low protein diets restricted in arginine (a precursor of ornithine) have been tried in an attempt to lower plasma ornithine levels, and hopefully arrest or reverse the course of the disease (Weleber & Kennaway, 1981; Berson, Shih & Sullivan, 1981; Kaiser-Kupfer *et al.*, 1981; Valle *et al.*, 1981). Unfortunately, the dietary approach has not been overly successful, although in a few cases, where compliance was exceptionally good, there was some evidence of improved visual performance (Weleber & Kennaway, 1981; Kaiser-Kupfer *et al.*, 1981). Not only is it difficult to maintain so harsh a dietary regimen, but there is a question as to whether hyperornithemia is the main factor in the pathogenesis of the degenerative changes. Hyperornithemia can occur without evidence of chorioretinal degeneration (Shih, Efron & Moser, 1969). Moreover, fundus changes similar to those of gyrate atrophy have been reported in a patient with normal ornithine levels and normal OAT activity in cultured skin fibroblasts, but who had excessive urinary excretion of proline, hydroxyproline and glycine (Hayaska *et al.*, 1982). Because ornithine may serve as a precursor for proline, these authors contend that a disturbance of proline metabolism rather than hyperornithemia is involved in the pathogenesis of the disease (Hayasaka *et al.*, 1985). It is apparent that more in-depth investigations are necessary to resolve current uncertainties. Nevertheless, this disorder provides an instructive example of a possibly metabolically-induced chorioretinal degeneration that may be responsive to dietary modification.

12.4.7 Animal models of nightblinding diseases

Within the animal kingdom, several vertebrate species are known to be afflicted with inherited forms of retinal degeneration. The degree to which any of these animal 'models' is homologous with the human condition is unknown, but there is much to be learned from an understanding of the various disease entities and the mechanisms by which they promote retinal degeneration. In canines, for example, the photoreceptor appears to be the primary target of a variety of genetically-mediated disorders grouped collectively under the rubric of progressive retinal atrophy (PRA). These are divided usually into two types depending upon the age (or stage of development) at which morphological and/or functional abnormalities are first seen.

Early-onset diseases

This type of disease, in which the photoreceptor outer segments fail to develop normally (rod–cone dysplasia), occurs in Irish setters (Aguirre & Rubin, 1975; Aguirre, 1976) and collies (Wolf, Vainisi & Santos-Anderson, 1978). Affected animals show early signs of night blindness and gross abnormalities in the ERG when tested within the first few weeks of life (Buyukmihci, Aguirre & Marshall, 1980); they are often blind by one year of age. In such cases, cytoplasmic disruption of the photoreceptors occurs prior to or soon after birth and a defect in cyclic nucleotide metabolism has been implicated as the causal factor (Schmidt & Lolley, 1973; Woodford *et al.*, 1980; Aguirre *et al.*, 1982). Although the sequence of events that initiates the degenerative process has yet to be defined, the toxicity of elevated levels of guanosine 3′, 5′-monophosphate (cyclic G,P) has been demonstrated experimentally (Lolley *et al.*, 1977; Ulshafer & Hollyfield, 1983; Kalmus, Dunson & Kalmus, 1982).

A similar abnormality in cGMP metabolism has been described in a type of retinal degeneration that occurs in at least 15 different substrains of the C_3H mouse (Farber & Lolley, 1974). The retinal degeneration (*rd*) gene, located on chromosome 5, is expressed early in post-natal life, and as in the Irish setter and collie, there is arrested photoreceptor cell development. The retina appears morphologically normal at birth, and although visual cells begin to form outer segments and ribbon synapses, neither end of the cell develops to full maturity. Electrophysiologically, the b-wave is smaller than normal at 14 days and is not recordable at one month of age. Biochemical studies of *rd* mice have shown that cGMP levels begin to rise above normal between 6–8 days of age, i.e. about 2–3 days before any pathological sign can be detected (Farmer & Lolley, 1974). The activity of cyclic GMP-phosphodiesterase (PDE), the enzyme that normally hydrolyzes cGMP is known to be below normal, and Farber & Shuster (1985) have suggested that an inability to dephosphorylate rhodopsin could lead to a defect in the photic activation of the PDE.

The retinal diseases associated with the dog and mouse models described above are transmitted as autosomal recessive traits in which the defect is expressed as an elevation in the retinal levels of cGMP. At present, there is no human subtype of retinitis pigmentosa or other degenerative disease in which elevated levels of cGMP have been detected. Because of the early age of onset, patients with Leber's amaurosis congenita, a genetic subtype of RP with diffuse photoreceptor disease may prove suitable candidates for studies of cGMP metabolism.

However, not all early-onset retinal diseases are associated with elevated levels of cGMP. For example, the PRA in the Norwegian elkhound begins with a selective rod dysplasia (Aguirre & Rubin, 1971) that leads to severe night blindness and absence of rod-mediated ERG responses within the first 7 weeks after birth. By 3 months of age, histological evidence of disorganization and shortening of rod cells is apparent. Because the cones are spared until much later (Aguirre, 1978), severe visual problems do not become apparent until the animals are 1–3 years of age.

Another early-onset retinal dystrophy unrelated to a rise in cGMP is seen in the *rds* mouse, so named because the rate of retinal degeneration is considerably slower than in the *rd* mouse. The aberrant photoreceptor cell differentiation results from an autosomal recessive gene located on chromosome 17; i.e. the trait is non-allelic with the *rd* gene, and crosses between the two strains result in normal off-spring. In homozygous *rds* mutants, the photoreceptor outer segments do not begin to form, and the gradual loss of remaining visual cell structures progresses from the peripheral to central retina; at about 1 year of age all the visual cells have deteriorated. An abnormality in disc synthesis and/or assembly has been reported in this condition (Sanyal, Chader & Aguirre, 1985), and unlike the *rd* mouse, the levels of cGMP are lower than normal at the earliest stages of the disease (Cohen, 1983).

Retinal diseases of late-onset

In addition to the early-onset diseases, where developmental abnormalities are evident, there are a number of animal models in which the photoreceptor degeneration occurs apparently after the visual cells have developed normally. The miniature poodle (Aguirre *et al.*, 1982) and Abyssinian cat models (Narfstrom, 1985) of PRA are good examples of the later-onset diseases with fairly slow rates of progression. These disorders, in which the rods of the mid-periphery are first to be affected, are generally considered to bear a closer resemblance to human RP. In the miniature poodle, for example, photoreceptor development is normal as judged electrophysiologically and ultrastructurally, and although the ERG response amplitudes are reduced at 7–8 months, degenerative changes in the photoreceptors are not obvious until the animals are 3–5 years of age (Aguirre *et al.*, 1982). The diseased visual cell outer segments appear disoriented, and vesiculated lamellar discs are evident in both rods and cones. The rate and extent of the degeneration is greater for rods, and there is evidence that a defect in disc assembly, resulting in an abnormally slow rate of renewal, is a fundamental feature of the disease process (Aguirre & O'Brien, 1986).

The RCS rat

The various canine, feline, and mouse models of diffuse degenerative disease described above involve autosomal recessive disorders in which the genetic abnormality is expressed primarily, if not exclusively, within the photoreceptor cells. A very different situation occurs in the recessively-inherited disease studied extensively in the Royal College of Surgeons (RCS) strain of rats. In the rat model, the abnormal gene is expressed as a defect in the phagocytic activity of the pigment epithelium (Herron *et al.*, 1969), and the diffuse photoreceptor degeneration appears secondarily. The failure of the RPE to phagocytize shed outer segment discs results in an extracellular accumulation of membranous debris that causes the destruction of the visual cells. The view that the RPE is the primary site of the *rdy* (retinal dystrophy) gene action has since been confirmed in experiments on rat chimeras in which the retina contains a mixture of mutant and genetically normal RPE cells (Mullen & LaVail, 1976), in studies using RCS pigment epithelial cells in culture (Edwards & Szamier, 1977), and by *in vivo* and *in vitro* studies on organ explants (Tamai & O'Brien, 1979). However, despite the clear demonstration of a genetic trait expressed in the RPE and leading to widespread visual cell degeneration, no human retinal disorder or other animal disease has been found which is attributable to a similar defect.

Nevertheless, there is an interesting postscript to the studies on the RCS rat. An early study by Dowling & Sidman (1962) had shown that raising *rdy* animals in darkness slowed the rate of photoreceptor degeneration and probably delayed the onset of the disease. Thus, during the first 60 days post-natally, both the histological and electroretinographic changes were less severe in the dark-reared animals. This finding was the impetus for a clinical study in which humans with RP were occluded moncularly for 6–8 h per day over a 5 year period, and the functional status of the two eyes were compared periodically; no modification in the progression of the disease or other beneficial effect could be demonstrated (Berson, 1980). In fact, subsequent studies have shown that the beneficial effects of dark rearing are unique to the pink-eyed (albino) RCS rats, and are not seen in pigmented rats or any of the mouse models of retinal dystrophy (LaVail, 1980).

12.5 Summary

We have described in this chapter some of the retinal anomalies associated with defective night vision, and considered the various ways in which they induce in man and animals functional abnormalities of the rod mechanism. Emphasis has been placed on the use of photochemical, electrophysiological and psychophysical tests to diagnose and categorize these disorders, and to provide quantitative data on the severity of the defect and the degree to which it changes with time. In addition, we have used several selected cases to illustrate how these methods can afford some insight into the identity of the affected cellular elements and the molecular basis of the functional disorder. Advances in our knowledge of the histochemistry, pharmacology, and molecular genetics of these night-blinding abnormalities should bring about a greater understanding of the underlying disturbances and far better approaches to their clinical management.

Acknowledgements

We are indebted to Jane Zakevicius and Adrienne Adelman for their valuable assistance in the preparation of the manuscript. Research in our laboratories is supported by a grant (EY 06516) from the National Eye Institute, USPHS, a center grant from the National Retinitis Pigmentosa Foundation Fighting Blindness, and an unrestricted award from Research to Prevent Blindness, Inc.

13

Aided vision at low luminances

A. van Meeteren

13.1 Introduction

13.1.1 The scope of this chapter

This chapter on aided vision at low luminances begins with a short general summary of the limitations of the naked eye. It appears that improvements can only be expected from devices that catch more light, such as the classical night-glasses and the modern image intensifiers. Next it is demonstrated that the effect of catching more light upon the basic detection of differences in luminance is adequately described by the De Vries–Rose fluctuation theory.

Night vision devices are predominantly built for observations in the field, where artificial illumination is not available or undesirable. As a practical performance measure the *range* of such instruments is defined as the distance required for 50% correct identifications of a set of real objects.

As logical ancestors, night-glasses will be treated first. The function of night-glasses simply is angular magnification with preservation of retinal illuminance. Thus, what can be seen through night-glasses follows straightforwardly from what can be seen by the naked eye. Some corrections must be made to account for optical losses. The 'twilight number', introduced as a performance measure in the German literature, applies exclusively to the gain in visual acuity.

In image intensifiers each photon that is detected by the photo-cathode of the intensifier-tube gives rise to a package of photons entering the user's eye. Retinal illuminance is the product of photon-catch and intensification. Just as for night-glasses the function of image intensifiers can be characterized as a transformation of the retinal image, be it more in the abstract sense, not of retinal illuminance, but of the underlying photon-catch. As predicted by the fluctuation theory visual performance with image intensifiers is primarily determined by the photon-catch. This is clearly demonstrated by measurements in which photon-catch and intensification are varied independently. These measurements also answer the question of the minimum required intensification for optimal performance. Again, some corrections must be made to account for optical and electro-optical losses.

Image intensifiers have been built and used in various designs, including helmet-mounted goggles, over the last 30 years. Their application, mainly but not exclusively for military observations in the field, will not be described in this chapter. Attempts have been made to introduce image intensifiers as a clinical aid for patients with retinitis pigmentosa (see Chapter 12 for clinical details), who lack scotopic vision. As far as we know this has not worked out practically.

Presently, image intensifiers are pushed aside from some applications by thermal imaging devices, which do not need any light at all, and as such are beyond the scope of this chapter, although they can practically replace vision at low luminance by making things 'visible'.

13.1.2 Limitations of the naked eye

The gradual decline of visual performance at lower luminances is inherent in the nature of light. When there is little light there is little to be seen. There is no abrupt breakdown. In fact it will be shown in Section 13.1.3 that the eye's scotopic sensitivity for light is constant over a luminance range of more than five decades. In the first instance this suggests that the only way to obtain better performance is to channel more light into the eye. However, one might wonder whether spatial or temporal redistribution of the available amount of light could be of any help.

The possibilities of angular magnification or minification can be judged from the data presented in Fig. 13.1. Contrast sensitivity defined as the reciprocal of the threshold contrast is plotted here for increment discs as a function of angular diameter with luminance as parameter. For detailed descriptions of the underlying threshold measurements we refer to the original paper of Blackwell (1946). These data are chosen from a much more extensive literature by which they are backed up in general. The curves represent Piper's law for objects with visible size, and Ricco's law for small objects, seen as 'point sources'. We now may apply angular magnification to the curves in Fig. 13.1 in a thought-experiment. The

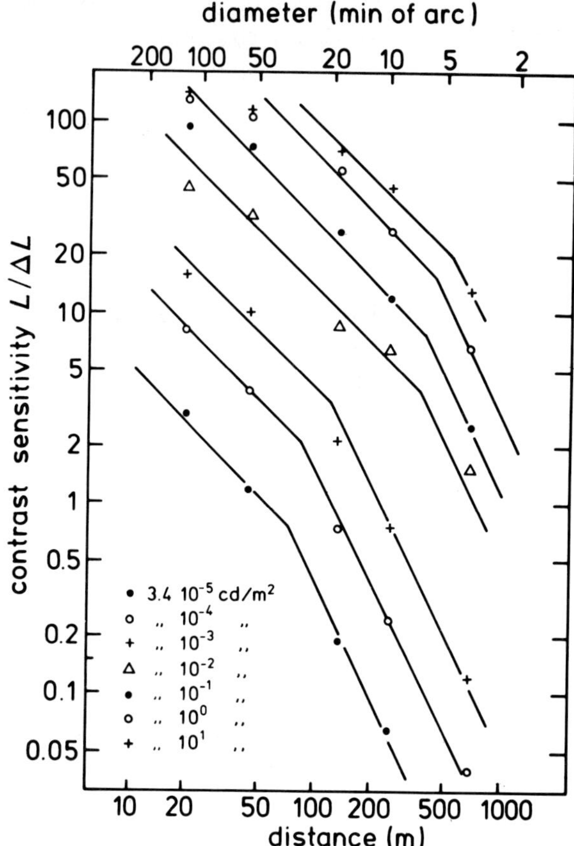

Fig. 13.1. Contrast sensitivity $L/\Delta L$ for a disc of 0.7 m diameter as a function of distance in meters (lower scale) or visual angle (upper scale) with background luminance as parameter. Data derived from the measurements reported by Blackwell (1946). Curves are according to Piper's law for objects with visible size, and Ricco's law for 'point sources'.

curves then are shifted to the right, i.e. towards better performance. However, when the angular magnification is not accompanied by more light, it will result in lower luminance and as a consequence the curves will be shifted downwards, and finally end up in the original position. Thus, the detection of single objects cannot be improved by angular magnification as such. Similarly, when such objects are switched on and off in time, there is no gain in shortening or prolongation, if not coupled with more light.

Angular magnification is more successful with regard to resolution as Fig. 13.2 demonstrates. In Fig. 13.2 contrast sensitivity for sine wave

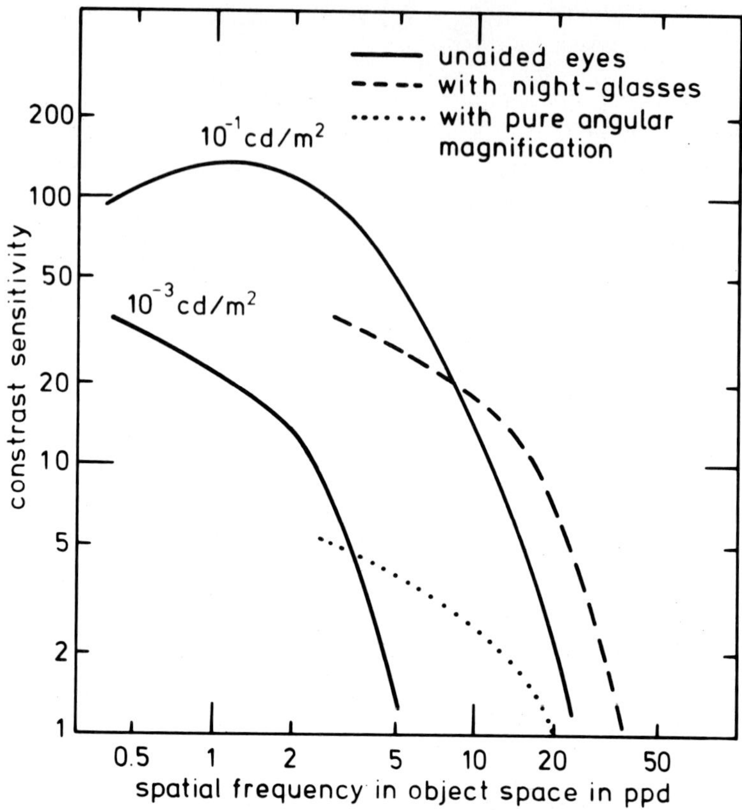

Fig. 13.2. Contrast sensitivity for sine wave gratings as a function of spatial frequency. The effect of angular magnification is to shift the contrast sensitivity function of the unaided eye towards higher spatial frequencies in object space. This shift is followed by a downward shift when angular magnification is not coupled with a corresponding gain in photon-catch.

gratings is plotted as a function of spatial frequency for the naked eye and for a hypothetical device with pure angular magnification, not accompanied by more light. In this case the decay of contrast sensitivity at higher spatial frequencies, caused by the eye's optical and neural blurring (van Meetren & Vos, 1972) is partly by-passed by projecting the image upon the retina with a greater size. Such a device certainly can be built, but its performance would lag far behind night-glasses, as we will see in Section 13.2.1, while its construction would require about the same effort.

Summarizing, in order to aid vision at low luminances, it is necessary to catch more light.

13.1.3 De Vries–Rose fluctuation theory

The predominant interest of catching more light is clearly explained by the fluctuation theory of De Vries (1943) and Rose (1948). This theory also explains why the decline of visual performance at lower luminances is as gradual as it is: visual performance follows the limit put by the quantal character of the light (see Chapter 4 for more details), more in particular by the inherent statistics of the photon-catch. This is an ultimate limit, beyond which no device can reach. The most interesting question is how close the eye comes to this ultimate limit.

The De Vries–Rose theory can be considered as an early application of the general statistical detection theory (Swets, 1964). Let a flux of ϕ photons per second per min^2 of arc enter the eye and let $\eta \cdot \phi$ of them be effectively absorbed in retinal receptor cells. Let there further be an increment $\Delta\phi$ over an area of α^2 min^2 of arc during a time interval of t seconds. Thus, the total number of extra photons absorbed is $\eta \cdot \Delta\phi \cdot \alpha^2 \cdot t$. The average number of background photons in the same area and time is $\eta \cdot \phi\alpha^2 \cdot t$. Repeated countings of this number would reveal a standard deviation equal to $(v \cdot \phi \cdot \alpha^2 \cdot t)^{1/2}$, caused by the Poisson-process. It is assumed that in order to detect the extra photons their number must exceed a threshold proportional to these fluctuations:

$$\eta \cdot \Delta\phi \cdot \alpha^2 t \geq k \cdot (\eta \cdot \phi \cdot \alpha^2 \cdot t)^{1/2} \tag{13.1}$$

So, for the contrast sensitivity $S = \phi/\Delta\phi$ one finds:

$$S = \frac{1}{k} \cdot (\eta\phi\alpha^2 t)^{1/2} \tag{13.2}$$

Thus, the De Vries–Rose theory of ideal detection limited by photon noise, predicts some very simple relations. First, contrast sensitivity will increase with the square root of luminance, as the photon density ϕ is directly proportional to luminance. This square root relation is confirmed experimentally by a vast body of data, among others by the data of Fig. 13.1 (see also Fig. 1.3). Second, contrast sensitivity will be proportional to the diameter of the disc, when measured for circular discs upon uniform backgrounds. Note that this prediction is identical with Piper's law, mentioned above, and confirmed by the data of Fig. 13.1. Third, contrast sensitivity will be proportional to the square root of the presentation time t. Obviously, these predictions must break down for extremely small and big discs as well as extremely short and long presentation times because of the physical limits of any conceivable sampling mechanism (also see Chapter 1 for an explanation based on neural filters).

In the threshold condition of (13.1) it is presupposed that photons are counted over the whole area α^2, i.e. that the signal is summated energetically over the whole object. However, it is more likely that direct summation is limited to built-in units of limited size. Perhaps, the visual system has the disposal of a set of such units, matching different sizes. If this is what De Vries and Rose suggested, they must in modern parlance be recognized as the first 'channel' theorists. Alternatively spatial integration over larger areas may be accomplished by two consecutive processes: direct summation over small sampling areas, followed by probability summation. Of course, this may also be the way of temporal integration. It should be realized then, that the two alternatives lead to the same effects of α^2 and t in (13.2). More importantly the probability summation model predicts these effects no matter the origin of the noise in the sampling units. Thus, experimental confirmation of the area and time effects predicted by (13.2) does not exclusively support the fluctuation theory.

The main evidence supporting the fluctuation theory as a valid description of vision at low luminances is the square root relation between contrast sensitivity and luminance, which has been confirmed experimentally again and again. There are exceptions to this rule. At higher light levels De Vries–Rose behaviour turns into Weber behaviour, where contrast-constancy is the rule. The transition depends on the size and duration of the test object. As Barlow (1972) remarked, there is little or no De Vries–Rose behaviour for large objects and long durations. Blackwell (1972) considered this as evidence against the fluctuation theory. However, it seems to us that these exceptions are logical. Once contrast sensitivity is high enough it is stabilized. Obviously, the strategy of the visual system is to start the consolidation of contrast sensitivity in the lower spatial and temporal frequency ranges. Against a background of 'Weberized' lower frequencies contrast sensitivity for small and flashed detail may still follow upwards the limit put by photon noise. Rose (1973) speculated that this perhaps may be so even in broad daylight for difficult tasks like hitting a tennis ball.

For quantitative predictions of visual performance according to the fluctuation theory the quantum efficiency factor η in (13.2) must be determined. Starting from (13.2), η can be estimated psychophysically in conditions where k, α^2 and t are known. For α^2 and t one may substitute the actual sizes of the stimuli only if one has made sure that total integration is really established in the conditions of the measurements. The factor k, related to the threshold criterion, can be reconstructed from the fraction of false positive responses when empty presentations are mixed with the stimuli. Surveying practically the whole available literature, Clark Jones (1959) came to values of η in the order of 1–2%. This was confirmed by van Meeteren (1973, 1978) and Engstrom (1974), who by-passed the need to know k, α^2 and t, in a comparison of unaided vision with vision through an ideal image intensifying device, whose photon catch was accurately known. This method will be further explained below in Section 13.3.1.

The question of how close the eye comes to the ultimate limit put by the fluctuations in the detected photon flux now can be answered by a comparison of η's psychophysical value with its direct physiological evaluation. Summarizing the existing literature, van Meeteren (1978) concluded that at least 12% of the photons entering the eye start off the required chain of events in a receptor cell. Thus, it appears that there is a gap of about a factor of 10 between the functional and the physiological values of the quantum efficiency. This discrepancy has been put forward as evidence against the De Vries–Rose theory (Hood & Finkelstein, 1986). Is it still correct to state that vision is limited by photon noise if sensitivity is lower than it could have been in view of the fraction of photons absorbed? We certainly think so (also see Chapters 1 and 4 for opposing view). Contrast sensitivity is proportional to the square root of luminance over five decades and increases over this range by a factor 300. The deficiency of the retina, discussed above, reduces the contrast sensitivity by a factor of 3, i.e. only 1% of its total range. Thus, the human eye follows the photon-noise limit over a wide range of luminances, be it at a certain distance. This distance probably is caused by internal noise inherent in the design of the photoreceptors and by the thresholding inherent in the generation of nerve spikes (see also Chapter 4).

13.1.4 Definition of visual performance

Visual observation devices serve to perform real tasks, such as the detection, recognition, and identification of real objects, relevant to the user. As a practical performance measure for night vision devices to be used in the field, van Meeteren (1977) introduced the range at which 50% correct identifications of a set of real objects could be made. He further developed a recipe to proceed from the prediction or measurement of elementary functions, like contrast sensitivity and resolution, to the prediction of the range in the above sense.

The concepts of detection, recognition and identification cannot be

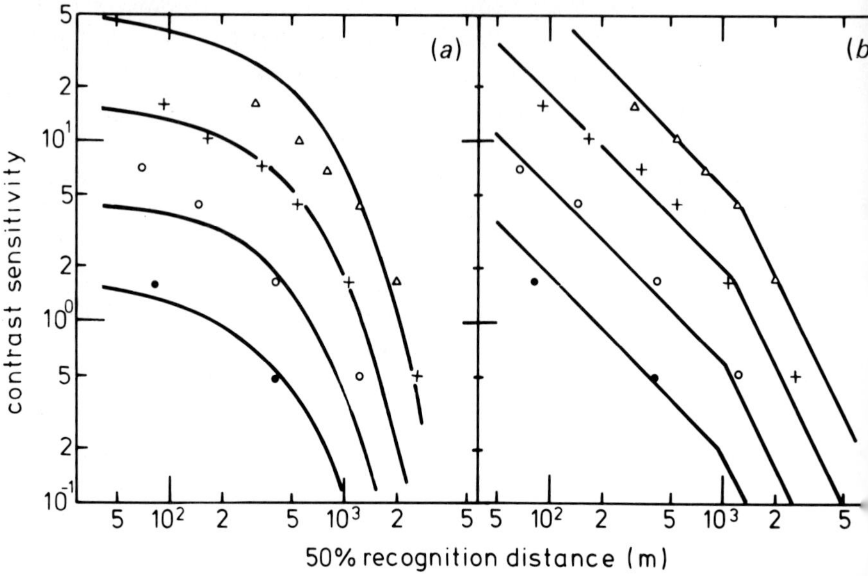

Fig. 13.3. Contrast sensitivity for 50% correct recognition of a set of six military vehicles as a function of distance with background luminance as parameter (3.2×10^{-6}, 3.2×10^{-5}, 3.2×10^{-3} cd/m^2). The curves in (*a*) are contrast sensitivity functions for sine wave gratings shifted along the axes to get the best fitting. The curves in (*b*) represent contrast sensitivity for a circular disc of 0.7 m diameter. See text.

used with regard to individual objects. These concepts are only meaningful with respect to a certain set of alternative objects. The difficulty of identifying one of the objects depends heavily on its similarity with the other objects in the set. As a consequence, every attempt to quantify performance must start from some well-defined realistic set of objects. In the context of his work van Meeteren (1977) for example used a set of 6 different military vehicles. The scenery was simulated indoors by slide-projection in order to obtain better controllability of conditions than possibly might be achieved in field experiments. The basic photographs were made at the location of a preceding field experiment, that served to verify and calibrate the simulation approach.

In a series of experiments, identification scores were measured as a function of distance and contrast reduction. Fig. 13.3 illustrates the results of such measurements for one of the image intensifiers investigated in this way. Contrast sensitivity, defined as the reciprocal of the threshold contrast required for 50% correct identifications of the objects is plotted here as a function of simulated distance. The original contrast of the objects was defined more or less arbitrarily as the average contrast of a number of relevant features. The apparent contrast could be reduced by projecting a veiling luminance over the entire scenery. The curves in Fig. 13.3*a* represent contrast sensitivity functions for sine wave gratings, and the curves in Fig. 13.3*b* represent contrast sensitivity for a circular disc according to Piper's law and Ricco's law. In both cases the array of curves has been shifted along the horizontal and the vertical axes in order to obtain the best fitting with the recognition data points. Obviously, recognition is best predicted on the basis of 'single object detection'. More specifically it appears that 50% correct identification of the set of objects is visually equivalent to the detection of a circular disc with a diameter of 0.7 m and a contrast of 2.0, with $k = 4$ as the value of the detection criterion (or 'signal-to-noise ratio') in (13.2).

In view of the aperiodic nature of the objects it is not surprising that recognition is not very well represented by the detection of sine wave gratings. More generally, this result calls attention for the low ecological validity of sine wave gratings.

13.2 Night-glasses

13.2.1 The gain in photon-catch

The function of night-glasses is angular magnification with preservation of retinal illuminance. Fig. 13.4 illustrates how the objective lens of a telescope, if sufficiently large, collects a factor m^2 more light than the unaided eye. This compensates exactly for the rarification of light over the image plane, as caused by the angular magnification m. As a consequence the contrast sensitivity functions of the unaided eye are simply shifted by ideal night-glasses towards higher spatial frequencies in object space conformably to the angular magnification. Fig. 13.5 shows the experimental verification of this simple prediction rule for vision through a pair of 7×50 night-glasses. The sine wave gratings were projected in this experiment on a white screen and observed from a distance of 4 m with the naked eyes and from a distance of 28 m through the binocular night-glasses. Due to optical losses the results remain slightly behind the ideal, as will be discussed in Section 13.2.2.

As Fig. 13.2 clearly demonstrates, the lion's share of the performance gain provided by night-glasses rests upon the gain in photon-catch. However, night-glasses cannot intensify the retinal illuminance. Their gain is provided exclusively in the form of angular magnification. This

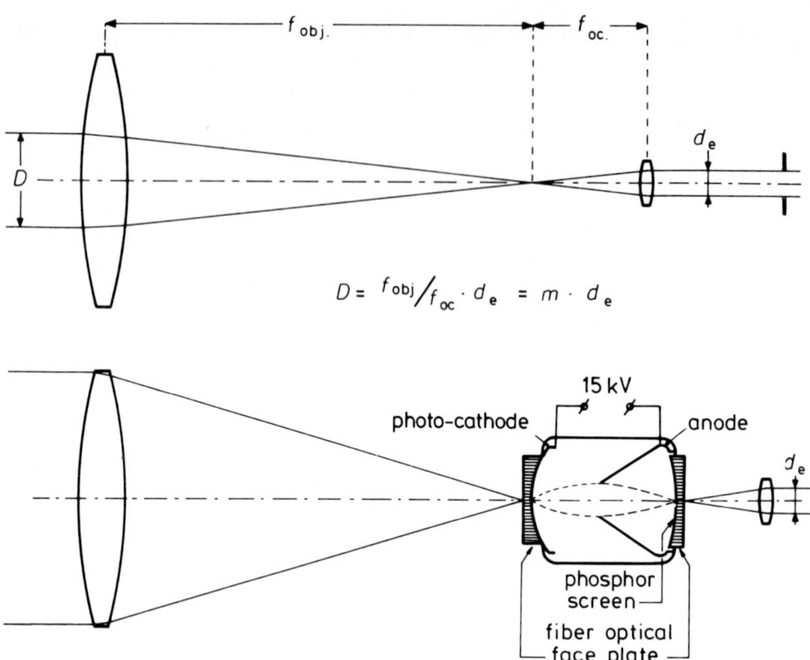

Fig. 13.4. Schematic diagram of a telescope with and without an image intensifier tube. Note that the effective diameter D of the entrance pupil is at best equal to $m \cdot d_e$, in the absence of the intensifier tube, where m is the angular magnification and d_e is the diameter of the pupil of the observer's eye. The intensifier tube breaks through this relation of entrance pupil and angular magnification. Note also the light losses by diffuse scattering of the phosphor screen, which have to be compensated for by the intensification of the tube.

nevertheless enables a visual performance that normally belongs to a higher luminance level as Fig. 13.2 illustrates. Thus, night-glasses bring about a functional gain in the luminance required for a certain visual performance. Although night-glasses cannot intensify the retinal illuminance, they in fact do intensify point sources, which are not visibly magnified, while their total amount of light is increased by a factor m^2. This is why more stars can be seen with greater astronomical telescopes.

It has been assumed so far that the exit pupil of the night-glasses just fills the pupil of the observer's eye. Only then the retinal illuminance will be the same as in unaided vision. Otherwise it will be reduced by a factor $D^2/(d_e^2 \cdot m^2)$, where D is the diameter of the entrance pupil of the night-glasses, m is the angular magnification and d_e is the diameter of the pupil of the eye. Thus choosing a larger magnification simultaneously results in a lower retinal illuminance. The best trade-off between more

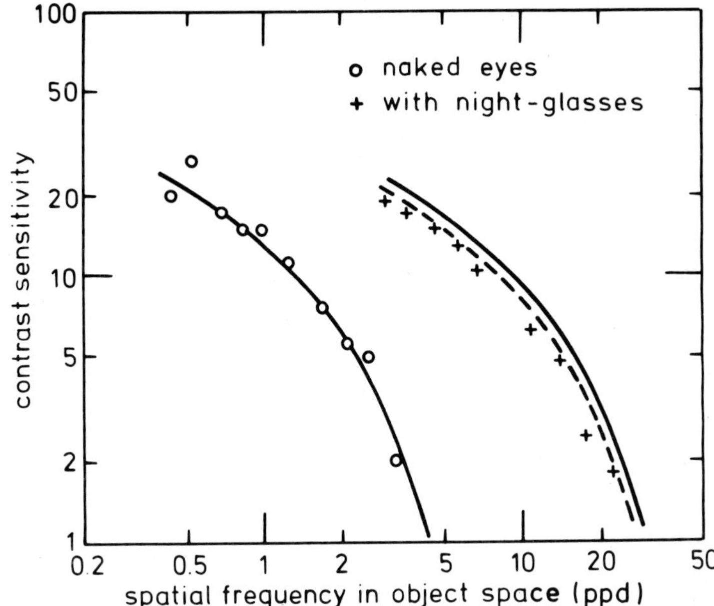

Fig. 13.5. Contrast sensitivity for sine wave gratings as a function of spatial frequency in object space, measured with and without a pair of 7 × 50 night-glasses at a luminance level of 3.5×10^{-4} cd/m². The right-most uninterrupted curve is obtained by shifting the contrast sensitivity function of the unaided eyes over a factor 7 corresponding to the angular magnification. After correction for imaging errors and straylight the interrupted curve predicts the contrast sensitivity function for vision through the night-glasses.

angular magnification and lower retinal illuminance has been discussed extensively in the German literature. According to Kühl (1927), visual acuity is roughly proportional to $E^{1/4}$ at low luminances, where E indicates the retinal illuminance. Thus the gain G_r in resolving power is:

$$G_r = m \cdot \left[\left(\frac{D^2}{d_e^2 \cdot m^2}\right)\right]^{1/4} = \sqrt{\left(\frac{mD}{d_e}\right)} \qquad (13.3)$$

The term $\sqrt{mD}$ became known as Dämmerungszahl or Twilight number. Equation (13.3) is supported experimentally (Köhler & Leinhos, 1957). According to (13.3), the resolution of a 10 × 50 telescope can be about 20% better at low luminances than the resolution of a 7 × 50 telescope, although the photon-catches are the same. This reflects the additional effect of pure angular magnification shown also in Fig. 13.2.

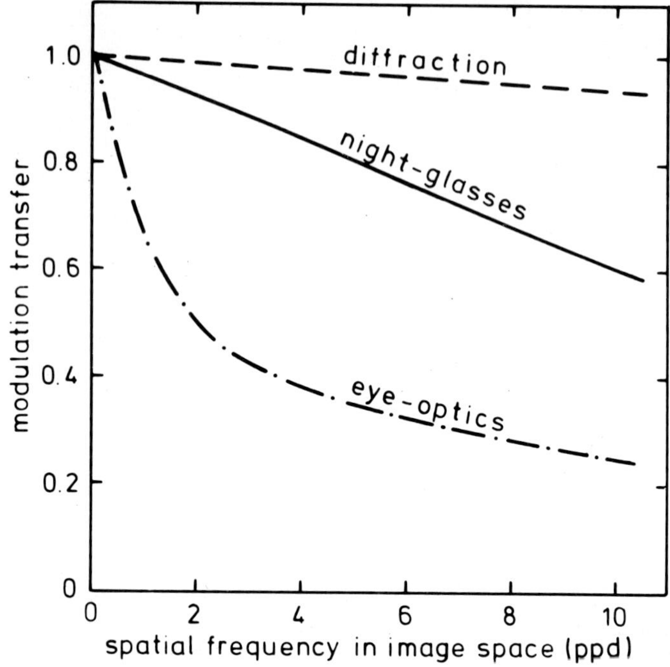

Fig. 13.6. Modulation transfer functions of a hypothetical diffraction limited pair of 7 × 50 night-glasses, an actual pair of 7 × 50 night-glasses, and the eye optics, all for a pupil of 7 mm in image space. For the combined effect of telescope and eye-optics see text.

13.2.2 Optical losses

A small fraction of the possible performance gain of night-glasses is unavoidably wasted by optical imperfections, such as aberrations, straylight, and light-losses. Fig. 13.6 shows the MTF (modular transfer function) for the night-glasses investigated in Fig. 13.5. There is a difficulty in the use of MTFs for direct viewing optical devices. Strictly speaking one should specify the wave aberrations of telescopes instead of their MTFs and evaluate the possible interactions with the wave aberrations of the human eye. This is a cumbersome way. It seems to be more realistic to characterize direct viewing instruments by an effective MTF, defined as the ratio of the contrast sensitivities for aided and unaided vision. In practice a satisfactory estimation of the effective MTF may be obtained from the nominal MTF, when the letter is divided by the diffraction limited MTF (van Meeteren, 1969). A second source of contrast reduction is instrumental straylight. As this factor depends upon

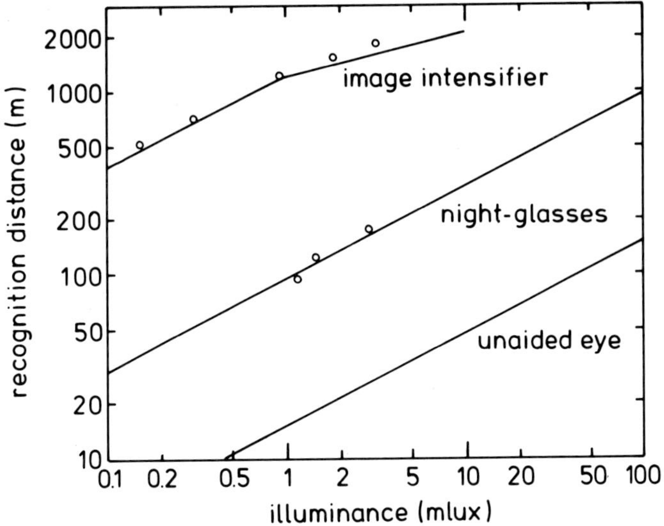

Fig. 13.7. Recognition distance as a function of target illuminance for the unaided eye, vision through a pair of 7 × 50 night-glasses, and vision through on image intensifier (HV 5 × 80). Recognition distance is defined as the distance at which a set of 6 military objects can be recognized 50% correctly. The curves represent model-predictions. All data refer to a clear atmosphere.

the light distribution in object space it does not make sense to include it in the MTF. In the conditions of the experiment described above, straylight reduced contrast by a factor 0.96. The interrupted curve in Fig. 13.5 is derived from the 'perfect' curve after multiplication with the effective MTF and accounting for the stray light.

About 20% of the light is lost in coated binoculars. In the measurements shown in Fig. 13.5 this loss was anticipated by increasing the luminance in object space accordingly. In practice it implies a reduction of contrast sensitivity with a factor $(0.80)^{1/2} = 0.9$ according to the fluctuation theory. Taking all losses together in a conservative estimation about 10% of the gain in photon-catch is sacrificed in its material realization.

13.2.3 *Field performance*

Fig. 13.7 gives an impression of the field performance of the 7 × 50 telescope introduced above, as an example of night-glasses in general. The range, as defined in Section 13.14 is plotted here as a function of target illuminance in the field, expressed in mlux. Only a few recognition experiments have been made so far with night-glasses. The curve represents the detection of the representative circular disc, introduced in Section 13.1.4. For comparison, a similar curve is plotted in Fig. 13.7 for the range of the naked eye. All ranges presented in Fig. 13.7 refer to a clear atmosphere.

13.3 Image intensifying devices

13.3.1 The gain in photon-catch

The basic form of an image intensifying device is illustrated in Fig. 13.4. The telescope shown in the upper part of Fig. 13.4 is simply cut, as it were, in the focal plane and an image intensifier tube is inserted. The scenery in object space is imaged upon the photo-cathode-end of the tube. The intensified image is displayed upon a phosphor-screen at the other end and can be observed through an ocular lens. Once detected by the photocathode photons are converted into free electrons, which are accelerated by a high voltage electric field and hit a phosphor screen with sufficient energy to evoke a light flash of about 1000 photons, the image is preserved by electrostatic focusing. Higher intensifications can be obtained by cascading a number of tubes or by other types of tubes (Biberman & Nudelman, 1971).

The gain in photon-catch provided by an image-intensifying device consists of three components. First, just as for night-glasses, the entrance pupil catches much more light than the pupil of the unaided eye. Second, the quantum efficiency of the photo-cathode is considerably higher. Third, the spectral sensitivity function of the photo-cathode is much wider, as Fig. 13.8 illustrates. For the spectral composition of night-light in the field the effective spectral window of a typical photo-cathode is about 4 times greater than for unaided scotopic vision. The quantum efficiency at the top of the spectral sensitivity function of a typical photo-cathode can be about 0.08, i.e. 8 times higher than in unaided scotopic vision (see below). The entrance pupil of an image intensifier finally can be made about 100 times greater than the pupil of the eye. Taking all factors together the gain in photon-catch can be in the order of 1000–10000. For more detailed discussions the reader is referred to the textbook of Biberman & Nudelman (1971), or van Meeteren (1973).

In the early days of the development of image intensifiers one has been fairly uncertain about the gain in performance that could be expected. The spectral window of photo-cathodes was not very much wider

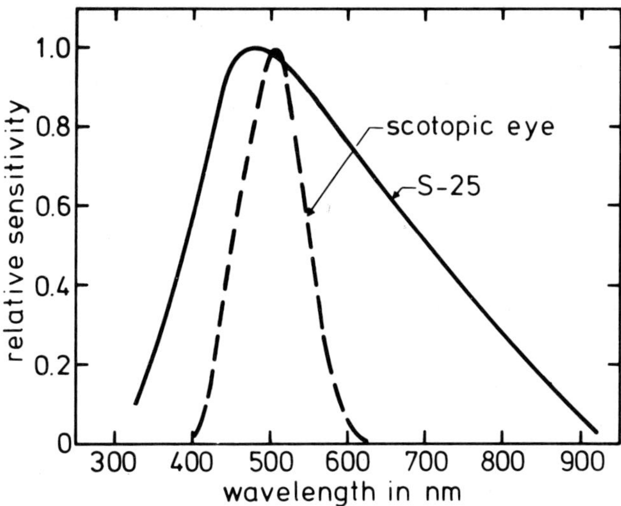

Fig. 13.8. Spectral windows of the scotopic human eye, and of the S-25 photon-cathode of typical image intensifier tubes.

initially, and many visuologists believed that the quantum efficiency of scotopic vision was as high as 0.05–0.20. Thus, the prospects were that image intensifiers could at best just compete with conventional night-glasses. In retrospect, actual performance with image intensifiers has made clear that the effective quantum efficiency of unaided scotopic vision is more in the order of 0.01. In fact the quantum efficiency can be determined straightforwardly by a direct comparison of unaided vision with vision through a well-calibrated ideal image intensifying device. Fig. 13.9 demonstrates this method. Contrast sensitivity for a sine wave grating of 2 ppd (periods per degree) was measured as a function of the number of photons per min^2 of arc per second entering the pupil of the naked eye on the one hand, and as a function of the number of specks per min^2 of arc per second displayed by an ideal image intensifier set-up on the other hand. Each speck represents an original photon and the statistics of the specks are identical to the Poisson-statistics of the original photons. For each speck a package of 500 photons enters the pupil of the observer's eye. This intensification is sufficient to make sure that each speck is effectively detected by the observer's eye. The number of specks was counted electronically and accurately known. We now can read from Fig. 13.9 that the number of photons per in min^2 of arc per second entering the unaided eye must be 100 times higher than the number of specks per min^2 of arc per second in order to obtain the same contrast

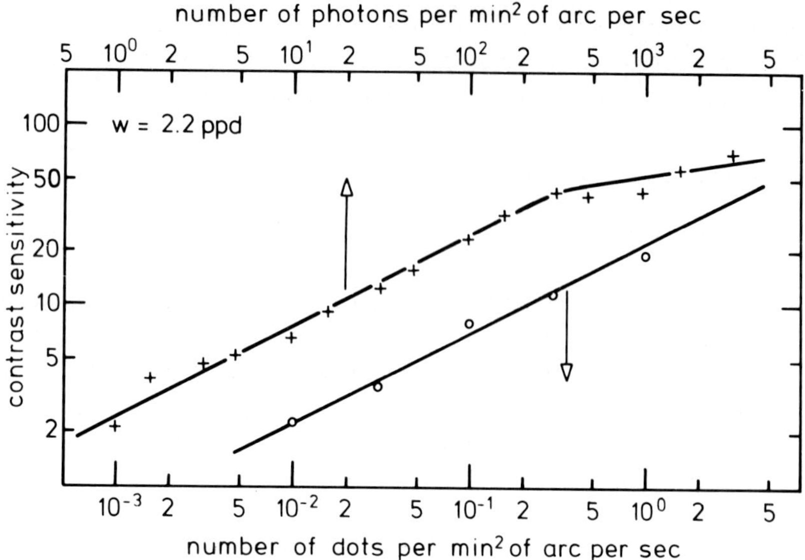

Fig. 13.9. Contrast sensitivity for unaided scotopic vision in peripheral fixation, 7° nasal as a function of the number of photons entering the pupil per min^2 of arc per second (upper curve, upper scale), and for vision to speck-images as a function of speck-density (lower curve, lower scale). By comparison it can be concluded that the functional quantum efficiency of scotopic vision is about 1%.

sensitivity. Note that contrast sensitivity is proportional to the square root of photon- and speck-density respectively, in agreement with the fluctuation theory. The validity of the fluctuation theory moreover is unambiguously supported for speck-vision, by the fact that the intensity of the specks, and thus retinal illuminance, can be varied without effect upon contrast sensitivity. Obviously, the effective or functional quantum efficiency of unaided scotopic vision is about 0.01, since about 100 photons must enter the eye on the average in order to result in one event that is counted in the same way as one speck.

For conventional night-glasses we have seen that the gain in photon-catch is coupled with angular magnification. As one may conclude immediately from Fig. 13.4 this is different for image intensifiers. Here, photon-catch and angular magnification are not coupled and can be manipulated independently. Thus in terms of Fig. 13.2 the contrast sensitivity function of the naked eye can now be shifted either to the right or upwards or both, on the understanding that the product of the shift factors is equal to the square root of the gain in photon-catch. It is even possible to transfer angular minification, realized electronically within the intensifier tube, into an upward shift of contrast sensitivity. This freedom of design has resulted in a wide variety of instruments including goggles and driving periscopes with unit magnification.

13.3.2 The required intensification

The intensification must be sufficient to make sure that each photon detected by the photo-cathode of an image intensifier is finally detected by the retina. Van Meeteren & Boogaard (1973) investigated the effect of the intensity of the specks, representing the original photons detected by the photo-cathode, upon contrast sensitivity measured with sine wave gratings. Fig. 13.10 summarizes the results for foveal fixation of the speck-images. For a more detailed description of these measurements we refer to the original paper. Starting from low intensifications contrast sensitivity at first increases when the number of photons per speck entering the artificial pupil is raised, and finally levels off. In the first stage the average number of photons per speck is too low to ascertain the detection of each speck. As the intensity of the specks is raised, more of them can be detected and contrast sensitivity increases. Finally, all specks are detected. Further intensification does not yield more specks. Thus, the signal-to-noise ratio, and, as a consequence, the contrast sensitivity level off. This is the most simple explanation of the experimental data which is further supported by the square root relation of contrast sensitivity and speck-density at the final level.

Remarkably, the required minimal intensification depends upon the density of the specks. At the lowest realistic speck-densities about 500 photons per speck must enter the pupil, in agreement with the absolute foveal threshold for a single flash (Marriot, 1963). However, at higher speck-densities, specks apparently help each other to pass the threshold. At a speck-density of about 20 specks per min^2 of arc per second, 30 photons per speck are enough. Similar measurements were made for peripheral fixation of the speck-images, 7° nasal, indicating that about 150 photons per speck are necessary in that condition, independent of speck-density.

To stay on the safe side the intensification should be either adjustable or as high as 500, expressed in the number of photons entering the pupil of the observer's eye for each originally detected photon. Note that the number of photons per speck ejected by the phosphor screen of the display must be very much higher: most of the light is scattered into directions other than the pupil of the observer's eye.

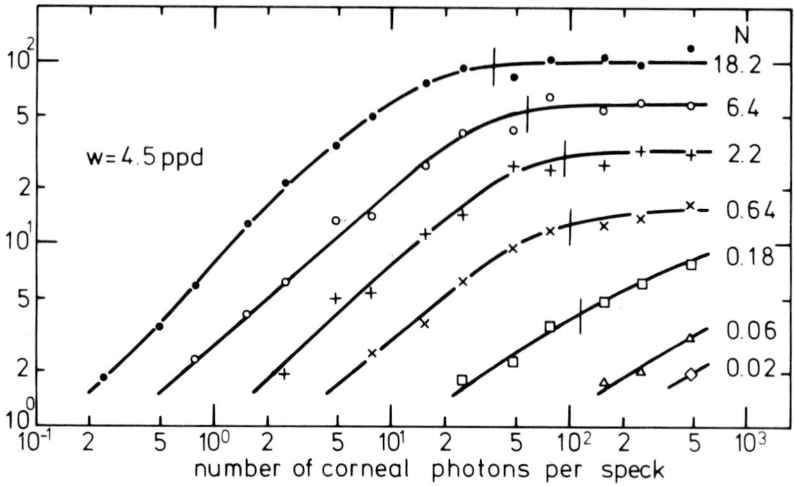

Fig. 13.10. Contrast sensitivity as a function of speck-intensity, with speck-density as parameter. The speck-intensity is expressed in the number of photons per speck entering the observer's eye. The speck-density is expressed in the number of specks per second per min^2 of arc. The speck-intensity at which speck-images can just be distinguished from normal images is indicated by vertical bars.

Van Meeteren & Boogaard (1973) have also measured contrast sensitivity for foveal observation of speck-images of sine wave gratings as a function of spatial frequency. The form of these contrast sensitivity functions was the same as for unaided foveal vision, indicating that intensified images, even in conditions where the noise is visible as such, are spatially processed in the normal way.

13.3.3 Optical and electro-optical losses

Again, a small fraction of the possible performance gain of image intensifiers will be lost due to optical imperfections, such as aberrations, straylight and light-losses especially in the objective lens. However, the electro-optical losses of the intensifier tube are more predominant. Fig. 13.11 shows the MTF of an early type of image intensifier, to be called SSS from here on, together with the MTF of the eye-optics. This MTF is almost completely determined by the imaging quality of the cascade of three image intensifier tubes in this device. Note the striking difference in the positions of the MTF of the instrument relative to the eye optics in Fig. 13.6 and Fig. 13.11.

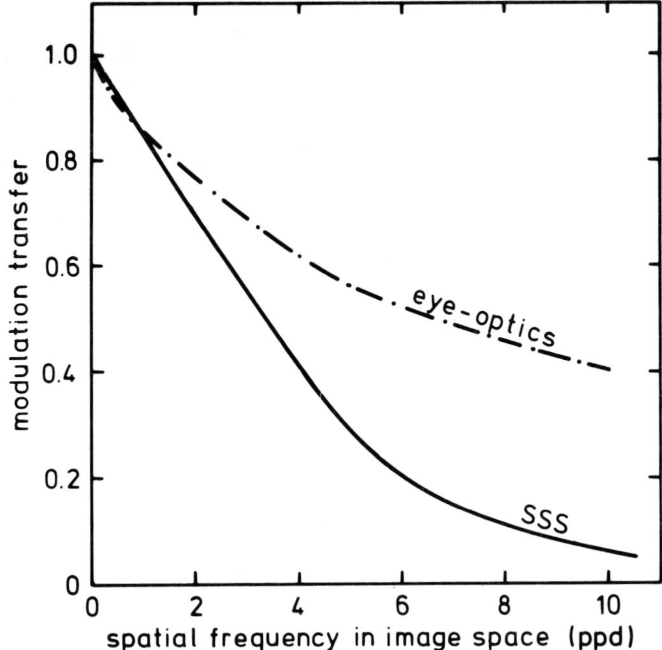

Fig. 13.11. Modulation transfer function of one of the first available image intensifiers (SSS), compared with the modulation transfer function of the eye-optics, both for a pupil of 5 mm diameter in image space. For the combined effect the two MTFs simply can be multiplied.

One may assume that the MTFs of more modern intensifier tubes are much better. Considerable amounts of straylight may also occur in image intensifiers, partly arising in the intensifier tubes. In the center of a small black test object upon a uniform illuminated background the luminance of the straylight proved to be 20% of the background luminance. This implies that straylight coming from bright parts of the scenery (the sky for example) may reduce contrast considerably in dark parts. Taking all losses together, Van Meeteren (1973) estimated that about 60% of the gain in photon-catch was lost due to optical and electro-optical imperfections of the SSS.

Fig. 13.12 shows contrast sensitivity functions for the SSS, measured with sine wave gratings as a function of spatial frequency in object space and with luminance in object space as parameter. The curves are predictions. Starting from the gain in photon-catch contrast sensitivity was first predicted with the aid of the data presented in Fig. 13.10 for a spatial frequency of 4 ppd. Next, foveal contrast transfer functions were

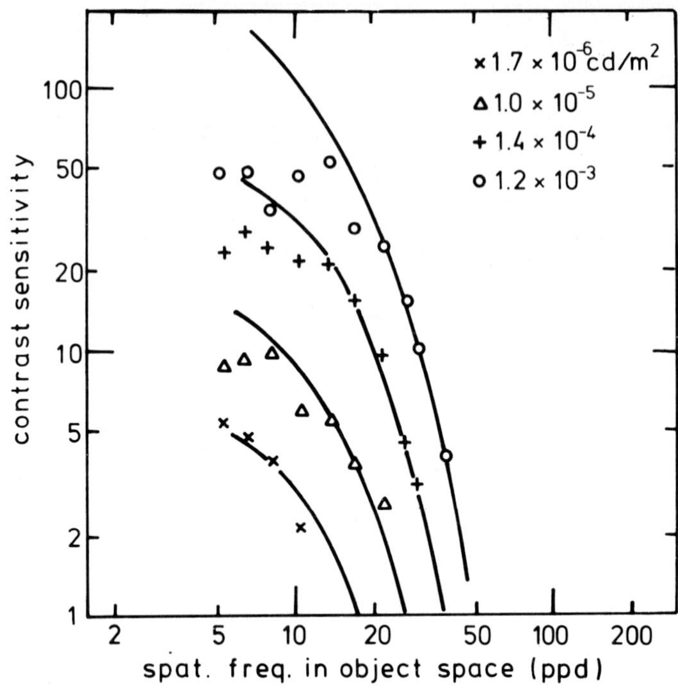

Fig. 13.12. Contrast sensitivity functions for vision through one of the first available image intensifiers (SSS). The measurements were made with a sine wave field of 3° × 3° in image space and a 3 mm artificial pupil. Curves are predictions based upon the sensitivity of the photocathode, and accounting for the MTF of the device.

applied to extrapolate contrast sensitivity for lower and higher spatial frequencies. Finally, the contrast sensitivity functions obtained in this way were corrected for the MTF of the SSS. The predicted curves in Fig. 13.12 agree satisfactorily with the experimental data points, except in the combined condition of high luminance and low spatial frequency, where contrast sensitivity remains markedly behind its predicted level. Contrast sensitivity is limited to about 50 in vision through this device. This might quite well be due to the visible chicken-wire structure of the phosphor screen in this older instrument. Contrasts lower than 0.02 apparently get lost against this background.

13.3.4 Field performance

To give an impression of field performance relative to night-glasses and the unaided eye the range of a typical handheld image intensifier, to be

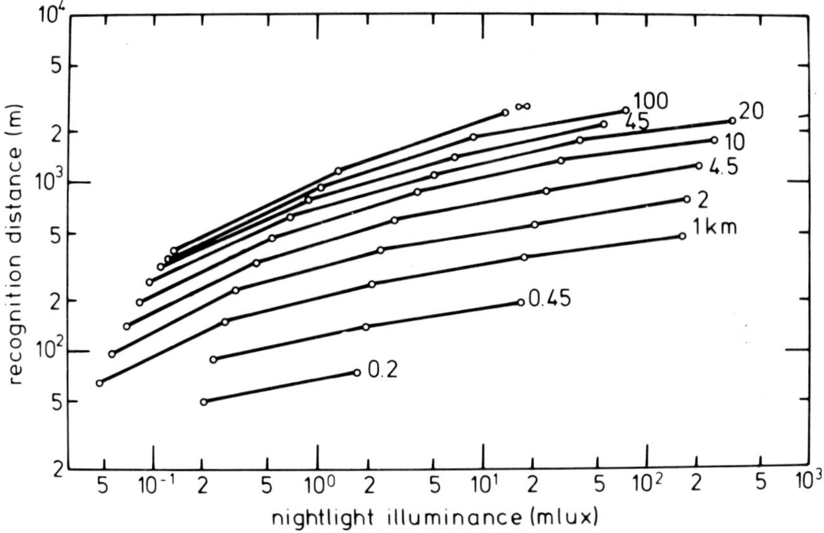

Fig. 13.13. The range of an image intensifier (HV 5 × 80) as a function of target illuminance in different atmospheric conditions. Atmospheric straylight is characterized here by the meteorological range in kilometers. See text.

called HV 5 × 80 from here on, is also plotted in Fig. 13.7. The data points represent indoor simulation measurements as described in Section 13.1.4. The curve represents the detection of the representative circular disc, introduced in Section 13.1.4. Note that all data in Fig. 13.7 apply to a clear atmosphere.

The effect of atmospheric straylight upon target contrast can be very complicated (Middleton, 1952), and precise reconstructions are hardly feasible. However, the main effect is exponential extinction of contrast as a function of distance. In order to evaluate this main effect, van Meeteren (1977) made some simplifying assumptions with regard to all secondary parameters. For details one is referred to the original paper. As soon as contrast reductions are known as a function of distance, the range follows from contrast sensitivity data, such as shown in Fig. 13.3. Fig. 13.13 illustrates the results of this procedure for the HV 5 × 80 image intensifier. The range is plotted here as a function of the light level for a number of different atmospheric conditions, characterized by the distance R, expressed in kilometers, over which the contrast of an object against the horizon sky is reduced by a factor 50.

It is not easy to verify the range, predicted here on the basis of indoor simulation experiments, directly in field trials. Van Meeteren (1977) has only been able to measure the recognition score at one distance during three nights with about the same target illuminance and atmospheric conditions in a real field experiment. Performance proved to be lower than in the indoor simulation, roughly by a factor 1.5 in terms of contrast sensitivity. A number of differences between the indoor simulation measurements and the field trial can be kept responsible for this 'field degradation effect'. As a consequence, one should be very careful with predictions of field performance in the absolute sense, partly because it is impossible to account for all factors of influence. However, relative performances of different devices, as well as the effects of a number of important parameters, can be judged adequately on the basis of indoor simulation experiments and the prediction rules that have emerged from this approach.

Returning to Fig. 13.13, it finally deserves attention that the rate of increase of the range with target illuminance is lower according as atmospheric conditions are worse. Obviously, image intensifiers do not provide a remedy for bad atmospheric visibility. As such they are true visual instruments. One of the advantages of the modern thermal imaging devices is their better penetration of haze and fog, but as remarked already in the introduction, these are not visual instruments and fall beyond the scope of this chapter.

References

Chapter 1

Aguilar, M. & Stiles, W. S. (1954) Saturation of the rod mechanism of the retina at high levels of stimulation. *Optica Acta* **1**, 59–65.

Aho, A.-C. Donner, K., Hyden, C., Larsen, L. U. & Reuter, T. (1988) Low retinal noise in animals with low body temperature allows high visual sensitivity. *Nature* **334**, 348.

Alexander, K. R. & Fishman, G. A. (1984) Rod–cone interaction in flicker perimetry. *Br. J. Opthal.* **68**, 303–9.

Alexander, K. R. & Kelly, S. A. (1984) The influence of cones on rod saturation with flashed backgrounds. *Vision Res.* **24**, 504–11.

Barlow, H. B. (1957) Increment thresholds at low intensities considered as signal noise discriminations. *J. Physiol.* **136**, 469–88.

(1958*a*) Temporal and spatial summation in human vision at different background intensities. *J. Physiol.* **141**, 337–50.

(1958*b*) Intrinsic noise of cones. In *Visual problems of colour*, Vol. 2, pp. 617–30.

(1962) Measurements of the quantum efficiency of discrimination in human scotopic vision. *J. Physiol.* **160**, 169–88.

(1965) Optic nerve impulses and Weber Law. *Cold Spring Harbor Symp. Quart. Biol.* **30**, 539–46.

(1972) Dark and light adaptation: *Psychophysics*. Vol. VII/4 *Visual Psychophysics*, *Handbook of Sensory Physiology* (eds. Jameson & Hurvich).

(1977) Retinal and central factors in human vision limited by noise. In *Photoreception in vertebrates* (eds. Barlow, H. B. & Fatt, P.). Academic Press, London.

Bauer, G. M. Frumkes, T. E. & Nygaard, R. W. (1983) The signal/noise characteristics of rod–cone interaction. *J. Physiol.* **337**, 101–19.

Baylor, D. A., Nunn, B. J. & Schnapf, J. L. (1984) The photocurrent, noise and spectral sensitivity of rods of the monkey *Macaca Fascicularis*. *J. Physiol.* **357**, 575–607.

Berg, T. van den & Spekreijse, H. (1977) Interaction between rod and cone signals studied with temporal sinewave stimulation. *J. opt. Soc. Am.* **67**, 1210–7.

Benimoff, N. I., Schneider, S. I & Hood, D. C. (1982) Interactions between rods and cone channels above threshold: a test of various models. *Vision Res.* **22**, 1133–40.

Bisti, S., Clement, R., Maffei, L. & Mecacci, L. (1977) Spatial frequency and orientation tuning curves of visual neurones of the cat: effects of mean luminance. *Expl Brain Res.* **27**, 335–45.

Blakemore, C. & Campbell, F. W. (1969) On the existence of neurones in the human visual system selectively sensitive to the orientation and size of retinal images. *J. Physiol.* **203**, 2377–80.

Blick, D. W. & MacLeod, D. I. A. (1978) Rod threshold: influence of neighbouring cones. *Vision Res.* **18**, 1611–16.

Bouman, M. A. (1950) Peripheral contrast thresholds of the human eye. *J. opt. Soc. Am.* **40**, 825–32.

Bouman, M. A. (1952) Peripheral contrast thresholds for various and different wavelengths for adopting fields and test stimulus. *J. opt. Soc. Am.* **42**, 820–31.

Bouman, M. A., Vos, J. J. & Walraven, P. L. (1963) Fluctuation theory of luminance and chromaticity discrimination. *J. opt. Soc. Am.* **53**, 121–8.

Braddick, O. J. (1974) A short range process in apparent motion. *Vision Res.* **14**, 519–27.

Bradley, A. & Ohzawa, I. (1986) A comparison of contrast detection and discrimination. *Vision Res.* **26**, 991–7.

Brindley, G. S. (1962) Beats produced by simultaneous stimulation of the human eye with intermittent or alternating electric current. *J. Physiol.* **164**, 157–67.

Brindley, G. S. (1970) *Physiology of the retina and visual pathway*. Edward Arnold Books, London.

Buck, S. L. & Makous, W. (1981) Rod–cone interactions on large and small backgrounds. *Vision Res.* **21**, 1181–7.

Buck, S. L., Peeples, D. R. & Makous, W. (1979) Spatial patterns of rod–cone interaction. *Vision Res.* **19**, 775–82.

Campbell, F. W. & Green, D. G. (1965) Optical and retinal factors affecting visual resolution. *J. Physiol.* **181**, 576–93.

Campbell, F. W. & Gubisch, R. W. (1967) The effect of chromatic aberration on visual acuity. *J. Physiol.* **192**, 345–58.

Campbell, F. W. & Robson, J. G. (1968) Application of Fourier analysis to the visibility of gratings. *J. Physiol.* **197**, 551–66.

Cohn, T. E. (1976) Quantum fluctuation limit in foveal vision. *Vision Res.* **16**, 573–9.

Coletta, N. J. & Adams A. J. (1984) Rod–cone interactions in flicker detection. *Vision Res.* **24**, 1333–40.

Coletta, N. J. & Adams, A. J. (1984) Loss of flicker sensitivity on dim backgrounds in normal and dichromatic observers. *Invest. Ophthal. Visual Sci.* **26**, 187.

Coletta, N. J. & Adams, A. J. (1986) Spatial extent of rod–cone and cone–cone interactions for flicker detection. *Vision Res.* **26**, 917–26.

Conner, J. D. (1982) The temporal properties of rod vision. *J. Physiol.* **332**, 139–55.

Conner, J. D. & MacLeod, D. I. A. (1977) Rod photoreceptors detect rapid flicker. *Science* **195**, 698–9.

De Vries, H. (1943) The quantum character of light and its bearing upon threshold of vision, the differential sensitivity and visual acuity of the eye. *Physica* **10**, 553–64.

Doesschate, J. Ten (1944) Ueber den Zusammenhang der Sehscaerife mid der Unlerschiedsschuelle von Helligkeitsempfindurgen. *Ophthalmologia* **108**, 187–209.

Donner, K. O. & Rushton, W. A. H. (1959) Rod–cone interaction in the frog's retina analysed by the Stiles–Crawford effect and by dark adaptation. *J. Physiol.* **149**, 303–17.

Drum, B. (1982) Summation of rod and cone responses at absolute threshold. *Vision Res.* **22**, 823–6.

D'Zmura, M. & Lennie, P. (1986) Shared pathways for rod and cone vision. *Vision Res.* **26**, 1273–80.

Enroth-Cugell, C. & Robson, J. G. (1966) The contrast sensitivity of retinal ganglion cells of the cat. *J. Physiol.* **187**, 517–52.

Enroth-Cugell, C. & Shapley, R. M. (1973*a*) Adaptation and dynamics of cat retinal ganglion cells. *J. Physiol.* **223**, 271–309.

Enroth-Cugell, C. & Shapley, R. M. (1973*b*) Flux, not retinal illumination is what cat retinal ganglion cells really care about. *J. Physiol.* **233**, 311–26.

Frumkes, T. E. & Eysteinsson, T. (1988) The cellular basis for suppressive rod–cone interaction. *Visual Neurosci.* **1**, 263–73.

Frumkes, T. E., Sekular, M. D., Barris, M. C., Reiss, E. H. & Chalupa, L. M. (1973) Rod–cone interaction in human scotopic vision. I: Temporal analysis. *Vision Res.* **13**, 1269–82.

Frumkes, T. E., Sekular, M. & Reiss, E. (1972) Rod–cone interaction in human scotopic vision. *Science* **175**, 913–14.

Georgeson, M. A. & Sullivan, G. (1975) Contrast constancy: deblurring in human vision by spatial frequency channels. *J. Physiol.* **252**, 627–56.

Goldberg, S. H. & Frumkes, T. E. (1983) A distal retinal locus for rod–cone interaction. *Invest. Ophthal. Visual Sci.* (*Suppl.*) **24**, 187.

Goldberg, S. H., Frumkes, T. E. & Nygaard, R. W. (1983). Inhibitory influence of unstimulated rods in the human retina: evidence provided by examining cone flicker. *Science* **221**, 180–2.

Graham, C. H., Brown, R. H. & Mote, F. A. (1939) The relation of size of stimulus and intensity in the human eye. Intensity thresholds for white light. *J. exp. Psycho*. **24**, 555–73.

Graham, N. (1972) Spatial frequency channels in the human visual system: effect of luminance and pattern drift rate. *Vision Res.* **12**, 53–68.

Hallett, P. E. (1969) Quantum efficiency and false positive rate. *J. Physiol.* **202**, 421–36.

Hallett, P. E., Marriott, F. H. & Rodgers, F. C. (1962) The relation of visual threshold to retinal position and area. *J. Physiol.* **160**, 362–73.

Hecht, S., Shlaer, S., Smith, E. L., Haig, C. & Peskin, J. C. (1948) The visual functions of the completely colour blind. *J. Gen. Physiol.* **31**, 459–472.

Hess, R. F. & Howell, E. R. (1988) Detection of low spatial frequencies: a single filter or multiple filters. *Ophthal. Physiol. Opt.* **8**, 378–85.

Hess, R. F. & Mullen, K. T. (1982) Suppression of the central cone signal under mesopic conditions. *Invest. Opthal. Visual Sci.* (*Suppl.*) **22(3)**, 16.

Hess, R. F. & Nordby, K. (1986*a*) Spatial and temporal limits of vision in the achromat. *J. Physiol.* **371**, 365–85.

Hess, R. F. & Nordby, K. (1986*b*) Spatial and temporal properties of human rod vision in the achromat. *J. Physiol.* **371**, 387–406.

Hess, R. F., Nordby, K. & Pointer, J. S. (1987) Regional variation of contrast sensitivity across the retina of the achromat: sensitivity of human rod vision. *J. Physiol.* **388**, 101–19.

Hess, R. F. & Plant, G. T. (1985) Temporal frequency discrimination in human vision. Evidence for an additional mechanism in the low spatial, high temporal region. *Vision Res.* **25**, 1493–1500.

Hubel, D. H. & Wiesel, T. N. (1977) Functional architecture of macaque monkey visual cortex. (Ferrier Lecture). *Proc. R. Soc. Lond. B* **198**, 1–59.

Ikeda, H. (1965) Temporal summation of positive and negative flashes in the visual system. *J. opt. Soc. Am.* **55**, 1527–34.

Kolb, H. (1977) The organization of the outer plexiform layer in the retina of the cat: electron microscopic observations. *J. Neurocytel*, **6**, 131–53.

Kranda, K. & Kulikowski, J. J. (1976) Adaptation to coarse gratings under scotopic and photopic conditions. *J. Physiol.* **257**, 35.

Lamar, E. S., Hecht, S., Shlaer, S. & Hendley, C. D. (1947) Size shape and contrast in detection of targets by daylight vision. I. Data and analytical description. *J. opt. Soc. Am.* **37**, 531–45.

Lamb, T. D. (1984) Photoreceptor adaptation – vertebrates. In *Molecular mechanism of photoreception.* (ed. Stieve, H.) pp. 267–86. Springer-Verlag, Berlin.

Latch, M. & Lennie, P. (1977) Rod–cone interaction in light adaptation. *J. Physiol.* **269**, 517–34.

Legge, G. E. (1981) A power law for contrast discrimination. *Vision Res.* **21**, 457–67.

Levine, M. W. & Frishman, L. J. (1984) Interactions between rod and cone channels: a model that includes inhibition. *Vision Res.* **24**, 513–6.

Lillywhite, P. G. & Laughlin, S. B. (1979) Transducer noise in a photoreceptor. *Nature* **277**, 569–72.

Lillywhite, P. G., Hess, R. F. & Parker, A. (1982) How effective is contrast constancy. *Invest. Opthal. Visual Sci.* (*Suppl.*) **22**, 207.

van Loo J. A. & Enoch, J. M. (1975) The scotopic Stiles–Crawford effect. *Vision Res.* **15**, 1005–9.

MacLeod, D. I. A. (1972) Rods cancel cones in flicker. *Nature* **144**, 285–94.

Makous, W. & Peeples, D. R. (1979) Rod–cone interaction: reconciliation with Flamant and Stiles. *Vision Res.* **19**, 695–8.

Meeteren, A. van (1973) Visual aspects of image intensification. Thesis, Utrecht.

Moore, B. C. J., Glasberg, B. R., Hess, R. F. & Birchall, J. P. (1985). Effects of flanking noise bands on the rate of growth of loudness of tones in normal and recruiting ears. *J. acoust. Soc. Am.* **77**, 1505–13.

Nachmias, J. & Sansbury, R. V. (1974) Grating contrast: discrimination may be better than detection. *Vision Res.* **14**, 1039–42.

Nelson, R. (1977) Cat cones have rod input: a comparison of the response properties of cones and horizontal cell bodies in the retina of the cat. *J. comp. Neurol.* **172**, 109–36.

van Nes, F. L. & Bouman, M. A. (1967) Spatial modulation transfer in the human eye. *J. opt. Soc. Am.* **57**, 401–6.

van Nes, F. L., Koenderink, J. J., Nas, H. & Bouman, M. A. (1967) Spatiotemporal modulation transfer in the human eye. *J. opt. Soc. Am.* **57**, 1082–8.

Ohzawa, I., Sclar, G. & Freeman, R. D. (1985) Contrast gain control in the cat visual system. *J. Neurophysiol.* **54**, 651–67.

Orban, G. A., Wolf, J. de & Maes, H. (1984) Factors influencing velocity coding in the human visual system. *Vision Res.* **24**, 33–39.

Pandey Vimal, R. L. & Wilson, H. R. (1987) Spatial frequency discrimination: Scotopic and photopic conditions compared. *Invest. Ophthal. Visual Sci.* (*Suppl.*) **28**, 360.

Piper, H. (1903) Überdie Abhangigkeit des Reizwertes leuchtender objekte von ihrer Flachen-bezu. *Winkelgrasse Z. psych. u. Physiol. d. Sinnesorg* **32**, 98–112.

Rashbass, C. (1970) The visibility of transient changes in luminance. *J. Physiol.* **210**, 165–86.

Riccò, A. (1877) Relazzione fra il minimo angelo visuale e l'intensitàluminosa. *Annali Ottalmologia* **6**, 373–479.

Robson, J. G. (1966) Spatial and temporal contrast sensitivity functions of the visual system. *J. opt. Soc. Am.* **56**, 1141–2.

Rodieck, R. W. & Rushton, W. A. H. (1976) Cancellation of rod signals by cones and cone signals by rods in the cat retina. *J. Physiol.* **254**, 775–785.

Rose, A. (1942) Quantum and noise limitations of the visual process. *J. opt. Soc. Am.* **43**, 715–25.

Rose, A. (1948) The sensitivity performance of the human eye on an absolute scale. *J. opt. Soc. Am.* **38**, 196–208.

Ross, J. & Campbell, F. W. (1978) Why do we not perceive photons? *Nature* **257**, 541–2.

Sakitt, B. (1971) Configuration dependence of scotopic spatial summation. *J. Physiol.* **216**, 513–29.

Schultze, M. (1866) Zur Anatomie und Physiologie der Retina. *ARCH mikr. Anat.* **2**, 175–286.

Shapley, R. & Enroth-Cugell, C. (1984) Visual adaptation and retinal gain control. *Prog. Ret. Res.* **3**, 263–346.

Sharpe, L. T., Stockman, A. & MacLeod, D. I. A. (1989) Rod flicker perception: scotopic duality, phase lags and destructive interference. *Vision Res.* **29**, 1539–59.

Spillmann, L. & Conlon, J. E. (1972) Photochromatic internal during dark adaptation as a function of background illuminance. *J. opt. Soc. Am.* **62**, 182–5.

Stabell, B. Nordby, K. & Stabell, U. (1987) Light-adaptation of the human rod system. *Clin. Vision Sci.* **2**, 83–91.

Sterling, P., Freed, M. & Smith, R. G. (1986) Microcircuitary and functional architecture of the cat retina. *TINS* **9**, 186–92.

Stiles, W. S. (1939) The directional sensitivity of the retina and the spectral sensitivities of rods and cones. *Proc. R. Soc. Lond. B* **127**, 64–105.

Stiles, W. S. & Crawford, B. H. (1933 The luminous efficiency of rays entering the eye pupil at different points. *Proc. R. Soc. Lond. B* **112**, 428–50.

Stromeyer III, C. F. & Julesz, B. (1972) Spatial frequency masking in vision. Critical bands and spread of masking. *J. opt. Soc. Am.* **62**, 1221–32.

Stromeyer III, C. F. Klein, S., Dawson, B. M. & Spillmann, L. (1982) Low spatial frequency channels in human vision: adaptation and masking. *Vision Res.* **22**, 225–33.

Teich, M. C. *et al.* (1978) Refractoriness in the maintained discharge of cat retinal ganglion cells. *J. opt. Soc. Am.* **68**, 368–402.

Teich, M. C. *et al.* (1982) Multiplication noise in the human visual system at threshold: The rule of non-Poisson quantum fluctuations. *Biol. Cyb.* **44**, 157–65.

Tolhurst, D. J. (1975) Reaction times in the detection of gratings by human observers: a probabilistic mechanism. *Vision Res.* **15**, 1143–9.

Tolhurst, D. J., Movshon, J. A. & Thompson, I. D. (1981) The dependence of response amplitude and variance of cat visual cortical neurones on stimulus contrast. *Exp. Brain Res.* **41**, 414–9.

Troy, J. B., Enroth-Cugell, C. & Robson, J. G. (1987) Do x and y retinal ganglion cells signal contrast? *I.E.E.E. Conference of the ISMC* **3**, 1070–4.

Virsu, V. (1974) Dark adaptation shifts apparent spatial frequency. *Vision Res.* **14**, 433–5.

Watson, A. B. (1979) Probability summation over time. *Vision Res.* **19**, 515–22.

Watson, A. B. & Nachmias, J. (1977) Patterns of temporal interaction in the detection of gratings. *Vision Res.* **17**, 893–902.

Watson, A. B. & Robson, J. G. (1981) Discrimination at threshold: labelled detectors in human vision. *Vision Res.* **21**, 1115–22.

Wilson, H. R. & Bergen, J. R. (1979) A four mechanism model for threshold spatial vision. *Vision Res.* **19**, 19–32.

Wooten, B. & Butler, T. (1976) Possible rod–cone interaction in dark adaptation. *J. opt. Soc. Am.* **66**, 1429–30.

Chapter 2

Adelson, E. H. (1982) Saturation and adaptation in the rod system. *Vision Res.* **22**, 1299–1312.

Aguilar, M. & Stiles, W. S. (1954) Saturation of the rod mechanism of the retina at high levels of stimulation. *Optica Acta* **1**, 59–65.

Aho, A,-C., Donner, K., Hyden, C., Larsen, L. O. & Reuter, T. (1988) Low retinal noise in animals with low body temperature allows high visual sensitivity. *Nature* **334**, 348–50.

Aho, A.-C., Donner, K., Hyden, C., Reuter, T. & Orlov, O. Y. (1987) Retinal noise, the performance of retinal ganglion cells, and visual sensitivity in the dark-adapted frog. *J. opt. Soc. Am.* **A 4**, 2321–9.

Alexander, K. R. (1974) Sensitization by annular surrounds: the effect of test stimulus size. *Vision Res.* **14**, 1107–13.

Alexander, K. R. & Fishman, G. A. (1984) Rod–cone interaction in flicker perimetry. *Br. J. Ophthal.* **68**, 303–9.

Alexander, K. R. & Fishman, G. A. (1985) Rod-cone interacton in flicker perimetry: evidence for a distal retinal locus. *Documenta Ophth.* **60**, 3–36.

Alexander, K. R. & Fishman, G. A. (1986) Rod influence on cone flicker detection: variation with retinal eccentricity. *Vision Res.* **26**, 827–34.

Alexander, K. R. & Kelly, S. A. (1984) The influence of cones on rod saturation with flashed backgrounds. *Vision Res.* **24**, 507–11.

Alexander, K. R., Kelly, S. A. & Morris, M. A. (1986) Background size and saturation of the rod system. *Vision Res.* **26**, 299–312.

Alpern M. (1971) Rhodopsin kinetics in the human eye. *J. Physiol.* **217**, 447–71.

Alpern, M., Ching, C. C. & Kitahara, K. (1983) The directional sensitivity of retinal rods. *J. Physiol.* **343**, 577–92.

Alpern, M. & Ohba, N. (1972) The effect of bleaching and backgrounds on pupil size. *Vision Res.* **12**, 943–51.

Alpern, M. & Pugh, E. N. Jr (1974) The density and photosensitivity of human rhodopsin in the living retina. *J. Physiol.* **237**, 341–70.

Andrews, D. P. & Butcher, A. K. (1971) Rod threshold and patterned rhodopsin bleaching, the pigment epithelium as an adaptation pool. *Vision Res.* **11**, 761–85.

Arden, G. B. & Weale, R. A. (1954) Variations of the latent period of vision. *Proc. R. Soc. Lond.* B **143**, 258–67.

Aulhorn, E. (1964) Über die Beziehung zwischen Lichtsinn und Sehschärfe. *Albrecht v Graefes Arch. Ophthal.* **167**, 4–74.

Autrum, H. (1943) Über kleinste Reize bei Sinnesorganen. *Biol. Zbl.* **63**, 200–35.

Baker, H. D. (1963) Initial stages of dark and light adaptation. *J. opt. Soc. Am.* **53**, 98–103.

Barlow, H. B. (1956) Retinal noise and absolute threshold. *J. opt. Soc. Am.* **46**, 634–39.

(1957) Increment thresholds at low intensities considered as signal/noise discriminations. *J. Physiol.* **136**, 469–88.

(1958) Temporal and spatial summation in human vision at different background intensities. *J. Physiol.* **141**, 337–50.

(1962) Measurements of the quantum efficiency of discrimination in human scotopic vision. *J. Physiol.* **160**, 169–88.

(1977) Retinal and central factors in human vision limited by noise. In *Photoreception in vertebrates* (eds. Barlow, H. B. & Fatt, P.), pp. 337–58, Academic Press, London.

(1988) The thermal limit to seeing. *Nature* **334**, 296–7.

Barlow, H. B. & Andrews, D. P. (1967) Sensitivity of receptors and receptor 'pools'. *J. opt. Soc. Am.* **57**, 837–8.

Barlow, H. B., Fitzhugh, R. & Kuffler, S. W. (1957) Change of organization in the receptive fields of the cat's retina during dark adaptation. *J. Physiol.* **137**, 338–54.

Barlow, H. B., Kaushal, T. P., Hawken, M. & Parker, A. J. (1987) Human contrast discrimination and the threshold of cortical neurons. *J. opt. Soc. Am.* **A 4**, 2366–71.

Barlow, H. B. & Levick, W. R. (1969) Changes in the maintained discharge with adaptation level in the cat retina. *J. Physiol.* **202**, 699–718.

Barlow, H. B. & Levick, W. R. (1976) Threshold setting by the surround of cat retinal ganglion cells. *J. Physiol.* **259**, 737–57.

Barlow, H. B., Levick, W. R. & Yoon, M. (1971) Responses to single quanta of light in retinal ganglion cells of the cat. *Vision Res.* Suppl. no. 3, 87–101.

Barlow, H. B. & Sakitt, B. (1973) Doubts about scotopic interactions in stabilized vision. *Vision Res.* **13**, 523–24.

Barlow, R. B. Jr & Silbaugh, T. H. (1989) Is photoreceptor noise caused by thermal isomerization of rhodopsin? *Invest. Ophthal. Visual Sci.* **30** (suppl.), 61.

Barris, M. C. & Frumkes, T. E. (1978) Rod–cone interaction in human scotopic vision. IV–Cones stimulated by contrast flashes influence rod threshold. *Vision Res.* **18**, 801–8.

Bauer, G. M., Frumkes, T. E. & Holstein, G. R. (1983*a*) The influence of rod light and dark adaptation upon rod–cone interaction. *J. Physiol.* **337**, 121–35.

Bauer, G. M., Frumkes, T. E. & Nygaard, R. W. (1983*b*) The signal-to-noise characteristics of rod–cone interaction. *J. Physiol.* **337**, 101–19.

Baumgardt, E. (1959) Visual spatial and temporal summation. *Nature* **184**, 1951–2.

(1960) Mesure pyrometrique du seuil visuel absolu. *Optica Acta* **7**, 305–16.

(1972) Threshold quantal problems. In *Handbook of sensory physiology*, Vol. VII/4: Visual psychophysics (eds. Jameson, D. & Hurvich, L. M.), Chapter 2, pp. 29–55. Springer-Verlag, Heidelberg.

Baumgardt, E. & Hillmann, B. M. (1961) Duration and size as determinants of peripheral retinal response. *J. opt. Soc. Am.* **51**, 340–4.

Baumgardt, E. & Smith, S. W. (1965) Facilitation effect of background light on target detection: a test of theories of absolute threshold. *Vision Res.* **5**, 299–312.

Baylor, D. A. (1987) Photoreceptor signals and vision. *Invest. Ophthal. Visual Sci.* **28**, 34–49.

Baylor, D. A. Fuortes, M. G. F. & O'Bryan, P. M. (1971) Receptive fields of single cones in the retina of the turtle. *J. Physiol.* **214**, 265–94.

Baylor, D. A. & Hodgkin, A. L. (1974) Changes in time scale and sensitivity in turtle photoreceptors. *J. Physiol.* **242**, 729–58.

Baylor, D. A., Lamb, T. D. & Yau, K.-W. (1979) The membrane current of single rod outer segments. *J. Physiol.* **288**, 589–611.

Baylor, D. A., Matthews, G. & Yau, K.-W. (1980) Two components of electrical dark noise in toad retinal rod outer segments. *J. Physiol.* **309**, 591–621.

Baylor, D. A., Nunn, B. J. & Schnapf, J. L. (1984) The photocurrent, noise and spectral sensitivity of rods of the monkey Macaca Fascicularis. *J. Physiol.* **357**, 575–607.

Belgum, J. H. & Copenhagen, D. R. (1988) Synaptic transfer of rod signals to horizontal and bipolar cells in the retina of the toad (*Bufo marinus*). *J. Physiol.* **396**, 667–80.

Benimoff, N. I., Schneider, S. & Hood, D. C. (1982) Interactions between rod and cone channels above threshold: a test of various models. *Vision Res.* **22**, 1133–40.

van den Berg, T. J. T. P. & Spekreijse, H. (1977) Interaction between rod and cone signals studied with temporal sine wave stimulation. *J. opt. Soc. Am.* **67**, 1210–7.

Blackwell, H. R. (1946) Contrast thresholds of the human eye. *J. opt. Soc. Am.* **36**, 624–43.

Blakemore, C. B. & Rushton, W. A. H. (1965) Dark adaptation and increment threshold in a rod monochromat. *J. Physiol.* **181**, 612–28.

Blick, D. W. & MacLeod, D. I. A. (1978) Rod threshold: influence of neighboring cones. *Vision Res.* **18**, 1611–6.

Bouger, M. (1760). *Traite d'Optique sur la Graduation de la Lumiere*. De la Calle, Paris.

Bouman, M.A. (1953). Visual thresholds for line-shaped targets. *J. opt. Soc. Am.* **43**, 209–11.

Bouman, M. A. & Blokhuis, E. W. M. (1952) The visibility of black objects against an illuminated background. *J. opt. Soc. Am.* **42**, 525–8.

Bouman, M. A. & van der Velden, H. A. (1948) The two-quanta hypothesis as a general explanation for the behavior of threshold values and visual acuity for the several receptors of the human eye. *J. opt. Soc. Am.* **38**, 570–81.

Bowmaker, J. K. & Dartnall, J. J. A. (1980) Visual pigments of rods and cones in a human retina. *J. Physiol.* **298**, 501–11.

Boycott, B. B. & Dowling, J. E. (1969) Organization of the primate retina: light microscopy. *Phil. Trans. R. Soc. Lond.* B **255**, 109–84.

Brindley, G. S. (1970) Physiology of the Retina and Visual Pathway (2nd edn.) Williams and Wilkins, Baltimore.

Buck, S. L. & Makous, W. (1981) Rod–cone interaction on large and small backgrounds. *Vision Res.* **21**, 1181–7.

Buck, S. L., Peeples, D. R. & Makous, W. (1979) Spatial patterns of rod–cone interaction. *Vision Res.* **19**, 775–82.

Burgess, A. E., Barlow, H. B., Jennings, R. J. & Wagner, R. F. (1981) Efficiency of human visual signal discrimination. *Science* **214**, 93–4.

Burkhardt, D. A. & Berntson, G. G. (1972) Light adaptation and excitation: lateral spread of signals within the frog retina. *Vision Res.* **12**, 1095–12.

Buss, C. M., Hayhoe, M. M. & Stromeyer, C. F. III (1982). Lateral interactions in the control of visual sensitivity. *Vision Res.* **22**, 693–709.

Cabello, J. & Stiles, W. S. (1950) Sensibilidad de bastognes y conos en la parafovea. *Anales Real soc. Espan. Fis. Quim.* A **46**, 251–82.

Chen, B., MacLeod, D. I. A. & Stockman, A. (1987) Improvement in human vision under bright light: grain or gain? *J. Physiol.* **394**, 17–38.

Cicerone, C. M. & Green, D. G. (1980) Dark adaptation within the receptive field centre of rat retinal ganglion cells. *J. Physiol*, **301**, 535–48.

Cicerone, C. M. & Green, D. G. (1981) Signal transmission from rods to ganglion cells in rat retina after bleaching a portion of the receptive field. *J. Physiol.* **314**, 213–24.

Cleland, B. G. & Enroth-Cugell, C. (1968). Quantitative aspects of sensitivity and summation in the rat retina. *J. Physiol.* **198**, 17–38.

Cohn, T. E. (1974) A new hypothesis to explain why the increment threshold exceeds the decrement threshold. *Vision Res.* **14**, 1277–9.

(1976) Quantum fluctuation limit in foveal vision. *Vision Res.* **16**, 573–9.

Cohn, T. E. (1981) Absolute threshold: analysis in terms of uncertainty. *J. Opt. Soc. Am.* **71**, 783–5.

Cohn, T. E. & Lasley, D. J. (1986) Visual sensitivity. *Ann. Rev. Psychol.* **37**, 495–521.

Cohn, T. E., Weissman, B. & Wasilewsky, P. (1972) Why the increment threshold exceeds the decrement threshold. *Am. J. Optom.* **49**, 893.

Coletta, N. J. & Adams, A. J. (1984) Rod-cone interaction in flicker detection. *Vision Res.* **24**, 1333–40.

Conner, J. D. (1982) The temporal properties of rod vision. *J. Physiol.* **332**, 139–55.

Conner, J. D. & MacLeod, D. I. A. (1977) Rod photoreceptors detect rapid flicker. *Science* **195**, 698–9.

Copenhagen, D. R., Donner, K. & Reuter, T. (1987) Ganglion cell performance at absolute threshold in toad retina: effects of dark events in rods. *J. Physiol.* **393**, 667–80.

Copenhagen, D. R. & Green, D. G. (1985) The absence of spread of adaptation between rod photoreceptors in turtle retina. *J. Physiol.* **259**, 251–81.

Craik, K. J. W. (1938) The effect of adaptation on differential brightness discrimination. *J. Physiol.* **92**, 406–21.

Craik, K. J. W. & Vernon, M. D. (1941) The nature of dark adaptation. *Br. J. Psychol.* **32**, 62–81.

Crawford, B. H. (1940) The effect of field size and pattern on the change of visual sensitivity with time. *Proc. R. Soc. Lond.* B. **129**, 94–106.

(1947) Visual adaptation in relation to brief conditioning stimuli. *Proc. R. Soc. Lond.* B. **134**, 283–302.

Curcio, C. A., Hendrickson, A. E. & Kalina, R. E. (1985) Topographical distribution of human photoreceptors. *Invest. Ophthal. Visual Sci.* **26** (suppl.), 261.

Curcio, C. A., Sloan, K. R., Packer, O., Hendrickson, A. E. & Kalina, R. E. (1987) Distribution of cones in human and monkey retina: individual variability and radial asymmetry. *Science* **236**, 579–82.

Dartnall, H. J. A. (ed.) (1972) Photosensitivity. In *Handbook of sensory physiology*, Vol. VII/I, Photochemistry of vision, pp. 122–45. Springer-Verlag, Berlin.

de Groot, J. J. & Gebhard, J. W. (1952) Pupil size as determined by adapting luminance. *J. opt. Soc. Am.* **42**, 492.

de Monasterio, F. M. (1978) Center and surround mechanisms of opponent-colour X and Y ganglion cells of retina of macaques. *J. Neurophysiol.* **41**, 1418–34.

Denton, E. J. & Pirenne, M. H. (1954) The absolute sensitivity and functional stability of the human eye. *J. Physiol.* **123**, 417–42.

Derrington, A. M. & Lennie, P. (1982) The influence of temporal frequency and adaptation level on receptive field organization of retinal ganglion cells in cat. *J. Physiol.* **333**, 343–66.

Detwiler, P. B., Hodgkin, A. L. & McNaughton, P. A. (1980) Temporal and spatial characteristics of the voltage response of the rods in the retina of the snapping turtle. *J. Physiol.* **300**, 213–50.

Donner, K. (1987) Adaptation-related changes in the spatial and temporal summation of frog retinal ganglion cells. *Acta physiol. scand.* **131**, 479–87.

(1989) The absolute sensitivity of vision: can a frog become a perfect detector of light-induced and dark rod events? *Physica Scripta* **39**, 133–40.

Dowling, J. E. (1967) The site of visual adaptation. *Science* **155**, 273–9.

(1987) *The retina: an approachable part of the brain.* Harvard University Press, Cambridge, Massachusetts.

Dowling, J. E. & Boycott, B. B. (1966) Organization of the primate retina: electronmicroscopy. *Proc. R. Soc. Lond.* B. **166**, 80–111.

Dowling, J. E. & Ripps, H. (1972) Adaptation in skate photoreceptors. *J. gen. Physiol.* **60**, 698–719.

Drum, B. (1982) Summation of rod and cone responses at absolute threshold. *Vision Res.* **22**, 823–6.

D'Zmura, M. & Lennie, P. (1986) Shared pathways for rod and cone vision. *Vision Res.* **26**, 1273–80.

Easter, S. S. Jr (1968) Adaptation in the goldfish retina. *J. Physiol.* **195**, 273–81.

Ehrenstein, W. H. & Spillmann, L. (1983) Time thresholds for increments and decrements in luminance. *J. opt. Soc. Am.* **73**, 419–26.

Enoch, J. M. (1978) Quantitative layer-by-layer perimetry. *Invest. Ophthal. Visual Sci.* **17**, 208–57.

Enoch, J. M. & Sunga, R. A. (1969) Development of quantitative perimetric tests. *Documenta ophth.* **26**, 215–29.

Enroth-Cugell, C., Hertz, B. G. & Lennie, P. (1977) Convergence of rod and cone signals in the cat's retina. *J. Physiol.* **269**, 297–318.

Enroth-Cugell, C. & Lennie, P. (1975) The control of retinal ganglion cell discharge by receptive field surrounds. *J. Physiol.* **247**, 551–78.

Enroth-Cugell, C., Lennie, P. & Shapley, R. M. (1975) Surround contribution to light adaptation in cat retinal ganglion cells. *J. Physiol.* **247**, 579–88.

Enroth-Cugell, C. & Robson, J. G. (1966) The contrast sensitivity of retinal ganglion cells of the cat. *J. Physiol.* **187**, 517–22.

Enroth-Cugell, C. & Shapley, R. M. (1973) Adaptation and dynamics of cat retinal ganglion cells. *J. Physiol.* **233**, 271–309.

Essock, E. A., Lehmkuhle, S., Frascella, J. & Enoch, J. M. (1985) Temporal modulation of the background affects the sensitization response of X- and Y-cells in the dLGN of cat. *Vision Res.* **25**, 1007–19.

Fach, C. C., Sharpe, L. T. & Stockman, A. (1989) The field adaptation of the 'isolated' rod visual system. *Invest. Opthal. Visual Sci.* **30** (suppl.), 455.

Fach, C. C., Sharpe, L. T. & Stockman, A. (1990) (In preparation.)

Fain, G. L. (1976) Sensitivity of toad rods: dependence on wave-length and background illumination. *J. Physiol.* **261**, 71–101.

Famiglietti, E. V. & Kolb, H. (1975) A bistratified amacrine cell and synaptic circuitry in the inner plexiform layer of the retina. *Brain Res.* **84**, 293–300.

Fechner, G. T. (1860) *Elemente der Psychophysik*. Breitkopf and Hartel, Leipzig.

Fiorentini, A., Bayly, E. J. & Maffei, L. (1972) Peripheral and central contributions to psychophysical spatial interactions. *Vision Res.* **12**, 253–8.

Flamant, F. & Stiles, W. S. (1948) The directional and spectral sensitivities of the retinal rods to adapting fields of different wave-lengths. *J. Physiol.* **107**, 187–202.

Foster, D. H. (1976) Rod–cone interaction in the after-flash effect. *Vision Res.* **16**, 393–6.

Foster, D. H. & Mason, R. J. (1977) Interaction between rod and cone systems in dichoptic visual masking. *Neurosci. Lett.* **4**, 39–42.

Frishman, L. J. & Levine, M. W. (1983) Statistics of the maintained discharge of cat retinal ganglion cells. *J. Physiol.* **339**, 475–94.

Frumkes, T. E. & Holstein, G. R. (1979) Rod–cone interrelationships at light onset and offset. *J. opt. Soc. Am.* **69**, 1727–30.

Frumkes, T. E., Naarendorp, F. & Goldberg, S. H. (1986) The influence of cone adaptation upon rod mediated flicker. *Vision Res.* **26**, 1167–76.

Frumkes, T. E., Sekuler, M. D., Barris, M. C., Reiss, E. H. & Chalupa, L. M. (1973) Rod–cone interaction in human scotopic vision–I. Temporal analysis. *Vision Res.* **13**, 1269–82.

Frumkes, T. E., Sekuler, M. D. & Reiss, E. H. (1972) Rod–cone interaction in human scotopic vision. *Science* **175**, 913–14.

Frumkes, T. E. & Temme, L. A. (1977) Rod–cone interaction in human scotopic vision–II. Cones influence rod increment thresholds. *Vision Res.* **17**, 673–9.

Fuld, K. (1978) A sensitization effect with rectilinear stimuli. *Vision Res.* **18**, 1045–51.

Fulton, A. B. & Rushton, W. A. H. (1978) The human rod ERG: correlation with psychophysical responses in light and dark adaptation. *Vision Res.* **18**, 793–800.

Fuortes, M. G. F. & Hodgkin, A. L. (1964) Changes in time scale and sensitivity in the ommatidia of Limulus. *J. Physiol.* **172**, 230–63.

Geisler, W. S. (1979) Initial-image and afterimage discrimination in the human rod and cone systems. *J. Physiol.* **294**, 165–79.

(1980) Increment threshold and detection latency in the rod and cone systems. *Vision Res.* **20**, 981–94.

Gildemeister, M. (1914) Über die Wahrnehmbarkeit von Lichtlücken. *Z. Sinnesphysiol.* **48**, 256–67.

Gouras, P. (1965) Primate retina: duplex function of dark adapted retinal ganglion cells. *Science* **147**, 1593–4.

Gouras, P. (1967) The effects of light-adaptation on rod and cone receptive field organization of monkey ganglion cells. *J. Physiol.* **192**, 747–60.

Gouras, P. & Link, K. (1966) Rod and cone interaction in dark-adapted monkey ganglion cells. *J. Physiol.* **184**, 499–510.

Graham, C. H., Brown, R. M. & Mote, F. A. (1939) The relation of size of stimulus and intensity in the human eye: I. Intensity threshold for white light. *J. exp. Psychol.* **24**, 555–73.

Green, D. G. (1986) The search for the site of visual adaptation. *Vision Res.* **26**, 1417–29.

Green, D. G., Dowling, J. E., Siegel, I. M. & Ripps, H. (1975) Retinal mechanisms of visual adaptation in the skate. *J. gen. Physiol.* **65**, 483–502.

Green, D. G., Tong, L. & Cicerone, C. M. (1977) Lateral spread of light adaptation in the rat retina. *Vision Res.* **17**, 479–86.

von Grünau, M. W. (1986) The fluttering heart and spatio-temporal characteristics of color processing. III. Interactions between the systems of the rods and the long wavelength cones. *Vision Res.* **16**, 397–401.

Hallett, P. E. (1963) Spatial summation. *Vision Res.* **3**, 9–24.

(1969) Quantum efficiency and false positive rate. *J. Physiol.* **202**, 421–36.

(1987) Quantum efficiency of dark-adapted human vision. *J. opt. Soc. Am.* A. **4**, 2330–5.

Hallett, P. E., Marriott, F. H. C. & Rodger, F. C. (1962) The relationship of visual threshold to retinal position and area. *J. Physiol.* **160**, 364–73.

Hayhoe, M. M. (1979) After-effects of small adapting fields. *J. Physiol.* **296**, 141–58.

Hayhoe, M. M., Benimoff, N. I. & Hood, D. C. (1987) The time-course of multiplicative and subtractive adaptation processes. *Vision Res.* **27**, 1981–96.

Hayhoe, M. M. & Levin, M. (1987) Spatial basis of subtractive adaptation. *Invest. Ophthal. Visual Sci.* **28** (suppl.), 357.

Hayhoe, M. M., MacLeod, D. I. A. & Bruch, T. (1976) Rod–cone independence in dark adaptation. *Vision Res.* **16**, 591–600.

Hayhoe, M. M. & Smith, M. (1989) The role of spatial filtering in sensitivity regulation. *Vision Res.* **29**, 457–69.

Hecht, S., Shlaer, S. & Pirenne, M. H. (1942) Energy, quanta and vision. *J. gen. Physiol.* **25**, 819–40.

Herrick, R. M. (1956) Foveal luminance discrimination as a function of the duration of the decrement or increment in luminance. *J. comp. physiol. Psychol.* **49**, 437–43.

Hess, R. F. & Nordby, (1986) Spatial and temporal properties of human rod vision in the achromat. *J. Physiol.* **371**, 387–406.

Hood, D. C. & Finkelstein, M. A. (1986) Sensitivity to light. In *Sensory processes and perception, handbook of perception and human performance* (eds. Boff, K. R., Kaufman, L. & Thomas, J. P., pp. (5)1–(5)66. John Wiley, New York.

Hubel, D. H. & Wiesel, T. N. (1960) Receptive fields of optic nerve fibers in the spider monkey. *J. Physiol.* **154**, 572–80.

Ikeda, M. & Urakubo, M. (1969) Rod–cone interrelation. *J. opt. Soc. Am.* **59**, 217–22.

Ingling, C. R. Jr, Lewis, A., Loose, D. & Myers, K. (1977) Cones change rod sensitivity. *Vision Res.* **17**, 555–63.

Kelly, D. H. (1961) Visual responses to time-dependent stimuli. I. Amplitude sensitivity measurements. *J. opt. Soc. Am.* **51**, 422–9.

Kleinschmidt, J. & Dowling, J. E. (1975) Intracellular recordings from Gecko photoreceptors during light and dark adaptation. *J. gen. Physiol.* **66**, 617–48.

Kohlrausch, A. (1922) Untersuchungen mit farbigen Schwellenprüflichtern über den Dunkeladaptationsverlauf des normalen Auges. *Pflügers Arch. ges. Physiol.* **196**, 113–17.

Kolb, H. (1970) Organisation of the outer plexiform layer of the primate retina: electron microscopy of Golgi-impregnated cells. *Phil. Trans. R. Soc. Lond.* B **258**, 261–83.

(1977) The organization of the outer plexiform layer in the retina of the cat: electron microscopic observations. *J. Neurocytol.* **6**, 131–53.

Kolb, H & Nelson, R. (1981) Amacrine cells of the cat retina. *Vision Res.* **21**, 1625–33.

Kolb, H. & Nelson, R. (1983) Rod pathways in the retina of the cat. *Vision Res.* **23**, 301–12.

Kolb, H., Nelson, R. & Mariani, A. (1981) Amacrine cells, bipolar cells, and ganglion cells of the cat retina: a Golgi study. *Vision Res.* **21**, 1081–114.

Krauskopf, J. & Reeves, A. (1980) Measurement of the effect of photon noise on detection. *Vision Res.* **20**, 193–6.

von Kries, J. (1894) Über den Einfluß der Adaptation auf Licht- und Farbenempfindung und über die Funktion der Stäbchen. *Ber. naturf. Ges. Freiburg im Breisgau* **9** (2), 61–70.

(1896) Über die Funktion der Netzhautstäbchen. *Z. Psychol.* **9**, 81–123.

(1929) Zur Theorie des Tages- und Dämmerungssehens. In *Handbuch der normalen und pathologischen Physiologie*, Vol. XII (1), Receptionsorgane 2 (Photoreceptoren I) (eds. Bethe, A., von Bergmann, G., Emden, G. & Ellinger A.), pp. 679–713. Springer, Berlin.

Lamb, T. D. (1987) Sources of noise in photoreceptor transduction. *J. opt. Soc. Am.* **A 4**, 2295–300.

Latch, M. & Baker, H. D. (1976) An alternative to rod–cone interaction in dark adaptation. *The Association for Research in Vision and Ophthalmology, Spring Meeting, Sarasota, Florida, April 26–30, 1976*, Abstract, p. 108.

Latch, M. & Lennie, P. (1977) Rod–cone interaction in light adaptation. *J. Physiol.* **269**, 517–34.

Lennie, P. (1979) Scotopic increment thresholds in retinal ganglion cells. *Vision Res.* **19**, 425–30.

Lennie, P. Hertz, B. G. & Enroth-Cugell, C. (1976) Saturation of rod pools in cat. *Vision Res.* **16**, 935–40.

Lennie, P. & MacLeod, D. I. A. (1973) Background configuration and rod threshold. *J. Physiol.* **233**, 143–56.

Levine, M. W. & Frishman, L. J. (1984) Interactions between rod and cone channels: a model that includes inhibition. *Vision Res.* **24**, 513–16.

Levine, M. W., Frishman, L. J. & Enroth-Cugell, C. (1987) Interactions between the rod and the cone pathways in the cat retina. *Vision Res.* **27**, 1093–104.

Levine, M. W. & Shefner, J. M. (1981) Distance-independent interactions between the rod and the cone systems in goldfish retina. *Exp. Brain Res.* **44**, 353–61.

Lillywhite, P. G. (1981) Multiplicative intrinsic noise and the limits to visual performance. *Vision Res.* **21**, 291–6.

Lillywhite, P. G. & Laughlin, S. B. (1979) Transducer noise in a photoreceptor. *Nature* **277**, 569–72.

Linsenmeier, R. A., Frishman, L. J., Jakiela, H. G. & Enroth-Cugell, C. (1982) Receptive field properties of X and Y cells in the cat retina derived from contrast sensitivity measurements. *Vision Res.* **22**, 1173–83.

MacLeod, D. I. A. (1972) rods cancel cones in flicker. *Nature* **235**, 173–4.

(1978) Visual sensitivity. *A. Rev. Psychol.* **29**, 613–45.

MacLeod, D. I. A., Chen, B. & Crognale, M. (1984) Local adaptation vs. neural pools in rod vision. *Invest. Ophthal. Visual Sci.* **25** (suppl.), 53.

MacLeod, D. I. A., Chen, B. & Crognale, M. (1989) Spatial organization of sensitivity regulation in rod vision. *Vision Res.* **29**, 965–78.

Maffei, L. (1968) Inhibitory and facilitatory spatial interactions in retinal receptive fields. *Vision Res.* **8**, 1187–94.

Makous, W. & Boothe, R. (1974) Cones block signals from rods. *Vision Res.* **14**, 285–94.

Makous, W. & Peeples, D. (1979) Rod–cone interaction: reconciliation with Flamant and Stiles. *Vision Res.* **19**, 695–8.

Mariani, A. P. (1982) Biplexiform cells: ganglion cells of the primate retina that contact photoreceptors. *Science* **216**, 1134–6.

(1988) Amacrine cells of the rhesus monkey retina. *Invest. Ophthal. Visual Sci.* **29** (suppl.), 198.

Markoff, J. I. & Sturr, J. F. (1971) Spatial and luminance determinants of the increment threshold under monoptic and dichoptic viewing. *J. opt. Soc. Am.* **61**, 1530–7.

Markstahler, U. & Sharpe, L. T. (1989) Increment threshold sensitivity of the rod visual system: the effect of target size and duration (unpublished observations).

Marrocco, R. T. (1972) Responses of monkey optic fibers to monochromatic lights. *Vision Res.* **12**, 1167–74.

Matthews, H. R., Murphy, R. L. W., Fain, G. L. & Lamb, T. D. (1988) Photoreceptor light adaptation is mediated by cytoplasmic calcium concentration. *Nature* **334**, 67–9.

McCann, J. J. (1972) Rod–cone interactions: different color sensations from identical stimuli. *Science* **176**, 1255–7.

McCann, J. J. & Benton, J. L. (1969) Interaction of the long-wave cones and the rods to produce color sensation. *J. opt. Soc. Am.* **59**, 103–7.

McKee, S. P. & Westheimer, G. (1970) Specificity of cone mechanisms in lateral interactions. *J. Physiol.* **206**, 117–28.

van Meeteren, A. (1978) On the detective quantum efficiency of the human eye. *Vision Res.* **18**, 257–67.

van Meetteren, A. & Barlow, H. B. (1981) The statistical efficiency for detecting sinusoidal modulation of average dot density in random figures. *Vision Res.* **21**, 765–77.

van Meeteren, A. & Vos, J. J. (1972) Resolution and contrast sensitivity at low luminances. *Vision Res.* **12**, 825–33.

Meister, M., Pine, J. & Baylor, D. A. (1989) Multielectrode recording from the vertebrate retina. *Invest. Ophthal. Visual Sci.* **30** (suppl.), 68.

Metz, J. W. & Brown, J. L. (1970) *Integration of responses between different types of cones and between rods and cones*. Technical Report No. 11, Department of Psychology, Kansas State University.

Nakatani, K. & Yau, K.-W. (1988) Calcium and light adaptation in retinal rods and cones. *Nature* **334**, 69–71.

Nelson R. (1977) Cat cones have rod input: a comparison of the response properties of cones and horizontal cell bodies in the retina of the cat. *J. comp. Neurol.* **172**, 109–35.

(1982) AII amacrine cells quicken time course of rod signals in the cat retina. *J. Neurophysiol.* **47**, 928–47.

Nelson, R. & Kolb, H. (1984) Amacrine cells in scotopic vision. *Opthal. Res.* **16**, 21–6.

Niemeyer, F. & Gouras, P. (1973) Rod and cone signals in S-potentials of the isolated perfused cat eye. *Vision Res.* **13**, 1603–12.

Nordby, K. & Sharpe, L. T. (1988) The directional sensitivity of the photoreceptors in the human achromat. *J. Physiol.* **399**, 267–81.

Norman, R. A. & Perlman, I. (1979) Evaluating sensitivity changing mechanisms in light-adapted photoreceptors. *Vision Res.* **19**, 391–4.

van Norren, D. & Vos, J. J. (1974) Spectral transmission of the human ocular media. *Vision Res.* **14**, 1237–44.

Nygaard, R. W. & Frumkes, T. E. (1985) Frequency dependence in scotopic flicker sensitivity. *Vision Res.* **25**, 115–27.

Oehler, R. (1985) Spatial interactions in the rhesus monkey retina: a behavioural study using the Westheimer paradigm. *Exp. Brain Res.* **59**, 217–25.

Osterberg, G. (1935) Topography of the layer of rods and cones in the human retina. *Acta ophthal.* (Suppl.) **6**, 1–102.

Parinaud, H. (1881) Des modifications pathologiques de la perception de la lumiere, des couleurs, et des formes, et des differentes especes de sensibilite oculaire. *C. r. Séanc. Soc. Biol.* **33**, 222.

Patel, A. S. & Jones, R. W. (1968) Increment and decrement visual thresholds. *J. gen. Physiol.* **58**, 696–9.

Penn, R. & Hagins, W. A. (1972) Kinetics of the photocurrent of retinal rods. *Biophysical J.* **12**, 1073–94.

Pirenne, M. H. (1967). *Vision and the eye* (2nd edn.), Chapter 12. Chapman and Hall, London.

Pirenne, M. H. & Marriott, F. H. C. (1959) The quantum theory of light and the psycho-physiology of vision. In *Psychology: a study of a science*, Vol. 1 (ed. Koch, S.), pp. 288–361. McGraw-Hill, New York.

Polyak, S. L. (1941) *The retina.* University Press, Chicago.

Purpura, K., Kaplan, E. & Shapley, R. (1989) Contrast gain difference between primate P and M retinal ganglion cells enhanced at low light levels. *Proc. natn. Acad. Sci. U.S.A.* (In press.)

Purpura, K., Tranchina, D., Kaplan, E. & Shapley, R. M. (1988) Light adaptation of monkey retinal ganglion cells: modelling changes in gain and dynamics. *Invest. Ophthal. Visual Sci.* **29** (suppl.), 297.

Ramon y Cajal, S. (1893) La rétine des vertébrés. *La Cellule* **9**, 119–257. (Translated, by Maguire, D. & Rodieck, R. W. in Rodieck, R. W., *The vertebrate retina: principles of structure and function*, pp. 773–904.)

Ransom-Hogg, A. & Spillmann, L. (1980) Perceptive field size in fovea and periphery of the light- and dark-adapted retina. *Vision Res.* **20**, 221–8.

Raviola, E. & Gilula, N. B. (1973) Gap junctions between photoreceptor cells in the vertebrate retina. *Proc. natn. Acad. Sci. U.S.A.* **70**, 1677–81.

Reuter, T., Donner, K. & Copenhagen, D. R. (1986). Does the random distribution of discrete photoreceptor events limit the sensitivity of the retina? *Neurosci. Res. Suppl.* **4**, 163–80.

Ripps, H. & Weale, R. A. (1969) Flash bleaching of rhodopsin in the human retina. *J. Physiol.* **200**, 151–9.

Robson, J. G. & Troy, J. B. (1987) Nature of the maintained discharge of Q, X, and Y retinal ganglion cells of the cat. *J. opt. Soc. Am.* A **4**, 2301–7.

Rodieck, R. W. & Rushton, W. A. H. (1976) Cancellation of rod signals by cones, and cone signals by rods in the cat retina. *J. Physiol.* **254**, 775–85.

Rose, A. (1942) The relative sensitivities of television pickup tubes, photographic film and the human eye. *Proc. Inst. Radio Eng., New York*, **30**, 293–300.

(1948) The sensitivity performance of the human eye on an absolute scale. *J. opt. Soc. Am.* **38**, 196–208.

(1973) *Vision, human and electronic.* Plenum Press, New York.

Rushton, W. A. H. (1956) The rhodopsin density in the human rods. *J. Physiol.* **134**, 30–46.

(1963) Increment threshold and dark adaptation. *J. opt. Soc. Am.* **53**, 104–9.

(1965*a*) The sensitivity of rods under illumination. *J. Physiol.* **178**, 141–60.

(1965*b*) *Visual adaptation. The Ferrier Lecture, 1962. Proc. R. Soc. Lond.* B. **162**, 20–46.

(1972*a*) *Visual pigments in man.* In *Photochemistry of vision, handbook of sensory physiology*, VII/1 (ed. Dartnall, H. J. A.) pp. 364–94. Springer-Verlag, Berlin.

(1972*b*) Light and dark adaptation. *Invest. Opthal.* **11**, 503–17.

Rushton, W. A. H. & Westheimer, G. (1962) The effect upon the rod threshold of bleaching neighbouring rods. *J. Physiol.* **164**, 318–29.

Said, F. S. & Weale, R. A. (1959) The variation with age of the spectral transmissivity of the living human crystalline lens. *Gerontologica* **3**, 213–31.

Saito, H. & Fukada, Y. (1986) Gain control mechanisms in X- and Y-type retinal ganglion cells of the cat. *Vision Res.* **26**, 391–408.

Sakitt, B. (1971) Configuration dependence of scotopic spatial summation. *J. Physiol.* **216**, 513–29.

(1972) Counting every quantum. *J. Physiol.* **223**, 131–50.

(1976) Psychophysical correlates of photoreceptor activity. *Vision Res.* **16**, 129–40.

Sakmann, B. & Fileon, M. (1972). Light adaptation of the late receptor potential in the cat retina. In *Advances in experimental medicine and biology*, Vol. 24, *The visual system–neurophysiology, biophysics and their clinical applications* (ed. Arden, S. B.), pp. 87–93. Plenum Press, New York.

Schneck, M. E., Volbrecht, V. J. & Adams, A. J. (1989) Rod saturation on steady and flashed backgrounds in rod monochromats. *Invest. Ophthal. Visual Sci.* **30** (suppl.), 455.

Scholtes, A. M. W. & Bouman, M. A. (1977) Psychophysical experiments on spatial summation at threshold level of the human peripheral retina. *Vision Res.* **17**, 867–73.

Schultze, M. (1866) Zur Anatomie und Physiologie der Retina. *Arch. mikrosk. Anat. EntwMech.* **2**, 175–286.

Schwartz, E. A. (1975) Rod–rod interaction in the retina of the turtle. *J. Physiol.* **246**, 617–38.

Shapley, R. M. (1986) The importance of contrast for the activity of single neurons, the VEP and perception. *Vision Res.* **26**, 45–61.

Shapley, R. M. & Enroth-Cugell, C. (1984) Visual adaptation and retinal gain control. In *Progress in retinal research*, Vol. 3 (eds. Oborne, N. O. & Chader, G. J.), Chap. 9, pp. 263–346. Pergamon Press, London.

Sharpe, L. T., Fach, C. & Nordby, K. (1988) Temporal summation in the achromat. *Vision Res.* **28**, 1263–9.

Sharpe, L. T., Fach, C., Nordby, K. & Stockman, A. (1989*a*) The increment threshold of the rod visual system and Weber's law. *Science* **244**, 354–6.

Sharpe, L. T. Stockman, A. & MacLeod, D. I. A. (1989*b*) Rod flicker perception: Scotopic duality, phase lags and destructive interference. *Vision Res.* **29**, 1539–59.

Sharpe, L. T., Whittle, P. & Nordby, K. (1990). (In preparation.)

Shefner, J. M. & Levine, M. W. (1977) Interactions between rod and cone systems in the goldfish retina. *Science* **198**, 750–3.

Short, A. D. (1966) Decremental and incremental visual thresholds. *J. Physiol.* **185**, 646–54.

Smith, R. A. Jr. (1973) Luminance-dependent changes in mesopic visual contrast sensitivity. *J. Physiol.* **230**, 115–35.

Smith, R. G., Freed, M. A. & Sterling, P. (1986) Microcircuitry of the dark-adapted cat retina: functional architecture of the rod–cone network. *J. Neurosci.* **6**, 3505–17.

Spillmann, L. & Coderre, J. (1973) Increment thresholds for striped and uniform fields as a function of background level. *J. opt. Soc. Am.* **63**, 601–5.

Spillmann, L. & Conlon, J. E. (1972) Photochromatic interval during dark adaptation and as a function of background luminance. *J. opt. Soc. Am.* **62**, 182–5.

Spillmann, L. & Seneff, S. (1971) Photochromatic intervals as a function of retinal eccentricity for stimuli of different size. *J. opt. Soc. Am.* **61**, 267–70.

Stabell, B., Nordby, K. & Stabell, U. (1987) Light-adaptation of the human rod system. *Clin. Vision Sci.* **2**, 83–91.

Stabell, U. & Stabell, B. (1975*a*) Scotopic contrast hues triggered by rod activity. *Vision Res.* **15**, 1115–8.

Stabell, U. & Stabell, B. (1975*b*) The effect of rod activity on colour matching functions. *Vision Res.* **15**, 1119–24.

Steinberg, R. H. (1969*a*) Rod and cone contributions to S-potentials from the cat retina. *Vision Res.* **9**, 1319–29.

Steinberg, R. H. (1969*b*) Rod–cone interaction in S-potentials from the cat retina. *Vision Res.* **9**, 1331–44.

Steinberg, R. H. (1969*c*). The rod after-effect in S-potentials from the cat retina. *Vision Res.* **9**, 1345–55.
Steinberg, R. H. (1971) Incremental responses to light recorded from pigment epithelial cells and horizontal cells of the cat retina. *J. Physiol.* **217**, 93–110.
Sterling, P. (1983) Microcircuitry of the cat retina. *A. Rev. Neurosci.* **6**, 149–85.
Sterling, P., Freed, M. & Smith, R. G. (1986) Microcircuitry and functional architecture of the cat retina. *Trends Neurosci.* **9**, 186–92.
Sternheim, C. E. & Glass, R. A. (1975) Evidence for cone and rod contributions to common 'adaptation pools'. *Vision Res.* **15**, 277–81.
Stiles, W. S. (1939) The directional sensitivity of the retina and the spectral sensitivities of the rods and cones. *Proc. R. Soc. Lond.* B. **127**, 64–105.
Stiles, W. S. & Crawford, B. F. (1933) The luminous efficiency of rays entering the eye pupil at different points. *Proc. R. Soc. Lond.* B. **112**, 428–50.
Stockman, A., Sharpe, L. T., Fach, C. C. & Nordby, K. (1990) (Submitted to *Nature*.)
Sturr, J. F. & Teller, D. Y. (1973) Sensitization by annular surrounds: dichoptic properties. *Vision Res.* **13**, 909–18.
Tamura, T., Nakatani, K. & Yau, K.-W. (1989) Light adaptation in cat retinal rods. *Science* **245**, 755–8.
Tan, K. E. W. P. (1971) *Vision in the Ultraviolet.* Thesis, University of Utrecht, The Netherlands.
Teich, M. C., Prucnal, P. R., Vannucci, G., Breton, M. E. & McGill, W. J. (1978) Non-Poisson nature of the effective noise in the visual system near threshold. *J. opt. Soc. Am.* **68**, 1454.
Teich, M. C., Prucnal, P. R., Vannucci, G., Breton, M. E. & McGill, W. J. (1982) Multiplication noise in the human visual system at threshold: the role of non-Poisson quantum fluctuations. *Biol. Cybernet.* **44**, 157–65.
Teller, D. Y., Andrews, D. P. & Barlow, H. B. (1966) Local adaptation in stabilized vision. *Vision Res.* **6**, 701–5.
Teller, D. Y. & Gestrin, P. J. (1969) Sensitization by annular surrounds: sensitization and dark adaptation. *Vision Res.* **9**, 1481–90.
Teller, D. Y., Matter, C. F. & Phillips, W. D. (1970) Sensitization by annular surrounds: spatial summation properties. *Vision Res.* **10**, 549–61.
Teller, D. Y., Matter, C. F., Phillips, W. D. & Alexander, K. (1971) Sensitization by annular surrounds: sensitization and masking. *Vision Res.* **11**, 1445–58.
Tong, L. & Green, D. G. (1977) Adaptation pools and excitation receptive fields of rat retinal ganglion cells. *Vision Res.* **17**, 1233–6.
Trezona, P. W. (1970) Rod participation in the blue mechanism and its effect on colour matching. *Vision Res.* **10**, 317–32.
Tulunay-Keesey, U. & Jones, R. M. (1977) Spatial sensitization as a function of delay. *Vision Res.* **17**, 1191–9.
Tulunay-Keesey, U. & Vassilev, A. (1974) Foveal spatial sensitization with stabilized vision. *Vision Res.* **14**, 101–5.
Valeton, M. J. & Van Norren, D. (1983) Light adaptation of primate cones: an anaysis based on extracellular data. *Vision Res.* **23**, 1539–47.
Veringa, F. & Roelofs, J. (1966) Electro-optical stimulation in the human retina. *Nature* **211**, 321–2.

de Vries, H. (1943) The quantum character of light and its bearing upon threshold of vision, the differential sensitivity and visual acuity of the eye. *Physica* **10**, 553–64.

Wald, G. (1945) Human vision and the spectrum. *Science* **101**, 653–8.

Walraven, J. & Valeton, J. M. (1984) Visual adaptation and response saturation. In *Limits in perception* (eds. van Doorn, A. J., van de Grind, W. A. & Koenderink, J. J.), pp. 401–29. VNU Science Press, Utrecht.

Weale, R. A. (1958) Retinal summation and human visual threshold. *Nature* **181**, 154–6.

Weber, E. H. (1834) *De pulsu, resorptione auditu et tactu annotationes anatomicae et physiologicae.* C. F. Koehler, Leipzig.

Werblin, F. S. (1974) Control of retinal sensitivity. II. Lateral interaction at the outer plexiform layer. *J. gen. Physiol.* **63**, 62–87.

(1977) Synaptic interactions mediating bipolar response in the retina of the tiger salamander. In *Vertebrate photoreception* (eds. Barlow, H. B. & Fatt, P.), pp. 205–30. Academic Press, London.

Werblin, F. S. & Copenhagen, D. R. (1974) Control of retinal sensitivity. III. Lateral interations at the inner plexiform layer. *J. gen. Physiol.* **63**, 88–110.

Westheimer, G. (1965) Spatial interaction in the human retina during scotopic vision. *J. Physiol.* **181**, 881–94.

(1967) Dependence of the magnitude of the Stiles–Crawford effect on retinal location. *J. Physiol.* **192**, 309–15.

(1968) Bleached rhodopsin and retinal interaction. *J. Physiol.* **195**, 97–105.

(1970) Rod–cone independence for sensitizing interaction in the human retina. *J. Physiol.* **206**, 109–16.

Westheimer, G. & Wiley, R. W. (1970) Distance effects in human scotopic retinal interaction. *J. Physiol.* **206**, 129–34.

Whitten, D. N. & Brown, K. T. (1973) Photopic suppression of monkeys' rod receptor potential, apparently by a cone-initiated lateral inhibition. *Vision Res.* **13**, 1629–58.

Whittle, P. (1986) Increments and decrements: luminance discrimination. *Vision Res.* **26**, 1677–91.

Whittle, P. & Challands, P. D. C. (1969) The effect of background luminance on the brightness of flashes. *Vision Res.* **9**, 1095–110.

Wiesel, T. N. & Hubel, D. H. (1966) Spatial and chromatic interactions in the lateral geniculate body of the rhesus monkey. *J. Neurophysiol.* **29**, 1115–56.

Willmer, E. N. (1950) Low threshold rods and the perception of blue. *J. Physiol.* **111**, 17P.

Wooten, B. R. & Butler, T. W. (1976) Possible rod–cone interaction in dark adaptation. *J. opt. Soc. Am.* **66**, 1429–30.

Wooten, B. R., Fuld, K. & Spillmann, L. (1975) Photopic spectral sensitivity of the peripheral retina. *J. opt. Soc. Am.* **65**, 334–42.

Wu, S. M. & Yang, X.-L. (1989) Light enhances rod–cone coupling in the tiger salamander retina. *Invest. Ophthal. Visual Sci.* **30** (suppl.), 62.

Wyszecki, G. & Stiles, W. S. (1982) *Color science* (2nd edn.), Wiley, New York.

Yang, X.-L. & Wu, S. M. (1989) Modualtion of rod–cone coupling by light. *Science* **244**, 352–4.

Yonemura, D. & Kawasaki, K. (1979) New approaches to ophthalmic electro-diagnosis by retinal oscillatory potential, drug-induced responses from retinal pigment epithelium and cone potential. *Doc Ophthal.* **48**, 163–222.

Zrenner, E., Nelson, R. & Mariani, A. (1983) Intracellular recordings from a biplexiform ganglion cell in macaque retina, stained with horseradish peroxidase. *Brain Res.* **262**, 181–5.

Zwas, F. & Alpern, M. (1976) The density of human rhodopsin in the rods. *Vision Res.* **16**, 121–7.

Chapter 3

Aguilar, M. and Stiles, W. S. (1945) Saturation of the rod mechanism of the retina at high levels of stimulation. *Optica Acta* **1**, 59–65.

Aho, A.-C., Donner, K., Hyden, C., Larsen, L. O. & Reuter, T. (1988) Low retinal noise in animals with low body temperature allows high visual sensitivity. *Nature* **334**, 348–50.

Alpern M. Rushton, W. A. & Torri, S. (1970) The attenuation of rod signals by backgrounds. *J. Physiol.* **206**, 209–27.

Ashmore, J. F. & Falk, G. (1980) Responses of rod bipolar cells in the dark-adapted retina of dogfish. *J. Physiol.* **300**, 115–50.

Barlow, H. B. (1958) Temporal and spatial summation in human vision of different background intensities. *J. Physiol.* **141**, 337–50.

Barlow, H. B. & Andrews, D. P. (1973) The site at which rhodopsin bleaching raises scotopic threshold. *Vision Res.* **13**, 903–8.

Barlow, H. B., FitzHugh, R. & Kuffler, S. W. (1957) Change of organization in the receptive fields of the cat's retina during dark-adaptation. *J. Physiol.* **137**, 338–54.

Barlow, H. B. & Levick, W. R. (1976) Threshold setting by the surround of cat retinal ganglion cells. *J. Physiol.* **259**, 737–57.

Baylor, D. A., Fuortes, M. G. F. & O'Bryan, P. M. (1971) Receptive fields of cones in the retina of the turtle. *J. Physiol.* **214**, 165–94.

Baylor, D. A. & Hodgkin, A. L. (1973) Detection and resolution of visual stimuli by turtle photoreceptors. *J. Physiol.* **234**, 163–98.

Baylor, D. A. & Hodgkin, A. L. (1974) Changes in time scale and sensitivity in turtle photoreceptors. *J. Physiol.* **242** 729–58.

Baylor, D. A., Nunn, B. J. & Schnapf, J. L. (1984) The photocurrent, noise and spectral sensitivity of rods of the monkey *Macaca Fascicularis. J. Physiol.* **357**, 575–607.

Bilotta, J. & Abramov, I. (1987) Spatio-spectral interactions in goldfish ganglion cells. *Invest. Opthal. Visual Sci.* **28** (Suppl.), 404.

Bisti, S., Clement, R., Maffei, L. & Mecacci, L. (1977) Spatial frequency and orientation tuning curves of visual neurons in the cat: effects of mean luminance. *Exp. Brain Res.* **27**, 335–45.

Campbell, F. W., Cooper, G. F. & Enroth-Cugell, C. (1969) The spatial selectivity of the visual cells of the cat. *J. Physiol.* **203**, 223–45.

Campbell, F. W. & Rushton, W. A. H. (1955) Measurement of scotopic pigments in the living human eye. *J. Physiol.* **130**, 131–47.

Cleland, B. G. & Enroth-Cugell, C. (1968) Quantitative aspects of sensitivity and summation in the cat retina. *J. Physiol.* **198**, 17–38.

Cooper, G. F. & Robson, J. G. (1968) Successive transformations of spatial information in the visual system. *IEEE Nat. Phys. Lab. Conf. Proc.* **42**, 134–43.

Copenhagen, D. R. & Green, D. G. (1985) The absence of spread of adaptation between rod photoreceptors in turtle retina. *J. Physiol.* **369**, 161–82.

Copenhagen, D. R. & Owen, W. G. (1976) Functional characteristics of laternal interactions between rods in the retina of the snapping turtle. *J. Physiol.* **259**, 251–82.

Copenhagen, D. R. & Owen, W. G. (1980) Current–voltage relations in the rod photoreceptor network of the turtle retina. *J. Physiol.* **308**, 159–84.

Diatch, D. Y. & Green, D. G. (1969) Contrast sensitivity of the human peripheral retina. *Vision Res.* **9**, 947–52.

Derrington, A. M. & Lennie, P. (1982) The influence of temporal frequency and adaptation level on receptive field organization of retinal ganglion cells in cat. *J. Physiol.* **333**, 343–66.

Detwiler, P. B. & Hodgkin, A. L. (1979) Electrical coupling between cones in turtle retina. *J. Physiol.* **291**, 75–100.

DeValois, R. L., Albrecht, D. G. & Thorell, L. G. (1982) Spatial frequency selectivity of cells in macaque visual cortex. *Vision Res.* **22**, 545–59.

DeValois, R. L. & Morgan, H. (1974) Psychophysical studies of monkey vision III. Spatial luminance contrast sensitivity tests of macaque and human observers. *Vision Res.* **14**, 75–81.

Dowling, J. E. (1987) *The retina: an approachable part of the brain.* Harvard University Press, Cambridge, Massachusetts.

Dowling, J. E. & Ripps, H. (1970) Visual adaptation in the retina of the skate. *J. Gen. Physiol.* **56**, 491–520.

Dowling, J. E. & Ripps, H. (1971) S-potentials in the skate retina: Intracellular recordings during light and dark adaptation. *J. Gen. Physiol.* **58**, 163–89.

Dowling, J. E. & Ripps. H. (1972) Adaptation in skate photoreceptors. *J. Gen. Physiol.* **60**, 698–719.

Easter, S. S. (1968) Adaptation in goldfish retina. *J. Physiol.* **195**, 273–81.

Enroth-Cugell, C. & Lennie, P. (1975) The control of retinal ganglion cell discharge by receptive field surrounds. *J. Physiol.* **247**, 551–768.

Enroth-Cugell, C. & Robson, J. G. (1966) The contrast sensitivity of retinal ganglion cells of the cat. *J. Physiol.* **187**, 517–52.

Enroth-Cugell, C. & Shapley, R. M. (1973) Flux, not retinal illumination, is what cat retinal ganglion cells really care about. *J. Physiol.* **233**, 311–26.

Fain, G. (1975) Quantum sensitivity of rods in the toad retina. *Science* **187**, 838–41.

Falzett, M., Nussdorf, J. D. & Powers, M. K. (1988) Responsivity and absolute sensitivity of retinal ganglion cells in goldfish of different sizes, when measured under 'psychophysical' conditions. *Vision Res.* **28**. 223–37

Fesenko, E. E., Kolenikov, S. S. & Lyubarsky, A. L. (1985) Induction by cyclic

GMP of cationic conductance in plasma membrane of retinal rod outer segment. *Nature* **313**, 310–13.

Fung, B. K.-K., Hurley, J. B. & Stryer, L. (1981) Flow of information in the light-triggered cyclic nucleotide cascade of vision. *Proc. Natl. Acad. Sci. USA* **77**, 2500–4.

Fuortes, M. G. F. & Hodgkin, A. L. (1964) Changes in time scale and sensitivity in the ommatidia of *Limulus*. *J. Physiol.* **172**, 239–63.

Grabowski, S. R., Pinto, L. H. & Pak, W. L. (1972) Adaptation in retinal rods of axolotl: intracellular recordings. *Science* **176**, 1240–2.

Graham, N. (1972) Spatial frequency channels in the human visual system: Effects of luminance and pattern shift rate. *Vision Res.* **12**, 53–68.

Green, D. G. (1986) The search for the site of visual adaptation. *Vision Res.* **26**, 1417–29.

Green, D. G., Dowling, J. E., Siegel, I. M. & Ripps, H. (1975) Retinal mechanisms of visual adaptation in the skate. *J. Gen. Physiol.* **65**, 483–502.

Green, D. G., Tong, L. & Cicerone, C. M. (1977) Lateral spread of light adaptation in the rat retina. *Vision Res.* **17**, 479–86.

Green, D. G. & Powers, M. K. (1982) Mechanisms of light adaptation in rat retina. *Vision Res.* **22**, 209–16.

Hecht, S. (1924) The visual discrimination of intensity and the Weber–Fechner Law. *J. Gen. Physiol.* **7**, 235–67.

Hecht, S., Shlaer, S. & Pirenne, M. H. (1942) Energy, quanta, and vision. *J. Gen. Physiol.* **25**, 819–40.

Hess, R. F. & Howell, E. R. (1988) Detection of low spatial frequencies; a single filter or multiple filters. *Ophthal. Physiol. Otd.* **8**, 378–85.

Hess, R. F. & Lillywhite, P. G. (1980) Effect of luminance on contrast coding in cat visual cortex. *J. Physiol.* **300**, 56.

Hood, D. C. & Finkelstein, M. A. (1986) Sensitivity to light, in *Handbook of Perception and Human Performance*, Vol. 1 (K. R. Boff, L. Kaufman and J. P. Thomas, eds.), John Wiley and Sons, new York, pp. 5–1 to 5–66.

Hood, D. C. & Grover, B. G. (1974) Temporal summation of light by a vertebrate visual receptor. *Science* **184**, 1003–5.

Hubel, D. H. & Wiesel, T. N. (1961) Integrative action in the cat's lateral geniculate body. *J. Physiol.* **155**, 385–98.

Jakeila, H. G., Enroth-Cugell, C. & Shapley, R. (1976) Adaptation and dynamics in X-cells and Y-cells of the cat retina. *Exp. Brain Res.* **24**, 335–42.

Kaplan E., Marcus, S. & So, Y. T. (1979) Effects of dark adaptation on spatial and temporal properties of receptive fields in cat lateral geniculate nucleus. *J. Physiol.* **294**, 561–80.

Kaplan, E. H. & Shapley, R. M. (1986) The primate retina contains 2 types of ganglion cells, with high and low contrast sensitivity. *Proc. Natl. Acad. Sci. USA* **83**, 2755–7.

Kleinschmidt, J. & Dowling, J. E. (1975) Intracellular recordings from Gecko photoreceptors during light and dark adaptation. *J. Gen. Physiol.* **66**, 617–48.

Koch, K.-W. & Stryer, L. (1988) Highly cooperative feedback control of retinal rod guanate cyclase by calcium ions. *Nature* **334**, 64–6.

Koenderink, J. J., Bouman, M. A., Bueno de Mesquita, A. E. & Slappendel, S. (1978) Perimetry of contrast detection thresholds of moving sine wave patterns. IV. The influence of the mean retinal luminance. *J. Opt. Soc. Am.* **68**, 860–5.

Kuffler, S. W. (1953) Discharge patterns and functional organization of mammalia retina. *J. Neurophysiol.* **16**, 37–68.

Linsenmeier, R. A. & Jakeila, H. G. (1979) Non-linear spatial summation in cat retinal ganglion cells at different background levels. *Exp. Brain Res.* **36**, 301–9.

Lipetz, L. E. (1961) A mechanism of light adaptation. *Science* **133**, 639–40.

MacLeod, D. I. A. (1978) Visual sensitivity. *A. Rev. Psychol.* **29**, 613–45.

Maffei, L. & Fiorentini, A. (1972) Retinogeniculate convergence and analysis of contrast. *J. Neurophysiol.* **35**, 65–72.

Matthews, G. (1983) Physiological characteristics of single green rod photoreceptors from toad retina. *J. Physical.* **342**, 347–59.

Matthews, H. R., Murphy, R. L. W., Fain, G. L. & Lamb, T. D. (1988). Photoreceptor light adaptation is mediated by cytoplasmic calcium concentration. *Nature* **334**, 67–9.

Movshon, J. A. & Lennie, P. (1979) Pattern selective adaptation in visual cortical neurons. *Nature* **278**, 850–1.

Movshon, J. A., Thompson, I. D. & Tolhurst, D. J. (1978) Spatial and temporal contrast sensitivity of neurons in areas 17 and 18 of the cat's visual cortex. *J. Physiol.* **283**, 79–99.

Naka, K. I. & Rushton, W. A. H. (1968) S-potential and dark adaptation in fish. *J. Physiol.* **194**, 259–69.

Nakatani, K. & Yau, K.-W. (1988) Calcium and light adaptation in retinal rods and cones. *Nature* **334**, 69–71.

Normann, R. A., Perlman, I., Kolb, H., Jones, J. & Daly, S. J. (1984) Direct excitatory interactions between cones of different spectral types in turtle retina. *Science* **224**, 625–7.

Normann, R. A. & Werblin, F. S. (1974) Control of retinal sensitivity. 1. Light and dark adaptation of vertebrate rods and cones. *J. Gen. Physiol.* **63**, 37–61.

Ohzawa, I., Sclar, G. & Freeman, R. D. (1982) Contrast gain control in the cat visual cortex. *Nature* **298**, 266–7.

Ohzawa, I., Sclar, G. & Freeman, R. D. (1985) Contrast gain control in the cat visual system. *J. Neurophysiol.* **54**, 651–67.

Pasternak, T. & Merigan, W. H. (1981) The luminance dependence of spatial vision in the cat. *Vision Res.* **21**, 1333–9.

Powers, M. K. & Easter, S. S. (1978) Behavioral confirmation of the 'silent period' during adaptation to bright lights. *Vision Res.* **18**, 1075–7.

Pugh, E. N. & Altman, J. (1988) A role for calcium in adaptation. *Nature* **334**, 16–17.

Purpura, K., Kaplan, E. & Shapley, R. M. (1986) The effect of mean luminance on the contrast gain of P and M cells in the macaque retina. *Soc. Neurosci. Abstr.* **12**, 7.

Purpura, K., Kaplan, E. & Shapley, R. M. (1987) Macaque M and P retinal

ganglion cells differ in gain control as well as gain. *Invest. Ophthal. Visual Sci.* **28** (Suppl.), 240.
Raynauld, J.-P., LaViolette, J. R. & Wagner, H.-J. (1979) Goldfish retina: A correlate between cone activity and morphology of horizontal cell in cone pedicles. *Science* **204**, 1436–8.
Rushton, W. A. H. (1961) Rhodopsin measurement and dark-adaptation in a subject deficient in cone vision. *J. Physiol.* **156**, 193–205.
Rushton, W. A. H. (1965*a*) Visual adaptation (The Ferrier Lecture). *Proc. R. Soc. Lond.* B **162**, 20–46.
Rushton, W. A. H. (1965*b*) The sensitivity of rods under illumination. *J. Physiol.* **178**, 141–60.
Rushton, W. A. H. & Westheimer, G. (1962) The effect upon rod threshold of bleaching neighboring rods. *J. Physiol.* **164**, 318–29.
Sackman, B. & Creutzfeldt, O. D. (1969) Scotopic and mesopic light adaptation in the cat's retina. *Pfluger Arch.* **313**, 168–85.
Schwartz, E. A. (1975) Rod–rod interaction in the retina of the turtle. *J. Physiol.* **246**, 617–38.
Shapley, R. W. & Enroth-Cugell, C. (1984) Visual adaptation and retinal gain control. In N. O. Osborne and G. J. Chader (eds.), *Progress in retinal research* Vol. 3, pp. 263–346. Elmsford, New York: Pergamon.
Shapley, R. M. & Lennie, P. (1985) Spatial frequency analysis in the visual system. *A. Rev. Neurosci.* **8**, 547–83.
Tolhurst, D. J. & Movshon, J. A. (1975) Spatial and temporal contrast sensitivity of striate cortical neurons. *Nature* **257**, 674–5.
van Meeteren, A. & Vos, J. J. (1972) Resolution and contrast sensitivity at low luminances. *Vision Res.* **12**, 825–33.
Virsu, V., Lee, B. B. & Creutzfeldt, O. D. (1977) Dark adaptation and receptive field organisation of cells in the cat lateral geniculate nucleus. *Exp. Brain Res.* **27**, 35–50.
Witkovsky, P., Nelson, J. and Ripps, H. (1973). Action spectra and adaptation properties of carp photoreceptors. *J. Physiol.* **71**, 401–23.
Yau, K.-W. & Nakatani, K. (1985) Light-induced reduction of cytoplasmic free calcium in retinal rod outer segment. *Nature* **313**, 579–82.

Chapter 4

Auerbach, E. & Peachey, N. S. (1984) Interocular transfer and dark adaptation to long-wave test lights. *Vision Res.* **24**, 1043–8.
Barlow, H. B. (1956) Retinal noise and absolute threshold. *J. opt. Soc. Am.* **46**, 634–9.
(1957) Increment thresholds at low intensities considered as signal/noise discriminations. *J. Physiol.* **136**, 469–88.
(1977) Retinal and central factors in human vision limited by noise. In *Vertebrate photoreception* (eds. Barlow, H. B. & Fatt, P.), pp. 337–58. Academic Press, New York.
Barlow, H. B., Levick, W. R. & Yoon, M. (1971) Responses to single quanta of light in retinal ganglion cells of the cat. *Vision Res.* Suppl. **3**, 87–101.

Baylor, D. A., Nunn, B. J. & Schnapf, J. L. (1984) The photocurrent, noise and spectral sensitivity of rods of the monkey Macaca fascicularis. *J. Physiol.* **357**, 575–607.

Blake, R. & Fox, R. (1973) The psychophysical inquiry into binocular summation. *Perception Psychophysics* **14**, 161–85.

Bolanowski, Jr., S. J. & Doty, R. W. (1987) Perceptual 'blankout' of monocular homogeneous fields (Ganzfelder) is prevented with binocular viewing. *Vision Res.* **27**, 967–82.

de Weert, C. M. M. (1984) Limits in vision with two eyes. In *Limits in perception* (eds. van Doorn, A. J., van de Grind, W. A. & Koenderink, J. J.), pp. 235–82. VNU Science Press BV, Utrecht.

Ginsburg, K. S., Johnsen, J. A. & Levine, M. W. (1984) Common noise in the firing of neighbouring ganglion cells in goldfish retina. *J. Physiol.* **351**, 433–50.

Hecht, S., Shlaer, S. & Pirenne, M. H. (1942) Energy, quanta, and vision. *J. Gen. Physiol.* **25**, 819–40.

Lillywhite, P. G. (1981) Multiplicative intrinsic noise and the limits to visual performance. *Vision Res.* **21**, 291–6.

Lillywhite, P. G. & Laughlin, S. B. (1979) Transducer noise in a photoreceptor. *Nature* **277**, 569–72.

Makous, W. & Sanders, R. K. (1978) Fluctuations of relative sensitivity of opposite eyes during fusion. *J. opt. Soc. Am.* **68**, 1365.

Makous, W., Teller, D. & Boothe, R. (1976) Binocular interaction in the dark. *Vision Res.* **16**, 473–6.

Massof, R. W. (1987) Relation of the normal-deviate vision receiver operating characteristic curve slope to d′. *J. opt. Soc. Am.* A **4**, 548–50.

Mastronarde, D. N. (1983*a*) Correlated firing of cat retinal ganglion cells. I. Spontaneously active input to X- and Y-cells. *J. Neurophysiol.* **49**, 303–24.

(1983*b*) Correlated firing of cat retinal ganglion cells. II. Responses of X- and Y-cells to single quantal events. *J. Neurophysiol.* **49**, 325–49.

(1983*c*) Interactions between ganglion cells in cat retina. *J. Neurophysiol.* **49**, 350–65.

Pelli, D. G. (1985) Uncertainty explains many aspects of visual contrast detection and discrimination. *J. opt. Soc. Am.* A **2**, 1508–32.

Pirenne, M. H. (1943) Binocular and uniocular threshold of vision. *Nature* **152**, 698–9.

Prucnal, P. R. & Teich, M. C. (1982) Multiplication noise in the human visual system at threshold: 2. Probit estimation of parameters. *Biological Cybernetics* **43**, 87–96.

Pulos, E. & Makous, W. (1982) Changes of visual sensitivity caused by on- and off-transients. *Vision Res.* **22**, 879–87.

Reeves, A., Peachey, N. S. & Auerbach, E. (1986) Interocular sensitization to a rod-detected test. *Vision Res.* **26**, 1119–27.

Rozhkova, G. I., Nikolayev, P. P. & Shchadrin, V. E. (1982) Perception of stabilized retinal stimuli in dichoptic viewing conditions. *Vision Res.* **22**, 293–302.

Sakitt, B. (1971) Configuration dependence of scotopic spatial summation. *J. Physiol.* **216**, 513–29.

(1972) Counting every quantum. *J. Physiol.* **223**, 131–50.
(1974) Canonical Ratings. *Perception Psychophysics* **16**, 478–88.
Shannon, C. E. & Weaver, W. (1949) *The mathematical theory of communication.* University of Illinois Press, Urbana.
Teich, M. C., Prucnal, P. R., Vannucci, G., Breton, M. E. & McGill, W. J. (1982) Multiplication noise in the human visual system at threshold: 1. Quantum fluctuations and minimum detectable energy. *J. opt. Soc. Am.* **72**, 419–31.
van Meeteren, A. (1978) On the detective quantum efficiency of the human eye. *Vision Res.* **18**, 257–67.
Wales, R. & Fox, R. (1970) Increment detection thresholds during binocular rivalry suppression. *Perception Psychophysics* **8**, 90–4.
Zacks, J. L. (1970) Temporal summation phenomena at absolute threshold: Their relation to visual mechanisms. *Science* **170**, 197–9.
Zuidema, P., Roest, W., Bouman, M. A. & Koenderink, J. J. (1984) Detection of light and flicker at low luminance levels in the human peripheral visual system. I. Psychophysical experiments. *J. opt. Soc. Am.* A **1**, 764–74.

Chapter 5

Aguilar, M. & Stiles, W. S. (1954) Saturation of the rod mechanism of the retina at high levels of stimulation. *Optica Acta* **1**, 59–65.
Alpern, M. (1971) Rhodopsin kinetics in the human eye. *J. Physiol.* **217**, 447–71.
Alpern, M. & Campbell, F. W. (1963) The behaviour of the pupil during dark adaptation. *J. Physiol.* **165**, 5*P*–7*P*.
Alpern, M., Rushton, W. A. H. & Torii, S. (1970) The attenuation of rod signals by bleachings. *J. Physiol.* **207**, 449–61.
Andrews, D. P. & Butcher, A. K. (1971) Rod threshold and patterned rhodopsin bleaching; the pigment epithelium as an adaptation pool. *Vision Res.* **11**, 761–5.
Barlow, H. B. (1956) Retinal noise and absolute threshold. *J. opt. Soc. Am.* **46**, 634–9.
(1957) Increment thresholds at low intensities considered as signal/noise discriminations. *J. Physiol.* **136**, 469–88.
(1964) Dark-adaptation: a new hypothesis. *Vision Res.* **4**, 47–58.
(1972) Dark and light adaptation: Psychophysics. In *Handbook of sensory physiology VII/4* (eds. Jameson, D. & Hurvich, L. M.), pp. 1–28. Springer, Berlin.
Barlow, H. B. & Andrews, D. P. (1973) The site at which rhodopsin bleaching raises the scotopic threshold. *Vision Res.* **13**, 903–8.
Barlow, H. B. & Sakitt, B. (1973) Doubts about scotopic interactions in stabilized vision. *Vision Res.* **13**, 523–4.
Barlow, H. B. & Sparrock, J. M. B. (1964) The role of after images in dark adaptation. *Science* **144**, 1309–14.
Baumann, C. & Bender, S. (1973) Kinetics of rhodopsin bleaching in the isolated human retina. *J. Physiol.* **235**, 761–73.
Bastian, B. L. & Fain, G. L. (1979) Light adaptation in toad rods: requirement for an internal messenger which is not calcium. *J. Physiol.* **297**, 493–520.

Baylor, D. A. (1987) Photoreceptor signals and vision. *Invest. Ophthal. Visual Sci.* **28**, 34–49.

Baylor, D. A. & Hodgkin, A. L. (1974) Changes in time scale and sensitivity in turtle photoreceptors. *J. Physiol.* **242**, 729–58.

Baylor, D. A., Lamb, T. D. & Yau, K.-W. (1979*a*) The membrane current of single rod outer segments. *J. Physiol.* **288**, 589–611.

Baylor, D. A., Lamb, T. D. & Yau, K.-W. (1979*b*) Responses of retinal rods to single photons. *J. Physiol.* **288**, 613–34.

Baylor, D. A., Matthews, G. & Yau, K.-W. (1980) Two components of electrical dark noise in toad retinal rod outer segments. *J. Physiol.* **309**, 561–91.

Baylor, D. A., Nunn, B. J. & Schnapf, J. L. (1984) The photocurrent, noise and spectral sensitivity of rods of the monkey, *Macaca fascicularis. J. Physiol.* **357**, 575–607.

Blakemore, C. B. & Rushton, W. A. H. (1965*a*) Dark adaptation and increment threshold in a rod monochromat. *J. Physiol.* **181**, 612–28.

Blakemore, C. B. & Rushton, W. A. H. (1965*b*) The rod increment threshold during dark adaptation in normal and rod monochromat. *J. Physiol.* **181**, 629–40.

Bonds, A. B. & MacLeod, D. I. A. (1974) The bleaching and regeneration of rhodopsin in the cat. *J. Physiol.* **242**, 237–53.

Bownds, M. D., Dawes, J., Miller, J. & Stahlman, M. (1972) Phosphorylation of frog photoreceptor membranes induced by light. *Nature* **237**, 125–7.

Campbell, F. W. & Rushton, W. A. H. (1955) Measurement of the scotopic pigment in the living human eye. *J. Physiol.* **130**, 131–47.

Cocozza, J. D. & Ostroy, S. E. (1987) Factors affecting the regeneration of rhodopsin in the isolated amphibian retina. *Vision Res.* **27**, 1085–91.

Cornwall, M. C., Fein, A. & MacNichol, E. F. (1990) Cellular mechanisms which underlie bleaching and background adaptation. *J. Gen. Physiol.* (In press.)

Crawford, B. H. (1937) The change of visual sensitivity with time. *Proc. R. Soc. Lond.* B**123**, 68–89.

(1946) Photochemical laws and visual phenomena. *Proc. R. Soc. Lond.* B**133**, 63–75.

(1947) Visual adaptation in relation to brief conditioning stimuli. *Proc. R. Soc. Lond.* B**134**, 283–302.

Donner, K. O. & Hemilä, S. (1975) Kinetics of long-lived rhodopsin photoproducts in the frog retina as a function of the amount bleached. *Vision Res.* **15**, 985–95.

Donner, K. O. & Hemilä, S. (1978) Excitation and adaptation in the vertebrate rod photoreceptor. *Med. Biol.* **56**, 52–63.

Dowling, J. E. (1960) Chemistry of visual adaptation in the rat. *Nature* **188**, 114–8.

Ernst, W. (1968) The dependence of critical flicker frequency and the rod threshold on the state of adaptation of the eye. *Vision Res.* **8**, 889–900.

Fain, G. L. (1975) Quantum sensitivity of rods in the toad retina. *Science* **187**, 838–41.

Fain, G. L. (1976) Sensitivity of toad rods: dependence on wavelength and background. *J. Physiol.* **261**, 71–101.

Fain, G. L., Lamb, T. D., Matthews, H. R. & Murphy, R. L. W. (1989) Cytoplasmic calcium as the messenger for light adaptation in salamander rods. *J. Physiol.* **416**, 215–43.

Geisler, W. S. (1980) Comments on the testing of two prominent dark-adaptation hypotheses. *Vision Res.* **20**, 807–11.

Gold, G. H. (1981) Photoreceptor coupling: its mechanism and consequences. In *Current topics in membrances and transport* **15** (ed. Miller, W. H.), pp. 59–89. Academic, New York.

Grabowski, S. R., Pinto, L. H. & Pak, W. L. (1972) Adaptation in retinal rods of axolotl: intracellular recordings. *Science* **176**, 1240–3.

Green, D. G., Dowling, J. E., Siegel, I. M. & Ripps, H. (1975) Retinal mechanisms of visual adaptation in the skate. *J. gen. Physiol.* **65**, 483–502.

Hagins, W. A., Penn, R. D. & Yoshikami, S. (1970) Dark current and photocurrent in retinal rods. *Biophys. J.* **10**, 380–412.

Hecht, S., Haig, C. & Chase, A. M. (1937) The influence of light adaptation on the subsequent dark adaptation of the eye. *J. gen. Physiol.* **20**, 831–50.

Hecht, S., Shlaer, S. & Pirenne, M. H. (1942) Energy, quanta, and vision. *J. gen. Physiol.* **25**, 819–40.

Hodgkin, A. L. & Nunn, B. J. (1988) Control of light-sensitive current in salamander rods. *J. Physiol.* **403**, 439–71.

Jones, G. J., Crouch, R. K., Wiggert, B., Cornwall, M. C. & Chader, G. J. (1989) Retinoid requirements for recovery of sensitivity after visual-pigment bleaching in isolated photoreceptors. *Proc. Nat. Acad. Sci. U.S.A.* **86**, 9606–10.

Koch, K.-W. & Stryer, L. (1988) Highly cooperative feedback control of retinal rod quanylate cyclase by calcium ions. *Nature* **334**, 64–6.

Kühn, H. & Dryer, W. J. (1972) Light-dependent phosphorylation of rhodopsin by ATP. *FEBS Lett.* **20**, 1–6.

Kühn, H., Hall, S. W. & Wilden, U. (1984) Light-induced binding of 48 kDa protein to photoreceptor membranes is highly enhanced by phosphorylation of rhodopsin. *FEBS Lett.* **176**, 473–8.

Lamb, T. D. (1980) Spontaneous quantal events induced in toad rods by pigment bleaching. *Nature* **287**, 349–51.

(1981) The involvement of rod photoreceptors in dark adaptation. *Vision Res.* **21**, 1773–82.

(1984*a*) Electrical response of photoreceptors. In *Recent advances in phsyiology* **10** (ed. Baker, P. F.), pp. 29–65. Churchill Livingstone, Edinburgh.

(1984*b*) Effect of temperature changes on toad rod photocurrents. *J. Physiol.* **346**, 557–78.

(1986*a*) Photoreceptor adaptation – vertebrates. In *The molecular mechanism of photoreception* (ed. Stieve, H.), pp. 267–86. Dahlem Konferenzen. Springer, Berlin.

(1986*b*) Transduction in vertebrate photoreceptors: the roles of cyclic GMP and calcium. *Trends Neurosci.* **9**, 224–8.

Lamb, T. D., McNaughton, P. A. & Yau, K.-W. (1981) Spatial spread of activation and background desensitization in rod outer segments. *J. Physiol.* **319**, 463–96.

Langer, H. (1973) (ed.) *Biochemistry and physiology of visual pigments*. Springer, Berlin.

Liebman, P. A. & Pugh, E. N. Jr (1980) ATP mediates rapid reversal of cGMP phosphodiesterase activation in visual receptor membranes. *Nature* **287**, 734–6.

Lisman, J. (1985) The role of metarhodopsin in the generation of spontaneous quantum bumps in ultraviolet receptors of *Limulus* median eye. *J. gen. Physiol.* **85**, 171–87.

MacLeod, D. I. A. (1978) Visual sensitivity. *A. Rev. Psychol.* **29**, 613–45.

MacLeod, D. I. A., Chen, B. & Crognale, M. (1989) Spatial organization of sensitivity regulation in rod vision. *Vision Res.* **29**, 965–78.

Matthews, H. R., Fain, G. L., Murphy, R. L. W. & Lamb, T. D. (1990) Light adaptation in cone photoreceptors of the salamander: a rule for cytoplasmic calcium. *J. Physiol.* **420**, 447–69.

Matthews, H. R., Murphy, R. L. W., Fain, G. L. & Lamb, T. D. (1988) Photoreceptor light adaptation is mediated by cytoplasmic calcium concentration. *Nature* **334**, 67–9.

Nakatani, K. & Yau, K.-W. (1988) Calcium and light adaptation in retinal rods and cones. *Nature* **334**, 69–71.

Nordby, K., Stabell, B. & Stabell, U. (1984). Dark-adaptation of the human rod system. *Vision Res.* **24**, 841–9.

Normann, R. A. & Perlman, I. (1979) The effect of background illumination on the photoresponses of red and green cones. *J. Physiol.* **286**, 509–24.

Pepperberg, D. R., Brown, P. K., Lurie, M. & Dowling, J. E. (1978) Visual pigment and photoreceptor sensitivity in the isolated skate retina. *J. gen. Physiol.* **71**, 369–96.

Perlman, J. I., Nodes, B. R. & Pepperberg, D. R. (1982) Utilization of retinoids in the bullfrog retina. *J. gen. Physiol.* **80**, 885–913.

Pugh, E. N. Jr (1975*a*) Rhodopsin flash photolysis in man. *J. Physiol.* **248**, 393–412.

(1975*b*) Rushton's paradox: rod dark adaptation after flash photolysis. *J. Physiol.* **248**, 413–31.

(1988) Vision: physics and retinal physiology. In *Stevens handbook of experimental psychology* (ed. Stevens, S. F.) (2nd edn), pp. 75–163. Wiley.

Pugh, E. & Altman, J. (1988) A role for calcium in adaptation. *Nature*. **334**, 16–17.

Pugh, E. N. Jr & Cobbs, W. H. (1986) Visual transduction in vertebrate rods and cones: a tale of two transmitters, calcium and cyclic GMP. *Vision Res.* **26**, 1613–43.

Ripps, H., Mehaffey, L. & Siegel, I. M. (1981) Rhodopsin kinetics in the cat retina. *J. gen. Physiol.* **77**, 317–34.

Rushton, W. A. H. (1961*a*) Dark-adaptation and the regeneration of rhodopsin. *J. Physiol.* **156**, 166–78.

(1961*b*) Rhodopsin measurement and dark-adaptation in a subject deficient in cone vision. *J. Physiol.* **156**, 193–205.

(1965*a*) Bleached rhodopsin and visual adaptation. *J. Physiol.* **181**, 645–55.

(1965*b*). The Ferrier Lecture, 1962. Visual adaptation. *Proc. R. Soc. Lond.* B**162**, 20–46.

Rushton, W. A. H. & Powell, D. S. (1972) The early phase of dark adaptation. *Vision Res.* **12**, 1083–93.

Rushton, W. A. H. & Westheimer, G. (1962) The effect upon the rod threshold of bleaching neighbouring rods. *J. Physiol.* **164**, 318–29.

Schnapf, J. L., Kraft, T. W., Nunn, B. J. & Baylor, D. A. (1987) Spectral sensitivity and dark adaptation in primate photoreceptors. *Invest. Ophthal. Visual Sci.* **28** (suppl.), 50.

Shapley, R. & Enroth-Cugell, C. (1984) Visual adaptation and retinal gain controls. In *Progress in retinal research* **3** (eds. Osborne, N. N. & Chader, G. J.), pp. 263–346. Pergamon, Oxford.

Sharpe, L. T., Fach, C., Nordby, K. & Stockman, A. (1989) The incremental threshold of the rod visual system and Weber's law. *Science* **244**, 354–6.

Sitaramayya, A. (1986) Rhodopsin kinase prepared from bovine rod disk membranes quenches light activation of cGMP phosphodiesterase in a reconstituted system. *Biochemistry* **25**, 5460–8.

Sharpe, L. T., van Norren, D. & Nordby, K. (1988) Pigment regeneration, visual adaptation and spectral sensitivity in the achromat. *Clin. Vision Sci.* **3**, 9–17.

Sitaramayya, A. & Liebman, P. A. (1983) Phosphorylation of rhodopsin and quenching of cGMP phosphodiesterase activation by ATP at weak bleaches. *J. biol. Chem.* **258**, 12 106–9.

Stabell, B., Stabell, V. & Nordby, K. (1986) Dark-adaptation in a rod monochromat: effect of stimulus size, exposure time and retinal eccentricity. *Clin. Vision Sci.* **1**, 75–80.

Stiles, W. S. & Crawford, B. H. (1932) Equivalent adaptation levels in localized retinal areas. In *Report of a joint discussion on vision*, pp. 194–211. Physical Society of London, Cambridge University Press, Cambridge. (Reprinted in Stiles, W. S. (1978) *Mechanisms of colour vision.* Academic, London).

Stryer, L. (1986) Cyclic GMP cascade of vision. *A. Rev. Neurosci.* **9**, 87–119.

Tamura, T., Nakatani, K. & Yau, K.-W. (1989) Light adaptation in cat retinal rods. *Science* **245**, 755–8.

Torre, V., Matthews, H. R. & Lamb, T. D. (1986) Role of calcium in regulating the cyclic GMP cascade of phototransduction in retinal rods. *Proc. Nat. Acad. Sci. U.S.A.* **83**, 7109–13.

Westheimer, G. (1968) Bleached rhodopsin and retinal interaction. *J. Physiol.* **195**, 97–105.

Wilden, U., Hall, S. W. & Kühn, H. (1986) Phosphodiesterase activation by photoexcited rhodopsin is quenched when rhodopsin is phosphorylated and binds the intrinsic 48 kDa protein of rod outer segments. *Proc. Nat. Acad. Sci. U.S.A.* **83**, 1174–8.

Williams, T. P. (1970) An isochromic change in the bleaching of rhodopsin. *Vision Res.* **10**, 525–33.

Chapter 6

Barlow, H. B. (1972) Dark and light adaptation: psychophysics. In *Handbook of sensory physiology*, vol. VII/4 (eds. Jameson, D. & Hurvich, L. M.), pp. 1–28. Springer, Berlin.

(1977) Retinal and central factors in human vision limited by noise. In *Vertebrate photoreception* (eds. Barlow, H. B. & Fatt, P., pp. 337–51. Academic Press, London.

Barlow, H. B., Levick, W. R. & Yoon, M. (1971) Responses to single quanta of light in retinal ganglion cells of the cat. *Vision Res.* **11**, 87–101.

Barlow, R. B., Jr. & Kaplan, E. (1977) Properties of visual cells in the lateral eye of *Limulus in situ.* Intracellular recordings. *J. gen. Physiol.* **69**, 203–20.

Barlow, R. B., Jr., Kaplan, E., Renninger, G. H. & Saito, T. (1987) Circadian rhythms in *Limulus* photoreceptors. *J. gen. Physiol.* **89**, 353–78.

Batra, R. & Barlow, R. B. (1981) Efferent control of pattern vision in *Limulus* lateral eye. *Soc. Neurosci. Abstr.* **8**, 49.

Baylor, D. A., Matthews, G., & Yau, K.-W. (1980) Two components of electrical dark noise in toad retinal rod outer segments. *J. Physiol.* **309**, 591–621.

Buchner, E. (1984) Behavioural analysis of spatial vision in insects. In *Photoreception and vision in invertebrates* (ed. Ali, M. A.), pp. 561–621. Plenum, New York.

Cohn, T. E. (1983) Receiver operating characteristics analysis of photoreceptor sensitivity. *IEEE Trans. on Systems, Man and Cybernetics* **13**, 873–81.

Doujak, F. (1985) Can a shore crab see a star? *J. exp. Biol.*, pp. 385–93.

Dubs, A., Laughlin, S. B. & Srinivasan, M. V. (1981) Single photon signals in fly photoreceptors and first order interneurones at behavioural threshold. *J. Physiol.* **317**, 317–34.

Exner, S. (1891) *De Physiologie der facettirten Augen von Krebsen und Insecten.* Franz Deuticke, Leipzig-Vienna.

Fermi, G. & Reichardt. W. (1963) Optomotorische Reaktionen der Fliege *Musca domestica. Kybernetik* **2**, 15–28.

Fuortes, M. G. F. & Yeandle, S. (1964) Probability of occurrence of discrete potential waves in the eye of *Limulus. J. gen. Physiol.* **47**, 443–63.

Gotz, K. G. (1964) Optomotorische Untersuchungg des visuellen Systems einiger Augenmutanten der Furchtfliegele *Drosophila*, *Kybernetik* **2**, 77–92.

Hamdorf, K. (1979) The physiology of invertebrate visual pigments. In *Handbook of sensory physiology*, vol. VII/6A (ed. Autrum, H.), pp. 146–224. Springer, Berlin.

van Hateren, J. H. (1984) Waveguide theory applied to optically measured angular sensitivities of fly photoreceptors. *J. comp. Physiol.* **154**, 761–71.

Hausen, K. (1984) The lobula complex of the fly: structure, function and significance in visual behaviour. In *Photoreception and vision in invertebrates* (ed. Ali, M. A.), pp. 523–59. Plenum, New York.

Hecht, S., Shlaer, S. & Pirenne M. (1942) Energy, quanta and vision. *J. gen. Physiol.* **25**, 819–40.

Horridge, G. A. (1978) The separation of visual axes in compound eyes. *Proc. R. Soc. Lond.* B. **285**, 1–59.

Howard, J. (1983) Variations in the voltage response to single quanta of light in the photoreceptors of *Locusta migratoria*. *Biophys. Struct. Mech.* **9**, 341–8.

Kaplan, E. & Barlow, R. B., Jr. (1976) Energy, quanta, and *Limulus* vision. *Vision Res.* **16**, 745–51.

Katz, B. & Miledi, R. (1972) The statistical nature of the acetylcholine potential and its molecular components. *J. Physiol.* **224**, 665–99.

Kelly, D. S. (1972) Flicker. In *Handbook of sensory physiology*, vol. VII/4 (eds. Jameson, D. & Hurvich, L. M.), pp. 273–302. Springer, Berlin.

Kirschfeld, K. (1965) Discrete and graded receptor potentials in the compound eye of the fly *Musca*. In *The functional organization of the compound eye* (ed. Bernhard, C. G.), pp. 291–307. Pergamon, Oxford.

(1974) The absolute sensitivities of lens and compound eyes. *Z. Naturf.* **29**c, 592–6.

(1976) The resolution of lens and compound eyes. In *Neural principles in vision* (eds. Zettler, F. & Weiler, R.), pp. 354–70. Springer, Berlin.

Lamb, T. D. (1981) The involvement of rod photoreceptors in dark adaptation. *Vision Res.* **12**, 1773–82.

Land, M. F. (1981) Optics and vision in invertebrates. In *Handbook of sensory physiology*, vol. VII/6B (ed. Autrum, H.), pp. 471–592. Springer, Berlin.

Laughlin, S. B. (1975) Receptor function in the apposition eye. In *Photoreceptor optics* (eds. Snyder, A. W. & Menzel, R.), pp. 479–98. Springer, Berlin.

(1976) The sensitivities of dragonfly photoreceptors and the voltage gain of transduction. *J. comp. Physiol.* **111**, 221–47.

(1981) Neural principles in the peripheral visual systems of invertebrates. In *Handbook of sensory physiology*, vol. VII/6B (ed. Autrum, H.), pp. 133–280. Springer, Berlin.

Laughlin, S. B. & Lillywhite, P.G. (1982) Intrinsic noise in locust photoreceptors. *J. Physiol.* **332**, 25–45.

Lillywhite, P. G. (1977) Single photon signals and transduction in an insect eye. *J. comp. Physiol.* **122**, 189–200.

(1981) Multiplicative intrinsic noise and the limits to visual performance. *Vision Res.* **21**, 291–6.

Lillywhite, P. G. & Dvorak, D. R. (1981) Responses to single photons in a fly optomotor neurone. *Vision Res.* **21**, 279–90.

Lillywhite, P. G. & Laughlin, S. B. (1979) Transducer noise in a photoreceptor. *Nature Lond.* **277**, 569–72.

Lisman, J. (1985) The role of metarhodopsin in the generation of spontaneous quantum bumps in the ultraviolet receptors of *Limulus* median eye. *J. gen. Physiol.* **85**, 171–87.

Paulsen, R. & Bentrop, J. (1984) Reversible phosphorylation of opsin induced by irradiation of blowfly retinae *J. comp. Physiol*, A **155**, 39–45.

Pick, B. & Buchner, E. (1979) Visual movement detection under light- and dark-adapted conditions in the fly *Musca domestica*. *J. comp. Physiol.* **134**, 45–54.

Reichardt, W. E. (1970) The insect eye as a model for analysis of uptake, transduction, and processing of optical data in the nervous system. In *The neurosciences: second study programme* (ed. Schmitt, F. O.), pp. 494–511. Rockefeller University Press, New York.

Rose, A. (1977) Vision: human versus electronic. In *Vertebrate photoreception* (eds. Barlow, H. B. & Fatt, P.), pp. 1–12. Academic Press, London.

de Ruyter van Steveninck, R. R. (1986) Real-time performance of a movement-sensitive neuron in the blowfly visual system. Ph.D. Thesis, Rijksuniversiteit te Groningen, Holland.

Scholes, J. H. (1964) Discrete sub-threshold potentials from the dimly lit insect eye. *Nature, Lond.* **202**, 572–3.

Scholes, J. H. & Reichardt, W. (1969) The quantal content of optomotor stimuli and the electrical responses of receptors in the compound eye of the fly *Musca. Kybernetik* **6**, 74–80.

Snyder, A. W. (1979) Physics of vision in compound eyes. In *Handbook of sensory physiology*, vol. VII/6A (ed. Autrum, H.), pp. 226–313. Springer, Berlin.

Snyder, A. W., Laughlin, S. B. & Stavenga, D. G. (1977) Spatial information capacity of compound eyes. *J. comp. Physiol.* **116**, 183–207.

Snyder, A. W., Stavenga, D. G. & Laughlin, S. B. (1977) Information capacity of eyes. *Vision Res.* **17**, 1163–75.

Srinivasan, M. V. & Dvorak, D. R. (1980) Spatial processing of visual information in the movement-detecting pathway of the fly. *J. comp. Physiol.* **140**, 1–23.

Srinivasan, M. V., Laughlin, S. B. & Dubs, A. (1982) Predictive coding: a fresh view of inhibition in the retina. *Proc. R. Soc. Lond.* B **216**, 427–59.

Stavenga, D. G. (1979) Pseudopupils of compound eyes. In *Handbook of sensory physiology*, vol. VII/6A (ed. Autrum, H.), pp. 357–439. Springer, Berlin.

Stern, J., Chinn, K. Robinson, P. & Lisman J. (1985) The effects of nucleotides on the rate of spontaneous quantum bumps in *Limulus* ventral photoreceptors. *J. gen. Physiol.* **85**, 157–69.

Teich, M. C., Prucnal, P. R., Vannucci, G., Breton, M. E. & McGill, W. J. (1982) Multiplication noise in the human visual system at threshold: 1. Quantum fluctuations and minimum detectable energy. *J. opt. Soc. Am.* **72**, 419–31.

Vogt, K. (1977) Ray path and reflection mechanisms in crayfish eyes. *Z. Naturf.* **32**c, 466–8.

Walcott, B. (1975) Anatomical changes during light adaptation in insect compound eyes. In *The compound eye and vision of insects* (ed. Horridge, G. A.). Oxford University Press, Oxford.

Wehner, R. (1981) Spatial vision in arthropods. In *Handbook of sensory physiology*, vol. VII/6C (ed. Autrum, H.), pp. 287–616. Springer, Berlin.

Weiss, G. H. & Yeandle, S. (1975) Distribution of response times in visual sense cells following weak stimuli. *J. theor. Biol.* **55**, 519–28.

Williams, D. S. (1983) Changes in photoreceptor performance associated with the daily turnover of photoreceptor membrane. *J. comp. Physiol.* **150**, 509–19.

Wilson, M. (1975) Angular sensitivity of light and dark adapted locust retinula cells. *J. comp. Physiol.* **97**, 323–8.

Wood, R. W. (1911) *Physical optics* (2nd edn) Macmillan, New York.

Yeandle, S. (1958) Evidence of quantized slow potentials in the eye of *Limulus. Am. J. Opthal.* **46**, 82–7.

(1977) Remarks on the noise of invertebrate photoreceptors. In *Vertebrate photoreception* (eds. Barlow, H. B. & Fatt, P.), pp. 355–8. Academic Press, London.

Zettler, F. (1969) Die Abhangigkeit des Ubertragungsverhaltens von Frequenz und Adaptationzustand, gemessen am einzelnen Lichtrezeptor von *Calliphora erythrocephala. Z. vergl. Physiol.* **64**, 432–49.

Chapter 7

Albert, M. L., Reches, A. & Silverberg, R. (1975) Hemianopic colour blindness. *J. Neurol. Neurosurg. Psychiat.* **38**, 546–9.

Alpern, M. (1974). What is it that confines in a world without color? *Invest. Ophthal.* **13**, 648–74.

Alpern, M., Falls, H. F. & Lee, G. B. (1960) The enigma of typical total monochromacy. *Am. J. Ophthal.* **50**, 996–1012.

Alpern M., Lee, G. B. & Spivey, B. E. (1965) π_1-cone monochromatism. *Arch. Ophthal.* **74**, 334–7.

Alpern, M., Lee, G. B., Maaseidvaag, F. & Miller, S. (1971) Colour vision in blue-cone 'monochromacy'. *J. Physiol.* **212**, 211–33.

Auerbach, E. (1974) Electroretinographical and psychophysical studies in achromats. In *Colour vision deficiencies II, modern problems in ophthalmology* (ed. Verriest, G.), vol. 13, pp. 169–76. S. Karger, Basel.

Auerbach, E. & Kripke, B. (1974) Achromatopsia with amblyopia. II: A psychophysical study of 5 cases. *Documenta Ophthal.* **37**, 119–44.

Auerbach, E. & Merin, S. (1974) Achromatopsia with amblyopia. I: A clinical and electroretinographical study of 39 cases. *Documenta Ophthal.* **37**, 79–117.

Baumgardt, E. & Magis, C. (1954) Sur un cas exceptionnel d'achromatopsie. *J. Physiol. (Paris)* **46**, 237–40.

Baylor, D. A., Nunn, B. J. & Schnapf, J. L. (1984) The photocurrent, noise and spectral sensitivity of rods of the monkey *Macaca fascicularis. J. Physiol.* **357**, 575–90.

Bell, J. (1926) *Eugenics Laboratory Memoirs No. XXIII.* The Treasure of Human Inheritance, Vol. II. Anomalies and Diseases of the Eye. Part II: Colour-Blindness, pp. 224 and 257. Cambridge University Press, London.

Berson, E. L., Sandberg, M. A., Rosner, B. & Sullivan, P. L. (1983) Color plates to help identify patients with blue cone monochromatism. *Am. J. Ophthal.* **95**, 741–7.

Bjerrum, J. (1904) Et Tilfælde af medfødt total Farveblindhed med Bemærkninger om Stav- og Tapfunktion. *Hospitalstidende* **12** (47), 1145–58.

Björk, A., Lindblom, U. & Wadensten, L. (1956) Retinal degeneration in hereditary ataxia. *J. Neurol. Neurosurg. Psychiat.* **19**, 186–93.

Blackwell, H. R. & Blackwell, O. M. (1957) Blue mono-cone monochromacy: A new color vision defect. *J. Opt. Soc. Am.* **47**, 338.

Blackwell, H. R. & Blackwell, O. M. (1961) Rod and cone receptor mechanisms in typical and atypical congenital achromatopsia. *Vision Res.* **1**, 62–107.

Böhm (1857) *Der Nystagmus und dessen Heilung*, 141.

Boyle, R. (1688) *Some uncommon observations about vitiated sight*. J. Taylor, London.

Colburn, J. E. (1897) Congenital nystagmus. *Am. J. Ophthal.* **14**, 237–47.

Cole, L. J. (1919) An early family history of color blindness. *J. Hered.* **10**, 372.

Crerar, J. W. & Ross, J. A. (1953) John Dalton, F.R.S., D.S.L. LL.D., Captain Huddart, F.R.S., and the Harris family. Historical notes on congenital colour blindness. *Br. J. Ophthal.* **37**, 181–4.

Critchley, M. (1965) Acquired anomalies of colour perception of central origin. *Brain* **88**, 711–24.

Crone, R. A. (1955) Clinical study of colour vison. *Br. J. Ophthal.* **39**, 170–3.

(1956) Combined forms of congenital color defects: a pedigree with atypical total color blindness. *Br. J. Ophthal.* **40**, 462.

(1965) Inkomplette Achromatopsie mit rohrförmigen Gesichtsfeldern. *Ber. Deut. Ophthal. Ges.* **66**, 176–80.

Dalton, J. (1798) Extraordinary facts relating to the vision of colours; with observations (read in October 1794). *Mem. Lit. Phil. Soc. Manchester* **5**, 28–45.

Damasio, A. R., Yamada, T., Corbett, J. & McKee, J. (1980) Central achromatopsia: Behavioral, anatomic and physiologic aspects. *Neurology* **30**, 1064–71.

Daw, N. W. & Enoch, J. M. (1973) Contrast sensitivity Westheimer function and Stiles–Crawford effect in a blue cone monochromat. *Vision Res.* **13**, 1669–80.

Descartes, R. (1638) La dioptrique. In R. Descartes, *Discourse de la methode*. J. Maire, Leyden.

Deutman, A. F. (1971) *The hereditary dystrophies of the posterior pole of the eye.* Van Gorcum, Assen.

Dodt, E., van Lith, G. H. M. & Schmidt, B. (1967) Electroretinographic evaluation of the photopic malfunction in a totally colour blind. *Vision Res.* **7**, 231–41.

Donders, F. (1871) Einige Mitteilungen verschiedenen Inhaltes. *Klin. Monats. Augenheilkunde* **9**, 468–77.

Dong, Tai-Huo & Jin, Wem-Ying (1989) The discoveries of color specification, color blindness and the opponent theory of color vision in the ancient Chinese literature. Manuscript submitted to the *6th Congress of the Association Internationale de la Couleur*, Buenos Aires, Argentina, 13–17 March, 1989.

Dubois-Poulsen, A. (1982) Colour vision in brain lesions. *Documenta Ophthal. Proceedings Series* **33**, 420–39 (ed. Verriest, G.). Dr. W. Junk, the Hague.

Dugacki, V. (1977) Prvi nas znanstventi traktat o fizoloskoj optici. (Our first known treatise on physiological optics.) *Jugosl. oftalm. arh.* **3**(4), 17–22.

Duke-Elder, S. (1964) Normal and abnormal development. Part 2: Congenital deformities. In *System of opthalmology*, Vol. III (ed. Duke-Elder). Henry Kimpton, London.

Duveen, D. I. & Klickstein, H. S. (1954) John Dalton's autopsy. *J. Hist. Med.* **9**, 360–2.

Earle, P. (1845) On the inability to distinguish colors. *Am. J. Med. Sci.* **9**, 346.

Falls, H. F., Wolter, J. R. & Alpern, M. (1965) Typical total monochromacy. *Arch. Ophthal.* **74**, 610–16.

von Feuerbach, A. (1834) *Kaspar Hauser:* An account of an individual kept in a dungeon, separated from all communication with the world, from early childhood to about the age of seventeen. Simpkin & Marshall, London.

Fick, A. E. (1874) Zur Theorie der Farbenblindheit. *Verh. phys.-med. Ges. (Würzburg)* **5**, 158–62.

Fincham, E. F. (1953) Defects of the colour-sense mechanism as indicated by the accommodation reflex. *J. Physiol.* **121**, 570–80.

Franceschetti, A. (1928) Die Bedeutung der Einstellungsbreite am Anomaloskop für die Diagnose der enzelnen Typen der Farbensinnstörungen, nebst Bemerkungen über ihren Vererbungsmodus. *Schweiz. med. Wochensch.* **58**, 1273–9.

(1939) Sur la forme incomplete de l'achromatopsie totale. *Bull. mem., Soc. fr. ophthal.* **52**, 135–9.

Franceschetti, A., Jaeger, W., Klein, D., Ohrt, V. & Rickli, H. (1958) Étude patho-physiologique de la grande famille d'achromates de l'île de Fur (Danemark). Déscription d'une nouvelle famille avec achromatopsie totale chez le fils âiné et achromatopsie incomplète chez le frère cadet. *XVIII Concilium ophthalmologicum, Belgica*, Vol. II, pp. 1582–8.

Franceschetti, A., Jaeger, W., Klein, D., Ohrt, V. & Rickli, H. (1959) New facts resulting from a pathophysiological and genetic study of the large family of achromats of the island of Fur (Denmark). *Abstr. Rep. 18th internat. Congr. Ophthal. Sept. Brussels, Exc. Med., 12, 9*, nr. **88**, p. C111.

François, J., De Rouck, A. & De Laey, J. J. (1976) Progressive cone dystrophies. *Ophthalmologica* **173**, 81–101.

François, J., De Rouck, A., Verriest, G., De Laey, J. J. & Cambie, E. (1974) Progressive generalized cone dysfunction. *Ophthalmologica* **169**, 255–84.

François, J., Verriest, G. & De Rouck, A. (1955*a*) L'achromatopsie congénitale. *Bull. Soc. belg. Ophthal.* **110**, 170–254.

François, J., Verriest, G. & De Rouck, A. (1955*b*) L'achromatopsie congénitale. *Documenta Ophthal.* **9**, 338–424.

François, J., Verriest, G., De Rouck, A. & Humblet, M. (1956) Dégénérescense maculaire juvenile avec atteinte predominante de la vision photopique, *Ophthalmologica* **131**, 393–402.

François, J., Verriest, G., Matton-Van Leuven, M. T., De Rouck, A. & Manavian, D. (1966) *Am. J. Ophthal.* **61**, 1101–8.

Fuortes, M. G. F., Gunkel, R. D. & Rushton, W. A. H. (1961) Increment thresholds in a subject deficient in cone vision. *J. Physiol.* **156**, 179–92.

Galezowski, X. (1868) *Du diagnostic des Maladies des yeux par la Chromatoscopie rétinienne: Procédé d'une Étude sur les Lois physiques et physiologiques des Couleurs.* J.-B. Baillière et fils, Paris.

Gibson, I. M. (1962) Visual mechanisms in a cone-monochromat. *J. Physiol.* **161**, 10P–11P.

Glickstein, M. & Heath, G. G. (1975) Receptors in the monochromat eye. *Vision Res.* **15**, 633–6.

Goodman, G., Ripps, H. & Siegel, I. M. (1963) Cone dysfunction syndromes. *Arch. Ophthal.* **70**, 214–31.

Goodman, G., Ripps, H. & Siegel, I. M. (1966) Progressive cone degeneration. In *Clinical electroretinography* (eds. Burian, H. M. & Jacobson, J. H), pp. 363–72. Pergamon, Oxford.

Green, D. G. (1972) Visual acuity in the blue cone monochromat. *J. Physiol.* **222**, 419–26.

Green, G. L. & Lessel, S. (1977) Acquired cerebral dyschromatopsia. *Arch. Ophthal.* **95**, 121–8.

Grützner, P. (1964) Der normale Farbensinn und seine Abweichungen. *Ber. Deut. Ophthal. Ges.* **66**, 161.

Hansen, E, Seim, T. & Olsen, B. T. (1978) Transient tritanopia experiments in blue cone monochromacy. *Nature*, **276**, 390–1.

Harrison, R., Hoefnagel, D. & Hayward, J. N. (1960) Congenital total colour blindness, a clinico-pathological report. *Arch. Ophthal.* **64**, 685–92.

Hecht, S., Shlaer, S., Smith, E. L., Haig, C. & Peskin, J. C. (1938) The visual functions of a completely colorblind person. *Am. J. Physiol.* **123**, 94–5.

Hecht, S., Shlaer, S., Smith, E. L., Haig, C. & Peskin, J. C. (1948) The visual functions of the completely colorblind. *J. gen. Physiol.* **31**, 459–72.

Hering, E. (1891) Untersuchung eines total Farbenblinden. *Pflügers Arch. ges. Physiol.* **49**, 563–608.

Hess, C. & Hering, E. (1898) Untersuchungen and total Farbenblinden. *Plügers Archiv für die gesamte Physiologie* **71**, 105–27.

Hess, R. F., Mullen, K. T., Sharpe, L. T. & Zrenner, E. (1989*a*) The photoreceptors in atypical achromatopsia. *J. Physiol.* **417**, 123–49

Hess, R. F., Mullen, K. T. & Zrenner, E. (1989*b*) Human photopic vision with only short wavelength cones: Post-receptoral properties. *J. Physiol.* **417**, 150–69.

Heywood, C. A., Wilson, B. & Cowey, A. (1987) A case study of cortical colour 'blindness' with relatively intact achromatic discrimination. *J. Neurol. Neurosurg. Psychiat.* **50**, 22–9.

Hirschberg, J. (1982) *The history of ophthalmology*, Vol. 1, pp. 59–134. (Translated by Blodi, F.) J. P. Wayenborgh, Bonn.

Hohki, R. (1938) Über vier Familien mit 'Achromatopsia totalis' und ihre Vererbung. *Chuogankaiho* **30**/10, 2–18.

Holm, E. & Lodberg, C. V. (1940) A family with total colour-blindness. *Acta Ophthal.* **18**, 224–58.

Holmgren, F. (1878) Über die Farbenblindheit in Schweden. *Centralbl. prak. Augenheil.* **2**, 201.

D'Hombres-Firmas (1849) Observation d'achromatopsie. *C. r. Acad. Sci.*, 2e partie, **25**, 175–9.

Huddart, J. (1777) An Account of Persons who could not distinguish Colours. (By Mr Joseph Huddart in a Letter to the Rev. Joseph Priestley, LL.D. F.R.S.) *Phil. Trans. R. Soc. Lond.* **67**, 260–5.

Hugens, C. (1690, 1912) *Treatise on Light, in which are explained the causes of that which occurs in reflexion, & in refraction. And particularly in the strange refraction of Iceland crystal.* (Rendered into English by S. P. Thompson.) Macmillan and Co, London.

Ikeda, H. & Ripps, H. (1966) The electroretinogram of a cone monochromat. *arch. Opthal.* **75**, 513–7.

Jaeger, W. (1950) Systematische Untersuchung über 'inkomplette' angeborene totale Farbenblindheit. *Albrecht von Graefes Arch. Klin. Exp. Ophthal.* **150**, 509–28.

(1951) Angeborene total Farbenblindheit mit Resten von Farbempfindung. *Klin. Monatsbl. Augenheil.* **118**, 228–88.

(1953) Typen der inkompletten Achromatopsie. *Ber. Deut. Ophthal. Ges.* **58**, 44–7.

Jaeger, W. & Krastel, H. (1981) Complete and incomplete congenital achromatopsia in one sibship. *Neurogenetics Neuro-ophthalmology*. (eds. Huber, A. & Klein, D.), pp. 241–5. North-Holland Biomedical, Elsevier.

Jaeger, W. & Krastel, H. (1983) Different types of congenital achromatopsia with residual cone functions: a new concept based on detection or remnant cone activities by large field examination of spectral sensitivity. *Festschrift Jules Francois: Retinal and Chorioretinal Pathology*, pp. 57–69. Aeolus, Amsterdam.

Jaeger, W. & Krastel. H. (1987) Normal and defective colour vision in large field. *Jap. J. Ophthal.* **31**, 20–40.

Kepler, J. (1604) *Ad Vitellionem Paralipomena, quibus Astronomiæ pars optica traditur, etc.* Cl. Marnium & Haer. J. Aubrii, Frankfurt.

(1611) *Dioptrice seu demonstratio eorum quæ visui & visibilibus propter conspicilla non ita pridem invent accidunt. Etc.* Augustæ Vindelicorum, Augsburg. In *Gesammelte Werke* (eds. von Dyck, W. & Casper, M.). München, Beck, 1937–1963, vol. 4.

König, A. (1894) Über den menschlichen Sehpurpur und seine Bedeutung für das Sehen. *Sitzungsber. könig̈. Preuss. Akad. Wissensch. (Berlin)*, pp. 577–98.

Krastel, H., Jaeger, W. & Blankenagel, A. (1981) Nachweis von Resten eines 'Rot-Rezeptors' unter chromatischer Adaptation bein Patienten mit zunächst typisch erscheinender angeborener totaler Farbenblindheit. *Ber. Deut. Ophthal. Gesell.* **78**, 717–26.

Krastel, H., Jaeger, W. & Blankenagel, A. (1983) Zapfenrestaktivitäten bei verschiedenen Typen angeborener totaler Farbenblindheit und das Konzept der inkompletten Achromatopsie. *Fortsch. Ophthal.* **79**, 499–502.

Kries, J. von (1897) Über das Sehen der total farbenblinden netzhautzone. *Centralb. Physiol.* **10**, 745–9.

(1924) Note. In H. von Helmholtz's (1909–1911) *Treatise on physiological optics* (translated from the 3rd German edition and edited by James P. C. Southall). Dover, New York (1962). Appendix to Vol. II, pp. 411–22.

Krill, A. E. (1977) *Congenital color vision defects. Krill's hereditary retinal and choroidal diseases.* Vol. II, *Clinical characteristics* (eds. Krill, A. E. & Archer, D. B.), pp. 355–90. Harper and Row, Hagerstown.

Krill, A. E. Deutman, A. F. & Fishman, M. (1973) The cone-degenerations. *Documenta Ophthal.* **35**, 1–80.

Krill, A. E. & Schneiderman, A. (1966) Retinal function studies, including the electroretinogram, in an atypical monochromat. *Clinical electroretinography (Supplement to Vision Res.)* **6**, 351–61.

Landolt, E. (1881) Achromatopsie totale. *Arch. opthal.* **1**, 144.

Larsen, H. (1918) Total Monochromasi. *Proc. Sess.* Det Oftalmologiske Selskab i København, (printed 1918 in) *Hospitalstidende* **61**, 1130–3.

(1921*a*) Demonstration mikroskopischer Präparate von einem monochromatischen Auge. *Klin. Monatsb. Augenheil.* **67**, 301–2.

(1921*b*) Demonstration mikroskopisher Präparate von einem monochromatischen Auge. *Ophthalmologica* **46**, 228–9.

Lascaratos, J. (1980) Ophthalmological treatment in the Aesclepeia. *Gr. Ann. Ophthal.* **17**, 143–54.

Lascaratos, J. & Marketos, S. (1988) Ophthalmological lore in the *Corpus Hippocraticum. Documenta Ophthal.* **68**, 35–45.

Leber, T. (1873) Über die Theorie der Farbenblindheit und über die Art und Weise, wie gewisse, der Untersuchung von Farbenblinden entnommenen Einwände gegen die Young–Helmholtz'sche Theorie sich mit derselben vereinigen lassen. *Klin. Monatsbl. Augenheil.* **11**, 467–73.

Lewis, S. D. & Mandelbaum, J. (1943). Achromatopsia: report of three cases. *Archiv Opthal.* **30**, 225–31.

Linksz, A. (1964) *An essay on color vision and clinical color vision tests.* Grüne & Stratton, New York.

van Lith, G. H. M. (1973) General cone dysfunction without achromatopsia. X. ISCERG Symposium, Los Angeles, 1972. *Documenta Ophthal. Proceedings Series* **2**, 175–80.

MacKay, G. & Dunlop, J. C. (1899) The cerebral lesions in a case of complete acquired colour-blindness. *Scot. med. surg. J.* **5**, 503–12.

Meadows, J. C. (1974) Disturbed perception of colours associated with localized cerebral lesions. *Brain* **97**, 615–32.

Miles, W. D. (1957) John Dalton's autopsy. *J. Hist. Med.* **12**, 263–4.

Mollon, J. D. (1985*a*) The identity of 'G. Palmer'. *Invest. Ophthal. Visual Sci.* **26**, 205.

(1985*b*) L'auteur énigmatique de la théorie trichromatique. In *Actes du 5eme Congrès de L'Association Internationale de la Couleur*, Tome 1, Paris: AIC, 1985.

(1989) Tho' she kneel'd in that place where they grew . . . The uses and origins of primate colour vision. *J. exp. Biol.* **146**, 21–38.

Mollon, J. D., Newcombe, F., Polden, P. G. & Ratcliff, G. (1980) On the presence of three cone mechanisms in a case of total achromatopsia. In *Color vision deficiencies V* (ed. Verriest, G.), Ch. 3, pp. 130–5. Hilger, Bristol.

Nagel, W. A. (1898) Beiträge zur Diagnostik, Symptomatologie und Statistik der angeborenen Farbenblindheit. *Arch. Augenheil.* **38**, 31–66.

(1907) Zwei Apparate für die augenärztliche Funktionsprüfung: Adaptometer und kleines Spektralphotometer (Anomaloscop). *Zeitschr. Augenheil.* **17**, 201–22.

Nagel, W. (1911) Adaptation, twilight vision and the duplicity theory. In H. von

Helmholtz's (1909–1911) *Treatise on physiological optics* (translated from the 3rd German ed. and edited by James P. C. Southall). Dover, New York (1962). Appendix to Vol. II, pp. 313–94.

Nathans, J., Davenport, C. M., Maumenee, I. H., Lewis, R. A., Hejtmancik, J. F., Litt, M., Lovrien, E., Weleber, R., Bachynski, B., Zwas, F., Klingaman, R. & Fishman, G. (1989) Molecular genetics of human blue cone monochromacy. *Science* **245**, 831–8.

Nettleship, E. (1880) On cases of congenital day-blindness with colour-blindness. *Saint Thomas Hospital Reports* **10**, 37.

Neuhann, T., Krastel, H. & Jaeger, W. (1978) Differential diagnosis of typical and atypical congenital achromatopsia. *Albrecht von Graefes Arch. Klin. Exp. Ophthal.* **209**, 19–28.

Newton, Isaac (1704) *Opticks: Or, a Treatise of the Reflexions, Refractions, Inflexions and Colours of Light; etc.* S. Smith & B. Walford, London. (Reprint: Dover, New York, 1952.)

Niemetschek, J. (1868) Über Farbenblindheit und Farbensehen. *Vierteljahrsch. prak. Heilkunde (Prague)* **100**, 224–38.

Nordby, K. & Sharpe, L. T. (1988) The directional sensitivity of the photoreceptors in the human achromat. *J. Physiol.* **399**, 267–81.

Okuzawa, Y. (1987) Looking for the roots of colour blindness. *Ophthalmology of Japan* **58**, 391–3.

Palmer, G. (1777) *Theory of colours and vision.* Printed for S. Leacroft, at the Globe, Charing-Cross, London. Excerpted in MacAdam, D. L. (ed.), *Sources of colour science*, 1970. MIT Press, Cambridge, Mass., p. 48.

Palmer, G. (1786) *Théorie de la Lumière applicable aux arts, et principalement à la peinture.* Hardouin et Gattey, Paris.

Pearlman, A. L., Birch, J., Phil, M. & Meadows, J. C. (1979) Cerebral colour blindness: an acquired defect in hue discrimination. *Ann. Neurol.* **5**, 253–61.

Pickford, R. W. (1957) Colour vision of achromat's parents. *Nature* **180**, 926–7.

Pinckers, A. (1972) An analysis of colour vision in 314 patients. *Mod. Prob. Ophthal.* **11**, 104–7.

Pitt, F. H. G. (1944) Monochromatism. *Nature* **154**, 466–8.

Platter, F. (1583) *De Corporis Humani Structura et Usu Libri III.* Apud Ludovicum König, Basel.

Playfair, L. (1899) Memoirs and correspondence (ed. Sir Wemyss Reid), p. 58. Harpe, New York.

Pokorny, J., Smith, V. C., Pinckers, A. J. L. G., & Cozijnsen, M. (1982) Classification of complete and incomplete autosomal recessive achromatopsia. *Albrecht von Graefes arch. Klin. Exp. Ophthal.* **219**, 121.

Pokorny, J., Smith, V. C. & Swartley R. (1970) Threshold measurements of spectral sensitivity in a blue monocone monochromat. *Invest. Ophthal. Visual Sci.* **9**, 807–13.

Pokorny, J., Smith, V. C. & Verriest, G. (1979) Congenital color defects. In *Congenital and acquired color vision defects* (eds. Pokorny, J., Smith, V. C., Verriest, G. & Pinckers, A. J. L. G.). Grune and Stratton, New York.

Polack, A. (1939) Anomalies du sens chromatique. In *Traite d'Ophthalmologie.*

Polyak, S. L. (1941) *The retina.* University of Chicago Press, Chicago.

(1957) *The vertebrate visual system* (ed. H. Kluver). University of Chicago Press, Chicago.

Priestley, Joseph (1772). *The history and present state of discoveries relating to vision, light, and colours.* J. Johnson, London.

Rayleigh, Lord (J. W. Strutt) (1881) Experiments on colour. *Nature* **25**, 64.

Reitner, A., Sharpe, L. T. & Zrenner, E. (1990) Is colour vision possible with only rods and blue-sensitive cones? (Submitted.)

Rozier, L'Abbé François (1779) *Obs. Phys. Hist. Nat. Arts* **13**, 86–7.

Sacks, O. & Wasserman, R. (1987) The case of the colorblind painter. *New York Rev. Books* **34** (18), 25–34.

Schoenhauer, A. (1812) Über das Sehen und die Farben. *Griesebach. Ausgabe* **6**, 81.

Schultze, M. (1866) Zur Anatomie und Physiologie der Retina. *Arch mikroskop. Anat. (und Entwicklungsmech.)* **2**, 175–286.

Seebeck, A. (1837) Über den bei mancher Personen vorkommenden Mangel an Farbensinn. *Ann. Phys. Chem. Leipzig* **42**, 177.

Sharpe, L. T. (1985) Color blindness. In *Physics in medicine & biology: medical physics, bioengineering and biophysics* (ed. McAinsh, T. F.), pp. 191–6. Pergamon, Oxford.

Sherman, P. D. (1981) *Colour vision in the nineteenth century.* Adam Hilger, Bristol.

Shindo, S. (1932) Two cases of congenital total colour-blindness. *Acta Soc. Ophthal. Jap.* **36**, 174.

Siegel, I., Graham, C., Ripps, H. & Hsia, Y. (1966) Analysis of photopic and scotopic function in an incomplete achromat. *J. opt. Soc. Am.* **56**, 699–704.

Sloan, L. L. (1954) Congenital achromatopsia: A report of 19 cases. *J. opt. Soc. Am.* **44**, 117–28.

(1958) The photopic retinal receptors of the typical achromat. *Am. J. Ophthal.* **46**, 81–6.

Sloan, L. L. & Brown, D. J. (1962) Progressive retinal degeneration with selective involvement of the cone mechanism. *Am. J. Ophthal.* **54**, 629–41.

Sloan, L. L. & Feiock, K. (1972) Acuity-luminance function in achromatopsia and in progressive cone degeneration: Factors related to individual differences in tolerance to bright light. *Invest. Ophthal. Visual Sci.* **11**, 862–8.

Sloan, L. L. & Newhall, S. M. (1942) Comparison of cases of atypical and typical achromatopsia. *Am. J. Ophthal.* **25**, 940–61.

Smith, V. C. & Pokorny, J. (1980) Cone dysfunction syndromes defined by colour vision. In *Colour vision deficiencies V*, Proceedings of the 5th International Symposium, London, 1979 (ed. Verriest, G.), pp. 69–82.

Smith, V. C., Pokorny, J. & Newell, F. W. (1978) Autosomal recessive incomplete achromatopsia with protan luminosity function. *Ophthalmologica* **177**, 197–207.

Smith, V. C., Pokorny, J. & Newell, F. W. (1979) Autosomal recessive incomplete achromatopsia with deutan luminosity. *Am. J. Ophthal.* **87**, 393–402.

Smith, V. C., Pokorny, J., Delleman, J. W., Cozijnsen, M., Houtman W. A. & Went, L. N. (1983) X-linked incomplete achromatopsia with more than one class of functional cones. *Invest. Ophthal. Vis. Sci.* **24**, 451–7.

Spivey, B. E. (1965) The X-linked recessive inheritance of atypical monochromatism. *Arch. Ophthal.* **74**, 327–33.

Spivey, B. E., Pearlman, J. T. & Burian, H. M. (1964) Electroretinographic findings (including flicker) in carriers of congenital X-linked achromatopsia. *Documenta Ophthal.* **18**, 367–75.

Spurzheim, S. (1825) *Phrenology or the doctrine of the mind and of the relations between its manifestations and the body.* London.

Steinmetz, R. D., Ogle, K. N. & Rucker, C. W. (1956) Some physiological considerations of hereditary macular degenerations. *Am. J. Ophthal.* **42**, 304–17 (October part II).

Stilling, J. (1878*a*) *Die prüfung des farbensinnes beim eisenbahn- und marinepersonal.* Fischer, Kassel.

(1878*b*) *Tafeln zur bestimmung der blau-gelbblindheit.* Fischer, Kassel.

Synder, C. (1967) *Our ophthalmic heritage.* Little, Brown & Co., Boston.

Trevor-Roper, P. D. (1960) *The eye and its disorders.* Blackwell Scientific, Oxford.

Turbervile, D. (1684) Two Letters from the great and experienced Oculist, Dr. Turbervile of Salisbury, to Mr. William Musgrave S.P.S. of Oxon, containing several remarkable cases in Physick, relating chiefly to the Eyes. *Phil. Trans. R. Soc. Lond.* **14** (First letter), 736–7.

Verrey, D. (1888) Hémiachromatopsie droite absolute. *Arch. opthal.* **8**, 289–300.

Verriest, G. (1971) Les courbes spectrales photopiques d'efficacité lumineuse relative dans les déficiences congénitales de la vision des couleurs. *Vision Res.* **11**, 1407–16.

Vierling, O. (1928) Über spektrale Wertbestimmung der Farben durch Schwellenmessung mit dem modifizierten Anomaloscope. *Zeitschr. Bahnärzte* **23**, 261–76.

Voigt, J. H. (1781) *Gothaisches Magazin Neuste Phys. Naturgesch.* (ed. Lichtenberg, J. C.) **2**, 57–81.

Vola, J. L., Riss, M. & Gosset, A. (1973) Les dyschromatopsies centrales dans les hémianopsies latérales homonymes. *Oto-Neuro-Ophthal.* **45**, 495–511.

Waardenburg, P. J. (1963) Achromatopsia congenita. In *Genetics and opthalmology* (eds. Waardenburg, P. J., Franceschetti, A. & Klein, D.) Vol. II, pp. 1695–718. Royal van Gorcum, Assen, Netherlands.

Walls, G. L. (1956) The G. Palmer story. *J. Hist. Med. All. Sci.* **XI**, 66–96.

Walls, G. L. & Heath, G. G. (1954) Typical total color blindness reinterpreted. *Acta Ophthal.* **32**, 253–97.

Wartmann, E. (1843) Memoir on Daltonism. *Mém. Soc. Phys. Hist. Nat. Genève* (English translation 1846 in *Taylor's Scientific Memoirs*, London, p. 158.)

Weale, R. A. (1953) Cone-monochromatism. *J. Physiol.* **121**, 548–69.

(1959) Photo-sensitive reactions in foveae of normal and cone-monochromatic observers. *Optica Acta* **6**, 158–74.

(1988) Leonardo and the eye. *Documenta Opthal.* **68**, 19–34.

Whisson (1778) An account of a remarkable imperfection of sight. *Phil. Trans. R. Soc. Lond.* **68**, 611–4.

Wilson, G. (1855) *Researches on Colour blindness.* Sutherland-Knox. Edinburgh.

Young, T. (1807) *A course of lectures on natural philosophy and the mechanical art* (republished 1845). P. Kelland, London.

Young, R. S. L. & Fishman, G. A. (1980). Loss of color vision and Stiles' pi-1 mechanism in a patient with cerebral infarction. *J. Opt. Soc. Am.* **70**, 1301–5.

Young, R. S. L. & Price, J. (1985) Wavelength discrimination deteriorates with illumination in blue cone monochromats. *Invest. Ophthal. Visual Sci.* **26**, 1543–9.

Zrenner, E., Magnussen, S. & Lorenz, B. (1988) Blauzapfenmonochromasie: Diagnose, genetische Beratung und optische Hilfsmittel. *Klin. Mbl. Augenheilk.* **193**, 510–7.

Chapter 8

Bjerrum, J. (1904) Et Tilfælde af medfødt total Farveblindhet med Bemærkninger om Stavog Tapfunktion. *Hospitaltidende (København)* **12**, 1145–58.

Krill, A. E. (1977) Congenital color vision defects. In *Krill's hereditary retinal and choroidal diseases, Vol. II, Clinical characteristics* (eds. Krill, A. E. & Archer, D. B.), pp. 355–90. Harper and Row, Hagerstown.

Larsen, H. (1918) Total Monochromasi. *Hospitaltidende (København)* **61**, 1030–3. (Proceedings of the 84th meeting of *Det oftalmologiske Selskab i København*, December 5, 1917.)

Sacks, O. & Wasserman, R. (1987) The Case of the Colorblind Painter. *New York Rev. Books* **34**(18), 25–34.

The following is a list of all the investigations of my visual system that have been published.

Greenlee, M. W., Magnussen, S. & Nordby, K. (1988) Spatial vision of the achromat: Spatial frequency and orientation specific adaptation. *J. Physiol.* **395**, 661–78.

Hess, R. F. & Nordby, K. (1986a) Spatial and temporal limits of vision in the achromat. *J. Physiol.* **371**, 365–85.

Hess, R. F. & Nordby, K. (1986*b*) Spatial and temporal properties of human rod vision in the achromat. *J. Physiol.* **371**, 387–406.

Hess, R. F., Nordby, K. & Pointer, J. S. (1987) Regional variation of contrast sensitivity across the retina of the achromat: Sensitivity of human rod vision. *J. Physiol.* **388**, 101–19.

Nordby, K. (1988) Sosiale mekanismer, stemplingseffekt m.v. ved synshandikap. *Skolepsykologi* **23**, 1–8 (ISSN 0333–0389). (Social mechanisms, stigma etc. connected with visual handicaps.)

(1990) Vision in a complete achromat: a personal account. In *Night vision: basic, clinical and applied aspects* (eds. Hess, R. F., Sharpe, L. T. & Nordby, K.). Cambridge University Press, Cambridge.

Nordby, K. & Sharpe, L. T. (1988) The directional sensitivity of the photoreceptors in the human achromat. *J. Physiol.* **399**, 267–81.

Nordby, K., Stabell, B. & Stabell, U. (1984) Dark-adaptation of the human rod system. *Vision Res.* **24**, 841–9.

Rosness, R. (1981) *Corticale konsekvenser av stavmonokramasi. En psykofysisk studie av orienteringsselektivitet*. (Master's Thesis, Institute of Psychology, University of Oslo, 1981) ISBN 82-569-0541-7, 83 pages, 12 figures.

Sharpe, L. T. (1990) The light-adaptation of the human rod visual system. In *Night vision: basic, clinical and applied aspects* (eds. Hess, R. F., Sharpe, L. T. & Nordby, K.). Cambridge University Press, Cambridge.

Sharpe, L. T., van de Berge, K., van der Tweel, L. H. & Nordby, K. (1988) The pupillary light reflex in a complete achromat. *Clin. Vision Sci.* **3**, 267–71.

Sharpe, L. T., Collewijn, H. & Nordby, K. (1986) Fixation, pursuit and optokinetic nystagmus in a complete achromat. *Clin. Vision Sci.* **1**, 39–9.

Sharpe, L. T., Fach, C. & Nordby, K. (1988) Temporal summation in the achromat. *Vision Res.* **28**, 1263–9.

Sharpe, L. T., Fach, C. Nordby, K. & Stockman, A. (1989) The incremental threshold of the rod visual system and Weber's law. *Science* **244**, 254–6.

Sharpe, L. T. & Nordby, K. (1990*a*). Total colour-blindness: an introduction. In *Night vision: basic, clinical and applied aspects* (eds. Hess, R. F., Sharpe, L. T. & Nordby, K.). Cambridge University Press, Cambridge.

Sharpe, L. T. & Nordby, K. (1990*b*) The photoreceptors in the achromat. In *Night vision: basic, clinical and applied aspects* (eds. Hess, R. F., Sharpe, L. T. & Nordby, K.). Cambridge University Press, Cambridge.

Sharpe, L. T., van Norren, D. & Nordby, K. (1988) Pigment regeneration, visual adaptation and spectral sensitivity in the achromat. *Clin. Vision Sci.* **3**, 9–17.

Skottun, B. C., Nordby, K. & Magnussen, S. (1980) Rod monochromat sensitivity to sine wave flicker at luminances saturating the rods. *Invest. Ophthal. Visual Sci.* **19**, 108–11.

Skottun, B. C., Nordby, K. & Magnussen, S. (1981) Photopic and scotopic flicker sensitivity of a rod monochromat. *Invest. Ophthal. Visual Sci.* **21**, 877–9.

Skottun, B. C., Nordby, K. & Rosness, R. (1982) Temporal summation in a rod monochromat. *Vision Res.* **22**, 491–3.

Stabell, B., Nordby, K. & Stabell, U. (1987) Light-adaptation of the human rod system. *Clin. Vision Sci.* **2**, 83–91.

Stabell, B., Stabell, U. & Nordby, K. (1986) Dark-adaptation in a rod monochromat: Effect of stimulus size, exposure time and retinal eccentricity. *Clin. Vision Sci.* **1**, 75–80.

Stabell, U., Stabell, B. & Nordby, K. (1986) Dark-adaptation of the human rod system: A new hypothesis. *Scand. J. Psychol.* **27**, 175–83.

Chapter 9

Alpern, M., Lee, G. B., Maaseidvaag, F. & Miller, S. (1971) Colour vision in blue-cone 'monochromacy'. *J. Physiol.* **212**, 211–33.

Blackwell, H. R. & Blackwell, O. M. (1957) Blue mono-cone monochromacy. A new color vision defect. *J. opt. Soc. Am.* **47**, 338 (Abstr.).

Blackwell, H. R. & Blackwell, O. M. (1961) Rod and cone receptor mechanisms in typical and atypical congenital achromatopsia. *Vision Res.* **1**, 62–107.

Crone, R. A. (1956) Combined forms of congenital color defects: a pedigree with atypical total color blindness. *Br. J. Ophthal.* **40**, 462–72.

(1965) Inkomplette Achromatopsie mit rohrförmigen Gesichtsfeldern. *Ber. Deut. Ophthal. Ges.* **66**, 176–80.

Feiock, K. B., Maumenee, I. H. & Sloan, L. L. (1977) Incomplete achromatopsia. Presented at the meeting of the Wilmer Residents Association, Baltimore, April 22, 1977.

Ferguson, W. J. W. & MacGregor, A. G. (1949) Four cases of congenital total colour blindness, with otosclerosis and hypertension as associated hereditary abnormalities. *Proc. ophthal. Soc. U.K.* **69**, 249–58.

Fleischman, J. A. & O'Donnell, F. E. (1981) Congenital X-linked incomplete achromatopsia. *Arch Ophthal.* **99**, 468–72.

Franceschetti, A., Jaeger, W., Klein, D., Ohrt, V. & Rickli, H. (1958) New facts resulting from a pathophysiological and genetic study of the large family of achromats of the island of Fur (Denmark). *Abstr. Rep. 18th Internat. Congr. Ophthalmol.* Sept. Brussels, *Excerpta Medica 12, 9*, nr. **88**, p. C111.

François, J., Verriest, G. & De Rouck, A. (1955) L'achromatopsie congénitale. *Bull. Soc. Belge Ophthal.* **110**, 170–254.

Goodman, G., Ripps, H. & Siegel, I. M. (1963) Cone dysfunction syndromes. *Arch. Ophthal.* **70**, 214–31.

Hansen, E. (1976) The value of tissue paper contrast tests. *Mod. Prob. Ophthal.* **17**, 179–84.

(1979) Typical and atypical monochromacy studied by specific quantitative perimetry. *Acta Ophthal.* **57**, 211–24.

Hansen, E., Frøyshov Larsen, I. & Berg, K. (1976) A familial syndrome of progressive cone dystrophy, degenerative liver disease, endocrine dysfunction and hearing defect. *Acta Ophthal.* **54**, 129–44.

Hansen, E., Seim, T. & Olsen, B. T. (1978) Transient tritanopia experiment in blue cone monochromacy. *Nature* **276**, 390–1.

Hess, R. F., Mullen, K. T., Sharpe, L. T. & Zrenner, E. (1989*a*) The photoreceptors in atypical achromatopsia. *J. Physiol.* **417**, 123–49.

Hess, R. F. Mullen, K. T. & Zrenner, E. (1989*b*) Human photopic vision with only short wavelength cones: post receptoral properties. *J. Physiol.* **417**, 151–72.

Holm, E. & Lodberg, C. V. (1940) A family with total colour-blindness. *Acta Ophthal.* **18**, 224–58.

Jaeger, W. (1953) Typen der inkompletten Achromatopsie. *Ber. Deut. Ophthal. Ges.* **58**, 44–7.

Jaeger, W. & Krastel, H. (1983) Different types of congenital achromatopsia with residual cone functions. A new concept based on detection of remnant cone activities by large field examination of spectral sensitivity. In *Festschrift Jules Francois.* Retinal and chorioretinal Pathology, pp. 57–69. Aeolus Press, Amsterdam.

Jan, J. E., Tze, W. J., Johnston, A. C. & Dunn, H. J. (1976) Familial congenital monochromatism, cataracts and sensorineural deafness. *Am. J. Disabled Child.* **130**, 1349–50.

Krastel, H., Grimm, H., Gøtz, M. L. & Bergdolt, K. (1981*a*) Der Grauglastest am Perimeter Gesichtsfeldbefunde bei herabgesetzter Beleuchtung. *Ber. Deut. Ophthal. Ges.* **78**, 1041–7.

Krastel, H., Jaeger, W. & Blankenagel, A. (1981*b*) Nachweis von Resten eines 'Rot-Rezeptors' unter chromatischer Adaptation bei Patienten mit zunächst typisch erscheinender angeborener totaler Farbenblindheit. *Ber. Deut. Ophthal. Ges.* **78**, 717–26.

Krill, A. E. (1965) Total color blindness and albinism. *Postgrad. Med.* **37**, 279–83.

(1968) The electroretinogram in congenital colour vision defects. In *The clinical value of electroretinography*. ISCERG Symp., Ghent 1966, pp. 205–14. Karges, Basel.

Mollon, J. D., Newcombe, F., Polden, P. G. & Ratcliff, G. (1980) On the presence of three cone mechanisms in a case of total achromatopsia. In *Color vision deficiencies V* (ed. Verriest, G.) Ch. 3, pp. 130–5. (Proc. 5. Symposium of the International Research Group on Colour Vision Deficiencies, London, 26–28 June 1979.) Adam Hilger, Bristol.

Neuhann, T., Krastel, H. & Jaeger, W. (1978) Differential diagnosis of typical and atypical congenital achromatopsia. *Albrecht von Graefes Arch. Klin. Exp. Ophthal.* **209**, 19–28.

Nordström, S. & Polland, W. (1980) Different expressions of one gene for congenital achromatopsia with amblyopia in northern Sweden. *Human Hered.* **30**, 122–8.

Norn, M. S. (1968) Achromatopsia. *Acta Ophthal.* **46**, 553–6.

Pitt, F. H. G. (1944) Monochromatism. *Nature* **154**, 466–8.

Sloan, L. L. (1954) Congenital achromatopsia: A report of 19 cases. *J. opt. Soc. Am.* **44**, 117–28.

Sloan, L. L. & Feiock, K. (1972) Acuity-luminance function in achromatopsia and in progressive cone degeneration: Factors related to individual differences in tolerance to bright light. *Invest. Ophthal. Visual Sci.* **11**, 862–8.

Smith, V. C. & Pokorny, J. (1980) Cone dysfunction syndromes defined by colour vision. In *Color vision deficiencies V* (ed. Verriest, G.), pp. 69–82. (Proc. 5. Symposium of the International Research Group on Colour Vision Deficiencies. London, 26–28 June 1979). Adam Hilger, Bristol.

Weale, R. A. (1953) Cone-monochromatism. *J. Physiol.* **121**, 548–69.

Weder, W. (1975) Spezielle Brillenverordnung bei Achromatopsie, *Klin. Monatsbl. Augenheil.* **166**, 380–3.

Young, R. S. L., Krefman, R. A. & Fishman, G. A. (1982) Visual improvement with red-tinted glasses in a patient with cone dystrophy. *Arch. Ophthal.* **100**, 268–71.

Chapter 10

Aguilar, M. & Stiles, W. S. (1954) Saturation of the rod mechanism of the retina at high levels of stimulation. *Optica Acta* **1**, 59–65.

Alexandridris, E. (1970) Spektrale Empfindlichkeit der Pupillenlichtreflexe eines Stäbchenmonochromaten. *Bericht über die 70. Zusammenkunft der*

Deutschen Ophthalmologischen Gesellschaft in Heidelberg 1969, pp. 580–3. J. F. Bergmann, Munich.

Alexandridis, E. & Dodt, E. (1967) Pupillenlichtreflexe und Pupillenweite einer Stäbchenmonochromatin. *Albrecht v. Graefes Arch. klin. exp. Ophthal.* **173**, 153–61.

Alpern, M. (1971) Effects of a bright light flash on dark adaptation of human rods. *Nature* **230**, 394–6.

(1974) What is it that confines in a world without color? *Invest. Ophthal.* **13**, 648–74.

Alpern, M., Ching. C. C. & Kitahara, K. (1983) The directional sensitivity of retinal rods. *J. Physiol.* **343**, 577–92.

Alpern, M., Falls, H. F. & Lee, G. B. (1960) The enigma of typical total monochromacy. *Am. J. Ophthal.* **50**, 996–1012.

Alpern, M., Lee, G. B., Maaseidwaag, F. & Miller, S. S. (1971) Colour vision in blue-cone monochromacy. *J. Physiol.* **212**, 211–33.

van Assen, E. C. H. (1960) The role of electroretinography in the diagnosis of total colour blindness. *Opthalmologica, Basel* **139**, 494–6.

Auerbach, E. & Kripke, B. (1974) Achromatopsia with amblyopia. II: A psychophysical study of 5 cases. *Documenta Ophthal.* **37**, 119–44.

Auerbach, E. & Merin, S. (1974) Achromatopsia with amblyopia. I: A clinical and electroretinographical study of 39 cases. *Documenta Ophthal.* **37**, 79–117.

Baker, H. D. & Donovan, W. J. (1982) Early dark adaptation, the receptor potential and lateral effects on the retina. *Vision Res.* **22**, 645–51.

Baloh, R. W., Yee, R. D. & Honrubia, V. (1980) Optokinetic asymmetry in patients with maldeveloped foveas. *Brain Res.* **186**, 211–16.

Barbel, I. (1938) Über angeborene Achromatopsie. *Vestn. Ofthal.* **13**, 598–612.

Barlow, H. B. (1958) Temporal and spatial summation in human vision at different background intensities. *J. Physiol.* **141**, 337–50.

Baylor, D. A., Nunn, B. J. & Schnapf, J. L. (1984) The photocurrent, noise and spectral sensitivity of rods of the monkey Macaca fascicularis. *J. Physiol.* **357**, 575–607.

Berson, E. L., Gouras, P. & Hoff, M. (1969) Temporal aspects of the electroretinogram. *Arch. Ophthal.* **81**, 207.

Best, F. (1917) Untersuchungen über die Dunkelanpassung des Auges mit Leuchtfarben (Mit Beitrag zur Bunt-farbenblindheit und Nachtblindheit). *Biol.* **68**, 119–46.

Blackwell, H. R. & Blackwell, O. M. (1961) Rod and cone receptor mechanisms in typical and atypical congenital achromatopsia. *Vision Res.* **1**, 62–107.

Blakemore, C. B. & Rushton, W. A. H. (1965) Dark adaptation and increment threshold in a rod monochromat. *J. Physiol.* **181**, 612–28.

Bunge, E. (1936) Totale Farbenblindheit, Hemeralopie, Tapetoretinal Degeneration bei zwei Geschwistern. *Klin. Monatsbl. Augenheil.* **97**, 243–51.

Conner, J. (1982) The temporal properties of rod vision. *J. Physiol.* **332**, 139–55.

Conner, J. & MacLeod, D. I. A. (1977) Rod photoreceptors detect rapid flicker. *Science* **195**, 698–9.

Crawford, B. H. (1937) The luminous efficiency of light entering the eye pupil at different points and its relation to brightness threshold measurements. *Proc. R. Soc. Lond.* B **124**, 81–96.

Daw, N. W. & Enoch, J. (1973) Contrast sensitivity, Westheimer function and Stiles-Crawford effect in a blue-cone monochromat. *Vision Res.* **13**, 1669–80.

Dell'Osso, L. F. & Daroff, R. B. (1975) Congenital nystagmus waveforms and foveation strategy. *Documenta Ophthal.* **39**, 155–82.

Dodt, E., van Lith, G. H. M. & Schmidt, B. (1967) Electroretinographic evaluation of the photopic malfunction in a totally colour blind. *Vision Res.* **7**, 231–41.

Dodt, E. & Wadensten, L. (1954) The use of flicker electroretinography in the human eye. Observations on some normal and pathological retinae. *Acta ophthal. (København)* **32**, 165–80.

Donner, K. O. & Rushton, W. A. H. (1959) Rod–cone interaction in the frog's retina analyzed by the Stiles–Crawford effect and by dark adaptation. *J. Physiol.* **149**, 303–17.

Elenius, V. & Heck, J. (1957) Relation of size of ERG to rhodopsin concentration in normal human beings and one total colour blind. *Nature* **180**, 810.

Elenius, V. & Zewi, M. (1958) Flicker electroretinography in 6 cases of total colour-blindness. *Acta Ophthal. (København)* **36**, 19–25.

Engelking, E. (1921) Über die Pupillenreaktion bei angeborenen Farbenblindheit, ein Beitrag zum Problem der pupillorischer Aufnahmenorgane. *Klin. Monatsbl. Augenheil. augenärzt. Fortbild.* **66**, 707–18.

(1922) Vergleichende Untersuchungen über die Pupillenreaktion bei der angeborenen totalen Farbenblindheit. *Klin. Monatsbl. Augenheil. augenärzt. Fortbild.* **69**, 177–8.

Fach, C. & Sharpe, L. T. (1988) Rod increment and flicker thresholds measured on backgrounds of different wave-length. *Invest. Ophthal. Visual Sci.* **29**, 59.

Falls, H. F., Wolter, J. R. & Alpern, M. (1965) Typical total monochromacy. *Arch. Ophthal.* **74**, 610–16.

Ferguson, W. & MacGregor, A. (1949) Four cases of congenital total colour-blindness, with otosclerosis and hypertension as associated hereditary conditions. *Trans. opthal. Soc. (United Kingdom)* **69**, 249–63.

Flamant, F. & Stiles, W. S. (1948) The directional and spectral sensitivities of the retinal rods to adapting fields of different wavelengths. *J. Physiol.* **107**, 187–202.

Franceschetti, A., Jaeger, W., Klein, D., Ohrt, V. & Rickli, H. (1958) Étude patho-physiologique de la grande famille d'achromates de l'île de Fur (Danemark). Déescription d'une nouvelle famille avec achromatopsie totale chez le fins aîné et achromatopsie incomplète chez le frère cadet. *XVIII Concilium ophthalmologicum, Belgica*, Vol. II, pp. 1582–8.

François, J., De Rouck, A. & Verriest, G. (1963) L'electroretinographie dans les dyschromatopsies et dans l'achromatopsie. *Opthalmologica* **146**, 87–100.

François, J., Verriest, G. & De Rouck, A. (1955) L'achromatopsie congenitale. *Documenta Ophthal.* **9**, 338–424.

François, J., Verriest, G. & De Rouck, A. (1956). Pathology of the x-wave of the human ERG-red blindness and other congenital functional abnormalities. *Br. J. Ophthal.* **40**, 439–43.

François, J., Verriest, G. & Renard, G. (1959) L'achromatopsie congenitale typique et son diagnostic clinique. *Arch. ophthal. (Paris)* **19**, 245–56.

Frey, R. G., Heilig, P. & Thayer, A. (1973) Die Dunkeladaptation der Achromaten. *Graefes Archiv* **186**, 55–65.

Fuortes, M. G. F., Gunkel, R. D. & Rushton, W. A. H. (1961) Increment thresholds in a subject deficient in cone vision. *J. Physiol.* **156**, 179–92.

Galezowski, X. (1868) *Du diagnostic des Maladies des Yeux par la Chromatoscopie rétinienne: Précéde d'une Etude sur les Lois Physiques et Physiologiques des Couleurs.* J. B. Baillière et Fils, Paris.

Glickstein, M. & Heath, G. G. (1975) Receptors in the monochromat eye. *Vision Res.* **15**, 633–6.

Goodman, G. & Bornschein, H. (1957) Comparative electroretinographic studies in congenital night blindness and total colour blindness. *Arch. Ophthal.* **58**, 174–82.

Goodman, G., Ripps, H. & Siegel, I. M. (1963) Cone dysfunction syndromes. *Arch. Ophthal.* **70**, 214–31.

Harrison, R., Hoefnagel, D. & Hayward, J. N. (1960) Congenital total color blindness, a clinicopathological report. *Arch. Ophthal.* **64**, 685–92.

Hayhoe, M. M., MacLeod, D. I. A. & Bruch, T. A. (1976) Rod–cone independence in dark adaptation. *Vision Res.* **16**, 591–600.

Hecht, S. & Mintz, E. U. (1939) The visibility of single lines at various illuminations and the retinal basis of visual resolution. *J. gen. Physiol.* **22**, 593–612.

Hecht, S. & Shlaer, S. (1936) Intermittent stimulation by light. V. The relation between intensity and cortical frequency for different parts of the spectrum. *J. gen. Physiol.* **19**, 965–79.

Hecht, S., Shlaer, S., Smith, E. L., Haig, C. & Peskin, J. C. (1938) The visual functions of a completely colourblind person. *Br. J. Physiol.* **123**, 94–5.

Hecht, S., Shlaer, S., Smith, E. L., Haig, C. & Peskin, J. C. (1948) The visual functions of the completely colourblind. *J. gen. Physiol.* **31**, 459–72.

Hess, C. (1902) Weitere Untersuchungen über totale Farbenblindheit. *Z. Physiol. Psychol. Sinnesorgane* **29**, 99–117.

Hess, C. & Hering, E. (1898) Untersuchungen an total Farbenblinden. *Pflügers Archiv ges. Physiol.* **71**, 105–27.

Hess, R. F., Mullen, K. T., Sharpe, L. T. & Zrenner, E. (1989) The photoreceptors in atypical achromatopsia. *J. Physiol.* **417**, 123–49.

Hess, R. F. & Nordby, K. (1986*a*) Spatial and temporal limits of vision in the achromat. *J. Physiol.* **371**, 365–85.

Hess, R. F. & Nordby, K. (1986*b*) Spatial and temporal properties of human rod vision in the achromat. *J. Physiol.* **371**, 387–406.

Hess, R. F. Nordby, K. & Pointer, J. S. (1987) Regional variation of contrast sensitivity across the retina of the achromat: Sensitivity of human rod vision. *J. Physiol.* **388**, 101–19.

Jaeger, W. & Krastel, H. (1981) Complete and incomplete congenital achromatopsia in one sibship. *Neurogenetics and Neeuro-opthalmology*. (eds. Huber, A. & Klein, D.), pp. 241–5. North-Holland Biomedical, Elsevier.

Jayle, G. E., Boyer, R. & Aubert, L. (1962) L'achromatopsie congenitale typique et son expression electro-retinographique. *Ann. Oculist* **195**, 193–204.

Keunen, J. E. E., van Meel, G. J. & van Norren, D. (1988) Rod densitometry in night blindness: a review and two puzzling cases. *Documental Ophthal.* **68**, 375–87.

Klingaman, R. L. (1977) A comparison of psychophysical and VECP increment threshold functions of a rod monochromat. *Invest. Ophthal. Visual Sci.* **16**, 870–3.

(1979) Light adaptation in a normal and a rod monochromat: psychophysical and VEP increment threshold. *Vision Res.* **19**, 825–9.

Kolycev, N. (1940) Zur frage der Achromasie. *Vestn. Oftalm.* **17**, 87.

König, A. (1894) Über den menschlichen Sehpurpur und seine Bedeutung für das Sehen. *Akad. Wissensch. (Berlin) Sitzungsber.*, pp. 577–98.

Krastel, H., Jaeger, W. & Blankenagel, A. (1983) Zapfenrestaktivitäten bei verschiedenen Typen angeborener totaler Farbenblindheit. *Fortsch. Ophthal.* **79**, 499–502.

Kries, J. von (1897*a*) Über das Sehen der total farben-blinde Netzhautzone. *Centralbl. Physiol.* **10**, 148–52.

(1897*b*) Über Farbensysteme. *Z. Physiol. Psychol. Sinnesorgane* **14**, 241.

Krill, A. E. (1966) The electroretinogram in congenital color vision defects. In *The clinical value of electroretinography, ISCERG Symposium, Ghent*, pp. 205–14. Karger, Basel.

(1972) Abnormal color vision. In *The assessment of visual function* (ed. Potts, A. M.), pp. 136–57. C. V. Mosby, Saint Louis.

(1977) Congenital color vision defects. In *Krill's hereditary retinal and choroidal diseases, Vol. II, Clinical characteristics* (eds. Krill, A. A. & Archer, D. B.), pp. 355–90. Harper and Row, Hagerstown, Penn.

Krill, A. E., Deutman, A. F. & Fishman, M. (1973) The cone-degenerations. *Documenta Ophthal.* **35**, 1–80.

Larsen, H. (1921*a*) Demonstration mikroskopischer Präparate von einem monochromatischen Auge. *Klin. Monatsbl. Augenheil.* **67**, 301–2.

(1921*b*) Demonstration mikroskopisher Präparate von einem monochromatischen Auge. *Opthalmologica* **46**, 228–9.

Lewis, S. D. & Mandelbaum, J. (1943) Achromatopsia: report of three cases. *Arch. Ophthal.* **30**, 225–31.

van Loo, J. A. & Enoch, J. M. (1975) The scotopic Stiles–Crawford effect. *Vision Res.* **15**, 1005–9.

Lowenstein, O. & Lowenfeld, I. E. (1969) The pupil. In *The eye, Vol. 3* (2nd edn) (ed. Davson, H.), pp. 255–337. Academic, New York.

MacLeod, D. I. A. (1972) Rods cancel cones in flicker. *Nature* **235**, 173–4.

(1974) Signals from rods and cones. Ph.D. dissertation: University of Cambridge.

Nagel, W. (1911) Adaptation, twilight vision and the duplicity theory. In H. von Helmholtz, *Treatise on physiological optics* appendix to Vol. II (translated from the 3rd German edition and edited by James P. C. Southall), Dover Publications, Ltd., New York, 1962, pp. 313–94.

von Noorden, G. K., Allen, L. & Burian, H. M. (1959) A photographic method for the determination of the behavior of fixation. *Am. J. Ophthal.* **48**, 511–14.

Nordby, K. & Sharpe, L. T. (1988) The directional sensitivity of the photoreceptors in the human achromat. *J. Physiol.* **399**, 267–81.

Nordby, K., Stabell, B. & Stabell, U. (1984) Dark adaptation of the human rod system. *Vision Res.* **24**, 841–9.

van Norren, D. & van der Kraats, J. (1981) A continuously recording retinal densitometer. *Vision Res.* **21**, 897–905.

Pabst, W. & Echte, K. (1962) Unterschiedsempfindlichkeitsschwelle bei Achromaten bestimmt mit hilf des Electroretinogramms. *Act Ophthal.* **70** (Suppl.), 168.

Peskin, J. (1954) Visual function of complete colorblinds. *J. appl. Physiol.* **6**, 660–6.

Pokorny, J., Smith, V. C., Pinckers, A. J. L. G. & Cozijnsen, M. (1982) Classification of complete and incomplete autosomal recessive achromatopsia. *Graefe's Arch. clin. exp. Opthal.* **219**, 121–30.

Polyak, S. L. (1941) *The retina.* University of Chicago Press, Chicago.

Ripps, H., Mehaffy, J. & Siegel, I. M. (1981) Rhodopsin kinetics in the cat retina. *J. gen. Physiol.* **77**, 317–34.

Rushton, W. A. H. (1961) Dark-adaptation and the regeneration of rhodopsin. *J. Physiol.* **156**, 166–78.

Sakitt, B. (1976*a*) Psychophysical correlates of photoreceptor activity. *Vision Res.* **16**, 129–41.

Sakitt, B. (1976*b*) Iconic memory. *Psychol. Rev.* **83**, 257–280.

Schappert-Kimmijser, J. (1958) Value of electroretinography in cases of doubtful diagnosis in the blind and partially sighted child. 138th meeting of the Netherlands Opthalmological Society (1956). *Ophthalmological (Basel)* **135**, 147–54.

Schultze, M. (1866) Zur Anatomie und Physiologie der Retina. *Arch. Mikrosk. Anatomie (Entwicklungs.)* **2**, 175–286.

(1867) Über Stäbchen und Zapfen der Retina. *Arch. Mikrosk. Anatomie (Entwicklungs.)* **3**, 215–47.

Sharpe, L. T., van den Berge, K., van der Tweel, L. H. & Nordby, K. (1988) The pupillary light reflex in a complete achromat. *Clin. Vis. Sci.* **3**, 267–71.

Sharpe, L. T., Collewijn, H. & Nordby, K. (1986) Fixation, pursuit and optokinetic nystagmus in a complete achromat. *Clin. Vis. Sci.* **1**, 39–49.

Sharpe, L. T., Fach, C. & Nordby, K. (1988*a*) Temporal summation in the achromat. *Vision Res.* **28**, 1263–9.

Sharpe, L. T., Fach, C., Nordby, K. & Stockman, A. (1989*a*) The incremental threshold of the rod visual system and Weber's law. *Science* **244**, 354–6.

Sharpe, L. T., van Norren, D. & Nordby, K. (1988*b*) Pigment regeneration, visual adaptation and spectral sensitivity in the achromat. *Clin. Vis. Sci.* **3**, 9–17.

Sharpe, L. T., Stockman, A. & MacLeod, D. I. A. (1989*b*) Rod flicker perception: scotopic duality, phase lags and destructive interference. *Vision Res.* **29**, 1539–59.

Skottun, B. C., Nordby, K. & Magnussen, S. (1980) Rod monochromat sensitivity to sine wave flicker at luminances saturating the rods. *Invest. Ophthal. Visual Sci.* **19**, 108–11.

Sloan, L. L. (1954) Congenital achromatopsia: A report of 19 cases. *J. opt. Soc. Am.* **44**, 117–28.

(1958) The photopic retinal receptors of the typical achromat. *Am. J. Ophthal.* **46**, 81–6.

Sloan, L. L. & Feiock, K. (1972) Acuity-luminance function in adaptation and in progressive cone degeneration: Factors related to individual differences in tolerance to bright light. *Invest. Ophthal. Visual Sci.* **11**, 862–8.

Sloan, L. L. & Newhall, S. M. (1942) Comparison of cases of atypical and typical achromatopsia. *Am. J. Opthal.* **25**, 940–61.

Smith, V. C., Pokorny, J. & van Norren, D. (1983) Densitometric measurement of human cone photopigment kinetics. *Vision Res.* **23**, 517–24.

Snyder, M. (1929) An experimental study of four cases of color-blindness. *Am. J. Psychol.* **41**, 398–411.

Stabell, B., Nordby, K. & Stabell, U. (1987) Light-adaptation of the human rod system. *Clin. Vis. Sci.* **2**, 83–91.

Stabell, U., Stabell, B. & Nordby, K. (1986) Dark-adaptation in a rod monochromat: Effect of stimulus size, exposure time and retinal eccentricity. *Clin. Vis. Sci.* **1**, 75–80.

Stiles, W. S. (1937) The luminous efficiency of monochromatic rays entering the eye pupil at different points and a new colour effect. *Proc. R. Soc. Lond.* B. **123**, 90–118.

(1939) The directional sensitivity of the retina and the spectral sensitivities of rods and cones. *Proc. R. Soc. Lond.* B **127**, 64–105.

Stiles, W. S., & Crawford, B. H. (1933) The luminous efficiency of rays entering the eye pupil at different points. *Proc. R. Soc. Lond.* B. **112**, 428–50.

Stockman, A., Sharpe, L. T., Fach, C. & Nordby, K. (1990) Self-cancelling rod flicker: slow and fast pathways in the human rod visual system. (Submitted)

van der Tweel, L. H. & Spekreijse, H. (1973) Psychophysics and electrophysiology of a rod achromat. *Documenta Ophthalmologica Proceedings Series, Xth I.S.C.E.R.G. Symposium*, pp. 163–73.

Vukovich, V. (1952) Das ERG des Achromaten. *Ophthalmological (Basel)* **124**, 354–9.

Waardenburg, P. J. (1930) Zu meiner Mitteilung über 'Kombination von angeborener Achromatopsie und Atrophia retina pigmentosa'. *Klin. Monatsbl. Augenheil.* **85**, 270–1.

(1963) Achromatopsia congenita. In *Genetics and ophthalmology*, *Vol. II* (eds. Waardenburg, P. J., Franceschetti, A. & Klein, D.), pp. 1695–1718. Royal van Gorcum, Assen, Netherlands.

Wadensten, L. (1954) Flicker electroretinography in some cases of total colourblindness. *Acta Ophthal. (København)* **32**, 743–4.

Walls, G. L. & Heath, G. G. (1954) Typical total color blindness reinterpreted. *Acta Ophthal.* **32**, 253–97.

Westheimer, G. (1967) Dependence of the magnitude of the Stiles–Crawford effect on retinal location. *J. Physiol.* **192**, 309–15.

Wølfflin, E. (1924) Über angeborene totale Farbenblindheit. *Klin. Monatsbl. Augenheil.* **72**, 1–8.

Wyszecki, G. & Stiles, W. S. (1982) *Color science: concepts and methods, quantitative data and formulas* (2nd edn.) John Wiley, New York.

Yee, R. D., Baloh, R. W. & Honrubia, V. (1981) Eye movement abnormalities in rod monochromacy. *Opthalmology* **88**, 1010–18.

Yee, R. D., Baloh, R. W. & Honrubia, V. & Jenkins, H. A. (1982) Pathophysiology of optokinetic nystagmus. In *Nystagmus and vertigo: clinical approaches to the patient with dizziness* (eds. Honrubia, V. & Brazier, M.), pp. 251–75. Academic Press, New York.

Yee, R. D., Farley, M. K., Bateman, J. B. & Martin, D. A. (1985) Eye movement abnormalities in rod monochromatism and blue-cone monochromatism. *Albrecht v. Graefe's Arch. klin. exp. Ophthal.* **223**, 55–9.

Yonemura, D. & Aoki, T. (1960) Electroretinal dark adaptation curve of one totally colour blind eye. *J. clin. Ophthal.* **14**, 429–32.

Chapter 11

Adelson, E. H. (1982) Saturation and adaptation in the rod system. *Vision Res.* **22**, 1299–1312.

Aguilar, M. & Stiles, W. S. (1954) Saturation of the rod mechanism of the retina at high levels of stimulation. *Optica Acta* **1**, 59–65.

Alpern M., Falls, H. & Lee, G. (1960) The enigma of typical total monochromacy. *Am. J. Ophthal.* **50**, 965–1012.

Barlow, H. B., Fitzhugh, R. & Kuffler, S. W. (1957) Change in organization in the receptive fields of the cat's retina during dark adaptation. *J. Physiol.* **137**, 338–54.

Baylor, D. A., Nunn, B. J. & Schnapf, J. L. (1984) The photocurrent, noise and spectral sensitivity of rods of the monkey *Macaca Fascicularis*. *J. Physiol.* **357**, 575–67.

Bisti, S., Clement, R., Maffei, L. & Mecacci, L. (1977) Spatial frequency and orientation tuning curves of visual neurones of the cat: effects of mean luminance. *Exp. Brain Res.* **27**, 335–45.

Blakemore, C. B. & Rushton, W. A. H. (1965) Dark adaptation and increment threshold in a rod monochromat. *J. Physiol.* **181**, 612–28.

Conner, J. D. (1982) The temporal properties of rod vision. *J. Physiol.* **332**, 139–55.

Conner, J. D. & MacLeod, D. I. A. (1977) Rod photoreceptors detect rapid flicker. *Science* **195**, 698–9.

Daw, N. W. & Enoch, J. M. (1973) Contrast sensitivity, Westheimer function and Stiles–Crawford effect in a blue cone monochromat. *Vision Res.* **13**, 1669–80.

D'Zmura, M. & Lennie, P. (1986) Shared pathways for rod and cone vision. *Vision Res.* **26**, 1273–80.

Enroth-Cugell, C. & Robson, J. G. (1966) The contrast sensitivity of retinal ganglion cells in the cat. *J. Physiol.* **187**, 517–52.

Enroth-Cugell, C. & Shapley, R. M. (1973) Flux, not retinal illumination is what cat retinal ganglion cells really care about. *J. Physiol.* **233**, 311–26.

Falls, H. F., Walter, J. R. & Alpern, M. (1965) Typical total monochromacy. *Arch. Ophthal.* **74**, 610–6.

Fuortes, M. G. F., Gunkel, R. D. & Rushton, W. A. H. (1961) Increment thresholds in a subject deficient in cone vision. *J. Physiol.* **156**, 179–92.

Glickstein, M. & Heath, G. G. (1975) Receptors in the monochromat eye. *Vision Res.* **15**, 633–6.

Gouras, P. & Link, K. (1966) Rod and cone interaction in dark-adapted monkey ganglion cells. *J. Physiol.* **182**, 499–510.

Graham, N. (1972) Spatial frequency channels in the human visual system: Effect of luminance and pattern drift. *Vision Res.* **12**, 53–68.

Green, D. G. (1972) Visual acuity in the blue cone monochromat. *J. Physiol.* **222**, 419–26.

Harrison, R., Hofnagel, D. & Hayward, J. N. (1960) Congenital total colour blindness. *Arch. Ophthal.* **64**, 685–92.

Hecht, S. & Shlaer, S. (1936) Intermittent stimulation by light. V. The relation between intensity and critical frequency for different parts of the spectrum. *J. gen. Physiol.* **19**, 965–79.

Hess, R. F. & Nordby, K. (1981) Rod monochromacy – spatio-temporal considerations. *Perception* **1**(1), 22.

Hess, R. F. & Nordby, K. (1986*a*) Spatial and temporal limits of vision in the achromat. *J. Physiol.* **371**, 365–85.

Hess, R. F. & Nordby, K. (1986*b*) Spatial and temporal properties of human rod vision in the achromat. *J. Physiol.* **371**, 387–406.

Hess, R. F., Nordby, K. & Pointer, J. S. (1987) Regional variation of contrast sensitivity across the retina of the achromat: sensitivity of human rod vision. *J. Physiol.* **388**, 101–19.

Hess, R. F. & Plant, G. T. (1985) Temporal frequency discrimination in human vision. Evidence for an additional mechanism in the low spatial, high temporal range. *Vision Res.* **25**, 1493–1500.

Kranda, K. & Kulikowski, J. J. (1976) Adaptation to coarse gratings under scotopic and photopic conditions. *J. Physiol.* **257**, 35.

Larsen, H. (1921*a*) Demonstration mikroskopischer praparate von einem monochromatische Auge. *Klin Monats fur Augen.* **67**, 301–2.

Larsen, H. (1921*b*) Demonstration mikroskopischer praparate von einem monochromatische Auge. *Ophthalmologia* **46**, 228–9.

Nordby, K. & Sharpe, L. T. (1988) The directional sensitivity of the photoreceptors in the human achromat. *J. Physiol.* **399**, 267–81.

Osterberg, G. (1935) Topography of the layer of rods and cones in the human retina. *Acta Ophthal. (Suppl.)* **6**, 1–102.

Perry, V. H. & Cowey, A. (1984) Retinal ganglion cells that project to the superior colliculus and pretectum in the Macaque monkey. *Neurosci* **12**, 1125–37.

Pointer, J. S. & Hess, R. F. (1989). The contrast sensitivity gradient across the human visual field: with exphasis on the low spatial frequency range. *Vision Res.* **29**, 1133–51.

Robson, J. G. & Graham, N. (1981) Probability summation and regional variation in contrast sensitivity across the visual field. *Vision Res.* **21**, 409–18.

Sakitt, B. (1976) Psychophysical correlates of photoreceptor activity. *Vision Res.* **16**, 129–40.

Sharpe, L. T., Stockman, A. & MacLeod, D. I. A. (1989) Rod flicker perception: scotopic duality, phase lags and destructive interference. *Vision Res.* **29**, 1539–59.

Watson, A. B. & Robson, J. G. (1981) Discrimination at threshold: labelled detectors in human vision. *Vision Res.* **21**, 1115–22.

Chapter 12

Aguirre, G. (1976) Inherited retinal degenerations in the dog. *Trans. Am. Acad. Ophthal. Otolaryngol.* **81**, 667–76.

(1978) Retinal degenerations of the dog. I. Rod dysplasia. *Exp. Eye Res.* **26**, 233–53.

Aguirre, G., Farber, D., Lolley, R., Fletcher, R. T. & Chader, G. J. (1978) Rod–cone dysplasia in Irish setters: A defect in cyclic GMP metabolism in visual cells. *Science* **201**, 1133–4.

Aguirre, G., Farber, D., Lolley, R., O'Brien, P., Alligood, S., Fletcher, T. & Chader, G. (1982) Retinal degenerations in the dog. III. Abnormal cyclic nucleotide metabolism in rod–cone dysplasia. *Exp. Eye Res.* **35**, 625–42.

Aguirre, G. & O'Brien, P. (1986) Morphological and biochemical studies of canine progressive rod–cone degeneration. *Invest. Opthal. Visual Sci.* **27**, 635–55.

Aguirre, G., O'Brien, P., Alligood, J. & Buyukmihci, N. (1982) Pathogensis of progressive rod–cone degeneration in the miniature poodle. *Invest. Ophthal. Visual Sci.* **23**, 610–30.

Aguirre, G. D. & Rubin, L. F. (1971) Progressive retinal atrophy (rod dysplasia) in the Norwegian elkhound. *J. Am. vet. Med. Ass.* **158**, 208–17.

Aguirre, G. D. & Rubin, L. F. (1975) Rod–cone dysplasia (progressive retinal atrophy) in Irish setters. *J. Am. vet. Med. Ass.* **166**, 157–64.

Alpern, M., Holland, M. G. & Ohba, N. (1972) Rhodopsin bleaching signals in essential night blindness. *J. Physiol.* **225**, 457–76.

Arden, G. B. & Fojas, M. R. (1962) Electrophysiological abnormalities in pigmentary degenerations of the retina. *Arch. Ophthal.* **68**, 369–89.

Armington, J. C. & Schwab, A. J. (1954) Electroretinogram in nyctalopia. *Arch. Ophthal.* **523**, 725–33.

Auerbach, E., Godel, V. & Rowe, H. (1969) An electrophysiological study of two forms of congenital night blindness. *Invest. Ophthal.* **8**, 332–45.

Bennett, N., Michel-Villaz, M. & Kuhn, H. (1982) Light-induced interaction between rhodopsin and the GTP-binding protein. *Eur. J. Biochem.* **127**, 97–103.

Berman, E. R., Horowitz, J., Segal, N., Fisher, S. & Feeney-Burns, L. (1980) Enzymatic esterification of vitamin A in the pigment epithelium of bovine retina. *Biochim. biophys. Acta* **630**, 36–46.

Berson, E. L. (1980) Light deprivation and retinitis pigmentosa. *Vision Res.* **20**, 1179–84.

Berson, E. L. (1982) Nutritional and retinal degenerations: Vitamin A, taurine, ornithine, and phytanic acid. *Retina* **2**, 236–55.

Berson, E. L., Gouras, P. & Hoff, M. (1969) Temporal aspects of the electroretinogram. *Arch. Ophthal.* **81**, 207–14.

Berson, E. L., Shih, V. E. & Sullivan, P. L. (1981) Ocular findings in patients with gyrate atrophy on pyridoxine and low-protein, low-arginine diets. *Opthalmology* **88**, 311–15.

Bhattacharya, S. S., Clayton, J. F., Harper, P. S., Hoare, G. W., Jay, M. R., Lyness, A. L. & Wright, A. F. (1985) A genetic linkage study of a kindred with X-linked retinitis pigmentosa. *Br. J. Ophthal.* **69**, 340–7.

Bok, D. & Heller, J. (1976) Transport of retinol from the blood to the retina: an autoradiographic study of the pigment epithelial cell surface receptor for plasma retinol-binding protein. *Exp. Eye Res.* **22**, 395–402.

Bridges, C. D. B. & Alvarez, R. A. (1982) Selective loss of 11-cis vitamin A in an eye with hereditary chorioretinal degeneration similar to sector retinitis pigmentosa. *Retina* **2**, 256–60.

Bridges, C. D. B., O'Gorman, S., Fong, S. L., Alvarez, R. A. & Berson, E. (1985) Vitamin A and interstitial retinol-binding protein in an eye with recessive retinitis pigmentosa. *Invest. Ophthal. Visual Sci.* **26**, 684–91.

Brown, G. C., Felton, S. M. & Benson, W. E. (1980) Reversible night blindness associated with intestinal bypass surgery. *Am. J. Ophthal.* **89**, 776–9.

Bunt-Milam, A. H., Kalina, R. E. & Pagon, R. A. (1983) Clinical–ultrastructural study of a retinal dystrophy. *Invest. Ophthal. Visual Sci.* **24**, 458–69.

Buyukmihci, N., Aguirre, G. & Marshall, J. (1980) Retinal degenerations in the dog. II. Development of the retina in rod–cone dysplasia. *Exp. Eye Res.* **30**, 575–91.

Campo, R. V. & Aaberg, T. M. (1982) Ocular and systemic manifestations of the Bardet-Biedl syndrome. *Arch. Ophthal.* **94**, 750–6.

Carr, R. E. (1969) The night-blinding disorders. *Int. Ophthal. Clincs* **9**, 971–1003.

Carr, R. E., & Gouras, P. (1965) Oguchi's disease. *Arch. Ophthal.* **73**, 646–56.

Carr, R. E., Margolis, S. & Siegel, I. M. (1976) Fluorescein angiography and vitamin A and oxalate levels in fundus albipunctatus. *Am. J. Ophthal.* **82**, 549–58.

Carr, R. E., & Ripps, H. (1967) Rhodopsin kinetics and rod adaptation in Oguchi's disease. *Invest. Ophthal.* **6**, 426–36.

Carr, R. E., Ripps, H. & Siegel, I. M. (1974) Visual pigment kinetics and adaptation in fundus albipunctatus. *Documenta Ophthal. Proc. Ser.* **9**, 193–9.

Carr, R. E., Ripps, H., Siegel, I. M. & Weale, R. A. (1966*a*) Rhodopsin and the electrical activity of the retina in congenital night blindness. *Invest. Ophthal.* **5**, 497–507.

Carr, R. E., Ripps, H., Siegel, I. M. and Weale, R. A. (1966*b*) Visual functions in congenital night blindness. *Invest. Ophthal.* **5**, 508–14.

Carroll, F. & Haig, C. (1952) Congenital stationary night-blindness without ophthalmoscopic or other abnormalities. *Trans. Am. Ophthal. Soc.* **50**, 193–209.

Chatzinoff, A., Nelson, E., Stahl, N. & Clahane, A. (1968) Eleven-cis vitamin A in the treatment of retinitis pigmentosa. *Arch. Ophthal.* **80**, 417–19.

Chew, J.-D., Halliday, F., Keith, G., Sheffield, L., Dickenson, P., Gray, R., Constable, I. & Denton, M. (1989) Linkage heterogeneity between X-linked retinitis pigmentosa and a map of 10 RFLP loci. *Am. J. Hum. Genet.* **45**, 401–11.

Cohen, A. I. (1983) Some cytological and initial biochemical observations on photoreceptors in retinas of rds mice. *Invest. Ophthal. Visual Sci.* **24**, 832–43.

Cutler, C. (1894) Drei ungewohnliche Falle von retinochoroioideal Degeneration. *Arch. Augenheilkd* **30**, 117.

Dewar, J. (1877) The physiologic action of light. *Nature* **15**, 433–5.

Donders, F. (1857) Beitraege Zur pathologischen anatomie des Auges: II. Pigmentbildung in der Netzhaut. *Arch. Ophthal.* **3**, 139–50.

Dowling, J. E. & Gibbons, I. R. (1961) The effect of vitamin A deficiency on the fine structure of the retina. In *The Structure of the Eye* (ed. Smelser, G. K.), pp. 85–99. Academic Press, New York.

Dowling, J. E., & Ripps, H. (1971) Aspartate isolation of receptor potentials in the skate retina. *Biol. Bull.*, **141**, 384–5.

Dowling, J. E. & Ripps, H. (1973) Effect of magnesium on horizontal cell activity in the skate retina. *Nature* **24**, 101–3.

Dowling, J. E. & Sidman, R. L. (1962) Inherited retinal dystrophy in the rat. *J. Cell Biol.* **14**, 73–109.

Dowling, J. E., & Wald, G. (1958) Vitamin A deficiency and night blindness. *Proc. nat. Acad. Sci. U.S.A.* **44**, 648–61.

Edwards, R. B. & Szamier, R. B. (1977) Defective phagocytosis of isolated rod outer segents by RCS rat retinal pigment epithelium in culture. *Science* **197**, 1001–3.

Farber, D. S. (1969) Analysis of slow transretinal potentials in response to light. Ph.D. Thesis, State University of New York, Buffalo, N.Y.

Farber, D. B. & Lolley, R. N. (1974) Cyclic guanosine monophosphate: Elevation in degenerating photoreceptor cells of the C3H mouse retina. *Science*, 186, 449–51.

Farber, D. B. & Shuster, T. A. (1985) A proposed sequence of events leading to photoreceptor degeneration in the rd mouse retina. In *Retinal degeneration: experimental and clinical studies* (ed. La Vail, M. M., Holyfield, J. G. & Anderson, R. E.), pp. 147–57, Alan R. Liss, Inc., New York.

Fesenko, E. E., Kolesnikov, S. S. & Lyubarsky, A. L. (1985) Induction by cyclic GMP of cationic conductance in plasma membrane of retinal rod outer segment. *Nature* **313**, 310–13.

Fishman, G. A. (1975) *The electroretinogram and electro-oculogram in retinal and choroidal disease.* Manual, 1st edn, American Academy of Ophthalmology and Otolaryngology, pp. 9–45, Rochester, Minnesota.

(1980) Hereditary retinal and choroidal disease; Electroretinogram and electro-oculogram findings. In *Principles and practice of ophthalmology*, vol. 2 (eds. Peyman, G. A., Sanders, D. R. & Goldberg, M. F.), pp. 857–904. W. B. Saunders Company, Philadelphia.

Fishman, G. A., Alexander, K. R. & Anderson, R. J. (1985) Autosomal dominant retinitis pigmentosa: A method of classification. *Arch Ophthal.* **103**, 366–74.

Fishman, G. A., Kumar, A., Joseph, M. E., Torok, N. & Anderson, R. J. (1983) Usher's syndrome: Ophthalmic and neuro-otologic findings suggesting genetic heterogeneity. *Arch. Ophthal.* **101**, 1367–74.

François, J., Verriest, G. & de Rouck, A. (1956) Electro-oculography as a functional test in pathological conditions of the fundus: I. First results. *Br. J. Ophthal.* **40**, 108–12.

Fuchs, E. (1896) Ueber Zewi der retinitis pigmentosa verwandte kornkheiten (retinitis punctata albescens und atrophia gyrate chorioideal et retinal). *Arch. Augenhelkd* **32**, 111–16.

Furakawa, T. & Hanawa, I. (1955) Effects of some common cations on electroretinogram of the toad. *Jap. J. Physiol.* **5**, 289–300.

Futterman, S. (1974) Recent studies on a possible mechanism for visual pigment regeneration. *Exp. Eye Res.* **18**, 89–96.

Futterman, S., Swanson, D. & Kalina, R. E. (1974) Retinol in retinitis pigmentosa: evidence that retinol is in normal concentration in serum and the retinol-blinding protein complex displays unaltered fluorescence properties. *Invest. Ophthal.* **13**, 798–801.

Goodman, G., Ripps, H. & Siegel, I. M. (1963*a*) Cone dysfunction syndromes. *Arch. Ophthal.* **70**, 214–31.

Goodman, G., Ripps, H. & Siegel, I. M. (1963*b*) Electroretinography in infants and children. *Int. Ophthal. Clinics* **3**, 777–802.

Gouras, P. & Carr, R. E. (1964) Electrophysiological studies in early retinitis pigmentosa. *Arch. Ophthal.* **72**, 104–10.

Gouras, P. & Carr, R. E. (1965) Light-induced DC responses of monkey retina before and after central retinal artery interruption. *Invest. Ophthal.* **4**, 310–7.

Green, D. G., Dowling, J. E., Siegel, I. M. & Ripps, H. (1975) Retinal mechanisms of visual adaptation in the skate. *J. gen. Physiol.* **65**, 483–502.

Hayasaka, S., Mizuno, K., Yabata, K., Saito, T. & Tada, K. (1982) Atypical gyrate atrophy of the choroid and retina associated with imonoglycinuria. *Arch. Ophthal.* **100**, 423–5.

Hayasaka, S., Saito, T., Nakajima, H., Tabahashi, O. Mizuno, K. & Tada, K. (1985) Clinical trials of vitamin B_6 and proline supplementation for gyrate atrophy of the choroid and retina. *B.J. Ophthal.* **69**, 283–90.

Herron, W. L., Riegel, B. W., Myers, O. E. & Rubin, M. L. (1969) Retinal dystrophy in the rat – a pigment epithelial disease. *Invest. Ophthal. Visual Sci.* **8**, 595–604.

Highman, V. N. & Weale, R. A. (1973) Rhodopsin density and visual threshold in retinitis pigmentosa. *Am. J. Ophthal.* **75**, 822–32.

Hock, P. A. & Marmor, M. F. (1983) Variability of the human c-wave. *Documenta Ophthal. Proc. Ser.* **37**, 151–7.

Hubbard, R. & Kropf, S. (1958) The action of light on rhodopsin. *Proc. natn. Acad. Sci. U.S.A.* **44**, 130–9.

Kaiser-Kupfer, M. I., de Monasterio, F., Valle, D., Walser, M. & Brusilow, S. (1981) Visual results of a long-term trial of a low-arginine diet in gyrate atrophy of choroid and retina. *Ophthalmology* **88**, 307–10.

Kalmus, G. W., Dunson, T. R. & Kalmus, K. C. (1982) The influence of cyclic nucleotides on macromolecular synthesis in cultured neural retinal cells. *Comp. Biochem. Physiol.* **72**C, 129–32.

Kaneko, A. & Shimazaki, H. (1975) Effects of external ions on the synaptic transmission from photoreceptors to horizontal cells in the carp retina. *J. Physiol.* **252**, 509–22.

Karpe, G. (1945) Basis of clinical electroretinography. *Acta Ophthal. Suppl.* **24**, 1–28.

Karwoski, C. J. & Proenza, L. M. (1980) Neurons, potassium, and glia in proximal retina of *Nectarus*. *J. gen. Physiol.* **75**, 141–62.

Kemp, C. M. & Faulkner, D. J. (1981) Rhodopsin measurement in human disease: fundus reflectometry using television. *Dev. Ophthal.* **2**, 130–4.

Kilbride, P. E., Read, J. S., Fishman, G. A. & Fishman, M. (1983) Determination of human cone pigment density difference spectra in spatially resolved regions of the fovea. *Vision Res.* **23**, 1341–50.

Kline, R. R., Ripps, H. & Dowling, J. E. (1978) Generation of b-wave currents in the skate retina. *Proc. natn. Acad. Sci. U.S.A.* **75**, 5727–31.

Kline, R. P., Ripps, H. & Dowling, J. E. (1985) Light-induced potassium fluxes in the skate retina. *Neuroscience* **14**, 225–35.

Kolb, H. & Gouras, P. (1974) Electron microscopic observations of human retinitis pigmentosa, dominantly inherited. *Invest. Ophthal.* **13**, 387–9.

Krachmer, J. H., Smith, J. L. & Tocci, P. M. (1966) Laboratory studies in retinitis pigmentosa. *Arch. Ophthal.* **75**, 661–4.

Krill, A. E. & Martin, D. (1971) Photopic abnormalities in congenital stationary night blindness. *Invest. Ophthal.* **10**, 625–36.

Krinsky, N. I. (1958) The enzymatic esterification of vitamin A. *J. biol. Chem.* **232**, 881–94.

Kuhn, H. & Chabre, M. (1983) Light-dependent interactions between rhodopsin and photoreceptor enzymes. *Biophys. Struct. Mech.* **9**, 231–4.

Kuhne, W. (1878) Zur Photochemie der Netzhaut. *Untersuchungen. Physiol.* Institute University Heidelberg. **1**, 1–14.

Kurstjens, J. H. (1965) Choroideremia and gyrate atrophy of the choroid and retina. *Documenta Ophthal.* **13**, 1–122.

Kuwabara, Y., Ishihara, K. & Akiya, S. (1963) Histopathological and electron microscopic studies of the retina of Oguchi's disease. *Acta Soc. Ophthal. Jap.* **67**, 1323–51.

Lai, Y. L., Wigert, B., Liu, Y. & Chader, G. (1982) Interphotoreceptor retinol-binding proteins: possible transport vehicles between compartments of the retina. *Nature* **298**, 848–9.

LaVail, M. M. (1980) Interaction of environmental light and eye pigmentation with inherited retinal degenerations. *Vision Res.* **20**, 1173–7.

Lewis, R. A., Nusbaum, R. L. & Ferrell, R. F. (1985) Mapping X-linked ophthalmic diseases: Provisional assignment of the locus for choroideremia to Xq13-q24. *Ophthalmology* **92**, 800–6.

Liebman, P. A. & Pugh, E. N., Jr. (1981) Control of rod disk membrane phosphodiesterase and a model of visual transduction. In *Current topics in membranes and transport*, vol. 15, pp. 157–70, Academic Press, New York.

Liou, G. I., Bridges, C. D. B., Fong, S. L., Alvarez, R. A. & Gonzalez-Fernandez, F. (1982) Vitamin A transport between retina and pigment epithelium – an interstitial protein carrying endogenous retinol (interstitial retinol-binding protein). *Vision Res.* **22**, 1457–67.

Lolley, R. N., Farber, D. B., Rayborn, M. & Hollyfield, J. G. (1977) Cyclic GMP accumulation causes degeneration of photoreceptor cells – simulation of an inherited disease. *Science* **196**, 664–6.

Lyness, A. L., Ernst, W., Quinlan, M. P., Clover, G. M., Arden, G. B., Carter, R. M., Bird, A. C. & Parker, J. A. (1985) A clinical, psychophysica, and electroretinographic survey of patients with autosomal dominant retinitis pigmentosa. *Br. J. Ophthal.* **69**, 326–39.

Main, A. N. H., Mills, P. R., Russell, R. I., Bronte-Stewart, J., Nelson, L. M. McLelland, A. & Shenkin, A. (1983) Vitamin A deficiency in Crohn's disease. *Gut* **24**, 1169–75.

Maraini, G., Fadda, G. & Gozzoli, F. (1975) Serum levels of retinol-binding protein in different genetic types of retinitis pigmentosa. *Invest. Ophthal.* **14**, 236–7.

Massof, R. W. & Finkelstein, D. (1979) Rod sensitivity relative to cone sensitivity in retinitis pigmentosa. *Invest. Ophthal. Visual Sci.* **18**, 263–72.

(1981) Two forms of autosomal dominant primary retinitis pigmentosa. *Documenta Ophthal.* **521**, 289–346.

Massoud, W. H., Bird, A. C. & Perkins, E. S. (1975) Plasma vitamin A and beta-carotene in retinitis pigmentosa. *Br. J. Ophthal.* **59**, 200–4.

Mauthner, L. (1871) Ein fall von choroideremia. *Naturwissenschaften* **2**, 191.

Mullen, R. J. & LaVail, M. M. (1976) Inherited retinal dystrophy: Primary defect in pigment epithelium determined with experimental rat chimeras. *Science* **192**, 799–801.

Musarella, M. A., Burghes, A., Anson-Cartwright, L., Mahtani, M. M., Argonza, R., Tsui, L.-C. & Worton, R. (1988) Localization of the gene for X-linked recessive type of retinitis pigmentosa (XLRP) to Xp 21 by linkage analysis. *Am. J. Hum. Genet.* **43**, 484–94.

Nakatani, K. & Yau, K. W. (1985) cGMP opens the light-sensitive conductance in retinal rods. *Biophys. J.* **47**, 356a.

Narfstrom, K. (1985) Retinal degeneration in a strain of Abyssinian cats: A hereditary, clinical, electrophysiological and morphological study. Linkoping University Medical Dissertations No. 208. Departments of Ophthalmology and Surgery, Linkoping, Sweden.

Newman, E. A. (1980) Current source-density analysis of the b-wave of frog retina. *J. Neurophysiol.* **43**, 1355–66.

Newman, E. A. & Odette, L. L. (1984) Model of electroretinogram b-wave generation: a test of the K^+ hypothesis. *J. Neurophysiol.* **51**, 164–82.

Nussbaum, R. L., Lewis, R. A., Lesko, J. G. & Ferrell, R. (1985) Choroideremia is linked to the restriction fragment length polymorphism DXYSl at Xq13–21. *Am. J. hum. Genet.* **37**, 473–81.

Oguchi, C. (1925) Zur Anatomie der sogenannten Oguchischen Krankheit *Albrecht v. Graefes Arch. Klin. Exp. Ophthal.* **115**, 234–45.

Ong, D. E., Page, D. L. & Chyutil, F. (1975) Retinoic acid binding protein: occurrence in human tumors. *Science* **190**, 60–1.

Ostroy, S. E. (1977) Rhodopsin and the visual process. *Biochim. biophys. Acta* **463**, 91–125.

Owens, D. A. & Leibowitz, H. W. (1976) Night myopia: Cause and a possible basis for amelioration. *Am. J. Optometry physiol. Optics* **53**, 709–17.

Pallin, O. (1969) The influence of the axial length of the eye on the size of the recorded b-potential in the clinical single-flash electroretinogram. *Acta Ophthal.* **202** (suppl), 3–57.

Partamian, L. G., Sidrys, L. A. & Tripathi, R. C. (1979) Iatrogenic night blindness and keratoconjunctval xerosis. *New England J. Medicine* **301**, 943–4.

Penn, R. D. & Hagins, W. A. (1969) Signal transmission along retinal rods and the origin of the electroretinographic a-wave. *Nature* **223**, 201–55.

Perlman, I. & Auerbach, E. (1981) The relationship between visual sensitivity and rhodopsin density in retinitis pigmentosa. *Invest. Ophthal. Visual Sci.* **20**, 758–65.

Perlman, I., Barzilai, D., Haim, T. & Schramek, A. (1983) Night vision in a case of vitamin A deficiency due to malabsorption. *B. J. Opthal.* **67**, 37–42.

Peterson, H. (1968) The normal b-potential in the single-flash clinical electroretinogram. *Acta Ophthal.* **99** (suppl.), 5–77.

Petersen, R. A., Petersen, V. S. & Robb, R. M. (1968) Vitamin A deficiency with xerophthalmia and night blindness in cystic fibrosis. *Am. J. Disabled Child.* **116**, 662–5.

Riggs, L. A. (1941) Continuous and reproducible records of the electrical activity of the human retina. *Proc. Soc. exp. Biol. Med.* **48**, 204–7.

(1954) Electroretinography in cases of night blindness. *Am. J. Ophthal.* **38**, 70–8.

Ripps, H. (1976) Night blindness and the retinal mechanisms of visual adaptation. *Ann. R. Coll. Surgeons England* **58**, 222–32.

(1982) Night blindness revisited: from man to molecules. The Proctor Lecture. *Invest. Ophthal. Visual Sci.* **23**, 588–609.

Ripps, H. Brin, K. P. & Weale, R. A. (1978) Rhodopsin and visual threshold in retinitis pigmentosa. *Invest. Ophthal. Visual Sci.* **17**, 735–45.

Ripps, H., Carr, R. E., Siegel, I. M. & Greenstein, V. C. (1984) Functional abnormalities in vincristine-induced night blindness. *Invest. Ophthal. Visual Sci.* **25**, 787–94.

Ripps, H., Mehaffey, L., Siegel, I. M. & Niemeyer, G. (1989) Vincristine-induced changes in the retina of the isolated arterially-perfused cat eye. *Exp. Eye Res.* **48**, 771–90.

Ripps, H., Shakib, M. & MacDonald, E. D. (1976) Peroxidase uptake by photoreceptor terminals of the skate retina. *J. Cell Biol.* **70**, 85–96.

Ripps, H., Siegel, I. M. & Mehaffey, L. III (1985) The cellular basis of visual dysfunction in hereditary retinal disorders. In *Cell and developmental biology of the eye: heredity and visual development* (eds. Sheffield, J. B. & Hilfer, S. R.), pp. 171–204, Springer-Verlag, New York.

Ripps, H. & Snapper, A. G. (1974) Computer analysis of photochemical changes in the human retina. *Computers Biol. Med.* **4**, 107–22.

Ripps, H. & Weale, R. A. (1965) Analysis of foveal densitometry. *Nature* **205**, 52–6.

Ripps, H. & Weale, R. A. (1969) Rhodopsin regeneration in man. *Nature* **222**, 775–7.

Ripps, H. & Witkovsky, P. (1985) Neuron-Glia Interaction in the Brain and Retina. In *Progress in retinal research*, vol. 4 (ed. Osborne, N. N. & Chader, G. J.) pp. 181–219. Pergamon Press, Oxford.

Rodrigues, M. M., Hackett, J., Gaskings, R., Wiggert, B., Lee, L., Redmond, M. & Chader G. J. (1986) Interphotoreceptor retinoid-binding protein in retinal rod cells and pineal gland. *Invest. Ophthal. Visual Sci.* **27**, 844–50.

Rushton, W. A. H. (1961) Rhodopsin measurement and dark adaptation in a subject deficient in cone vision. *Physiol.* **156**, 193–205.

Sanyal, S., Chader, G. & Aguirre, G. (1985) Expression of retinal degeneration slow (rds) gene in the retina of the mouse. In *Retinal degeneration: experimental and clinical studies* (eds. LaVail, M. M., Hollyfield, J. G. & Anderson, R. E.), pp. 239–56. Alan R. Liss, Inc., New York.

Schmidt, S. Y. & Lolley, R. N. (1973) Cyclic nucleotide phosphodiesterase. An early defect in inherited retinal degeneration of C_3H mice. *J. Cell Biol.* **57**, 117–23.

Schubert, G. & Bornschein, H. (1952) Beitrag zur Analyse des menschlichen Elektroretinogramms. *Ophthalmoligica* **123**, 396–412.

Shih, V. E., Efron, M. L. & Moser, H. W. (1969) Hyperornithinemia, hyperammonemia, and homocitrullinemia. A new disorder of amino acid metabolism associated ith myoclonic seizures and mental retardation. *Am. J. Diseases Child.* **117**, 83–92.

Sieving, P. A., Niffenegger, J. H. & Berson, E. L. (1986) Electroretinographic findings in selected pedigrees with choroideremia. *Am. J. Ophthal.* **101**, 361–7.

Sillman, A. J., Ito, H. & Tomita, T. (1969) Studies on the mass receptor potential of the isolated frog retina. II. On the basis of the ionic mechanism. *Vision Res.* **9**, 1443–51.

Simell, O. & Takki, K. (1973) Raised plasma-ornithine and gyrate atrophy of the choroid and retina. *Lancet* **1**, 1031–3.

Sloan, L. L. (1947) Rate of dark adaptation and regional threshold gradients of the dark-adapted eye: Physiologic and clinical studies. *Am. J. Ophthal.* **30**, 705–20.

Smith, F. R. & Goodman, D. S. (1971) The effect of diseases of the liver, thyroid and kidneys on the transport of vitamin A in human plasma. *J. clin. Invest.* **50**, 2426–36.

Sondheimer, S., Fishman, G. A. Young, R. & Vasquez, V. V. (1979) Dark adaptation testing in heterozygotes of Usher's syndrome. *Br. J. Ophthal.* **63**, 547–50.

Steinberg, R. H., Linsenmeier, R. A. & Griff, E. R. (1983) Three light-evoked responses of the retinal pigment epithelium. *Vision Res.* **23**, 1315–23.

Stiggelbout, W. (1972) The Bardet–Biedl syndrome. In *Handbook of clinical neurology*, vol. 13 (eds. Vinken, P. J. & Bruyn, G. W.), pp. 380–412. American Elsevier Publishing Company, Inc., New York.

Stryer, L. (1986) Cyclic GMP cascade of vision. *A. R. Neurosci.* **9**, 87–119.

Szamier, R. B. & Berson, E. L. (1977) Retinal ultrastructure in advanced retinitis pigmentosa. *Invest. Ophthal. Visual Sci.* **16**, 947–62.

Szamier, R. B., Berson, E. L., Klein, R. & Meyers, S. (1979) Sex-linked retinitis pigmentosa: ultrastructure of photoreceptors and pigment epithelium. *Invest. Opthal. Visual Sci.* **18**, 145–60.

Tamai, M. & O'Brien, P. J. (1979) Retinal dystrophy in the RCS rat. In vivo and in vitro studies of phagocytic action of pigment epithelium on the shed rod outer segments. *Exp. Eye Res.* **28**, 399–411.

Taumer, R., Wichmann, W., Rohde, N. & Rover, J. (1976) ERG of humans without C-wave. *Albrecht v. Graefes Arch. Klin. Exp. Opthal.* **198**, 275–89.

Tranchina, D., Gordon, J. & Shapley, R. M. (1984) Retinal light adaptation – evidence for a feedback mechanism. *Nature* **310**, 314–16.

Ulshafer, R. J. & Hollyfield, J. G. (1982) Cyclic nucleotides alter protein metabolism in the human and baboon retinas. In *Proceedings fourth international symposium on the structure of the eye* (ed. Hollyfield, J. G.), pp. 115–21, Elsevier, Holland.

Valle, D., Walser, M., Brusilow, S., Kaiser-Kupfer, M.I. & Takki, K. (1981) Gyrate atrophy of the choroid and retina. *Ophthalmology* **88**, 325–30.

Wagrcich, H., Lasky, M. A. & Alkan, B. (1961) Some biochemical studies in retinitis pigmentosa. *Clin. Chem.* **7**, 143–8.

Wald, G. (1945) Human vision and the spectrum. *Science* **101**, 653–8.

Witzel, D. A., Smith, E. L., Wilson, R. D. & Aguirre, G. D. (1978) Congenital stationary night blindness: an animal model. *Invest. Ophthal. Visual Sci.* **17**, 78–95.

Weleber, R. G. (1981) The effect of age on human cone and rod ganzfeld electroretinograms. *Invest. Ophthal. Visual Sci.* **20**, 392–9.

Weleber, R. G. & Kennaway, N. G. (1981) Clinical trial of vitamin B_6 for gyrate atrophy of the choroid and retina. *Ophthalmology* **88**, 316–24.

Wolf, D. E., Vainisi, S. J. & Santos-Anderson, R. (1978) Rod–cone dysplasia in the collie. *J. Am. vet. Med. Ass.* **173**, 1331–3.

Woodford, B. J., Chader, G. J., Farber, D. B., Liu, L., Fletcher, R. T., Santos-Anderson, R. & Tso, M. O. M. (1980) Cyclic nucleotides in inherited degeneration in collies. *Invest. Ophthal. Visual Sci. (suppl)* **19**, 249.

Yamanaka, J. (1924) Existiert die Pigmentverschiebung in Retinal-epithel in menschlichen Auge? Der erst Sektionsfall von sogenannter Oguchischer Krankheit. *Klin. Monatsbl. Augenheil* **73**, 742–52.

Yamanaka, J. (1969) Histological study of Oguchi's disease. *Am. J. Ophthal.* **68**, 19–26.

Chapter 13

Barlow, H. B. (1972) Dark and light adaptation: psychophysics. *Handbook of sensory physiolog. Vol. VII-4 Visual psychophysics*, Chapter I, pp. 1–28. Springer Verlag, Berlin.

Biberman, L. A. & Nudelman, S. (1971) *Photoelectronic imaging devices. Vol. 2. Devices and their evaluation.* Plenum Press, New York.

Blackwell, H. R. (1946) Contrast thresholds of the human eye. *J. opt. Soc. Am.* **36**, 624–43.

(1972) Luminance difference thresholds. *Handbook of sensory physiology, Vol. VII-4 Visual psychophysics*, Chapter 4, pp. 78–101. Springer Verlag, Berlin.

Clark Jones, R. (1959) Quantum efficiency of human vision. *J. opt. Soc. Am.* **49**, 645–53.

De Vries, H. (1943) The quantum character of light and its bearing upon threshold of vision, the differential sensitivity and visual acuity of the eye. *Physica* **10**, 553–64.

Engstrom, R. W. (1974) Quantum efficiency of the eye determined by comparison with a TV camera. *J. opt. soc. Am.* **64**, 1706–10.

Hood, D. C. & Finkelstein, M. A. (1986) Sensitivity to light. *Handbook of perception and human performance. Vol. I Sensory processes and perception.* John Wiley, New York.

Köhler, H. & Leinhos, R. (1957) Untersuchungen zu der Gesetzen des Fernrohrsehens. *Optica Acta* **4**, 88–101.

Kühl, A. (1927) Die visuelle Leistung von Fernrohren. *Z. Instrum.* **47**, 75–86.

Marriot, F. H. C. (1963) The foveal visual threshold for short flashes and small fields. *J. Physiol.* **169**, 416–23.

Middleton, W. E. K. (1952) *Vision through the atmosphere.* University of Toronto Press.

Rose, A. (1948) The sensitivity performance of the human eye on an absolute scale. *J. opt. Soc. Am.* **38**, 196–208.

(1973) *Vision: human and electronic.* Prentice Hall, New York.

Swets, J. A. (1964) *Signal detection and recognition by human observers.* John Wiley, New York.

van Meeteren, A. (1969) Modulation sensitivity in instrumental vision. In: *Nato Symposium on image evaluation*, pp. 279–91, Munich.

van Meeteren, A. (1973) *Visual aspects of image intensification.* Thesis, University of Utrecht. Also published as Report Institute for Perception, TNO, Soesterberg. The Netherlands.

van Meeteren, A. (1977) *Prediction of realistic visual tasks from image quality data.* SPIE Vol. 98 Assessment of Imaging systems (Sira Nov. 1978 London).

(1978) On the detective quantum efficiency of the human eye. *Vision Res.* **18**, 257–67.

van Meeteren, A. & Boogaard, J. (1973) Visual contrast sensitivity w [illegible] image intensifiers. *Optik* **37**, 179–91.

van Meeteren, A. & Vos, J. J. (1972) Resolution and contrast sen[illegible] luminances. *Vision Res.* **12**, 825–33.

Index

Page numbers in italic type refer to figures, those in bold to tables.

a-wave (ERG), *419*, 420
  achromatopsia, 376–7
  inherited night blindness, 430, 433, 436, *436*, 438, *439*
absolute dark light, 183, 203–5, *204*
  see also dark noise
absolute sensitivity, rods *see* absolute threshold
absolute threshold, 54, 57–61, **59**, **100**, 146, 180–2, *181*
  acromat, 57, *58*, 59–61, **60**, 70, **100**, 117, 345
  image intensifying devices, 467
  invertebrates, 245–6, 250
  noise, 146–8, 167–73, *169*, *170*, *171*
  non-Poisson noise, 160–7, *162*, *164*, *165*, *166*, *167*
  see also dark noise, neural noise, Poisson distribution, quantum efficiency
achromat, 4
  history, 253–67
acquired achromatopsia, 266
see also cerebral achromatopsia, progressive cone dysfunction
action potential generation, photoreceptors, 234
action spectrum, rod–cone interaction, 113–14, *113*
acuity
  achromats, 255, 258, 260, 269, 270–1, 275, 277–8
    complete, 292, 301, 304, 312–14, 316, 317, 321, *321*, 347, **354**, **355**, 356
    incomplete, 282, 283, 285, 362
  aids, 333, 461
  choroideremia, 444
  cerebral, 286–7
  progressive cone dysfunction, 287, 288, 353
  see also complete achromatopsia with normal visual acuity, spatial acuity, temporal acuity
adaptation, 125–7
  see also dark adaptation, light adaptation, physiology
adaptation pool, 80, 94, 122, 144, 177
  cone contribution, 108, 109–11, 114, 116
  local adaptation, 87, *87*, *88*, 91
  multiple-sized, 91–2
  physiological evidence, 88–91, 133–8, *137*
  site of, 80–2
  size of, 82–4, 403, 404
  spatial–temporal mechanisms, 15, *16*, *17*, 18, 84–6, *83*, **86**, 88–91
adaptation rate, achromat, 271
adenosine 5′-diphosphate (ADP), rhodopsin cycle, 219
adenosine 5′-triphosphate (ATP), rhodopsin cycle, 218, 219, *228*, 229
after image, dark adaptation, 179–80, 191, 192–3, 361, 391
Aguilar & Stiles, rod isolation, *50*, 51–4, *52*, 98, 117–18, 366–9, *367*
aided vision, 451–9, *453*, *454*, *458*
  see also image intensifying devices, night glasses
albinism, achromatopsia, 280, 320, 331
alpha break, dark adaptation, 357
amacrine cells, 28, 68, 82, 110, 111, 122–3
amblyopia, 331
  see also complete achromatopsia with reduced visual acuity
amphibians, 66–7, 194, 196
  see also frog, toad
amplification, noise, 64
angular magnification, aided vision, 452–4, *453*, *454*, 466–7
  see also night glasses

angular spacing photoreceptors, compound eyes, 238, 240
animal models, night blinding disease, 447–50
anomaloscope, introduction of, 265
anomalous trichromats, 255, **317**
antagonistic surround, amacrine cells, 122
Appaloosa Horse, 438
apposition compound eyes, 240–4, *241*, 245
Arago's phenomena, 338
arginine, gyrate atrophy, 44
arrestin, rhodopsin cycle, 218
arthropods, 223
  see also invertebrates
astigmatism, achromatopsia, 280, 293, 321
atmospheric conditions, image intensifying devices, 471–2, *471*
atypical achromatopsia *see* autosomal recessive incomplete achromatopsia, X-linked incomplete achromatopsia
auditory system, compared to visual, 37, 41
augenschwarz *see* dark light
autophagic vacuoles, retinitis pigmentosa, 442
autosomal recessive inheritance
  incomplete achromatopsia, 278, **279**, 280, 282–3, 285, 317, **317**, *318*, 319
  night blindness, animal models, 448, 449
  see complete achromatopsia with normal visual acuity, complete achromatopsia with reduced visual acuity, fundus albipunctatus, gyrate atrophy, Oguchi's disease
axolotl, 126
axon cells, rod–cone interaction, 110

b-wave (ERG), 81, 127, *128*, 129, 130–1, *130*, 132–3
  achromatopsia, 376–7, 419–20, *419*
  night blindness, 422, 430, *431*, 433, 436–7, *436*
background illuminance
  increment threshold, 103–6, *104*, 365
  saturation, 120–1
  spatial temporal summation, 84–5, 87, 90–1
  see also light adaptation, noise, physiology
bandpass temporal filtering, 26, 27
Bardet–Biedl syndrome, 441
Barlow's fluctuation theory, 77–9, *78*, 188–9, 210, 220
Bassen–Kornzweig syndrome, 441
bees, compound eyes, 243
Best's macular dystrophy, 422
binocular rivalry, 167–73, 176
binoptic effect, noise, 163–6, *164*, *165*, *166*, 167, *167*
  see also binocular rivalry
bipolar cells, 68, 81–2, 110, 420
bleaching, 62, 71, 80
  see also dark adaptation
blinking, achromatopsia, 292, 310–11, 320, 361
Block's Law for Thermal Summation, 24, 159
blue cone monochromacy *see* X-linked incomplete achromatopsia
blur perception and discrimination, 45–7, *46*
Boyle, R., 258, 260, 286–7
brain fever, achromatopsia, 278
Brewster, D., 265
brightness discrimination, rod–cone interaction, 108
Brodman's areas, achromatopsia, 285
Bufo *see* toad
butterflies, compound eyes, 243

c-wave (ERG), retinal pigment epithelium, 420–1
calcium, adaptation, 75, 132, 198–9
canines, night blinding disease, 447, 448, 449
carotenoids, vitamin A, 428
cat
  adaptation pool, 81, 82–3, 90
  amacrine cells, 28, 111, 122–3
  contrast sensitivity, 13–14, *13*, 15–16, *16*
  dark adaptation, 190, 216
  ganglion cells, 121, 138, 139–40, *139*, *140*, 141
  increment threshold, 88–90, *88*, *89*
  noise, absolute sensitivity, 64, 67, 68
  photoreceptor light adaptation, 73, 75–6
  rod–cone interaction, 102, 109–10
  saturation, 121
  subtractive filtering, 94
cellular adaptation *see* photoreceptor light adaptation
cellular retinoid-binding protein (CRBP), rhodopsin cycle, 427–8, 431
central cone achromatopsia, 275
centre–surround antagonism, 90, 91, 95–6
cerebral achromatopsia, 278, 285–7
cerebral infarction, achromatopsia, 278
cerebral pathology, achromatopsia, 331
cerebral palsy, achromatopsia, 319
channel theory, 456
chemical synaptic transmitter, 132, 234
  coupling, adaptation pool, 80, 136
choriocapillaris, 324, 445

choroid
  achromatopsia, 272, 324
  choroideremia, 444–5, *444*
  gyrate atrophy, 445–7, *446*
choroideremia, 422, 444–5, *444*
chromatic aberration, 282, 283, 284, 329
chromophore change *see* rhodopsin cycle
CIE (Commission International de L'Eclairage), scotopic luminosity function, *113*, 114, 341, 342, *344*, 345, 389, 437, *437*
circadian clock, 64, 229–30, 244, 249
Colardeau, C. P., 261–2, 268–9
cold blooded vertebrates, adaptation, 126, 135
  see also frog, toad
collie, night blinding disease, 447
colour discrimination, rod–cone interaction, 36
colour vision test, 325–8, *326*, *327*, *328*
complete achromatopsia with normal visual acuity, 278, **279**, 281–2, 316
complete achromatopsia with reduced visual acuity, 278, **279**, 280–1, 316, 317, **317**
  see also Nordby
complete achromats, 321–4, *322*, *323*, *324*, 334, 335
  colour vision tests, 325–8, *326*, *327*, *328*
  electrophysiological examinations, 324–5, 325
  heredity, 318–19
  see also Nordby
compound eye, 223–4
  neural sampling and processing, 245–50
  noise, 64, 226–35, *228*, *232*
  optical trade-offs, 239–45, *241*, *242*
  photoreceptor response, 224–6
  sampling and processing, 239
  transmission efficiency, 235–9, *236*
cone dystrophy syndrome, 316
  see also complete achromatopsia
cone-monochromates *see* complete achromatopsia with reduced visual acuity
cone progressive dystrophy, 324
cones
  achromats, 269, 270–1, 273, 274, 337–8
  compound eyes, 239
  degeneration, 324, 353, 360
  ERG, 421
  gain control, 177
  local adaptation, 87
  night blindness, 417
  retinal eccentricity, *30*, 31, *31*, 33
  spatial sensitivity, 19–20, 22–4, *23*
  temporal sensitivity, 26, *27*
  see also rod–cone interactions, rod only theory
congenital achromatopsia
  classification 278–80, **279**
  discovery of, 261, 266
  progressive, compared, 331–2
  see also autosomal recessive incomplete achromatiopsia, complete achromatopsia with normal visual acuity, complete achromatopsia with reduced visual acuity, X-linked incomplete achromatopsia
congenital stationary night blindness (CSNB), 423, *425*, *435*, 434–9, *436*, *437*, *439*
contact lens electrode, 418
contrast flash technique, 183
contrast, sensitivity, 4, 178
  aided vision, 457–9, *458*
  adaptation, 108, 127
  compound eye, 241
  method, compared increment threshold, 5–18, *5*, *7*, *10*, *12*
  retinal eccentricity, *30*, 31–4, *31*, *32*
  spatial sensitivity, 22–4, *23*
  suprathreshold, 37, 38, 39–41, *39*, *40*, *41*, 43–4, *44*, *45*
  temporal sensitivity, 26–9, *27*, *28*
  see also image intensifying devices, night glasses
Corpus Hippocraticum, Hippocrates, 256
cortical neurons, adaptation, 143–4, *143*, 145, 404
cortical trauma, achromatopsia, 278
coupling, photoreceptors, 135–7, *137*
  see also adaptation pooling
crabs, 226, 227, 246
Crawford–Westheimer effect, 92–5, 102, 121
crayfish, 244
critical flicker fusion (CFF) *see* flicker sensitivity
crustaceans, 223, 244
crypto-incomplete achromatopsia, 329
CSNB (Congenital stationary night blindness), 423, *425*, *435*, 436–9, *436*, *437*, *439*
Cynomolgus monkey, achromatopsia, 347

Dalton, J., 257, 262–5, 266, 269
Dämmerungszahl number, 461
dark adaptation, 178, 179–80, 193
  achromats, 270, 272, 273, 274, 276, 277, 391
    complete achromatopsia, 280, 323, *323*, 331, 336, *344*, 345, 349–50, *349*, **354**, **355**, 356–61, *358*, *359*, *360*

evolutionary aspects, 221–2
model of, 210–19, *212*, *214*, *215*, 220–1
night blindness, 417, 429–30, *431*
noise, 163–6, *164*, *165*, *166*, *167*, 224–5, 226–7
physiology, 62, 127, 138–40, 142, 194–210, *195*, *197*, *199*, *203*, *204*, *206*, *209*, 243, 246–7, 249
psychophysics, 93, 183–93, *184*, *185*, *186*, *187*, *188*, 219–20
pupillary reflex, 389
rod–cone interaction, *35*, 36–7, 103–4, 105, 108
see also fundus reflectometry
'Dark-glasses' model of adaptation, 131–2
dark noise, 6, 180–3, *181*
Barlow's equation, 77–9, *78*
De Vries–Rose square root law, 114, *115*
estimates of, 17–18, 65–6
invertebrates, 223, 224–5, 226–30, *228*, 235, 237, 238
Weber–Fechner fraction, 68–9, *69*
see also absolute sensitivity, neural noise, photon noise
Dartnall nomogram, 342–3, *343*
Daubeney–Huddart anomaly, 266
Day-rods
flicker sensitivity, 372
increment threshold, 362
theory, 271, 273, 277, 335, 338, 381
De Coloribus, Aristotle, 256
De Vries–Rose, fluctuation theory, 8, 9, *10*, 11–12, 13–14, 43, 85, 114, *115*, 365
aided vision, 451, 452, 455–7, 463, 466
physiology, 131
decrement threshold curve of rods, 55–7, *56*
degenerative achromats, 275
densitometry, 339
see fundus reflectometry
desensitization of rods
pigment depletion, 71, *72*
pupil constriction, 76–7
Weber–Fechner fraction, 68–71, *69*, **70**
see also adaptation pool, noise, photoreceptors – light adaptation, rod–cone interaction, subtractive filtering
Descartes, R., 257
detection sensitivity, 4–5, 54
achromat, 393–7, *395*, *396*
rod–cone interactions, 34–7, *35*
spatial acuity, *33*, 34
see also contrast sensitivity, increment threshold curve, spatial sensitivity, temporal sensitivity
deuteranomaly, **317**
deuteranopes, 254–5, 265, 281, 282, 283, 284, **317**
colour vision tests, 327, *328*
rod–cone interactions, 106, *107*, **107**, 108
dichromats, 307, **317**
see also deuteranopes, protanopes, tritanopes
dilator muscles, 387, 389
directional sensitivity, 4, 6, *50*, 120, 276, 348–53, *349*, *351*, **352**, 391
discrimination sensitivity, 54, 55
see also spatial sensitivity, suprathreshold sensitivity, temporal sensitivity
DNA fragment polymorphism, choroideremia, 445
dominant inheritance, night blindness, 434–5, *435*, 442
DOPT (optimal spatial displacement), motion sensitivity, 42
double stimuli, spatial summation, 20
Dowling–Rushton model, dark adaptation, 187, 219, 220
dragonflies, 243
dual-jerk nystagmus, achromatopsia, 383–4, *385*
duplicity theory, 3, 49, 51, 177
Duplizitätstheorie *see* duplicity theory
duration, target
absolute sensitivity, 57, *58*, 59–61, **60**, 62, 65–6
background, saturation, 119–20
increment threshold, 51, 70, **70**, 114–15, 182, 364, *365*, 455, 456
noise, 65–6, 79
saturation, 117
see also temporal sensitivity
dysplasia, of macular yellow, achromatopsia, 280

eccentric cell, invertebrates, 235, 237, 248–9
eccentricity
adaptation pool, 85, **86**, 90
dark adaptation, 357
detection sensitivity, **396**, 397, *399*, 400–4, *401*, *402*
increment threshold, 51–2, 93, 104, 364–5, *366*
saturation, achromat, 392, *394*
spatial sensitivity, 22, 23, *23*, 29–34, *30*, *32*, *33*
temporal sensitivity, 26, *27*, *31*, 33–4
see also fixation
eigengrau *see* dark noise

electrical coupling, receptors, 80, 136
electro-oculography (EOG), 421–2
  achromatopsia, 324
  night blindness, 422, 430, 433, 444, 445
electron microscope, 439
electroretinography (ERG), 418–21, *419*
  achromatopsia, 277, 317, 324–5, *325*, 331, 336, 376–80, *379*, *380*
  adaptation pool, 81
  compared EOG, 422
  dark adaptation, 184, 187
  night blinding diseases
    animal models, 447, 448
    progressive, 442, *443*, 444, 445, 447, 448
    stationary, 428, 430, *431*, 433, 434, 436, *436*, 438–9, *439*
envelope response, filters, 9
enzymes, rhodopsin, 201
equivalent background intensity, 191–3, 194, 200, 211, 219–20
equivalent Poisson noise *see* dark noise
ERG *see* electroretinography
erythroblastosis, 319
evolution
  achromatopsia, 255
  dark adaptation, 221–2
Extraordinary Facts Relating to the Vision of Colours: With Observations, Dalton, J., 257
eye movements
  Crawford–Westheimer effect, 93
  see also nystagmus

F-ratio, fly and man, 246
Farnsworth–Munsell 100 hue test, 291, 303, 326
Farnsworth Panel D-15 test, 326, *326*
Fechner fraction *see* Weber fraction
feedback
  bipolar cells, 81–2
  horizontal cells, 110, 136
  pupil constriction, 76
field adaptation *see* light adaptation
filtering, 4, 47–8
  neural filters, 173–4, 176
  see also contrast sensitivity, detection sensitivity, discrimination sensitivity, spatial sensitivity, temporal sensitivity
firefly, 244
fixation, achromatopsia, 272, 319, 320, 339, 382–3, *383*, *384*
flicker sensitivity
  achromatopsia, 270, 276, 324–5, *325*, 336, **354**, **355**, 356, 362, 368, 371–6, *371*, *373*, *374*, 421
  action spectrum, 113–14, *114*
  increment threshold, 73–5, *74*, 111–13, *112*
  invertebrates, 249
  rod–cone interaction, 28, *35*, 36–7, 109
  saturation, 120, 135
flies, 226, 235, *236*, 237–8, 245–6, 249
fluctuation theory, Barlow, 77–9, *78*, 188–9, 210, 220
48 kDa protein, 218, 201
Fourier optics, 240, 243
fovea, achromat, 271, 273, 274, 275, 323–4
  Nordby, Knut, 336, 337, 338
foveal fixation, complete achromatopsia, 280
Francis Galton Laboratory for National Eugenics, 266
frequency of seeing curve, invertebrates, 225, 237, 238
frog, 84, 89, 126, 134, 216
  absolute sensitivity, 64–5, 67
functional rod-monochromat *see* complete typical achromatopsia
fundus, picture, achromatopsia, 275, 283, 284, 323–4, *324*
fundus albipunctatus, 422, 429–31, *430*, *431*, 433
fundus reflectometry, 423, 424–6, *426*
  achromatopsia, 282, 339–44, *340*, *341*, *343*
  night blinding disease, 428–9, 430, *430*, 434, *435*, 436
Fur, Island of, Denmark, 267, 272

gain control
  photoreceptors, 71, 73–6, *74*, 177, 179, 200, 366
  see also adaptation pool
Galezowski, 269, 335–6
ganglion cells
  achromats, 403, 412
  adaptation pool, 15, 82–4, 88, 89–91, 137–8
  ERG, 420, 433
  increment threshold function, 129–30, *130*
  intensity response function, 127–9, *128*, 130–1, 132
  night blindness, 417
  noise, 65, 66–7, 68, 175
  response compression, 133
  rod–cone interaction, 101–2, 110, 111
  spatial sensitivity, 138–42, *139*, *140*, 144–5
  subtractive filtering, 94, 121
gap junctions, rod–cone interaction, 29, 81, 109, 110
Gaussian distribution

image, angular displacement, 247
noise, 149, 158, 160–1, 176
gecko, 73, 126
Gegenfarben, theory, 275
giant movement detector cell, 237–9
glasses, achromatopsia, 333
glaucoma, photophobia, 331
glycine, gyrate atrophy, 446
goldfish, adaptation pool, 84, 102, 135, 140, 175
Gothaisches Magazin für das Neuste aus der Physik und Naturgeschichte, Lichtenberg, J. C., 262
grating experiments *see* contrast sensitivity
guanine crystals, compound eye, 244
guanosine 5′-diphosphate (GDP), 427
guanosine 5′-monophosphate (GMP), 63–4, 447–8
guanosine 5′-triphosphate (GTD), 427
guanylate cyclase, phototransduction, 199
guinea pig, 198
gyrate atrophy, 445–7, *446*

Harris, J. and T., 259–61, 262, 263, 269
hearing defects, achromatopsia, 319
heat, quanta, 59, **59**
hemeralopia, 256
hemianopia, 286
Hering, E., 270
herpes encephalitis, achromatopsia, 285
Herschel, J., 264
heterozygous manifestation, achromatopsia, 281, 291, *292*
Hippocrates, 256
History and Present State of Discoveries Relating to Vision, Light and Colours, Priestly, J., 257
history, colour blindness, 253
Holmgren, F., 265
Holmgren wool skein test, 326
homozygous, achromatopsia, 291, *292*
horizontal cells
adaptation, 81, 96, 126, 136, 145
rod–cone interaction, 36, 110
Horseshoe crab *see Limulus*
Huddart, J., 259–61, 262, 263, 266, 269
hydroxyproline, gyrate atrophy, 446
hypermetropia, achromatopsia, 293, 312
hyperornithemia, gyrate atrophy, 445–7
hypersensitivity to light *see* light aversion
hypertension, achromatopsia, 319
hysteria, achromatopsia, 331

image intensifying devices, 148, 451–2, 457, *460*, *463*, 464–72, *465*, *466*, *468*, *469*, *470*, *471*
impulse quantization error, noise, 64
incomplete achromat, 278, 317–18, **317**, 321–3, *322*, 329, 336, 346
heredity, 318–19
tests, 325, 329, *330*, 377
see also autosomal recessive incomplete achromatopsia, X-linked incomplete achromatopsia
increment threshold curve, 51–5, *50*, *52*, *53*, 73–5, *74*, 127, 129–31, *130*, 180–3, *181*
achromatopsia, 270, 276, 336, 346, **354**, **355**, 356, 362–9, *363*, *365*, *366*, *367*
blur perception and discrimination, 45–7, *46*
compared contrast sensitivity, 5–18, *5*, *7*, *12*
compared decrement, 55–7, *56*
contrast discrimination, 43–4, *44*, *45*
noise, 65, 77–9, *78*
rod–cone interaction, 36, 98–100, *99*, **100**, 103–8, *104*, *107*, **107**, 111–13, *112*, 123
spatial sensitivity, 18–22, *20*, *21*, 44–5
spatial–temporal reorganisation, 88–90, *88*, *89*
temporal sensitivity, 24, *25*, 44–5
see also Crawford–Westheimer effect, De Vries–Rose, Weber–Fechner fraction
information theory, 146–7, 240
inhibition *see* lateral inhibitory influences
inner plexiform layer, feedback, 82
insects, 223, 227, 244
intensity–response, adaptation, 127–31, *128*, 132
interbreeding, achromatopsia, 259, 291
interstitial retinoid-binding protein (IRBP), 427, 431, 441
intestinal by-pass surgery, vitamin A, 428
intrinsic light *see* dark light
invertebrates, 223–4
neural sampling and processing, 245–50
optical trade-offs, 239–45, *241*, *242*
photoreceptor intrinsic noise, 226–35, *228*, *232*
photoreceptor response, 71, 73, 75, 224–6
transmission of signals, 223, 224, 235–9, *236*
Irish setter, night blinding disease, 447
Ishihara pseudoisochromatic plate test, 291, 305
isolation, rod and cones, 3–4
see also Aguilar & Stiles
isomerism, rhodopsin, 62, 201, 427, 441

jerk nystagmus, achromatopsia, 383–4, *385*, *386*
Jonathan I., 286–7, 305–6
juvenile macular degeneration, 288

Kepler, J., 257
kinetic adaptation *see* speed
Kohlrausch break, dark adaptation, 357

L-cone *see* long wave sensitivity
lamellae, cones, 239–40
Larsen, H., 272
lateral geniculate nucleus (LGN), adaptation, 91, 94, 137–8, 141, 142, 145
lateral inhibitory influences, 90, 121, 138–9, 142, 144–5, 247, 248–50
Leber's amaurosis congenita, 448
lens, compound eyes, 239, 240, 242, 243, 244
lenticular sclerosis, 418
Leptograpsis, 246
light adaptation, 3–4, 47–8, 49–51, 122–3, 125–7, 178, 180–3
  see also absolute threshold, adaptation pool, desensitization, detection sensitivity, discrimination sensitivity, noise, photoreceptors – light adaptation, physiology, rod–cone interactions, saturation, Stiles–Crawford effect, subtractive filtering
light aversion
  achromats, 278, 316–17, 319–20, 331, 333
  complete achromatopsia, 280, 281, 291, 292, *293*
  incomplete achromatopsia, 282, 283, 284
  progressive cone dysfunction, 287, 288
light sensitive channels, photoreceptor light adaptation, 73
Limulus, 64, 134, 223, 227, 229, 230, 235–7, 244–5, 248–9
lizards, saturation, 135
local adaptation, 87, *88*, *89*, 91
locust, 14, 64, 225–6, 230–4, *232*, 244, 248
long wave sensitivity, 106, 269, 272, 276, **279**, 378, *379*, *380*
  cerebral achromatopsia, 286
  complete achromatopsia with normal visual acuity, **279**, 281, 282
  incomplete achromatopsia, **279**, 283, 284
luminosity function, scotopic, 58–9

M-cones *see* middle wave sensitivity
Macaque monkey (*Macaca fascicularis*), 61, 73–5, *74*, 91, 118–19, 141
'Mach bands', invertebrates, 249
macular disorders, achromatopsia, 278, 282, 284, 286, 288, 331
  see also fovea
magnification, achromatopsia, 300, 312, 313, 333
magnocellular cell bodies, lateral geniculate nucleus, 91, 141, 142
malnutrition, night vision, 428
mammalian adaptation, 132
  see also monkey
meningitis, achromatopsia, 285
mesopic vision, 4
  achromats, 390
  retinal eccentricity, *30*, 31, 33, 34
  see spatial sensitivity, temporal sensitivity
metarhodopsin, 201, 427
  dark adaptation, 212, 216, 217–18, 219
  dark noise, 227, 228–9, *228*, 230
microvilli, compound eyes, 239, 244
middle wave sensitivity, 106, 276, **279**
  cerebral achromatopsia, **279**, 286
  complete achromatopsia, 281
  incomplete achromatopsia, **279**, 283, 284
minification, 452
Mizuo–Nakamura phenomenon, 432
modular transfer function (MFT)
  image intensifying devices, 468–70, *469*, *470*
  night glasses, 462–3, *462*
moiety, rhodopsin cycle, 427
monkey
  adaptation pool, 81, 134
  dark adaptation, 194–6, 200, 203
  increment threshold, 73–5, *74*
  noise, 65, 66, 148, 176, 209–10
  rod–cone interaction, 110, 111
  see also Macaque monkey
monochromates **317**
  see also complete archromatopsia with reduced visual acuity
monopolar cells, fly, *236*, 249
monotopic effect, noise, *162*, 163, 167
motion sensitivity *see* temporal sensitivity
mouse, night blinding disease, 447–8
movement, eye, achromatopsia, 382, **384**
  see also nystagmus
Muller cells, ERG, 420
multiplicative noise, 161, 225, 231, 233–4
Musca, *236*, 245–6
myopia, achromatopsia, 284, 312, 321

Nagel, W., 270

Nagel anomaloscope, 265, 327–8, *328*, 329
'network' adaptation, 133
neural noise, 14, 64–5, 114, *115*, 173–5, 176, 223
  synaptic noise, 64, 67, 68, 77, 79
neural sampling and processing, compound eyes, 243, 245–50
  see also post receptor
Newton, I., 257
Nielsen, M., 267, 272–3, 275
night blindness, 417–18, 429, 439–40, 450
  animal models, 447–50
  choroideremia, 422, 444–5, *444*
  congenital stationary night blindness, 423, *425*, 434–9, *435*, *436*, *437*, *439*
  fundus albipunctatus, 422, 429–31, *430*, *431*, 433
  gyrate atrophy, 445–7, *446*
  non-invasive tests, 418–26, *419*, *424*, *425*, *426*
  Oguchi's disease, 422, 431–3, *432*
  vitamin A, 427–9
  see also retinitis pigmentosa
night glasses, 451, 454, 459–64, *460*, *461*, *462*, *463*
night myopia, 418
noise, 15, 54, 178
  achromats, 352
  absolute threshold, 61, 63
  adaptation pool, 80, 81
  dark adaptation, 188–9, 203–21, *204*, *206*, *209*, *212*, *214*, *215*
  decrement threshold, 56–7
  image intensifying devices, 467, 468
  increment threshold, 54–5
  invertebrates, 223, 224–5, 242, *242*
  phototransducer, 63–4, 77, 79, 226, 230–5, *232*, 237
  saturation, 118
  suprathreshold, 37
  see also absolute threshold, dark noise, neural noise, photon noise, Poisson distribution
non-Poisson noise, 160–6, *162*, *164*, *165*, *166*, *167*
Nordby, Knut, achromatopsia – personal account
  biography, 290–314, *292*, *293*, *294*, 315
  rod vision, 304–14
  see also rod only theory
normal distribution curve *see* Gaussian distribution
Norway, achromatopsia, 280, 316
Norwegian elkhound, night blinding disease, 448
nuclear layer, test, 420, 422
  see also bipolar cells
nucleotide metabolism, night blinding disease, 447
nyctalopia, 422
nystagmus, 269, 272, 319, 320, 321, 331, 339
  complete achromatopsia, 280, 281, 291, 292, 301, 316, 317, 352, 361, 382–7, *385*, *386*
  incomplete achromatopsia, 282, 283, 284
  progressive cone dysfunction, 288

object agnosia, 285
Observations sur la Physique, sur l'Histoire Naturelle et sur les Arts, Rozier, F., 261
octopus type perimeters, 322
ocular media, quanta, 58, **59**, 62
OFF cells, ganglion, 139
Oguchi's disease, 422, 431–3, *432*
ommatidium *see* compound eye
ON cells, ganglion, 68, 139
opsin, rhodopsin cycle, 200, 201, 427
optic disc
  achromatopsia, 280, 324, *324*, 331
  retinitis pigmentosa, 440
optic nerve fibres, ERG, 420
optical losses
  image intensifying devices, 468–70, *469*, *470*
  night glasses, 462–3, *462*
Opticks, Newton, 256
optimal spatial displacement (DOPT), 42
optokinetic nystagmus (OKN), 384–7, *386*
optomotor response, flies, 245–6
ornithine α-aminotransferase (OAT), 446
Osterberg pseudoisochromatic plate test, 291, 305, 369

Palmer, G., 268–9
palmitate, rhodopsin, cycle, 428
parafoveal region, rod sensitivity, 29, 31, 36, 37
parvocellular cell bodies, lateral geniculate nucleus, 91, 141, 142
pedestal contrast, 43, *44*
pendular nystagnus, achromatopsia, 383–4, *385*, *386*
Philosophical Transactions of the Royal Society of London, 257, 259, 261, 263, 269
phosphenes, 257, 258
phosphodiesterase (PDE), 427, 448
phosphorylation, rhodopsin, 201, 218–19, 227, *228*, 229
photocathode *see* image intensifying devices
photochromatic glasses, achromatopsia, 310

photochromatic interval, rod-cone interaction, 105, 108–9
photoisomerization, 212–13, 217–18
photon noise, 64, 147–8
  dark adaptation, 196
  decrement threshold, 56–7
  increment threshold, 77–9, *78*, 92, 131
  invertebrates, 230, 231, *232*, 233, 243, 245, 248, 249–50
  see also dark noise
photons *see* De Vries–Rose fluctuation theory, image intensifying devices, night glasses
photophobia *see* light aversion
photopic function, 3
  ERG, 376–8, *379*, *380*
photopigment *see* rhodopsin
photoproducts *see* rhodopsin
photoreceptors
  dark adaptation, 62, 179, 200, 202–10, *203*, *204*, *206*, *209*
  light adaptation, 71, 73–6, *74*, 75, 126, 127–32, *128*, *130*, 135–6
  night blindness, 417, 429, 439, 445, 447–50
  response compression, 73, 75, 118, 120, 132–3, 134
  testing, 419–20, 422
  see also a-wave, dark noise, invertebrates, rhodopsin, transducer noise
phototactic jumping, frog, 67
phototransducer noise, 63–4, 77, 79, 226, 230–5, *232*, 237
physical noise, 113, *114*
physiology, visual adaptation, 73–5, *74*, 118–19, 125–7, 144–5
  luminance detection, effect of background light, 127–38, *128*, *137*
  spatial vision, effect of background light, 138–44, *139*, *140*, *143*
  see also photoreceptors – light adaptation
π-cone monochromacy *see* X-linked incomplete achromatopsia
pigment
  choroideremia, 444
  see also retinitis pigmentosa, rhodopsin, spectral sensitivity
Pipers Law, 19, 452, *453*, 455, 459
Platter, F., 256
Plexiform layer, 68
  adaptation pool, 81, 82
  rod–cone interaction, 110, 111
  subtractive filtering, 94, 122
point spread function, 238, 240, 248
Poisson distribution, noise, 14, 56–7, 77, 131, 148–9, 175
  aided vision, 455, 465
  invertebrates, 225, 233, 234, 237
  Sakitts experiment, 149–50, *150*, *151*, *152*, *154*, *155*, **156**, *157*
polyallelic inheritance, achromatopsia, 336
pooling, dark adaptation, 190
post receptor
  adaptation, 18, 28–9, 126, 127–31, *128*, *130*, 137–8, *137*, 144
  b-wave (ERG), 419–420
  connections, achromats, 278, 390, 394–5, 397
  invertebrates, 243, 245–50
  night blindness, 433, 437
  see also adaptation pool, cortical neurons, ganglion cells, lateral geniculate nucleus
potassium concentration, ERG, 420
Priest, J., 257
primate *see* monkey
probability summation, temporal filtering, 26
progressive cone/rod dysfunction, 33, 287–8, 331–2, 417
progressive night blinding disease, 429, 439–40
  see also choroideremia, gyrate atrophy, retinitis pigmentosa
progressive retinal atrophy (PRA), animal models, 447–9
proline, gyrate atrophy, 446
prosopagnosia, achromatopsia, 285
protan defects
  complete achromatopsia, 282
  incomplete achromatopsia, 283, 284, 317, **317**, *318*, 319
protanomaly, **317**
protanopia, 281, **317**, 327, 328, *328*
  early documented cases, 262–3, 265, 266, 269
  increment threshold, 106, *107*, **107**, 108
  saturation, 120
pseudo-isochromatic test charts, 265, 325–6, **326**
psychometric functions, binocular rivalry, 168–70, *169*, *170*, *171*
psychophysical testing, 4, 5
  night blinding disorders, 422–3, *424*, *425*
  see also dark adaptation, increment threshold curve, spatial sensitivity, spectral sensitivity, temporal sensitivity
pupil size, adaptation, 76–7, 179, 191, 192, 387–9, *388*
pupillary light reflex, 76–7, 179, 191, 192, 387–9, *388*
pupillary sphincter, 387, 389

pure rod theory *see* rod only theory
Purkinje shift, achromatopsia, 280, 282, 284, 329, 345
purple glasses, 333
pyridoxal phosphate (Vit B6), gyrate atrophy, 446

quanta, absolute threshold, 58–61, **59**, **60**
quantal fluctuation theory, 77–9, *78*, 114, 366
quantum efficiency, 61–3, **63**, 65, 455, 456–7
  invertebrates, 223, 224, 225–6, 230–5, 237, 238
  rod length, 423, 427
  see also De Vries–Rose, photon noise, rhodopsin

Rana temporaria, 67
Ransome, J. A., 264–5
rats, 73, 82, 127–9, *128*, *130*, 135
Rayleigh equation, 265, 283, 327, *328*
receiver operating characteristic curves, 149–56, *150*, *151*, *152*, *154*, *155*, 158, 160–1, 175, 234
receptor gain control *see* photoreceptor light adaptation
receptor loss theory, 268–9
receptor potential, 127, *128*, 129–30, *130*, 132
recessive inheritance *see* complete achromatopsia with reduced visual acuity, fundus albipunctatus, gyrate atrophy, Oguchi's disease, X-linked incomplete achromatopsia
rectangular stimuli, spatial summation, 20
red-blindness *see* protanopia
reflecting superposition eye, 244
reflection, visual adaptation, 178
refracting superposition eye, 244–5
refractive index, compound eyes, 240, *241*, 244–5
Refsum's syndrome, 441
regional sensitivity *see* eccentricity
reliability, vision, 54
residual cone theory, 271, 275–6, 335, 348, 352, 360, 362
resolution *see* spatial sensitivity
response compression, photoreceptors, 73, 75, 118, 120, 132–3, 134
retinal, rhodopsin cycle, 201, 202, *203*, 208
retinal degeneration gene, night blinding disease, 447
retinal densitometer, 126
retinal disorders, achromatopsia, 278
retinal eccentricity *see* eccentricity
retinal pigment epithelium, 420–1, 422, 427, 429, 430, 441, 444–5, *444*
retinal profile, use of, 423, *425*
retinal-S-antigen, 201, 218
retinal vessels, achromatopsia, 324, *324*
retinitis pigmentosa, 291, 422, 423, *424*, 440–3, *440*, *443*, 444, 452
  animals, 448, 449
  glasses, 310
retinol, rhodopsin cycle, 202
  see also vitamin A
retinol-binding protein, 428, 430, 441
Rhesus monkey, 81, 111, 123
rhodopsin
  absolute threshold, 58, **59**
  achromatopsia, 336
  cycle, 67, 200–2, 427–8
  dark adaptation, 184, 187, 190–1, 193, 202–3, *203*, 208, 211, 212–13, *212*, 216–19, 220–1
  disorders of, 433, 434, 441, 442
  invertebrates, 239, 240, 244
  light adaptation, 71, *72*, 126, 131
  saturation, 118, 122, 135
  see also dark noise, fundus reflectometry, quantum efficiency
rhodopsin filled cones, theory, 271, 276–8, 284, 335, 338, 381
  testing, 329, 346, 347, 348, 352, 353, 372
rhodopsin kinase, 201, 218
Ricco's Law, 18–22, *21*, 24, 159, 452, *453*, 459
rod–cone dysplasia, 447, 448
rod–cone interactions, 34–7, *35*
  achromat, 394–5
  adaptation pool, 109–11, 116
  background adaptation, 103–6, *104*
  detection threshold, 12, 13, 36, 98–102, *99*, **100**, 106–8, *107*, **107**, 114–16, *115*, **116**, 123
  flicker sensation, 36, 109
  photochromatic interval, 108–9
  subtractive pooling, 111–14, *112*, *113*
rod field adaptation *see* light adaptation
rod isolation, Aguilar & Stiles, *50*, 51–4, *52*, 98, 117–18, 366–7, *367*
rod monochromats *see* complete achromatopsia with reduced visual acuity
rod only theory, achromatopsia, 269–71, 273, 335–6
  evidence, 337–53, *340*, *341*, *343*, *344*, *349*, *351*, **352**
  psychophysics, 353–6, **354**, **355**, 380–1
    dark adaptation, 356–61, *358*, *359*, *360*
    electroretinogram, 376–80, *379*, *380*

rod only theory (*cont.*)
flicker sensitivity, 371–6, *371*, *373*, *374*
increment threshold, 362–9, *363*, *365*, *366*, *367*
spatial sensitivity, 369–70, *370*
rod response, ERG, 421
Rose–De Vries region *see* De Vries–Rose
Rozier L'Abbe, F., 261–2
Rushton's theory, 183–8, *184*, *185*, *186*, *187*, *188*, 189–91, 210, 219

S-cones *see* short wave sensitivity
salamander, 73, 81
saturation, 6, 8, 16, 55, 117–19, 122, 134–5, 181, *181*
acromatopsia, 55, 277, 278, 319, 391–3, *392*, *393*, *394*
complete achromatopsia with reduced visual acuity, 280, 310, 336, 346–8, 364, 370, 372, 382
subtractive filtering, 120–1
Schultze, M., 269, 335
scotma, achromats, 270, 271, 321, 323, 336, 338–9
scotopic conditions, achromat, 393–7, *395*, *396*
scotopic components (ERG), 376–8, *379*, *380*
scotopic function, duplex retina, 3
scotopization of vision, 318, 332
Scott, J., 261
Seebeck, A., 265
self inhibition, neural filtering, 248–9
short wave sensitivity, 106–8, *107*, **107**, 268, 275, **279**
cerebral achromatopsia, 286
complete achromatopsia, 281
electroretinography, 421
incomplete achromatopsia, 283, 284, 285
shrimp, 244
sinewave gratings *see* contrast sensitivity method
size, target
absolute sensitivity, 57, *58*, 59–61, **60**, 62, 65–6
dark adaptation, 189, 192
increment threshold, 10–11, 51, 70–1, **70**, 99–100, 114–16, 362–4, *363*, 456
saturation, 117, 119–20, 121
see also Crawford–Westheimer effect, Piper's Law, spatial sensitivity
skate, 73, 135, 433
Sloan achromatopsia test, 326, *327*
snapping turtle, 126, 136, *137*
SNR, signal levels, compound eyes, 242–3
sodium ion channels, invertebrates, 73
Some Uncommon Observations about Vitiated Sight, Boyle, R., 258
spatial acuity, 31, *33*, 34, 336, 369, *370*, 372, 398, 400, 403, 412
spatial sensitivity, 4, 5, 55, 111
achromatopsia, 274, 347, 369–70, *370*
mesopic, 397–412, *398*, *399*, *401*, *402*, *405*, *406*, *407*, *409*, *410*, *411*
saturation, 391–2, *392*, *393*
scotopic, 395–7, *395*, *396*
aided vision, 452, 453–4, *454*, 459, 469–70, *469*, *470*
dark adaptation, 191
detection sensitivity, 9–10, *10*, 13–14, 15, 18–24, *20*, *21*, *23*, 26, 29–34, *32*, *33*
discrimination sensitivity, 37–8, *38*, *40*, *41*, 42, 44–5
invertebrates, 239, 240–1, 247–8
noise, 159–60, 176
physiology, 138–45, *139*, *140*, *143*
see also Crawford–Westheimer effect
spatial sensitivity function, 397
spatial sensitivity profile, 397
spatial–temporal mechanisms, light adaptation, 15, *16*, *17*, 18, *83*, 84–6, **86**, 87, 88–91, *88*, *89*
spectral analysis, bleaching, 207
spectral equal brightness function, 306
spectral luminosity function, **279**
complete achromatopsia, 272, 280, 281, 327, *327*, 331, *332*
incomplete achromatopsia, 282, 283, 285, 329, *330*
see also CIE luminosity function
spectral sensitivity, 332, 345–6
CSNB, 437, *437*, 438, *438*
image intensifying devices, 464, *465*
rod and cones compared, 4, 6
see also spectral luminosity function
spectrophotometry, rhodopsin cycle, 217–18
speed response, adaptation, 127, 134
spike initiation, neural noise, 64
spike *see* transmission
spontaneous nystagmus, 383–4, *385*
square root relation *see* De Vries–Rose
squinting, achromatopsia, 292, *293*, *294*, 310, 311, 320, 361
Standard of Diagnosis and Treatment of Six Categories of Diseases, Wang-Ken-Tang, 259
Stargardt's disease, 288
stationary disorders, night blinding disease, 429

see also congenital stationary night blindness, fundus albipunctatus, Oguchi's disease
stearate, rhodopsin cycle, 428
Stiles–Crawford effect, dark adaptation, 191, 211, 219–20
directional sensitivity, *50*, 120, 276, 336, 348–53, *349*, *351*, **352**, 391
Stilling, J., 265
striate neurons, 42
subtractive filtering, 91, 92–8, *97*, 111–14, *112*, *113*, 119–21, 122
suction pipette technique, 194
summation area, 13, 15
superposition compound eyes, 240, *241*, 244–5
suprathreshold sensitivity, 15, 16, 37, 47, 390, 409–12, *410*, *411*
surround inhibition *see* lateral inhibitory influences
synapses, 136, 438–9
synaptic noise, 64, 67, 68, 77, 79

target *see* duration, size
telescopes *see* night glasses
temperature, quantum/spike ratio, 238
temporal acuity, 27, *28*, 29, 31, 398, 400, 403, 412
temporal sensitivity, 4, 5, 55, 92, 96–8, *97*, 101, 102
achromatopsia, 347
mesopic, 397–412, *398*, *399*, *401*, *405*, *406*, *407*, *409*, *410*, *411*
saturation, 391–2, *392*, *393*
scotopic, 395–7, *395*, *396*
aided vision, 452
dark adaptation, 191
detection sensitivity, 10–11, 13–14, 19, *20*, 24–9, *25*, *27*, *28*, *30*, 31, *31*, 33–4, *35*, 36
discrimination sensitivity, 37–8, *38*, *39*, 42, 44–5
ERG, 421
invertebrates, 237–9, 246–8
noise, 159–60, 176
physiology, 141–2
tests, 418
see also electro-oculography, electroretinography, fundus reflectometry, psychophysical testing
thermal imaging devices, 452, 472
thermal isomerization, 64, 66–8, 201, 203–5, 212–13, 216, 427
invertebrates, 227, 229
threshold *see* absolute threshold, increment threshold curve
tiger salamander, 81, 109
tissue paper contrast tests, 326–7
toad
absolute threshold, 67
dark adaptation, 194, 196–8, *197*, 200, 203, *204*, 205–9, *206*, *209*, 214
light adaptation, 73, 126, 134, 135, 136
noise, 227
topographic memory, 285
transducer noise, 63–4, 77, 79, 226, 230–5, *232*, 237
transducin, rhodopsin cycle, 427
transduction efficiency, **59**, 62
transmission of light, invertebrates, 223, 224, 235–9, *236*
transthyretin, rhodopsin cycle, 428
tritan defects, 282, 284
tritanomaly, **317**
tritanopia, **317**
tunnel vision, achromatopsia, 311, 321–2
Tubervile, D., 257–8, 260, 266, 269, 287
turtle, light adaptation, 73, 81, 134
'twilight number', aided vision, 451, 461
twilight vision, compared colour blindness, 270
typical achromatopsia *see* complete achromats
typical complete monochromats *see* complete achromatopsia with reduced visual acuity

unitary response, 8–9, 12, 14
Usher's syndrome, 441
Utrecht continuous recording densitometer, 339, 342

velocity discrimination, 42
vincristine induced night blindness, 438–9, *439*
visual evoked response (VER), achromatopsia, 324
visual fields, achromatopsia, 321–3, *322*, 331
visual purple, rods, 270
vitamin A, 427–9, 430, 441
vitamin B6, gyrate atrophy, 446
Voigt, J. H., 262
Vries, De–Rose *see* De Vries–Rose

Wang-Ken-Tang, 258–9
wasps, 243
wavelength
absolute sensitivity, 59
directional sensitivity, 351–2, *351*, **352**, 353
increment threshold, 51, 98–100, *99*, **100**, 103–6, *104*, 182, 364

Weber–Fechner fraction, 6–15, *7*, *10*, *12*, *13*, 44, 68–71, *69*, **70**, 125, 181–2, 366, 456
  adaptation pool, 81
  dark adaptation, 198, 199, *199*, 200, 211, 216
  rod–cone interaction, 114–16, *115*, **116**
  physiology, 131
  saturation, 117, 118, 121, 346
Weber law, dark adaptation, 211
Whisson, 261, 262, 263
Wilson, G., 265

X-cells, ganglion, 139–41, *139*, *140*
X-linked
  incomplete achromatopsia, 276, 277, 278, **279**, 283–5, 317, **317**, *318*, 353
    hereditary, 318–19
    myopia, 321
    prognosis, 334
    rod–cone interaction, 106–8, *107*, **107**
    testing, *326*, 328, *328*, 329, *330*
  retinitis pigmentosa, 442, 443
  see also choroideremia

Y-cells, ganglion, 139–41, *140*
Yellow Emperor's Canon of Internal Medicine, 254
Young, T., 264, 269